TUBERCULOSIS
Current Concepts and Treatment

Edited by
Lloyd N. Friedman, M.D.
Director, Intensive Care
Milford Hospital
Milford, Connecticut
and
Assistant Clinical Professor of Medicine
Pulmonary and Critical Care Section
Yale University School of Medicine
New Haven, Connecticut

CRC Press
Boca Raton Ann Arbor London Tokyo

Library of Congress Cataloging-in-Publication Data

Friedman, Lloyd N.
  Tuberculosis: Current concepts and treatment / Lloyd N. Friedman.
     p.   cm.
  Includes bibliographical references and index.
  ISBN 0-8493-4825-0
  1. Tuberculosis. I. Title.
  [DNLM: 1. Tuberculosis. WF 200 F911t 1994]
RC311.F85 1994
616.9′95—dc20
DNLM/DLC
for Library of Congress

94-1524
CIP

No claim to original U.S. Government works
International Standard Book Number 0-8493-4825-0
Library of Congress Card Number 94-1524
Printed in the United States of America 1 2 3 4 5 6 7 8 9 0
Printed on acid-free paper

DEDICATION

This book is dedicated to my wife, Kai, our new son, David, and our parents and siblings.

THE EDITOR

Lloyd N. Friedman, M.D., is an Assistant Clinical Professor of Pulmonary and Critical Care Medicine at the Yale University School of Medicine, New Haven, Connecticut. He is the Director of Intensive Care and the Chairman of the Quality Assurance Committee at Milford Hospital, Milford, Connecticut.

Dr. Friedman graduated in 1975 from Columbia University, New York, with a B.A. degree in biochemistry and obtained his M. D. degree in 1979 from Yale University. He completed an internship in Internal Medicine at Beth Israel Medical Center, New York in 1980, and residency training at Oregon Health Sciences University in 1983. He completed his fellowship training in Pulmonary and Critical Care Medicine at Yale University School of Medicine in 1988, and he was the recipient of a National Institutes of Health Training Grant in Clinical Investigation during the years 1988 and 1989.

Dr. Friedman began his work in tuberculosis in 1984 as Medical Director of HS Systems, Inc., New York, a diagnostic facility that performed medical evaluations for New York City welfare applicants, and has been studying the development of tuberculosis in a cohort of alcoholics and drug addicts who were screened at that time. He also has conducted research in the development of a rapid immunologic diagnostic test for tuberculosis.

Dr. Friedman is a member of the American Thoracic Society, and is a fellow of the American College of Chest Physicians. He is a member of the Connecticut Tuberculosis Elimination Advisory Committee, and is on the nomination committee of the Program Committee of the Mycobacteriology and Infectious Disease Assembly of the American Thoracic Society.

His current research interests include the epidemiology of AIDS and tuberculosis, and the use of skin testing and chemoprophylaxis in the control of tuberculosis.

PREFACE

Tuberculosis has become an extremely challenging disease. Within 4 years, the emphasis has changed from eliminating tuberculosis in the United States by the year 2010 to attempting to control the insidious and ominous increase in rates and drug resistance that have occurred in the United States and throughout the world. The AIDS epidemic is playing a major role in the recrudescence of tuberculosis, but also very important have been the underallocation of resources and manpower to help handle the problem in the homeless, alcoholics, migrant farm workers, foreign-born, prisoners, and other populations. The astonomical growth in the volume of literature reflects the attempt to address the major problems in the field of tuberculosis. The purpose of this book is to summarize the basic fund of knowlege and review the current important relevant issues.

Each author has written a detailed review of a selected topic, and a balanced account of the latest controversies. The reader will obtain a thorough understanding of the epidemiology, presentation, and treatment of multidrug-resistant tuberculosis, as well as environmental and public health issues. New diagnostic methods are discussed, with particular emphasis on the polymerase chain reaction and restriction fragment-length polymorphisms. There are comprehensive presentations of pulmonary and extrapulmonary tuberculosis as they occur in adults and children, as well as a special section on pregnancy, and a chapter on atypical mycobacteria. The influence of the human immunodeficiency virus on the epidemiology, transmission, pathophysiology, manifestations, and treatment of tuberculosis and atypical mycobacteria are reviewed, including the latest American Thoracic Society/Centers for Disease Control recommendations for diagnosis, treatment, and control of these conditions. There are 117 radiographs of mycobacterial disease in a special chapter devoted solely to radiology. Also, the complex and rapidly changing recommendations for skin testing and chemoprophylaxis are presented, as well as public health control issues, and the use of the BCG vaccine for prevention of disease.

Thus, the reader will receive a practical, thorough, and balanced review of the literature from a group of outstanding contributors with vast clinical and research experience.

CONTRIBUTORS

Joseph H. Bates, M.D.
Professor of Medicine and Microbiology
University of Arkansas College of Medicine
and
Chief, Medical Service
Little Rock Veterans Affairs Medical Center
Little Rock, Arkansas

George M. Cauthen, Sc.D.
Epidemiologist
Surveillance and Epidemiologic Investigations
   Branch
Division of Tuberculosis Elimination
Centers for Disease Control and Prevention
Atlanta, Georgia

George W. Comstock, M.D., Dr. P.H.
Alumni Centennial Professor of Epidemiology
School of Hygiene and Public Health
The Johns Hopkins University
Baltimore, Maryland

Anne McB. Curtis, M.D.
Professor of Diagnostic Radiology
Yale University School of Medicine
New Haven, Connecticut

Michael H. Cynamon, M.D.
Professor of Medicine
Infectious Disease Section
State University of New York Health Science
   Center at Syracuse
Veterans Affairs Medical Center
Syracuse, New York

Jerrold J. Ellner, M.D.
Professor of Medicine and Pathology
Case Western Reserve University of School of
   Medicine
Chief, Division of Infectious Diseases
University Hospitals of Cleveland
Cleveland, Ohio

Lloyd N. Friedman, M.D.
Director, Intensive Care
Milford Hospital
Milford, Connecticut
and
Assistant Clinical Professor
   of Medicine
Pulmonary and Critical Care Section
Yale University
School of Medicine
New Haven, Connecticut

Lawrence J. Geiter, M.P.H.
Chief, Clinical Research Branch
Division of Tuberculosis Elimination
Centers for Disease Control and Prevention
Atlanta, Georgia

Marian Goble, M.D.
Clinical Professor of Medicine
University of Colorado Health Sciences Center
Infectious Diseases Division
National Jewish Center for Immunology and
   Respiratory Medicine
Denver, Colorado

James L. Hadler, M.D., M.P.H.
Chief, Epidemiology Section
Division of Infectious Diseases
Connecticut Department of Health Services
Hartford, Connecticut

Sandra Handwerger, M.D.
Clinical Scholar, Assistant Professor
Rockefeller University
New York, New York

Robin E. Huebner, M.P.H., Ph.D.
Medical Epidemiologist
Clinical Research Branch
Division of Tuberculosis Elimination
Centers for Disease Control and Prevention
Atlanta, Georgia

John A. Jereb, M.D.
Medical Officer
Clinical Research Branch
Division of Tuberculosis Elimination
Centers for Disease Control and Prevention
Atlanta, Georgia

Gloria D. Kelly, B.A.
Information Resource Specialist
Surveillance and Epidemiologic Investigations
   Branch
Division of Tuberculosis Elimination
Centers for Disease Control and Prevention
Atlanta, Georgia

Sally P. Klemens, M.D.
Assistant Professor of Medicine
Infectious Disease Section
State University of New York Health Science
   Center at Syracuse
Veterans Affairs Medical Center
Syracuse, New York

Klaus-Dieter K. L. Lessnau, M.D.
Senior Fellow
Division of Pulmonary and Critical Care
    Medicine
Cabrini Medical Center
New York, New York

Edward A. Nardell, M.D.
Assistant Professor of Medicine
Harvard Medical School
The Cambridge Hospital
Cambridge, Massachusetts
    and
Tuberculosis Control Officer
Massachusetts Department of Public Health
Boston, Massachusetts

Elizabeth A. Rich, M.D.
Associate Professor of Medicine
Division of Pulmonary and Critical Care
    Medicine
University Hospitals of Cleveland
Cleveland, Ohio

Peter A. Selwyn, M.D., M.P.H.
Associate Director, AIDS Program
Associate Professor of Medicine, Epidemiology,
    and Public Health
Yale University School of Medicine
New Haven, Connecticut

Ronald W. Smithwick, M.S.
Senior Microbiologist
Mycobacteriology Laboratory
Division of Bacterial and Mycotic Diseases
Centers for Disease Control and Prevention
Atlanta, Georgia

Jeffrey R. Starke, M.D.
Associate Professor of Clinical Pediatrics
Section of Infectious Diseases
Baylor College of Medicine
Houston, Texas

Wilfredo Talavera, M.D.
Chief, Division of Pulmonary and Critical Care
    Medicine
Cabrini Medical Center
    and
Associate Professor of Clinical Medicine
New York Medical College
New York, New York

Richard J. Wallace, Jr., M.D.
John Chapman Professorship in Microbiology
Professor of Medicine
Chairman
Department of Microbiology
University of Texas Health Center at Tyler
Tyler, Texas

Paul W. Wright, M.D.
Professor of Family Medicine
University of Texas Health Center at Tyler
Tyler, Texas

CONTENTS

Chapter 1

The Epidemiology of Tuberculosis

John A. Jereb, M.D., George M. Cauthen, Sc.D., Gloria D. Kelly, B.A., and Lawrence J. Geiter, M.P.H.

CONTENTS

0-8493-4825-0/94/$0.00+$.50

I. GENERAL AND THEORETICAL CONSIDERATIONS

A. BASIC MODELING

Current tuberculosis epidemiology relies on a stepwise model, and it assumes an infectious cause of the disease as tendered by Koch and predecessors. A population can be divided into three groups, with a "step" between each group: an unexposed group, usually indistinguishable from a group that has been exposed but is uninfected; a group exposed and infected with *Mycobacterium tuberculosis* but not diseased; and a group diseased with tuberculosis (Figure 1-1). Persons who have recovered from tuberculosis with or without medical treatment compose another group. Persons who have had previous infection or disease have a poorly understood risk of reinfection with *M. tuberculosis*, and they also have a risk of relapse from endogenous reactivation (see Section I.F).

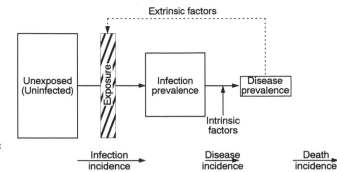

Figure 1-1 Basic epidemiologic model and indices for tuberculosis.

This stepwise infectious disease model is very useful as a conceptual aid for describing tuberculosis epidemiology, but it has limited direct application. It oversimplifies the actually seamless transition from exposure to infection to disease. Moreover, our incomplete knowledge of tuberculosis pathogenesis does not allow the model to predict accurately the outcome for an individual patient. The compartmentalized structure of the model makes calculating projections so complicated that computerized iterative approximations are required. Also, the distinctions between risk factors frequently are blurred. Delineating the associations between specific risks and specific steps in the model seldom is possible under operational research conditions.

B. TUBERCULOSIS INDICES

Prevalence and incidence are indices that summarize the epidemiologic status of both tuberculous infection and disease, and they commonly are expressed as ratios (rates) to adjust the absolute figures to a denominator population (prevalence rates) or to a population and time (incidence rates). These indices are useful for evaluating the status of tuberculosis in a population, but rarely are all indices available for the same population.

1. Infection

The standard method of measuring the prevalence of tuberculous infection is the tuberculin skin test survey.[1] Surveys give only an estimate of the true prevalence because the sensitivity and specificity of the tuberculin skin test are imperfect (see Chapter 13, this volume) and because most surveys are done on samples; sampling adds another source of variance. Nevertheless, tuberculin skin testing surveys are informative, and they are relatively quick, simple, and inexpensive. They are most useful in populations where the prevalence of tuberculous infection is comparatively high; if the prevalence is low, the predictive power of a positive result becomes vanishingly small.[2] Also, the usefulness is limited sometimes by regional differences in the prevalence of nonspecific tuberculin reactivity caused by sensitization to nontuberculous myco-

bacteria; this shortcoming is substantial in regions with warm, humid climates, and it requires analytical adjustments.[1-5] Administration of bacillus Calmette–Guérin (BCG) vaccine also causes variable response to tuberculin (see Chapters 13 and 15, this volume), and widespread use of BCG may complicate a skin testing survey.

a. Serial Tuberculin Skin Testing

Although a tuberculin skin test survey measures only the *prevalence* of infection, prevalence can be used in two ways to estimate *incidence* of infection. In the direct method, a defined population has serial tuberculin skin testing, and the annual change in the prevalence of reactivity reflects the acquisition of tuberculous infection. This method is limited by several factors: the problem of finding representative samples that can remain intact for extended periods, the relative inaccuracy of the tuberculin skin test in comparison to the small number of new infections expected each year, and the potential boosting of delayed T-cell hypersensitivity after repeated testing of persons who were infected in the remote past (see Chapter 13, this volume).

b. Annual Risk of Infection

An indirect method for measuring the incidence of infection uses a mathematical relationship between incidence and point prevalence: the prevalence of tuberculin reactivity for a birth cohort reflects the accumulation of tuberculous infection since birth. In the simplest model, the incidence rate of infection is assumed to be constant for the susceptible (uninfected) persons during the life of the cohort. Under these assumptions, the prevalence $p(t)$ at a given age t of the cohort and the annual risk of infection r are related by the expression[6-8]

$$p(t) = 1 - (1-r)^t, \quad \text{and thus } r = 1 - (1-p)^{1/t}$$

Figure 1-2 shows possible age and prevalence relationships for tuberculin reactivity in three populations. In curve A, the incidence rate of tuberculous infection is steady and high, and prevalence

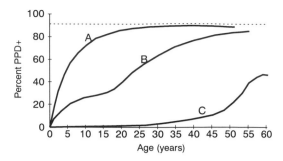

Figure 1-2 Hypothetical age distributions, tuberculin reactivity. (A) Constant, elevated annual risk of infection (ARI). (B) Time- and age-dependent ARI. (C) Declining ARI, currently very low.

accumulates very early in the life of each age cohort. This pattern was observed in studies of Alaskan natives in the 1950s.[9] A characteristic plateau, at 90–95%, is thought to be due to the inability of some infected persons to react to tuberculin, inherent immunity to tuberculous infection, or the reversion of reactivity (see Chapter 13, this volume). Because of this plateau, the best estimates for the incidence of infection in this population come from evaluating younger cohorts, who quickly acquire tuberculin reactivity. Curve C shows a population in which the prevalence of infection is low among young persons but high among old persons. Curve C represents countries that have reached extremely low incidence rates of tuberculosis; thus, rates for the recent transmission of infection are low. In these countries, the transmission of infection used to be common, so older individuals are likely to have been exposed and infected.[1,10,11] Curve B represents a population that has more complex tuberculosis indices.[12] Here, incidence rates of infection are different for each age cohort, either because of past fluctuations in the incidence rate of infection or because of social factors that change the likelihood of exposure depending on the age of the cohort, even though the infection rate at each age has not changed with time.

Most surveys to measure ARI evaluate school-aged children or military recruits. Observed values of ARI range from hundredths of a percent to thirty percent.[1,13-16] The World Health Organization (WHO) and the International Union Against Tuberculosis and Lung Diseases (IUATLD) advocate the ARI as a useful overall index to evaluate the tuberculosis situation in many regions.[6,8,17] Compared to other indices, the ARI is relatively insensitive to variations in survey methods, and it is easy to measure in areas where logistical problems make other indices unreliable, unavailable, or too expensive.[18]

2. Morbidity

The prevalence and incidence of active tuberculosis are the morbidity that a population suffers, and their magnitude determines the cost of health care and public health efforts as well as indirect costs, such as lost productivity and secondary tuberculosis cases.

a. Acid-Fast Bacillus Sputum Surveys

The simplest tuberculosis case definition is the detection of acid-fast bacilli (AFB) in the sputum smear of a patient who has respiratory symptoms; sometimes this is referred to as bacillary pulmonary tuberculosis. This case definition allows simple, fast case ascertainment with reasonable specificity. It has low technological requirements, because microscopy is the easiest and least expensive diagnostic technique to introduce in an area that does not have laboratory services.[19] Its specificity is good because bacillary tuberculosis usually is more common than nontuberculous mycobacterial pulmonary disease. However, this detection method is insensitive because it ignores a large proportion of tuberculosis morbidity; in developing countries, for every case of sputum smear-positive tuberculosis, there are an estimated 1.2 cases of AFB sputum smear-negative tuberculosis, pulmonary or extrapulmonary.[20,21] In addition, approximately 95% of tuberculosis in children younger than 10 years old cannot be detected by sputum smear examination.[2,20,22,23] Still, the sputum microscopy survey is a good method in some areas.[24] It provides important information, because bacillary tuberculosis is the most likely source of infection for new cases.

The prevalence of AFB sputum smear-positive tuberculosis disease influences the annual risk of infection directly.[20] It has been estimated that on average, 20 persons will acquire infection from a person with untreated, AFB smear-positive pulmonary tuberculosis during a 2-year span.[1] Because the first priority of a tuberculosis control program is to find and treat patients who have contagious tuberculosis,[1,14,17,20] the prevalence of contagious tuberculosis determines the initial needs of a new control program (see Chapter 14, this volume).

b. Other Methods of Case Detection

Chest radiography, laboratory isolation and identification of *M. tuberculosis* from clinical specimens, tuberculin skin test results, and the clinical decision to diagnose and treat tuberculosis increase the completeness of case ascertainment. Various combinations of these criteria are used by public health agencies in different countries to define cases. The recurrence of tuberculosis in a person may or may not be classified as a new case for counting. As new techniques for diagnosing tuberculosis become available, case detection may become more sensitive (see Chapters 4 and 5, this volume); this will have to be considered in interpreting longitudinal incidence rates.

3. Case Fatality Ratio and Mortality

Deaths due to tuberculosis can be expressed as a death rate for a given population or as a ratio of the number of deaths per 100 tuberculosis cases (case fatality ratio). Clearly, accurate death statistics are necessary to monitor the incidence of deaths due to tuberculosis.

a. Case Fatality

The factors that influence the unadjusted case fatality ratio are the effectiveness of the treatment program and the attributes of the patient population. Case fatality is very dependent on the availability and the timely use of adequate chemotherapy; it generally is higher for elderly patients and patients who have underlying illnesses.[1,25,26]

b. Mortality

Mortality data were the principal tuberculosis data collected systematically before the development of tuberculosis control programs, and our information about tuberculosis in the 19th and early 20th centuries comes from these data. Because a comprehensive tuberculosis control program that has good treatment results decreases the case fatality ratio, the death rate from tuberculosis now underestimates morbidity in some countries.[1,27,28]

C. REPORTING

Surveys directly measure the prevalence of tuberculosis, but some means of registering cases is required to measure the incidence. Serial surveys of a representative sample of a population can measure the incidence, but this method is expensive and usually not practical. Routinely, the registration of cases occurs when tuberculosis patients seek medical care. In countries where the health care delivery and the surveillance are separated, the counting of cases requires that each diagnosis of tuberculosis is reported to the public health authorities.

1. Case Notification Ratio

After the diagnosis of cases, reporting is the next step for keeping accurate tuberculosis statistics. The fraction of cases captured by a surveillance system is called the notification ratio or the coverage, and it is a function of the combined health care systems. "Coverage" connotes the ability to detect cases, whereas "notification" presupposes that cases are detected and refers to the completeness of surveillance.

2. Tuberculosis Diagnosed at or after Death

Late detection is a hallmark of tuberculosis. Numerous clinical and autopsy series have reported this problem throughout the world.[22,29-32] For example, a recent autopsy series in a Hong Kong hospital found that of patients who had tuberculosis when they died, 62% were diagnosed after death.[33] The autopsy series are sensitive and specific, but their results cannot be generalized, because deaths leading to autopsy are not representative of all deaths. Still, because some cases are not detected until autopsy, and because not all patients who die have an autopsy, the deaths of tuberculosis patients whose cases are undetected cases leads to the undercounting of tuberculosis cases.

Tuberculosis that is not diagnosed before the patient dies is a particular problem among the elderly.[29,34] Disseminated tuberculosis is relatively rare in the elderly, but when it does occur the symptoms are insidious and nonspecific; death may occur before the diagnosis is made.[26]

D. OUTBREAKS
1. Model of Concentric Circles

An important underlying pattern in tuberculosis outbreaks is that the risk of infection or disease increases as exposure to the person who has contagious tuberculosis (i.e., source case) increases.[13,35-39] This observation led to the method of "concentric circles" to organize the medical evaluation of persons exposed to tuberculosis (i.e., contacts). The group of contacts who were most exposed are evaluated first; decisions to evaluate groups who were less exposed are based on the results for the preceding group (see Chapter 14, this volume).

2. Source Cases

A common finding reported from outbreaks is the delayed detection of the source case.[37-46] One series attributed this delay both to the patient and the physician.[13] On average, the length of time required to diagnose tuberculosis was twice as long for source cases as it was for other tuberculosis cases. In countries with low incidence, unfamiliarity with tuberculosis can delay its diagnosis;[47,48] in Japan, outbreak-associated cases have increased as a fraction of morbidity.[48]

E. EXTRAPULMONARY TUBERCULOSIS

Although tuberculosis is a systemic disease that has protean symptoms, the distinction between pulmonary and extrapulmonary disease is important for diagnosis, morbidity, mortality, and surveillance. Extrapulmonary tuberculosis rarely is a public health threat because it is not transmissible in most settings; the infrequent reports of transmission from extrapulmonary sources imply iatrogenesis.[49,50] Still, in regions with declining tuberculosis incidence rates, extrapulmonary tuberculosis is becoming a larger fraction of cases.[10,15,51-53]

1. Surveillance

Extrapulmonary tuberculosis, where it exists, probably is detected in a smaller proportion of cases than is pulmonary tuberculosis. Extrapulmonary tuberculosis often is diagnosed late; tuberculous arthritis and osteitis are not diagnosed until an average of 10 months after symptoms begin.[54,55] Lethal forms, such as central nervous system disease or disseminated (miliary) disease, often are not diagnosed until after death, especially in the elderly[30,31,56] (see Section I.C.2).

F. REINFECTION

The basic infectious disease model did not include the reinfection of the populations who already have tuberculous infection or healed tuberculosis (Figure 1-1). Before the DNA fingerprinting of *M. tuberculosis*, it was difficult to confirm a case of reinfection, although phage typing has been used (see Chapter 5, this volume).[57,58] Data from outbreak investigations have implied reinfection;[59] one report showed evidence of reinfection from antimicrobial susceptibility patterns and phage typing,[60] and in another report, there is strong evidence of reinfection based on restriction fragment length polymorphism analysis.[61]

The relative contribution of reinfection to the incidence of tuberculosis is unknown. Some investigators have argued that the results of autopsy series demonstrate that reinfection in some populations is common and frequently leads to disease.[1] Models have been developed to estimate the incidence of exogenous reinfection and subsequent morbidity.[7] From these models, the incidence of exogenous reinfection and the reactivation of endogenous infection can be compared for each age group.

G. NATURAL TREND AND NATURAL HISTORY OF TUBERCULOSIS

The long-term trend of tuberculosis in a population and the clinical outcome of tuberculosis in untreated persons are unfortunate circumstances, but they are necessary standards to measure the efficacy of control programs. The outcome of untreated tuberculosis has global importance: only 46% of all the persons in the world who have tuberculosis are in any way reached by control programs,[21] and not all those who are reached will receive effective treatment. The rest of the persons will become chronically disabled (and possibly continue to spread infection), die, or sometimes recover.

1. Long-Term Trends

Since the 19th century, tuberculosis has been receding from the industrialized countries that previously had suffered high tuberculosis mortality rates. Some epidemiologists have attributed the sustained fall in rates to improvements in the human social milieu, presumably because less crowded housing decreased transmission and because a generally healthier population could better resist disease once infected with *M. tuberculosis*. Others, taking a guarded view,[62,63] have speculated that the complex balance between *M. tuberculosis* and the human species has reached a stage in which the human position is more favorable. In the most rigorous application of this approach, Grigg[10] concluded that a pandemic of tuberculosis had been started in Europe by sociologic or biological changes at a remote point in time. He argued that the fall of tuberculosis death rates represented the expected course of an epidemic "running its course" over a very long time. On average, tuberculosis is an indolent disease, and it has the ability to skip generations. According to this model, the epidemic slowly has selected a human population that survives because of inherited resistance to tuberculosis. The surviving population produces a new generation that has a higher fraction of persons who are resistant to the disease. The tuberculosis epidemic curve naturally takes the form of a "dampened wave" (Figure 1-3). This model predicts that the median age for tuberculosis patients will increase as the epidemic recedes and that the proportion of extrapulmonary tuberculosis will increase because of a changing host response to the infection.

H. MOLECULAR EPIDEMIOLOGY

To date, DNA fingerprinting (i.e., RFLP, see Chapter 5, this volume) has been used mostly to type strains of *M. tuberculosis* isolated from patients in outbreaks.[43,64-73] The technique is more specific and convenient than phage typing, and it can identify a strain independent of antimicrobial susceptibility results.[73,74] It is a powerful tool for clarifying and confirming the results of standard investigational methods. When the technique is available more widely, it should be possible to study reinfection caused by different strains of tuberculosis.[51]

DNA fingerprinting eventually may allow the development of a global epidemiologic history of *M. tuberculosis*. In countries where tuberculosis has been endemic for a long time, *M. tuberculosis* isolates have similar fingerprints that are different from isolates in other regions of the world.[75] Other potential applications include the isolation and characterization of strains that have altered virulence.

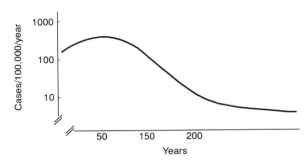

Figure 1-3 Theoretical time course of tuberculosis epidemic: under the "dampened wave" model.

II. GENERAL ASSOCIATIONS

A. AGE

All tuberculosis indices have an association with the age of the host. Infection and disease indices relate to age differently depending on the trend of tuberculosis in the population. If the indices are decreasing, then older populations bear more of the burden than if the indices are stable or increasing, when prevalence and incidence are high among adults from 20 to 40 years. Some of the relationships seen between age and tuberculosis must have underlying biological bases, but some also must be due to extrinsic social factors that influence the risk of infection and the general health of individuals.

1. Annual Risk of Infection

The ARI is weakly related to age and is more strongly influenced by the trends of tuberculosis incidence. However, for ascending age cohorts in a given year, the ARI increases slightly up to the age of about 20 years.[1]

2. Disease

For recently infected persons, the risk of disease has a complex association with age. Children younger than 4 years old are at high risk; disease develops in as many as 60% of newly infected, untreated children within the first year of infection (recalculated from old data[76] adapted to the current tuberculosis case definition in the United States). Children of grade school age are at lower risk — from 5–10%. The risk increases among young adults, and possibly again in the elderly.

For persons infected in the remote past, the risk of disease (i.e., the risk of endogenous reactivation) becomes lower.[77,78] Although it has been accepted that waning immunity in the elderly increases the risk of reactivation, this has been disputed by an analysis of age cohorts.[11] The estimated average risk of disease in an adult infected with *M. tuberculosis* is 5–15% distributed over a lifetime, and about half the risk is incurred within the first 2 years following infection.[1] The remaining risk is distributed over the rest of a lifetime.

3. Case Fatality

Although the age distribution for tuberculosis cases varies greatly among different populations, and the age-specific tuberculosis mortality rate mirrors the age distribution for cases,[79] there are distinct, age-specific variations in the case fatality ratio. The highest ratios are for the very old. The timely, correct use of chemotherapy is an overriding factor.

4. Extrapulmonary Tuberculosis

Age also plays a role in the proportion of cases of extrapulmonary disease. Extrapulmonary disease is more common among children less than 5 years old,[77] and this probably is a factor in the fatality for untreated tuberculosis in this group.[76,80]

B. GENDER

The differences in tuberculosis indices by gender vary with age and are not the same from population to population. Among adults, males are afflicted more often than females (at an approximate ratio of 2:1). Disease incidence rates by gender are very similar for young children, and among 15 to 25 year olds in populations that have endemic tuberculosis, the incidence is higher among females.[1,22,79] The ARI is slightly higher for males.[1] These differences probably have both biological and social roots.

C. RACE

Wherever different races coexist within an area reporting tuberculosis, the incidence rates differ by race. After tuberculosis was found to be an infectious disease, debates arose about possible links between race and inherited susceptibility to infection or disease.[81] It is plausible that some of the reasons for tuberculosis differences between races are purely biological.[82] As in most nature-versus-nurture debates, however, the differences would have to be fairly marked to be detectable by epidemiologic methods, because many confounding factors have unmeasurable effects on the contributory risks. Furthermore, in most situations, comparing racial groups is imprecise because these groups are heterogeneous. The diversity within each racial group likely increases the overlap of immunologic characteristics between groups.

Some studies in the United States have shown differences in infection rates between adult blacks and whites who may have been exposed to tuberculosis equally,[83] but confirming equal exposure is troublesome. In an example where exposure probably was equal, a point-source school outbreak of tuberculosis, infection rates were equal by race, but more of the infected black students had abnormal chest radiographs.[84] This result is similar to the findings of Brailey.[76] For more information, see Chapters 2 and 13, this volume.

D. OCCUPATION

Some occupations have been associated with increased tuberculosis indices. Three interdependent sources for the association can be postulated. First, workers may have come from populations for which rates of tuberculosis are high.[85] Second, there may be transmission of tuberculous infection in the work place. Third, a toxic contaminant in the work place may alter the host response to tuberculous infection.

1. Toxic Exposure — Silicosis

A confirmed example of an association between a harmful contaminant and tuberculosis is the increased rate and severity of tuberculosis among miners who have pulmonary silicosis.[86-89] A similar relationship for potters, whose occupational exposure to silica dust is high,[90] has been reported from England.[25] An incidence rate of more than 600 cases per 100,000 person-years has been reported for gold miners in South Africa.[91] For the gold miners, a high incidence of tuberculosis in the community, silicosis, and transmission in the work place may contribute.

2. Outbreaks

The transmission of tuberculosis in the work place can cause an outbreak. This occurred recently in the United States at a shipyard.[92] Such an outbreak, which might go undetected unless an association is made between the place of employment and the cases of tuberculosis, demonstrates the importance of thorough contact investigation.

3. Human Services

In human services, some employees are more likely to be exposed to tuberculosis because they work with groups among whom tuberculosis prevalence rates are higher. For example, exposure may occur in nursing homes,[93] prisons, and health care facilities.[39,44,45,49,50,68,70,71,94-97]

E. SPECIAL RISK GROUPS

The incidence of tuberculosis is increased among several socially defined groups.[98,99] Although these groups usually overlap other definable groups at risk for tuberculosis, e.g., socially disadvantaged persons, they have distinguishing features that challenge the delivery of health care (see Chapters 13 and 14, this volume).

1. Elderly in Nursing Homes

One such group is the elderly in nursing homes.[100] In addition to an elevated incidence rate attributable to common latent tuberculous infection,[11,101] the elderly in nursing homes have a high risk of exposure and new infection or possibly reinfection. Exposure risks are increased by the delayed diagnosis of contagious tuberculosis[40,93] (see Section I.C.2). Consequently, outbreaks occur.

2. Inmates of Correctional Facilities

Another group at risk is inmates of prisons and jails.[102] Prisons and jails may draw from groups for which tuberculosis incidence rates are increased, and they also draw from groups at risk for HIV infection.[103,104] The closed prison environment, ventilation that is possibly inadequate, and prolonged contact between inmates promote tuberculosis outbreaks.[105] In 1991 an extensive outbreak of multidrug-resistant tuberculosis in the New York State correctional system was attributed to delayed diagnosis of tuberculosis, the late recognition of drug resistance, the inadequate isolation of patients who had contagious tuberculosis, the interprison transfer of sick or newly infected inmates, and the high prevalence of HIV infection.[106] Jails are a special problem: inmates may stay in them long enough to become infected but not long enough for tuberculosis to incubate fully, and the jail might not be suspected as the site of transmission.

3. Migrant Farm Workers

Another group at risk is migrant farm workers.[107] It is difficult to administer a complete course of anti-tuberculosis chemotherapy to migrant farm workers because the patients and their contacts have to move seasonally. The prevalence of both HIV and tuberculous infection[108] and the incidence rate of tuberculosis[109] are increased among migrant farm workers.

4. Homeless Persons

Controlling tuberculosis among homeless persons is difficult because these persons can be hard to locate. Also, concurrent illnesses, substance abuse and subsequent HIV infection, and possible nonadherence to treatment are more prevalent among this group.[110-114] Measuring the incidence of tuberculosis among homeless persons in the United States was not possible previous to January 1993 because homelessness had not been reported in the Report of a Verified Case of Tuberculosis (RVCT). The prevalence rate of tuberculosis in one survey of homeless persons was 6%.[115] Erratic chemotherapy greatly increases the chance of drug resistance, which was found for 21% of homeless tuberculosis patients in one study.[116] The congregation of homeless persons in shelters is an opportunity for transmission and outbreaks,[59,43] and transmission may go undetected if symptoms of tuberculosis develop after newly infected persons have left the shelter. Homelessness has been reported as a risk factor in several other countries: Scotland,[117] South Africa,[118] and Japan.[119]

III. TUBERCULOSIS STATISTICS FOR THE WORLD

To estimate the global status of tuberculosis, projected indices are better than reported indices because some countries that have large tuberculosis burdens report erratically and others do not report at all. In 1992, WHO published estimated tuberculosis indices for the year 1990.[21] The estimated worldwide coverage for tuberculosis cases was 46%, which reflects the disparity between the tuberculosis problem and the capacity of current control programs to handle it.

A. INFECTION

In the 1992 WHO report,[21] the projected crude prevalence for infection was similar throughout the world; it ranged from 19.4% in the Eastern Mediterranean region to 43.8% in the Western Pacific region. Europe and the other industrialized nations (United States, Canada, Japan, Australia, and New Zealand) had a combined projected prevalence of 31.6%, although there have been no comprehensive tuberculin skin test surveys in these countries recently to support this high estimate. Overall, the prevalence rates were similar among areas, but the age-specific rates were much higher for younger age groups in countries that have high tuberculosis incidence rates.

1. Coinfection with HIV

The estimated number of persons infected with both *M. tuberculosis* and HIV was 3,053,000. Three-fourths of coinfected persons live in Africa. The estimated annual rate of tuberculosis for these persons was 10 per 100. Whether this potential increase of tuberculosis will be realized remains to be seen.[120,121]

B. MORBIDITY AND MORTALITY

For 1990, the projected incidence of tuberculosis in the world was 8,002,000. Only 392,000 cases, 5% of the projected incidence, were in persons in the industrialized nations, where the average incidence rate was 31 per 100,000 person-years. In the rest of the world, projected incidence rates ranged from 191 to 220. The global tuberculosis situation probably is worsening.[14]

1. Deaths

The projection for annual deaths due to tuberculosis ranged from 2,596,000 to 2,907,000, and 98.8% of the deaths were of persons in developing countries. The projected death rate from tuberculosis was approximately 30 times higher in the developing nations than in the industrialized nations; the case fatality ratio was four to five times higher (calculated).

2. Tuberculosis in China

About a quarter of tuberculosis cases in the world occur in China. A national survey done in China from 1984 through 1985 found a prevalence rate of 0.55%, and the calculated prevalence of active pulmonary disease was 5,700,000.[122] If chemotherapy were not being used, tuberculosis incidence would be about twice tuberculosis prevalence; the Chinese survey found more cases than would be estimated from the WHO projected incidence of 2,127,000.[21] This discrepancy suggests that existing programs may be prolonging the survival of tuberculosis patients but not curing them.

IV. TUBERCULOSIS IN THE UNITED STATES

Recent developments in the United States signal a new era in tuberculosis epidemiology. The new era is marked by a reversal of the long decline of incidence rates, an increase in tuberculosis in regions and demographic groups where HIV infection is prevalent, a decrease in the median age of persons who have tuberculosis, an increase in cases in children, an increase of cases in foreign-born persons, extensive outbreaks of multidrug-resistant tuberculosis in institutions housing HIV infected-persons, and perhaps a rising incidence of drug resistant tuberculosis.[34,98,99,123] Other industrialized nations report similar changes.

A. SURVEILLANCE

Tuberculosis is a reportable disease in all jurisdictions in the United States. The states and territories, the District of Columbia, and New York City have reported tuberculosis data to CDC since 1953 (Figure 1-4). At first, aggregate reports were submitted, but since 1985 most reporting areas have submitted individual case reports through an interactive system called the Report of a Verified Case of Tuberculosis (RVCT).

1. Case Definition

The RVCT case definition requires either a bacteriologic or a medical diagnosis of tuberculosis: either isolation of *M. tuberculosis* from a patient specimen or all four of the following factors:

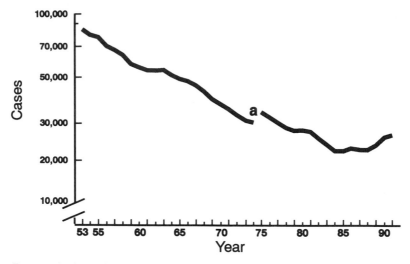

Figure 1-4 Reported tuberculosis cases, United States, 1953–1991. (a) Change in case definition.

1. completed diagnostic procedures,
2. evidence of tuberculous infection, usually a positive tuberculin skin test result,
3. abnormal, unstable chest radiographs or other diagnostic findings suggesting tuberculosis, and
4. medical decision to treat the patient with a full course of two or more antituberculosis medications.

Tuberculosis recurring in a patient at least 1 year after a previous diagnosis of tuberculosis is counted as a new case.

2. Verification

At CDC case reports are edited weekly to verify diagnoses and detect errors; suspected problems are referred to the reporting areas. Quarterly, the cumulative data are returned to the respective areas, which may correct or update case reports. At the end of the year, the data are reviewed by the respective areas before the national data are put into final form. Presently, these methods of verification are being revised.

The notification ratio (sensitivity) of the RVCT system is unknown. The Division of Tuberculosis Elimination, CDC, plans to study this and other parameters.

B. TUBERCULOSIS INCIDENCE, 1991

In 1991, the 50 states, the District of Columbia, and New York City reported 26,283 cases to CDC (Table 1-1), an increase of 2.3% (582) cases from the 1990 total of 25,701, which itself was an increase of 9.4% (2,206) from the total reported for 1989. The preliminary incidence in 1992 was 26,673 cases, another increase. The incidence rate in 1991 was 10.4 per 100,000 person-years; it was 10.3 in 1990 and 9.5 in 1989.

1. Incidence by State

All states reported at least six cases in 1991. California reported the most cases, 5,273; New York reported 4,430 and Texas reported 2,525. New York had the highest incidence rate: 24.5 cases per 100,000 person-years. Incidence rates in Hawaii and California were 17.7 and 17.4, respectively. Reported incidence rates increased in 14 states, remained unchanged in 6, and decreased in 30. Among states reporting over 100 cases in 1991, the largest relative increases in incidence rate were reported from Maryland (+16.3%), Arizona (+14.6%), and Georgia (+11.4%).

2. Incidence by City

New York City reported 3,682 cases in 1991, the most in any U.S. city; the incidence rate was the third highest, with 50.3 cases per 100,000 person-years. The highest city-specific rates were reported from Atlanta, Georgia, which had 76.4 per 100,000 person-years, and Newark, New Jersey, which had 71.8.

3. Incidence Rate Trend

In the United States, tuberculosis incidence rates decreased by about 6% annually for many years. In 1985, rates stabilized and then rose. Other low-incidence countries, such as Germany,[124-126] Czechoslovakia,[127,128] The Netherlands,[129] Japan,[48,130] Italy,[131] England,[132,133] Australia,[134,135] and New Zealand[136] also have reported a slowing or reversal of the downward trend.

4. Age Distribution

During several generations of declining tuberculosis indices in the United States, the age distribution of tuberculous infection increasingly shifted into older groups, and tuberculosis became a disease of

Table 1-1 **Reported cases of tuberculosis by sex, age group, race/ethnicity, and country of origin: United States, 1985 and 1991**

Characteristic	1985	1991	% Change
Totals	22,201	26,283	+18.4
Sex			
Male	14,496	17,069	+17.7
Female	7,704	9,214	+19.6
Unknown	1	0	—[a]
Age			
0–4	789	1,006	+27.5
5–14	472	656	+39.0
15–24	1,672	1,971	+17.9
25–44	6,758	10,263	+51.9
45–64	6,138	6,297	+2.6
65+	6,356	6,068	–4.5
Unknown	16	22	—[a]
Race/ethnicity			
White, non-Hispanic	8,453	7,709	–8.8
Black, non-Hispanic	7,592	9,536	+25.6
Hispanic	3,092	5,330	+72.4
Asian/Pacific Islander	2,530	3,346	+32.3
American Indian/Alaskan native	397	345	–13.1
Unknown/other	137	17	—[a]
Country of origin	(1986)[b]		
Foreign born	4,925	6,982	+41.8
U.S. born	17,712	19,161	+8.2
Unknown	131	140	—[a]

[a] Not calculated.

[b] Country of origin statistics presented for 1986, first year of uniform reporting, and 1991.

the elderly. With the recent resurgence of tuberculosis, this trend has reversed. In 1985 the median age of tuberculosis patients whose cases were reported to CDC was 49 years. This decreased to 44 years in 1990 and 43 years in 1991. The increase in cases among children younger than 5 years old[2] is most likely due to an increase in recent transmission, i.e., an increase in the ARI.

The ARI is not determined systematically for the United States presently. The best estimate of the average ARI, 0.06–0.09% (calculated), comes from the results of skin testing of Navy recruits from 1980 through 1986.[137] Still, the ARI for some groups must be much higher.[138]

The reversion to younger groups is not uniform across demographic strata. Although there has been a moderate increase among young, non-Hispanic white adults, the most marked incidence increases have occurred among nonwhite and Hispanic children and young adults; in these groups the incidence has nearly doubled from 1985 to 1991 (Figure 1-5). Among non-Hispanic whites the median age for reported tuberculosis cases decreased from 62 years to 59 years from 1985 to

1991; among non-Hispanic blacks it decreased from 43 years to 40 years; and among Hispanics it decreased from 36 years to 34 years. The median age of Hispanic tuberculosis patients born in the United States has been stable at 37 years; the downward age shift for all Hispanics in the United States is due to the increasing cases among foreign-born Hispanics, whose median age has been stable at 32 years.

5. Race or Ethnicity

For the RVCT, race is defined by local convention, and patients classify themselves. Increases in tuberculosis incidence rates have been greater in some racial or ethnic groups[98,99,139] (Table 1-1). From 1985 through 1991, increases were reported for Asian and Pacific Islanders and for Hispanics and non-Hispanic blacks. Incidences decreased among non-Hispanic whites and American Indians or Alaskan natives, but this downward trend has stagnated.

a. Incidence Rates by Race or Ethnicity

Relative incidence rates by race or ethnicity showed marked differences (Table 1-2). In 1991, the inci-

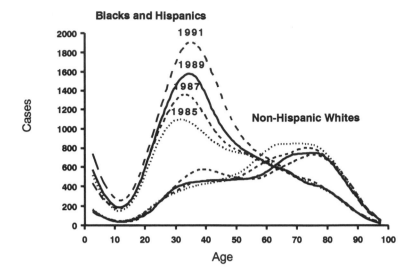

Figure 1-5 TB cases among blacks and Hispanics compared to non-Hispanic whites, United States, 1985, 1987, 1989, 1991.

Table 1-2 **Tuberculosis incidence rates by race, 1991**

Race	Rate[a]	Rate Ratio
White, non-Hispanic	4.1	1.0 (reference value)
Black, non-Hispanic	31.9	6.2
Hispanic	22.8	5.6
Asian/Pacific Islander	41.8	10.2
American Indian/ Alaskan native	16.3	4.0

[a]Per 100,000 person-years.

dence rate was highest among Asians or Pacific Islanders. Cases classified by race are very localized in the United States (Figures 1-6 to 1-8). Geographic concentration of cases warrants the development of targeted tuberculosis control programs.

b. Indigenous Peoples

Many countries that are socially stratified along racial or ethnic lines have reported differences in tuberculosis incidence by race or ethnicity. Examples include England,[140] the former Soviet Union,[141] and Israel.[142] Also, once-colonial countries usually report higher incidence rates for indigenous peoples, such as the American Indians and Alaskan natives in the United States.[16,143-145] In Australia, the incidence rate is 3 times higher for the aboriginal people[146] than for the descendants of European immigrants, in New Zealand it is 5 times higher for the Maori,[136] and in Canada it is 12 times higher for the Indians and Inuits.[47] A similar phenomenon has been reported from the northern re-

publics of the former Soviet Union.[147] Outbreaks among American Indians in the United States have contributed to the elevated incidence.[148]

6. Foreign Born Persons

Country of birth for patients who have tuberculosis in the United States has been reported uniformly to CDC since 1986. Reports of tuberculosis cases in foreign-born persons increased by 2,057 (+41.8%) from 1986 to 1991 (Table 1-1, Figure 1-9). For persons whose country of origin was reported (98.5–99.5% of cases), the fraction of cases in foreign born persons has increased steadily from 21.6% in 1986 to 26.6% in 1991. Exact incidence rates cannot be determined except for certain groups[149] because the population of foreign-born persons in the United States is not known.[150]

a. Incidence by State

The incidence of tuberculosis in foreign-born persons has great regional variation. Incidence among foreign-born persons is higher in states that have many immigrants from countries with higher tuberculosis incidence rates (parts of Asia, Central and South America, and Africa). In 1991, the largest fraction of cases in the foreign born, 155 (77%) of 201 cases, was in Hawaii. The greatest incidence, 3,198 (61.3%) of 5,220 cases for whom country of origin was reported, was in California, which also reported the largest increase of cases in foreign-born persons from 1986 to 1991 (1,240 cases or +63.3%). Other states reporting high incidence among foreign-born persons in 1991 were New York (810 cases), Texas (682), Florida (395), and Massachusetts (223).

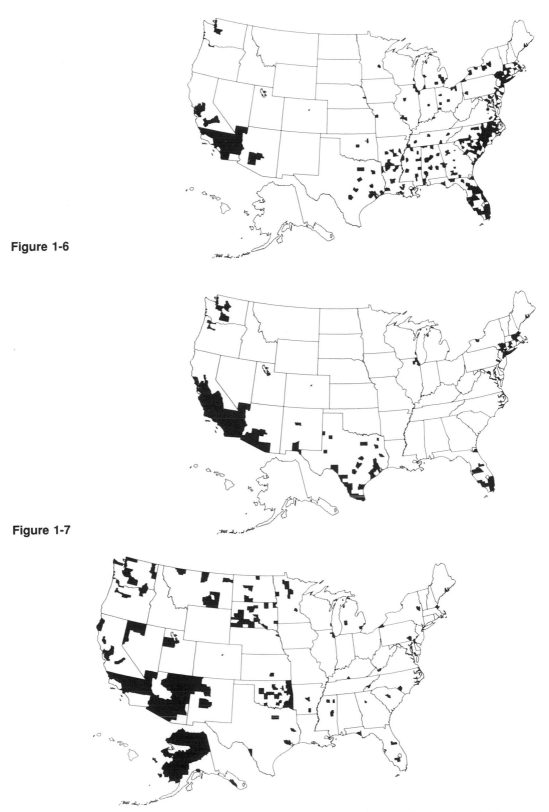

Figure 1-6

Figure 1-7

Figure 1-8 United States countries reporting 1 or more tuberculosis cases in American Indians and Alaskan natives; *N* = 147 (11.0%).

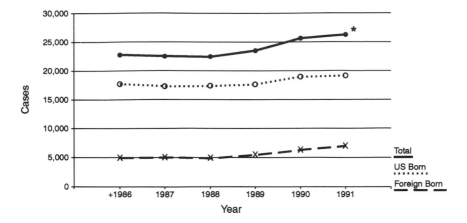

Figure 1-9 Tuberculosis cases by country of origin, United States, 1986–1991. (*) Includes about 1% without reported country of origin. (+) First year of uniform reporting of country of origin. Source: CDC.

b. Incidence by Race or Ethnicity

Tuberculosis incidence for Asians or Pacific Islanders and for Hispanics in the United States has been influenced strongly by cases in foreign born persons.[98] In 1991, 2,979 (89.6%) of 3,325 cases in Asian or Pacific Islanders and 2,952 (56.0%) of 5,276 cases in Hispanics for whom country of origin was reported were in foreign-born persons. The number of cases in U.S.-born Hispanics increased by 734 (+46.2%) between 1986 to 1991, whereas the number in foreign-born Hispanics increased by 1,367 (+86.2%).

c. Interval after Arrival

From 1986 through 1991, the reports for 75.2% of cases in foreign born persons specified the interval between arrival in the United States and the diagnosis of tuberculosis. This percentage has fluctuated little from year to year, and the distribution of duration in the United States before tuberculosis developed also has remained about the same. More than a quarter of cases (29.0%) occurred in persons who had been in the United States for less than 1 year. More than half (58.6%) occurred in persons within 5 years of immigration, and three quarters (74.7%) occurred within 10 years. Although some researchers have proposed that emotional and physical stress from relocation contributes to the development of tuberculosis soon after immigration, this remains conjectural. Davies has implicated falling vitamin D levels in the immigrants who came to a cloudy climate from their native sunny lands.[151,152] But researchers in Canada showed that the incidence rates for immigrants were slightly lower than the age-specific incidence rates in their countries of origin, regardless of the immigrants' duration in Canada.[153]

Other industrialized nations, including Australia,[134,135,154] New Zealand,[136] England,[132,140] Canada,[47,89,153,155] Japan,[156] Belgium,[157] Denmark,[158] Finland,[159] and Germany,[124] have reported large fractions of tuberculosis cases in foreign-born persons. In a study in British Columbia, Canada, tuberculosis developed in 5% of Vietnamese immigrants who were observed for as long as 6 years.[160] The corresponding average incidence rate is more than 800 per 100,000 person-years (calculated). In Switzerland, the tuberculosis prevalence rate was 0.17% for new immigrant workers and 1.4% for new refugees.[161] Nonindustrialized nations also have reported higher incidence of tuberculosis among immigrants.[162]

C. TUBERCULOSIS DEATHS

The primary source of information on tuberculosis deaths in the United States is the vital statistics from the National Center for Health Statistics. In 1989, the most recent year for which final results are available, 1,970 tuberculosis deaths were reported — an increase of 13.9% from the low figure of 1,729 reported in 1984 (Figure 1-10). Case fatality was highly dependent on age (Figure 1-11).

1. Case Fatality Ratio

The case fatality ratio in 1989 was 8.38 deaths per 100 tuberculosis cases; the lowest case fatality ratio in U.S. history was 7.08, recorded in 1981 and 1982. In a regression analysis of case fatality for 1982 through 1989, the odds ratio for a comparison of case fatalities from 1982 through 1989 was 1.32 after adjustment for age and race, i.e., tuberculosis patients matched on sex and age were 32% more likely to die of tuberculosis in 1989 than in 1982 (Table 1-3). Although the cause of this increase is unknown, it could be due to changing detection or reporting. This analysis must be interpreted with caution, because it is done on unlinked case and death data. Still, an increased case fatality rate might reflect the changing characteristics of patients, treatment, or pathogenesis.

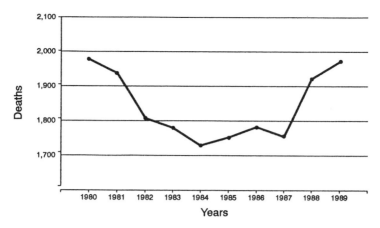

Figure 1-10 Tuberculosis deaths by year, United States, 1980–1989. Source: National Center for Health Statistics.

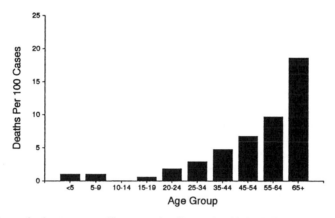

Figure 1-11 Tuberculosis age-specific case fatality ratio, United States, 1989. Sources: CDC; National Center for Health Statistics.

a. Case Fatality by Age

From 1982 to 1989, the case fatality ratio for tuberculosis in children less than 14 years old averaged 0.8 per 100. The ratio for children under 5 years was not significantly greater than the ratio for children 5 to 14 years; therefore, these age groups were combined to make the reference group. Age was the strongest determinant of case fatality (Table 1-3, Figure 1-11).

b. Case Fatality by Race or Ethnicity and Gender

The unadjusted case fatality ratio in 1989 was higher for non-Hispanic whites than for other racial or ethnic groups combined — 10.03 versus 6.81 deaths per 100 cases. This difference is attributable to the older age distribution in non-Hispanic white persons who have tuberculosis. After age adjustment, from 1982 through 1989 case fatality was lower for non-Hispanic whites than for other groups combined (Table 1-3). There was not a significant difference by sex after adjustment for age, race, and year.

2. Deaths Reported from Tuberculosis Control Programs

Death data also are available in the aggregate reports sent to CDC by tuberculosis control programs in the United States. Patients who die from any cause while receiving treatment for tuberculosis are reported at 3, 6, and 12 months after enrollment. The denominator is the number of patients who remain known to the programs, and the outcome for patients who leave the programs is unknown but likely to be different than for those who remain. The data are not categorized by age, race, sex, or cause of death. Most deaths occur during the first 3 months of treatment. In 1990, 8.9% of the patients who were observed for 3 months died, and 10.9% of those who were observed for 12 months died. These results have not changed notably from the previous 4 years.

3. Tuberculosis Diagnosed at Death

The incidence of tuberculosis diagnosed too late for successful treatment is underestimated for two rea-

Table 1-3 **Odds ratios for tuberculosis case fatality, adjusted for year, age, and race, logistic regression, 1982–1989**

Factor	Reference	Odds	95% Confidence Interval
1989	1982	1.32	1.25, 1.39
Age			
15–24	0–14	1.79	1.35, 2.37
25–44	0–14	5.28	4.14, 6.74
45–64	0–14	12.20	9.57, 15.55
65+	0–14	28.34	22.26, 36.08
Race			
Non-white	White	1.09	1.05, 1.13

sons. First, for RVCT reporting, a person in whom tuberculosis was diagnosed before death — even on the day before death — is correctly classified as alive at the time of diagnosis. Second, not all tuberculosis cases in persons who die are detected.

From 1985 through 1991, status (alive or dead) at the time of diagnosis was reported for more than 99% of tuberculosis patients. In 1991, 1248 (4.7%) of 26,263 cases for which status was known were reported as dead at the time of diagnosis. This figure has decreased from the most recent high of 1402 (6.2%) reported in 1987. Two reasons for the decline in tuberculosis diagnosed at death could be underdetection or underreporting. Another reason could be the downward shift of the age distribution of tuberculosis patients in the United States. The 25- to 44-year-old age group, which had the greatest increase in incidence, had the lowest fraction of cases diagnosed at death, 3.1%, whereas 11.4% of cases in persons 65 or older were diagnosed at death. These results agree with the observation that the diagnosis of tuberculosis is more likely to be missed in the elderly (see Section I.C.2).

D. EXTRAPULMONARY TUBERCULOSIS

At least since 1963, incidence has decreased more slowly for extrapulmonary than for pulmonary tuberculosis in the United States. This observation has never been completely explained.[10,51] Recently, the incidence has increased faster for extrapulmonary tuberculosis than for pulmonary. Some of this disparity may be caused by coinfection with HIV, which probably promotes the dissemination of tuberculosis and progression of disease at extrapulmonary foci. However, this cannot account for the observed increases in extrapulmonary tuberculosis in groups thought to have a low prevalence of HIV infection. Another factor may be ongoing transmission and the resulting primary tuberculosis. Several kinds of extrapulmonary tuberculosis (meningeal, miliary,

pleural, and bone and joint) are most frequent in the year after new infection.[77] Caution must be used in analyzing surveillance data on extrapulmonary tuberculosis, because ascertainment and reporting bias are possible. No surveys have been done to assess the validity of the RVCT system for reporting the site of disease.

1. Incidence

From 1985 through 1991, the site of active tuberculosis was specified in 99.95% of case reports in the United States; 77.8% of cases were pulmonary only, 17.2% were extrapulmonary only, and 5.0% were both extrapulmonary and pulmonary. In all, 22.2% (17.2% plus 5.0%) of reported cases had some extrapulmonary (only or both) component. Children had higher fractions of extrapulmonary (only or both) disease: 28.7% for those who were younger than 5 years old and 29.7% for those who were 5 to 14 years old. The fraction was also slightly higher for persons who were 25 to 44 years old, at 24.9%.

2. Increases in Extrapulmonary Tuberculosis

The disparities between the increases in pulmonary and extrapulmonary tuberculosis are marked. From 1985 through 1991, reported pulmonary (only) tuberculosis incidence increased from 17,622 to 20,142 cases (+14.3%), but extrapulmonary (only) incidence increased from 3595 to 4708 cases (+30.9%). Combined forms (cases of both pulmonary and extrapulmonary tuberculosis) had the largest relative increase, going from 981 to 1416 cases (+44.3%). Large increases in the "both" category could be attributed to the HIV epidemic, because this is the disease pattern reported in case series of tuberculosis patients coinfected with HIV.

a. Increases by Age

From 1985 through 1991, the 45- to 64-year-old age group had the greatest disparity in change: a decrease of 2.5% for pulmonary (only) tuberculosis versus an increase 27.4% for extrapulmonary (only or both). The 25- to 44-year-old age group also had a disparity: an increase of 47.4% for pulmonary versus an increase of 66% for extrapulmonary (only or both). The incidence for combined pulmonary and extrapulmonary (both) increased by 132% in the 25- to 44-year-old age group.

b. Increases by Race or Ethnicity

From 1985 through 1991, all racial or ethnic groups showed the disparity. It was more marked among Asians or Pacific Islanders: an increase of 29.5% for pulmonary (only) versus an increase of 40.6% for extrapulmonary (only or both) from 1985 through 1991. For Hispanics, the difference was

+66.0% versus +94.8%; for non-Hispanic blacks, it was +22.8% versus +35.0%.

c. Increases by Gender

From 1985 through 1991, the age-unadjusted fraction of extrapulmonary (only or both) tuberculosis was lower for males than for females, but the disparity between the increases of pulmonary and extrapulmonary disease was greater for males. For males, tuberculosis increased by 12.9% for pulmonary (only) versus 38.6% for extrapulmonary (only or both), whereas for females, the increases were 17.2% versus 26.8%.

E. CULTURE POSITIVITY

In 1991 a positive culture for *M. tuberculosis* was reported for 81.5% of cases, a figure not notably different from figures from the previous 6 years. Averaged from 1986 through 1991, the culture positivity was highest for persons 65 years and older (87.6%) and lowest for persons 5–14 years old (22.5%). By site of disease, culture positivity was highest for persons who had both extrapulmonary and pulmonary disease (85.5%), slightly lower for persons who had pulmonary disease only (83.5%), and lowest for persons who had extrapulmonary disease only (76.5%).

F. TUBERCULOSIS AND HIV INFECTION

As of June 1993, information about HIV infection or AIDS diagnosis is being incorporated into tuberculosis case reporting in the United States. Current data are limited to the results of targeted studies (see Section V).

Mathematical modeling suggests that the prevalence of coinfection with HIV and *M. tuberculosis* in the United States currently is between 40,000 and 100,000.[163] If tuberculosis develops in 8% of coinfected persons per year,[164,165] the predicted incidence of tuberculosis in HIV-infected persons would be 3200 to 8000 per year. Future data collection in the RVCT should allow the refinement of these projections.

V. INFECTION WITH HUMAN IMMUNODEFICIENCY VIRUS

Many studies have shown that infection with HIV increases the risk of tuberculosis,[166,167] although the analysis is confounded because groups at risk for exposure to HIV often overlap with groups at risk for exposure to tuberculosis.[41,110,111,168-172] Results support the theory that HIV infection facilitates the transition from tuberculous infection to tuberculosis, but no studies have demonstrated that HIV infection increases susceptibility to tuberculous infection. Investigations have taken several forms.

A. CASE SERIES AND CASE CONTROL STUDIES[173-182]

These studies emphasized the demographics and unexpected clinical features of tuberculosis in HIV-infected patients, and they showed an increased prevalence of HIV infection among some groups of tuberculosis patients, generally those at risk for HIV infection because of injecting drug use. These studies found that in HIV-infected persons, tuberculosis usually was diagnosed before other AIDS case-defining illnesses occurred, cavitary pulmonary tuberculosis was uncommon, extrapulmonary disease was common, and fatality was increased. Tuberculin reactivity was as low as 7% in persons who had more advanced HIV disease and lower CD4[+] T-lymphocyte counts.[168] Some series showed that HIV-infected pulmonary tuberculosis patients were less likely to have AFB smear-positive sputa than were pulmonary tuberculosis patients who were not HIV-infected,[175,181,183] but other studies did not;[179] contagiousness was similar for HIV-infected pulmonary tuberculosis patients and pulmonary tuberculosis patients without HIV infection.[168,184] Comparisons of tuberculosis patients with patients in matching control groups usually have shown a much higher prevalence of HIV infection among the tuberculosis patients, but the careful selection of controls is important. One study found an HIV prevalence of 26% among tuberculosis patients but a prevalence of 20% among the controls.[185] The overlap of risk factors for both infections probably is the confounder.

B. HIV OR AIDS REGISTRIES

In the United States, the AIDS registry, which from 1987 through 1992 recorded only extrapulmonary tuberculosis, has noted an approximately 3% prevalence of tuberculosis among patients whose AIDS cases were reported. In Italy, about 2% of patients whose cases were in the AIDS registry by the end of 1989 had tuberculosis (all forms) and the percentage was increasing.[186]

C. MATCHES BETWEEN REGISTRIES FOR TUBERCULOSIS AND AIDS

In the United States, cross-matches between tuberculosis registries and AIDS registries have found a significant number of tuberculosis patients who had cases listed in AIDS registries and AIDS patients who had cases listed in tuberculosis registries.[169] A match in a state prison system showed that 56% of inmates who had tuberculosis had cases listed in the HIV or AIDS registry.[103]

D. HIV SEROPREVALENCE SURVEYS

Seroprevalence surveys among tuberculosis patients have shown a high HIV seroprevalence, up to

50%.[168,187,188] However, some surveys have low rates of HIV seropositivity or no HIV seropositivity.[189-191] The independent prevalence of each infection and the distribution within groups at risk for both infections affect the group-specific prevalence of coinfection.

E. PROSPECTIVE STUDIES

Several prospective studies of patients who have asymptomatic coinfection with *M. tuberculosis* and HIV are under way. In one cohort, the annual incidence rate of tuberculosis was approximately 8% among HIV-infected injecting drug users who had positive tuberculin skin test results.[164,165]

F. TUBERCULOSIS OUTBREAKS AMONG HIV-INFECTED PERSONS

An early reported tuberculosis outbreak among HIV-infected persons was in an Italian hospital.[42] The rapid evolution of this outbreak, the high attack rates, and the severe morbidity have been repeated in similar outbreaks since then, and mortality was high in some. Evidence from these outbreaks suggests that tuberculosis has a shorter incubation period and a more fulminant clinical course among person who have HIV infection and later become infected with *M. tuberculosis* than among persons who have latent tuberculous infection and later become infected with HIV. Most of the reported outbreaks in the United States have been of drug-resistant tuberculosis.[69-72] This is partly because drug resistance is a marker for an outbreak, and perhaps because drug-resistant tuberculosis that is incompletely treated may remain contagious for a longer period. Most of the reported outbreaks have occurred in health care facilities, but other institutions where HIV-infected persons are congregated have reported outbreaks.[41,73,106,171] To date, over 200 patients have been involved, and the case–fatality ratio approaches 90%. These outbreaks can be attributed to the congregation of HIV-infected patients, failure to detect and effectively treat for tuberculosis, delayed AFB isolation precautions, and inadequate facilities for effective isolation. The rapid evolution of these outbreaks — in some, secondary cases appeared as soon as a month after exposure to a source case — means that several generations of transmission may take place before control measures are implemented. Because of the high attack rates, these tuberculosis outbreaks among HIV-infected persons have been larger than typical tuberculosis outbreaks among persons not infected with HIV.

G. POPULATION-BASED STUDIES

One study showed a positive correlation between HIV prevalence and tuberculosis incidence rate by geographic area in the United States.[192] This observation was of association, and thus causality was not proven.

H. INCREASED TUBERCULOSIS INCIDENCE IN AREAS WHERE AIDS IS EPIDEMIC

In some countries in Africa[79,120] and in the areas in the United States[98,167] that are most affected by the AIDS epidemic, tuberculosis incidence rates have been rising. A similar association is suspected in Italy, too.[186]

IV. DRUG-RESISTANT TUBERCULOSIS

A. WORLDWIDE

Surveys in developed countries have shown that the relative prevalence of drug-resistant tuberculosis is higher among immigrants.[123,193-195] Presumably, the immigrants who have drug-resistant disease have been given incomplete treatment previously and then had a relapse of tuberculosis, this time resistant to drugs (secondary resistance). Alternatively, they have been infected with *M. tuberculosis* that has primary resistance, because drug-resistant tuberculosis is commonly transmitted in their countries of origin. Estimates for the prevalence of drug-resistant tuberculosis compared to drug-sensitive tuberculosis throughout the world are variable (because of sampling differences) and sporadic, and most surveys were done more than 10 years ago.[196] Estimates from 1984 "World Atlas of Initial Drug Resistance"[196] (patients assumed to be previously untreated) show that in Madras, India in 1982, of 750 patients tested, the rates of resistance to INH and streptomycin were 22.3 and 16.8%, respectively. In Pakistan, from 1955 to 1978, of 1176 patients tested, the rates of resistance to INH and streptomycin were 31.8 and 36.7%, respectively. In East Africa, during 1978, of 876 patients tested, the rates of resistance to INH, streptomycin, and both were 5.0, 2.3, and 1.3%, respectively. In the African tribes (Tswana, Zulu, Xhosa, and Shangaan), from 1970 to 1982, of a total of 24,310 patients tested, the rates of resistance to INH, streptomycin, and both ranged from 17.8 to 32.9%, 4.6 to 12.5%, and 0 to 5.2%, respectively. The prevalence of resistance to a given antimicrobial medication probably depends on the local misuse of that medication, so large regional differences are to be expected. Furthermore, these rates certainly are different today. The collection of worldwide updated survey data is still under way.[197]

B. UNITED STATES

Antimicrobial susceptibility patterns of tuberculosis once were the focus of systematic surveys in the United States. When prevalence became very low and continued to decrease, surveillance for drug susceptibility patterns was stopped.[123,198] Large outbreaks of multidrug-resistant tuberculosis in several institutions raised the possibility that the prevalence of resistance was increasing (see Section V.F). In 1991, surveillance was renewed with more complete coverage than before, and drug resistance information is being incorporated in the RVCT. In April 1991 investigators in New York City studied 227 newly diagnosed, culture-positive tuberculosis patients not known to have been previously treated for tuberculosis. Of these patients, isoniazid resistance was found in 15%, rifampin resistance was found in 10%, and resistance to both isoniazid and rifampin was found in 7%. There were a total of 23% of patients with *M. tuberculosis* isolates that were resistant to at least one of 11 medications tested; resistance appeared to be primary. The percentage of patients resistant to at least one drug was twice that observed in New York City 10 years earlier. Of 239 previously treated patients, isoniazid resistance was found in 36%, rifampin resistance was found in 33%, and resistance to both isoniazid and rifampin was found in 30%. There were a total of 44% of patients with *M. tuberculosis* isolates that were resistant to at least one of 11 medications tested.[199] Overall resistance (primary and secondary) was less common with rifabutin (14%), streptomycin (13%), ethambutol (8%), and ethionamide (6%). These data demonstrate the importance of surveillance for drug-resistant tuberculosis, and they emphasize how urgent it is to implement the recently issued tuberculosis treatment and control guidelines.[200,201]

REFERENCES

1. Styblo, K., Epidemiology of tuberculosis, *Selected Papers, Royal Netherlands Tuberc. Assoc.*, 24, 1991.
2. Starke, J. R., Jacobs, R. F., Jereb, J., Resurgence of tuberculosis in children, *J. Pediatr.*, 120, 839, 1992.
3. Lind, A., Larsson, L. O., Bentzon, M. W., Magnusson, M., Olofson, J., Sjogren, I., Strannegard, I. L., Skoogh, B. E., Sensitivity to sensitins and tuberculin in Swedish children. I. A study of schoolchildren in an urban area, *Tubercle*, 72, 29, 1991.
4. Larsson, L. O., Skoogh, B. E., Bentzon, M. W., Magnusson, M., Olofson, J., Taranger, J., Lind, A., Sensitivity to sensitins and tuberculin in Swedish children. II. A study of preschool children, *Tubercle*, 72, 37, 1991.
5. Bleiker, M. A., Non-specific tuberculin sensitivity in school children in European countries [German; English abstract], *Zeit. Erkrankung. Atmungsorg.*, 173, 46, 1989.
6. Bleiker, M. A., The annual tuberculosis infection rate, the tuberculin survey and the tuberculin test, *Bull. Int. Union Tuberc. Lung Dis.*, 66, 53, 1991.
7. Sutherland, I., Svandova, E., Radhakrishna, S., The development of clinical tuberculosis following infection with tubercle bacilli, *Tubercle*, 63, 255, 1982.
8. Sutherland, I., On the risk of infection, *Bull. Int. Union Tuberculosis Lung Dis.*, 66, 189, 1991.
9. Comstock, G. W., Porter, M. E., Tuberculin sensitivity and tuberculosis among natives of the lower Yukon, *Public Health Rep.*, 74, 621, 1959.
10. Grigg, E. R. N., The arcana of tuberculosis, *Am. Rev. Tuberc. Pulmonary Dis.*, 78, 151, 1958.
11. Comstock, G. W., Frost revisited: the modern epidemiology of tuberculosis, *Am. J. Epidemiol.*, 101, 363, 1975.
12. Bi-Ya, Y., Status of TB control in selected developing countries: China, presented at World Congress on Tuberculosis, Bethesda, Maryland, November 17, 1992.
13. Veen, J., Tuberculosis in a low prevalence country: a wolf in sheep's clothing, *Bull. Int. Union Tuberc. Lung Dis.*, 66, 203, 1991.
14. Kochi, A., The global tuberculosis situation and the new control strategy of the World Health Organization, *Tubercle*, 72, 1, 1991.
15. Aditama, T. Y., Prevalence of tuberculosis in Indonesia, Singapore, Brunei Darussalam and the Philippines, *Tubercle*, 72, 255, 1991.
16. Comstock, G. W., Philip, R. N., Decline of the tuberculosis epidemic in Alaska, *Public Health Rep.*, 76, 19, 1961.
17. International Union against Tuberculosis, World Health Organization, Tuberculosis control, *Tubercle*, 63, 157, 1982.
18. Mayurnath, S., Vallishayee, R. S., Radhamani, M. P., Prabhakar, R., Prevalence study of tuberculous infection over fifteen years, in a rural population in Chingleput district (south India), *Indian J. Med. Res.*, 93, 74, 1991.
19. Smithwick, R. W., World Health Organization, *Laboratory Manual for Acid-Fast Microscopy*, 2nd ed., U.S. Department of Health, Education, and Welfare, Atlanta, 1976, 1.
20. Murray, C. J. L., Styblo, K., Rouillon, A., Tuberculosis in developing countries: burden, intervention and cost, *Bull. Int. Union Tuberc. Lung Dis.*, 65, 7, 1990.
21. Sudre, P., ten Dam, G., Kochi, A., Tuberculosis: a global overview of the situation today, *Bull. W.H.O.*, 70, 149, 1992.
22. Second East African/British Medical Research Council Kenya Tuberculosis Survey, Tuberculosis in Kenya: a second national sampling survey of drug resistance and other factors, and a comparison with the prevalence data from the first national sampling survey, *Tubercle*, 59, 155, 1978.

23. Snider, D. E., Jr., Rieder, H. L., Combs, D., Bloch, A. B., Hayden, C. H., Smith, M. H., Tuberculosis in children, *Pediatr. Infect. Dis. J.*, 7, 271, 1988.

24. Hafez, M. A., Mazumder, A., Begum, J., Tarafder, M. A., A study on the prevalence of tuberculosis in a rural community of Bangladesh, *Bangladesh Med. Res. Council Bull.*, 17, 23, 1991.

25. Cole, R. B., Respiratory tuberculosis in the potteries, *Ann. Occupation. Hyg.*, 33, 387, 1989.

26. King, D., Davies, P. D. O., Disseminated tuberculosis in the elderly: still a diagnosis overlooked, *J. R. Soc. Med.*, 85, 48, 1992.

27. Grzybowski, S., Natural history of tuberculosis, *Bull. Int. Union Tuberc. Lung Dis.*, 66, 193, 1991.

28. Stevens, R. G., Lee, J. A. H., Tuberculosis: generation effects and chemotherapy, *Am. J. Epidemiol.*, 107, 120, 1978.

29. Rieder, H. L., Kelly, G. D., Bloch, A. B., Cauthen, G. M., Snider, D. E., Tuberculosis diagnosed at death in the United States, *Chest*, 100, 678, 1991.

30. Chen, T. M., Lee, P. Y., Perng, R. P., Extrapulmonary tuberculosis: experience at Veterans General Hospital — Taipei, 1985 to 1987, *J. Formosan Med. Assoc.*, 90, 1163, 1991.

31. Yamada, H., Katoh, O., Hiura, K., Nakanishi, Y., Kuroki, S., Aoki, Y., Nakahara, Y., Yamaguchi, M., The present status of active tuberculosis in a general hospital: a study of 186 cases, *Jpn. J. Med.*, 30, 304, 1991.

32. Trnka, L., Dankova, D., The epidemiologic situation regarding tuberculosis and the effectiveness of tuberculosis surveillance in Bohemia in 1988 [Czech; English abstract], *Casopis Lekaru Ceskych*, 129, 166, 1990.

33. Lee, J. K., Ng, T. H., Undiagnosed tuberculosis in hospitalized patients — an autopsy survey, *J. R. Soc. Health*, 110, 141, 1990.

34. Bloch, A. B., Rieder, H. L., Kelly, G. D., Cauthen, G. M., Hayden, C. H., Snider, D. E., The epidemiology of tuberculosis in the United States, *Clinics Chest Med.*, 10, 297, 1989.

35. Lincoln, E. M., Epidemics of tuberculosis, *Adv. Tuberc. Res.*, 14, 157, 1965.

36. DiStasio, A. J., II, Trump, D. H., The investigation of a tuberculosis outbreak in the closed environment of a U.S. navy ship, 1987, *Military Med.*, 155, 347, 1990.

37. Hyge, T. V., Epidemic of tuberculosis in a state school, *Acta Tuberculosa Scand.*, 21, 1, 1947.

38. Gross, T. P., Silverman, P. R., Bloch, A. B., Smith, T. Y., Rogers, G. W., An outbreak of tuberculosis in rural Delaware, *Am. J. Epidemiol.*, 129, 362, 1989.

39. Ehrenkranz, N. J., Kicklighter, J. L., Tuberculosis outbreak in a general hospital: evidence for airborne spread of infection, *Ann. Intern. Med.*, 77, 377, 1972.

40. Taylor, D. R., Allison, G., Tuberculosis among long term hospital residents: report of a recent outbreak, *N. Z. Med. J.*, 104, 421, 1991.

41. Centers for Disease Control, Transmission of multidrug-resistant tuberculosis from an HIV-positive client in a residential substance-abuse treatment facility — Michigan, *Morbid. Mortal. Weekly Rep.*, 40, 129, 1991.

42. Di Perri, G., Danzi, M. C., DeChecchi, G., Pizzighella, S., Solbiati, M., Cruciani, M., Luzzati, R., Malena, M., Mazzi, R., Concia, E., Bassetti, D., Nosocomial epidemic of active tuberculosis among HIV-infected patients, *Lancet*, 2, 1502, 1989.

43. Centers for Disease Control, Tuberculosis among residents of shelters for the homeless — Ohio, 1990, *Morbid. Mortal. Weekly Rep.*, 40, 869, 1991.

44. Catanzaro, A., Nosocomial tuberculosis, *Am. Rev. Resp. Dis.*, 125, 559, 1982.

45. Craven, R. B., Wenzel, R. P., Atuk, N. O., Minimizing tuberculosis risk to hospital personnel and students exposed to unsuspected disease, *Ann. Intern. Med.*, 82, 628, 1975.

46. Gronauer, W., The epidemiologic significance of unrecognized lung tuberculosis in the present-day [German; English abstract], *Pneumologie*, 43, 20, 1989.

47. Enarson, D. A., Wade, J. P., Embree, V., Risk of tuberculosis in Canada: implications for priorities in programs directed at specific groups, *Can. J. Public Health*, 78, 305, 1987.

48. Aoki, M., Surveillance of tuberculosis in low prevalence countries where tuberculosis is in decline, *Bull. Int. Union Tuberc. Lung Dis.*, 66, 201, 1991.

49. Frampton, M. W., An outbreak of tuberculosis among hospital personnel caring for a patient with a skin ulcer, *Ann. Intern. Med.*, 117, 312, 1992.

50. Hutton, M. D., Stead, W. W., Cauthen, G. M., Bloch, A. B., Ewing, W. M., Nosocomial transmission of tuberculosis associated with a draining abscess, *J. Infect. Dis.*, 161, 286, 1990.

51. Rieder, H. L., Snider, D. E., Jr., Cauthen, G. M., Extrapulmonary tuberculosis in the United States, *Am. Rev. Resp. Dis.*, 141, 347, 1990.

52. Heng, B. H., Tan, K. K., Three decades of tuberculosis in Singapore, *Bull. Int. Union Tuberc. Lung Dis.*, 66, 125, 1991.

53. Garcia-Rodriguez, J. A., Garcia Sanchez, J. E., Gomez Garcia, A. C., Extrapulmonary tuberculosis in a university hospital in Spain, *Eur. J. Epidemiol.*, 5, 154, 1989.

54. Foley-Nolan, D., Deegan, R. I., Foley-Nolan, A. A., Barry, C., Coughlan, R. J., Hone, R., Skeletal tuberculosis, *Irish Med. J.*, 84, 72, 1991.

55. Agarwal, R. P., Mohan, N., Garg, R. K., Bajpai, S. K., Verma, S. K., Mohindra, Y., Clinicosocial aspect of osteoarticular tuberculosis, *J. Indian Med. Assoc.*, 88, 11, 1990.

56. Ibanez Martinez, J., Bautista Ojeda, M., D., Saez Torres, C., Jorda i Heras, M., Ayerza Lerchundi, M. A., Pachon Diaz, J., Multicenter study of tuberculosis in clinical autopsies in Andalucia, in the 1973–1988 period [Spanish; English abstract], *Rev. Clin. Espanola*, 188, 273, 1991.

57. Snider, D. E., Jr., Jones, W. D., Good, R. C., The usefulness of phage typing *Mycobacterium tuberculosis* isolates, *Am. Rev. Resp. Dis.*, 130, 1095, 1984.

58. Raleigh, J. W., Wichelhausen, R., Exogenous reinfection with *Mycobacterium tuberculosis* confirmed by phage typing, *Am. Rev. Resp. Med.*, 108, 639, 1973.

59. Nolan, C. M., Elarth, A. M., Barr, H., Saeed, M., Risser, D. R., An outbreak of tuberculosis in a shelter for homeless men. A description of its evolution and control, *Am. Rev. Resp. Dis.*, 143, 257, 1991.

60. Nardell, E., McInnis, B., Thomas, B., Weidhaas, S., Exogenous reinfection with tuberculosis in a shelter for the homeless, *N. Engl. J. Med.*, 315, 1570, 1986.

61. Small, P. M., Shafer, R. W., Hopewell, P. C., Singh, S. P., Murphy, M. J., Desmond, E., Sierra, M. F., Schoolnik, G. K., Exogenous reinfection with multidrug-resistant *Mycobacterium tuberculosis* in patients with HIV infection, *N. Engl. J. Med.*, 328, 1137, 1993.

62. Forst, W. H., How much control of tuberculosis?, *Am. J. Public Health*, 27, 759, 1937.

63. Wallgren, A., Combating tuberculosis in a Swedish city, *Irish J. Med. Sci.*, July, 1939.

64. Cave, M. D., Eisenach, K. D., McDermott, P. F., Bates, J. H., Crawford, J. T., IS6110: conservation of sequence in the *Mycobacterium tuberculosis* complex and its utilization in DNA fingerprinting, *Mol. Cell. Probes*, 5, 73, 1990.

65. Otal, I., Martin, C., Vincent-Levy-Frebault, V., Thierry, D., Gicquel, B., Restriction fragment length polymorphism analysis using IS6110 as an epidemiologic marker in tuberculosis, *J. Clin. Microbiol.*, 29, 1252, 1991.

66. Mazurek, G. H., Cave, M. D., Eisenach, K. D., Wallace, R. J., Jr., Bates, J., H., Crawford, J. T., Chromosomal DNA fingerprinting patterns produced with IS6110 as strain-specific markers for epidemiologic study of tuberculosis, *J. Clin. Microbiol.*, 29, 2030, 1991.

67. Ross, B. C., Raios, K., Jackson, K., Sievers, A., Dwyer, B., Differentiation of *Mycobacterium tuberculosis* strains by use of a nonradioactive southern blot hybridization method, *J. Infect. Dis.*, 163, 904, 1991.

68. Pearson, M. L., Jereb, J. A., Frieden, T. R., Crawford, J. T., Davis, B. J., Dooley, S. W., Jarvis, W. R., Nosocomial transmission of multidrug-resistant *Mycobacterium tuberculosis*: a risk to patients and health care workers, *Ann. Intern. Med.*, 117, 191, 1992.

69. Centers for Disease Control, Nosocomial transmission of multidrug-resistant tuberculosis among HIV-infected persons — Florida and New York, 1988–1991, *Morbid. Mortal. Weekly Rep.*, 40, 585, 1991.

70. Dooley, S. W., Villarino, M. E., Lawrence, M., Salinas, L., Amil, S., Rullen, J. V., Jarvis, W. R., Bloch, A. B., Cauthen, G. M., Nosocomial transmission of tuberculosis in a hospital unit for HIV-infected patients, *J. Am. Med. Assoc.*, 267, 2632, 1992.

71. Beck-Sague, C., Dooley, S. W., Hutton, M. D., Otten, J., Breeden, A., Crawford, J. T., Pitchenik, A. E., Woodley, C., Cauthen, G., Jarvis, W. R., Hospital outbreak of multidrug-resistant *Mycobacterium tuberculosis* infections. Factors in transmission to staff and HIV-infected patients, *J. Am. Med. Assoc.*, 268, 1280, 1992.

72. Edlin, B. R., Tokars, J. I., Grieco, M. H., Crawford, J. T., Williams, J., Sordillo, E. M., Ong, K. R., Kilburn, J. O., Dooley, S. W., Castro, K. G., Jarvis, W. R., Holmberg, S. D., An outbreak of multidrug-resistant tuberculosis among hospitalized patients with the acquired immunodeficiency syndrome, *N. Engl. J. Med.*, 326, 1514, 1992.

73. Daley, C. L., Small, P. M., Schecter, G. F., Schoolnik, G. K., McAdam, R. A., Jacobs, W. R., Jr., Hopewell, P. C., An outbreak of tuberculosis with accelerated progression among persons infected with the human immunodeficiency virus, *N. Engl. J. Med.*, 326, 231, 1992.

74. Godfrey-Faussett, P., Scott, J. A. G., Kelly, P., Stoker, N. G., DNA fingerprints of *Mycobacterium tuberculosis* do not change during the development of rifampicin resistance, in *World Congress on Tuberculosis Program and Abstracts*, Bethesda, Maryland, 1992, 32.

75. Van Soolingen, D., Hermans, P. W. M., De Haas, P. E. W., Soll, D. R., Van Embden, J. D. A., Occurrence and stability of insertion sequences in *Mycobacterium tuberculosis* strains: evaluation of an insertion sequence-dependent DNA polymorphism as a tool in the epidemiology of tuberculosis, *J. Clin. Microbiol.*, 29, 2578, 1991.

76. Brailey, M., Mortality in tuberculin-positive infants, *Milbank Memorial Fund Quart.*, 15, 36, 1937.

77. Wallgren, A., The time-table of tuberculosis, *Tubercle*, 29, 245, 1948.

78. Tuberculosis Vaccines Clinical Trials Committee of the British Medical Research Council, BCG and vole bacillus vaccines in the prevention of tuberculosis in adolescence and early adult life, *Bull. W.H.O.*, 46, 371, 1972.

79. Broekmans, J. F., Tuberculosis and HIV-infection in developing countries, *Trop. Geograph. Med.*, 43, S13, 1991.

80. Brailey, M., Factors influencing the course of tuberculous infection in young children, *Am. Rev. Tuberc.*, 36, 347, 1937.

81. Stocks, P., Fresh evidence on the inheritance factor in tuberculosis, *Ann. Eugen.*, 2, 6, 1927.

82. Crowle, A. J., Elkins, N., Relative permissiveness of macrophages from black and white people for virulent tubercle bacilli, *Infect. Immun.*, 50, 632, 1990.

83. Stead, W. W., Senner, J. W., Reddick, W. T., Lofgren, J. P., Racial differences in susceptibility to infection by *Mycobacterium tuberculosis*, *N. Engl. J. Med.*, 322, 422, 1990.

84. Hoge, C. W., Tuberculosis outbreak in an elementary school: report of epidemic assistance 90-63-2, Centers for Disease Control, 1990 (unpublished report).

85. Kistnasamy, B., Yach, D., Tuberculosis in commerce and industry in a Western Cape suburb, South Africa, 1987, *Am. J. Indust. Med.*, 18, 87, 1990.

86. Snider, D. E., Jr., The relationship between tuberculosis and silicosis, *Am. Rev. Resp. Dis.*, 118, 455, 1978.

87. Sherson, D., Lander, F., Morbidity of pulmonary tuberculosis among silicotic and nonsilicotic foundry workers in Denmark, *J. Occupation. Med.*, 32, 110, 1990.

88. Hong Kong Chest Service/Tuberculosis Research Centre, Madra/British Medical Research Council, A controlled clinical comparison of 6 and 8 months of antituberculosis chemotherapy in the treatment of patients with silicotuberculosis in Hong Kong, *Am. Rev. Resp. Dis.*, 143, 262, 1991.

89. Enarson, D. A., Fanning, E. A., Allen, E. A., Case-finding in the elimination phase of tuberculosis: high risk groups in epidemiology and clinical practice, *Bull. Int. Union Tuberc. Lung Dis.*, 65, 73, 1990.

90. Centers for Disease Control, Work related lung disease surveillance report, U.S. Department of Health and Human Services, Morgantown, WV, 1991, 7.

91. Cowie, R. L., Langton, M. E., Becklake, M. R., Pulmonary tuberculosis in South African gold miners, *Am. Rev. Resp. Dis.*, 139, 1086, 1989.

92. Mishu, B., Gensheimer, K., Bogden, G., Horan, J., Andrews, A., Bloch, A., Schaffner, W., Tuberculosis outbreak in a shipyard, in *Abstracts of the 1992 ICAAC*, Anaheim, California, 1992, 203.

93. Stead, W. W., Tuberculosis among elderly persons: an outbreak in a nursing home, *Ann. Intern. Med.*, 94, 606, 1981.

94. Calder, R. A., Duclos, P., Wilder, M. H., Pryor, V. L., Scheel, W.J., Mycobacterium tuberculosis transmission in an health clinic, *Bull. Int. Union Tuberc. Lung Dis.*, 66, 103, 1991.

95. Malasky, C., Jordan, T., Potulski, F., Reichman, L. B., Occupational tuberculous infections among pulmonary physicians in training, *Am. Rev. Resp. Dis.*, 142, 505, 1990.

96. Haley, C. E., McDonald, R. C., Rossi, L., Jones, W. D., Haley, R. W., Luby, J. P., Tuberculosis epidemic among hospital personnel, *Infect. Control Hosp. Epidemiol.*, 10, 204, 1989.

97. Kwan, S. Y., Yew, W. W., Chan, S. L., Nosocomial tuberculosis in hospital staff. The size of the problem in a Hong Kong chest hospital, *Chin. Med. J. — Peking*, 103, 909, 1990.

98. Bloch, A. B., Rieder, H. L., Kelly, G. D., Cauthen, G. M., Hayden, C. H., Snider, D. E., The epidemiology of tuberculosis in the United States, *Sem. Resp. Infect.*, 4, 157, 1989.

99. Rieder, H. L., Cauthen, G. M., Kelly, G. D., Bloch, A. B., Snider, D. E., Tuberculosis in the United States, *J. Am. Med. Assoc.*, 262, 385, 1989.

100. Centers for Disease Control, Prevention and control of tuberculosis in facilities providing long-term care to the elderly, *Morbid. Mortal. Weekly Rep.*, 39, RR-10, 1990.

101. Stead, W. W., Dutt, A. K., Tuberculosis in the elderly, *Sem. Resp. Infect.*, 4, 189, 1989.

102. Centers for Disease Control, Prevention and control of tuberculosis in correctional institutions: recommendations of the Advisory Committee for the elimination of tuberculosis, *Morbid. Mortal. Weekly Rep.*, 38, 313, 1989.

103. Braun, M. M., Truman, B. I., Maquire, B., DiFerdinando, G. T., Jr., Wormser, G., Broaddus, R., Morse, D. L., Increasing incidence of tuberculosis in a prison inmate population, association with HIV infection, *J. Am. Med. Assoc.*, 261, 393, 1989.

104. Salive, M. E., Vlahov, D., Brewer, T. F., Coinfection with tuberculosis and HIV-1 in male prison inmates, *Public Health Rep.*, 105, 307, 1990.

105. Centers for Disease Control, Tuberculosis transmission in a state correctional institution — California, 1990–1991, *Morbid. Mortal. Weekly Rep.*, 41, 927, 1992.

106. Centers for Disease Control, Transmission of multidrug-resistant tuberculosis among immunocompromised persons in a correctional system — New York, 1991, *Morbid. Mortal. Weekly Rep.*, 41, 507, 1992.

107. Centers for Disease Control, Prevention and control of tuberculosis in migrant farm workers, *Morbid. Mortal. Weekly Rep.*, 41(RR-10), 1, 1992.

108. Centers for Disease Control, HIV infection, syphilis, and tuberculosis screening among migrant farm workers — Florida, 1992, *Morbid. Mortal. Weekly Rep.*, 41, 723, 1992.

109. Ciesielski, S. C., Seed, J. R., Esposito, D. H., Hunter, N., The epidemiology of tuberculosis among North Carolina migrant farm workers, *J. Am. Med. Assoc.*, 265, 1715, 1991.

110. Lin, R. Y., Goodhart, P. T., Population characteristics of tuberculosis in an HIV/AIDS registry from an East Harlem hospital, *N.Y. State J. Med.*, 91, 239, 1991.

111. Brudney, K., Dobkin, J., Resurgent tuberculosis in New York City, *Am. Rev. Resp. Dis.*, 144, 745, 1991.

112. Centers for Disease Control, Tuberculosis control among homeless populations, *Morbid. Mortal. Weekly Rep.*, 36, 257, 1987.

113. Schieffelbein, C. W., Jr., Snider, D. E., Jr., Tuberculosis control among homeless populations, *Arch. Intern. Med.*, 148, 1843, 1988.

114. Torres, R. A., Mani, S., Altholz, J., Brickner, P. W., Human immunodeficiency virus infection among homeless men in a New York City shelter. Association with *Mycobacterium tuberculosis* infection, *Arch. Intern. Med.*, 150, 2030, 1990.

115. McAdam, J. M., Brickner, P. W., Scharer, L. L., Crocco, J. A., Duff, A. E., The spectrum of tuberculosis in a New York men's shelter clinic — 1982–1988, *Chest*, 97, 4, 799, 1990.

116. Pablos-Mendez, A., Raviglione, M. C., Battan, R., Ramos-Zuniga, R., Drug resistant tuberculosis among the homeless in New York City, *N.Y. State J. Med.*, 90, 351, 1990.

117. Wosornu, D., MacIntyre, D., Watt, B., An outbreak of isoniazid resistant tuberculosis in Glasgow, 1981–1988, *Resp. Med.*, 84, 361, 1990.

118. Ramphele, M. A., Heap, M., Health status of hostel dwellers. V. Tuberculosis notifications, *S. Afr. Med. J.*, 79, 714, 1991.

119. Toyota, E., Ootani, N., Matsuda, Y., Tajima, H., An approach to the control of the so-called vagrant patients with tuberculosis [Japanese; English abstract], *Kekkaku*, 65, 223, 1990.

120. Styblo, K., The impact of HIV infection on the global epidemiology of tuberculosis, *Bull. Int. Union Tuberc. Lung Dis.*, 66, 27, 1991.

121. Styblo, K., The global aspects of tuberculosis and HIV infection, *Bull. Int. Union Tuberc. Lung Dis.*, 65, 28, 1990.

122. Nationwide random survey on the epidemiology of pulmonary tuberculosis in China [Chinese; English abstract], *Chung-Hua Chieh Ho Ho Hu Hsi Tsa Chih*, 13, 67, 1990.

123. Villarino, M. E., Geiter, L. J., Simone, P. M., The multidrug-resistant tuberculosis challenge to public health efforts to control tuberculosis, *Public Health Rep.*, 107, 616, 1992.

124. Schilling, W., Tuberculosis epidemiology and surveillance, *Bull. Int. Union Tuberc. Lung Dis.*, 65, 40, 1990.

125. Schnorr, R., Hafa, U., Schilling, W., Tuberculosis among immigrants in East Germany [German; English abstract], *Zeit. Erkrankung. Atmungsorg.*, 175, 120, 1990.

126. Fille, M., Allerberger, F., Zangerle, R., Dierich, M. P., Reversal of the decline in the incidence of tuberculosis in the Austrian Tyrol and Vorarlberg in 1989, *Weiner Klin. Wochenschrift*, 104, 158, 1992.

127. Trnka, L., Dankova, D., Tuberculosis surveillance in the Czech Republic in 1989, *Czech. Med.*, 14, 87, 1991.

128. Trnka, L., Dankova, D., Tuberculosis surveillance in the Czech Republic in 1990 [Czech; English abstract], *Casopis Lekaru Ceskych*, 131, 107, 1992.

129. Broekmans, J. F., The point of view of a low prevalence country: The Netherlands, *Bull. Int. Union Tuberc. Lung Dis.*, 66, 179, 1991.

130. Kobayashi, M., Epidemiological study on tuberculosis in Tochigi Prefecture. II. The changes in tuberculosis incidence and analysis of relating factors [Japanese; English abstract], *Kekkaku*, 65, 1, 1990.

131. Acocella, G., Comaschi, E., Nonis, A., Rossanigo, C., Migliori, G. B., Past, present and future trends in tuberculosis epidemiology in a region of northern Italy: an analysis carried out through the application of a simulation model (Eskimo), *Giorn. Ital. Chemioter.*, 36, 11, 1989.

132. Watson, J., Epidemiological situation and surveillance of tuberculosis in England and Wales, *Bull. Int. Union Tuberc. Lung Dis.*, 65, 42, 1990.

133. Davies, P. D., The slowing of the decline in tuberculosis notifications and HIV infection, *Resp. Med.*, 83, 321, 1989.

134. Dawson, D., Anargyros, P., Blacklock, Z., Chew, W., Dagniz, H., Gow, G., Jackson, K., Sievers, A., Tuberculosis in Australia: an analysis of cases identified in reference laboratories in 1986–88, *Pathology*, 23, 130, 1991.

135. Dawson, D., Tuberculosis in Australia: an unfinished fight, *Med. J. Aust.*, 154, 75, 1991.

136. Stehr-Green, J. K., Tuberculosis in New Zealand, 1985–90, *N. Z. Med. J.*, 105, 301, 1992.

137. Cross, E. R., Hyams, K. C., Tuberculin skin testing in U.S. Navy and Marine Corps personnel and recruits, 1980–86, *Am. J. Public Health*, 80, 435, 1990.

138. Barry, M. A., Shirley, L., Grady, M. T., Etkind, S. W., Almeida, C., Bernardo, J., Lamb, G. A., Tuberculosis infection in urban adolescents: results of a school-based testing program, *Am. J. Public Health*, 80, 439, 1990.

139. Snider, D. E., Jr., Salinas, L., Kelly, G. D., Tuberculosis: an increasing problem among minorities in the United States, *Public Health Rep.*, 104, 646, 1989.

140. Teale, C., Cundall, D. B., Pearson, S. B., Time of development of tuberculosis in contacts, *Resp. Med.*, 85, 475, 1991.

141. Khauadamova, G. T., The risk of tuberculosis in the principal ethnic groups of Kazakhstan [Russian; English abstract], *Probl. Tuberkuleza*, (4), 22, 1991.

142. Dolberg, O. T., Alkan, M., Schlaeffer, F., Tuberculosis in Israel: a 10-year study of an immigrant society, *Israel J. Med. Sci.*, 27, 386, 1991.

143. Sugarman, J., Chase, E., Johannes, P., Helgerson, S. D., Tuberculosis among American Indians and Alaska Natives, 1985–1990, *IHS Prim. Provider*, 16, 186, 1991.

144. Rieder, H. L., Tuberculosis among American Indians of the contiguous United States, *Public Health Rep.*, 104, 653, 1989.

145. Rieder, H. L., Notes on the history of an epidemic, tuberculosis among North American Indians, *IHS Prim. Provider*, 14, 45, 1989.

146. Beilby, J., Reed, J., Baker, J., Wilson, K., Sansbury, M., Antic, R., Robinson, P. C., Tuberculosis surveillance in the South Australian Aboriginal community, *Med. J. Aust.*, 153, 149, 1990.

147. Tyryltin, M. A., Social factors and their effect on the epidemiology of tuberculosis in the Far North areas [Russian; English abstract], *Probl. Tuberkuleza*, (1), 12, 1990.

148. Centers for Disease Control, Tuberculosis outbreak on Standing Rock Sioux Reservation — North Dakota and South Dakota, 1987–1990, *Morbid. Mortal. Weekly Rep.*, 40, 204, 1991.

149. Powell, K. E., Brown, E. D., Farer, L. S., Tuberculosis among Indochinese refugees in the United States, *J. Am. Med. Assoc.*, 249, 1455, 1983.

150. Centers for Disease Control, Tuberculosis among foreign-born persons entering the United States, *Morbid. Mortal. Weekly Rep.*, 39(RR-18), 1, 1990.

151. Davies, P. D., A possible link between vitamin D deficiency and impaired host defence to *Mycobacterium tuberculosis*, *Tubercle*, 66, 301, 1985.

152. Davies, P. D., The role of vitamin D in tuberculosis, *Am. Rev. Resp. Dis.*, 139, 1571, 1989.

153. Enarson, D. A., Wang, J. S., Grzybowski, S., Case-finding in the elimination phase of tuberculosis in displaced people, *Bull. Int. Union Tuberc. Lung Dis.*, 65, 71, 1990.

154. Plant, A. J., Rushworth, R. L., Wang, Q., Thomas, M., Tuberculosis in New South Wales, *Med. J. Aust.*, 154, 86, 1991.

155. Orr, P. H., Manfreda, J., Hershfield, E. S., Tuberculosis surveillance in immigrants to Manitoba, *Can. Med. Assoc. J.*, 142, 453, 1990.

156. Yamagishi, F., Suzuki, K., Sasaki, Y., Mori, N., Yagi, T., Shirai, T., Satoh, N., Tougoh, N., Ihara, S., Pulmonary tuberculosis in youth [Japanese, English abstract], *Kekkaku*, 67, 427, 1992.

157. Toppet, M., Malfroot, A., Hofman, B., Casimir, G., Cantraine, F., Dab, I., Tuberculosis in children: a 13-year follow up of 1714 patients in a Belgian home care centre, *Eur. J. Pediatr.*, 150, 331, 1991.

158. Mortensen, J., Lange, P., Storm, H. K., Viskum, K., Tuberculosis in children in Copenhagen during 1975–1985 [Danish; English abstract], *Ugesdrift Laeger*, 152, 1226, 1990.

159. Tala, E., Tuberculosis in Scandinavia — Finland families' black sheep [Swedish; English abstract], *Nord. Med.*, 105, 320, 1990.

160. Wang, J. S., Allen, E. A., Enarson, D. A., Grzybowski, S., Tuberculosis in recent Asian immigrants to British Columbia, Canada: 1982–1985, *Tubercle*, 72, 277, 1991.

161. Ravessoud, M., Zellweger, J. P., Clinical presentation of tuberculosis among immigrants seen at the antituberculosis outpatient clinic in Lausanne [French; English abstract], *J. Suisse Med.*, 122, 1037, 1992.

162. Malik, S. K., Khalfan, S., The epidemiology of tuberculosis in Bahrain, *Tubercle*, 71, 51, 1990.

163. Cauthen, G. M., unpublished studies, 1992.

164. Selwyn, P. A., Hartel, D., Lewis, V. A., Schoenbaum, E. E., Vermund, S. H., Klein, R. S., Walker, A. T., Friedland, G. H., A prospective study of the risk of tuberculosis among intravenous drug users with human immunodeficiency virus infection, *N. Engl. J. Med.*, 320, 545, 1989.

165. Selwyn, P. A., Sckell, B. M., Alcabes, P., Friedland, G. H., Klein, R. S., Schoenbaum, E. E., High risk of active tuberculosis in HIV-infected drug users with cutaneous anergy, *J. Am. Med. Assoc.*, 268, 504, 1992.

166. Harries, A. D., Tuberculosis and human immunodeficiency virus infection in developing countries, *Lancet*, 335, 387, 1990.

167. Barnes, P. F., Bloch, A. B., Davidson, P. T., Snider, D. E., Jr., Tuberculosis in patients with human immunodeficiency virus infection, *N. Engl. J. Med.*, 423, 1644, 1991.

168. Pitchenik, A. E., Burr, J., Suarez, M., Fertel, D., Gonzalez, G., Moas, C., Human T-cell lymphotropic virus-III (HTLV-III) seropositivity and related disease among 71 consecutive patients in whom tuberculosis was diagnosed, *Am. Rev. Resp. Dis.*, 135, 875, 1987.

169. Centers for Disease Control, Tuberculosis and acquired immunodeficiency syndrome — New York City, *Morbid. Mortal. Weekly Rep.*, 36, 48, 1987.

170. Cayla, J. A., Jansa, J. M., Plasencia, A., Batalla, J., Parellada, N., Impact of the new AIDS definition on tuberculosis in Barcelona, *Bull. Int. Union Tuberc. Lung Dis.*, 66, 43, 1991.

171. Centers for Disease Control, Crack cocaine use among persons with tuberculosis — Contra Costa County, California, 1987–1990, *Morbid. Mortal. Weekly Rep.*, 40, 485, 1991.

172. Reichman, L. B., Felton, C. P., Edsall, J. R., Drug dependence, a possible new risk factor for tuberculosis disease, *Arch. Intern. Med.*, 139, 337, 1979.

173. Colebunders, R. L., Ryder, R. W., Nzilambi, N., Dikilu, K., Willame, J., Kaboto, M., Bagala, N., Jeugmans, J., Muepu, K., Francis, H. L., Mann, J. M., Quinn, T. C., Piot, P., HIV infection in patients with tuberculosis in Kinshasa, Zaire, *Am. Rev. Resp. Dis.*, 139, 1082, 1989.

174. Sunderam, G., McDonald, R. J., Maniatis, T., Oleska, J., Kapila, R., Reichman, L. B., Tuberculosis as a manifestation of the acquired immunodeficiency syndrome (AIDS), *J. Am. Med. Assoc.*, 256, 362, 1986.

175. Neumann, G., Lichterfeld, A., HIV infection and tuberculosis — results of a survey [German; English abstract], *Pneumologie*, 45, 565, 1991.

176. Theuer, C. P., Hopewell, P. C., Elias, D., Schecter, G. F., Rutherford, G. W., Chaisson, R. E., Human immunodeficiency virus infection in tuberculosis patients, *J. Infect. Dis.*, 162, 8, 1990.

177. Van Deutekom, H., Manos, G. E., Danner, S. A., Jansen, H. M., Coutinho, R. A., AIDS and tuberculosis: results of a retrospective study in 225 AIDS patients, *Bull. Int. Union Tuberc. Lung Dis.*, 65, 33, 1990.

178. Braun, M. M., Badi, N., Ryder, R. W., Baende, E., Mukadi, Y., Nsuami, M., Matela, B., Willame, J., Kaboto, M., Heyward, W., A retrospective cohort study of the risk of tuberculosis among women of childbearing age with HIV infection in Zaire, *Am. Rev. Resp. Dis.*, 143, 501, 1991.

179. Long, R., Scalcini, M., Manfreda, J., Carre, G., Philippe, E., Hershfield, E., Sekla, L., Stackiw, W., Impact of human immunodeficiency virus type 1 on tuberculosis in rural Haiti, *Am. Rev. Resp. Dis.*, 143, 69, 1991.

180. Heckbert, S. R., Elarth, A., Nolan, C. M., The impact of human immunodeficiency virus infection on tuberculosis in young men in Seattle-King County, Washington, *Chest*, 102, 433, 1992.

181. Elliott, A. M., Luo, N., Tembo, G., Halwiindi, B., Steenbergen, G., Machiels, L., Pobee, J., Nunn, P., Hayes, R. J., McAdam, K. P., Impact of HIV on tuberculosis in Zambia: a cross sectional study, *Br. Med. J.*, 301, 412, 1990.

182. Standaert, B., Niragira, F., Kadende, P., Piot, P., The association of tuberculosis and HIV infection in Burundi, *Aids Res. Human Retrovir.*, 5, 247, 1989.

183. Tomlinson, D. R., Moss, F., McCarty, M., Mitchell, D., Main, J., Harris, J. R., Karim, Q. N., Tuberculosis in HIV seropositive individuals — a retrospective analysis, *Int. J. STD AIDS*, 3, 38, 1992.

184. Manoff, S. B., Cauthen, G. M., Stoneburner, R. L., Bloch, A. B., Schultz, S., Snider, D. E., Jr., Risk of tuberculosis infection among contacts of tuberculosis patients with and without AIDS — New York City 1979–1985, presented at the annual meeting of the Tuberculosis and Surveillance Unit, International Union Against Tuberculosis and Lung Disease, October 16, 1989, Ghardaia, Algeria.

185. Kool, H. E., Bloemkolk, D., Reeve, P. A., Danner, S. A., HIV seropositivity and tuberculosis in a large general hospital in Malawi, *Trop. Geograph. Med.*, 42, 128, 1990.

186. Antonucci, G., Armignacco, O., Girardi, E., Ippolito, G., Angarano, G., Babudieri, S., Bini, A., Bottura, P., Costigliola, P., Cargnel, A., Chirianni, A., Crosato, I. M., DiPerri, G., Errante, I., Fantoni, M., Galli, M., Guarascio, P., Isabella, L., Libanore, M., Manzillo, E., Minoli, L., Pagano, G., Quirino, T., Salmaso, S., Santoro, D., Suter, F., Traverso, A., Vigevani, G. M., Tuberculosis and human immunodeficiency virus infection in Italy. Preliminary results from a multicenter study, *Chest*, 100, 586, 1991.

187. Onorato, I. M., McCray, E., Field Services Branch, Prevalence of human immunodeficiency virus infection among patients attending tuberculosis clinics in the United States, *J. Infect. Dis.*, 165, 87, 1992.

188. McCray, E., Onorato, I. M., Miller, B. I., Dondero, T. J., Bloch, A. B., Estimating HIV levels and trends among patients of tuberculosis clinics, *Public Health Rep.*, 105, 135, 1990.

189. Hellinger, J., Marlink, R., Kaptue, L., Zekeng, L., Essex, M., Are tuberculosis patients a "sentinel" population for HIV epidemic in Africa?, *Trans. R. Soc. Trop. Med. Hyg.*, 84, 292, 1990.

190. Trnka, L., Dankova D., Erban, J., Surveillance systems and public health priority actions, *Bull. Int. Union Tuberc. Lung Dis.*, 65, 37, 1990.

191. Kritski, A. L., Werneck, E. B., Medeiros, D., Study of association between active pulmonary tuberculosis and human immunodeficiency virus (HIV), at a sanitorium in Rio de Janeiro, Brazil. A prospective study, *Am. Rev. Resp. Dis.*, 137, 494, 1988.

192. Levin, V. R., Tuberculosis incidence and the seroprevalence of HIV infection in the United States, *Am. J. Prevent. Med.*, 7, 422, 1991.

193. Hershfield, E. S., Eidus, L., Helbecque, D. M., Canadian survey to determine the rate of drug resistance to isoniazid, PAS and streptomycin in newly detected untreated tuberculosis patients and retreatment cases, *Int. J. Clin. Pharmacol. Biopharm.*, 17, 387, 1979.

194. Zaman, R., Tuberculosis in Saudi Arabia: Initial and secondary drug resistance among indigenous and non-indigenous populations, *Tubercle*, 72, 51, 1991.

195. Riley, L. W., Arathoon, E., Loverde, V. D., The epidemiologic patterns of drug-resistant *Mycobacterium tuberculosis* infections: a community-based study, *Am. Rev. Resp. Dis.*, 139, 1282, 1989.

196. Kleeberg, H. H., Oliver, M. S., Tuberculosis Research Institute of the South African Medical Research Council, *A World Atlas of Initial Drug Resistance*, 2nd rev. ed., U.S. Department of Health and Human Services, Atlanta, 1984.

197. Committee on Bacteriology and Immunology, IUATLD news — meeting of the scientific committees, Paris, 13–14 October 1989, *Bull. Int. Union Tuberc. Lung Dis.*, 65, 1990.

198. Simone, P. M., Iseman, M. D., Drug-resistant tuberculosis: a deadly — and growing — danger, *J. Resp. Dis.*, 13, 960, 1992.

199. Frieden, T. R., Sterling, T., Pablos-Mendez, A., Kilburn, J. O., Cauthen, G. M., Dooley, S. W., The emergence of drug-resistant tuberculosis in New York City, *N. Engl. J. Med.*, 328, 521, 1993.

200. Centers for Disease Control and Prevention, Initial therapy for tuberculosis in the era of multidrug resistance: recommendations of the Advisory Council for the Elimination of Tuberculosis, *Morbid. Mortal. Weekly Rep.*, 42(RR-7), 1, 1993.

201. American Thoracic Society, Control of tuberculosis in the United States, *Am. Rev. Resp. Dis.*, 146, 1623, 1992.

CHAPTER 2

Pathogenesis of Tuberculosis

Elizabeth A. Rich, M.D. and Jerrold J. Ellner, M.D.

CONTENTS

I. OVERVIEW

Current thought on the pathogenesis of tuberculosis (TB) has been gleaned from experimental observations in infected animals and clinical observations in humans, pathologic and immunologic studies of the blood and tissues of infected animals and humans with TB, and microbiologic, biochemical, and molecular genetic studies of *Mycobacterium tuberculosis* (MTB) and its molecular constituents. There are corresponding levels of complexity to the understanding of TB. No one approach to elucidation of the pathogenesis of TB encompasses its entirety, but each is directed toward understanding how the host resists the disease.

This chapter begins with a brief review of the natural history of TB and virulence factors, and then focuses on the major new developments in the pathogenesis of TB. Native resistance to MTB will be discussed from the standpoint of animal studies; from *in vitro* studies of phagocytosis and T-cell-independent growth inhibition of MTB by mononuclear phagocytes and neutrophils and from genetic influences including resistance in mice and association of HLA phenotype with TB in humans. Acquired resistance to MTB will include discussions of T-cell-dependent macrophage activation and the role of CD4[+] and CD8[+] T cells, Th1 and Th2 type responses, and $\gamma\delta$ T cells in resistance to MTB. Pleural and alveolar T-lymphocytes will be considered separately. Other categories include the role of tumor necrosis factor-α (TNF-α) in resistance to MTB and in granuloma formation, modulation of macrophage effector function by growth-enhancing and macrophage-deactivating cytokines, Class II-restricted cytotoxicity and its role in protection and immunopathology, immune responses in human TB, and the role of direct stimulation of macrophages by mycobacterial products in regulation of T-cell responses in TB. The epidemic of dual infection by MTB and human immunodeficiency virus (HIV) requires that attention also be placed on the immunopathogenic mechanisms by which each impacts on the other (see Section X.D).

II. NATURAL HISTORY AND IMMUNOPATHOLOGY

Exposure to an individual with active pulmonary TB carries a substantial risk of acquiring infection with MTB (i.e., PPD skin test conversion in household contacts is approximately 25%). This risk results from the acquisition of MTB infection by inhalation of microdroplets (droplet nuclei) containing the organism.[1-4] Large droplets are deposited on the upper airways (trachea and bronchi) and removed by the mucociliary clearance mechanisms of this region. Animal and human studies demonstrate that smaller droplets (approximately 1–5 μm) that contain three or fewer bacilli reach the alveoli.[2-6] Because alveolar macrophages are the major immune effector cells lining the alveoli, the first defense against the MTB that reach alveoli is via phagocytosis and killing by these cells. For most persons exposed to MTB, either the bacilli are killed before infection is established or the bacilli grow to a limited extent within alveolar

macrophages with formation of small granulomas in the adjacent lung parenchyma (with occult hematogenous dissemination as below). Either no evidence of infection or infection but not disease thus is established, the latter evidenced by development of a positive PPD skin test within 4 to 6 weeks. Alternatively MTB may continue to replicate and disseminate as progressive primary TB.

By inference from animal studies and the natural history of TB, soon after the primary inoculation, the organism invades the bloodstream and lymphatics and is carried within lymphatics to the hilar lymph nodes. The organisms disseminate hematogenously to various organs including the lung and either are destroyed locally or persist in a latent phase within tissue macrophages often for years. Dormant foci most commonly include the apices of the lungs, the cortex of the kidneys, and the growing ends of long bones. A characteristic common to these regions is a high local concentration of oxygen that presumably helps the bacilli survive. It is of interest that *in vitro* studies confirm that higher levels of ambient oxygen increase intracellular growth.[7] In approximately 5% of cases, primary TB is not self-limited and progresses to clinical TB. Presumably patients with such progressive disease have a failure of acquired resistance to the growth of the bacillus.

The pathologic hallmark of TB is granuloma formation in various tissues.[8] Tuberculous granulomas are characterized by accumulations of blood-derived macrophages, epithelioid cells that are degenerating macrophages, multinucleated giant cells that are fused macrophages with nuclei around the periphery of the giant cell (Langhan's type giant cells), and T-lymphocytes around the periphery of the granuloma. Central caseation of granulomas is common. Thus, mononuclear phagocytes, a term referring to blood monocytes and tissue macrophages, and T-lymphocytes are the main cellular constituents of tuberculoid granulomas. Granulomas of other chronic infections such as fungal infections are similar architecturally. In tuberculous granulomas, acid fast bacilli (AFB) are found in the mononuclear phagocytes.[8] Whether the epithelioid cells and multinucleated giant cells are adapted for mycobacterial killing is not known, although activated macrophages may be more microbicidal than blood monocytes.[9,10]

Postprimary or reactivation TB is the most common manifestation of TB in adults. Reactivation may be either through activation of endogenous latent foci or less commonly through reinfection of an immunocompromised patient by new exposure to MTB. Medlar described the pathologic features of reactivation TB.[11] Pulmonary disease generally is localized to the apical and posterior segments of the upper lobes or the superior segment of the lower lobes. Caseous necrosis of granulomas is the pathologic hallmark of both primary and reactivation TB. In some granulomas, liquefaction of the caseated material occurs and it is believed that MTB thrives better in this liquefied material than in caseous material. Caseous necrosis and cavity formation likely result from sensitivity to tuberculoprotein since, as shown by Yamamura et al., cavity formation is prevented in rabbits by desensitizing the animals with a tuberculin-active peptide before infecting them.[12] Healing occurs by fibrosis and contraction of the affected structures. A characteristic feature of TB is the concurrent findings of caseation, liquefaction, cavity formation, and fibrosis in lungs and other organs of affected individuals assessed at autopsy. It is assumed that hydrolytic enzymes and oxygen radicals produced by macrophages and neutrophils mediate much of the tissue damage with resulting liquefaction of granulomas and cavity formation. Nevertheless, little is known about the cellular and molecular basis for the immunopathology in TB.

III. VIRULENCE FACTORS

There are three major types of virulence factors of mycobacteria that have been molecularly characterized: cord factor, sulfatides, and mycosides. Each of these is located in the outer layer of the complex mycobacterial cell wall. A review of the history, chemistry, and biologic activities of these factors can be found in the recent thorough reviews of Rastogi and David[13] and Rastogi.[14] The expression of virulence in guinea pigs and mice and the formation of compact parallel cords during culture were described by Middlebrook,[15] and were attributed to "cord factor" by Bloch.[16] Cord factor(s) later were determined to be α,α-trehalose-6,6'-dimycolates.[17] Cord factor coated onto *Bacillus subtilis* inhibits the migration of blood leukocytes and kills mice when injected intraperitoneally.[15] The toxic effects of cord factor have been attributed to interaction with mitochondrial membranes resulting in reduction in the activity of NAD-dependent microsomal enzymes in various tissues (lung, liver, spleen).[18,19] One problem with ascribing cord factor with a major role in virulence is its occurrence in nonpathogenic as well as pathogenic species of mycobacteria.[20]

Dubos and Middlebrook showed that INH-sensitive, virulent strains of tubercle bacilli also bind neutral red in alkaline solutions.[21] This property was attributed to a sulfolipid found in virulent strains. Goren determined the chemical structure of the sulfolipid to be phthioceranic and hydroxyphthioceranic esters of a sulfated trehalose.[22,23] These sulfolipids kill mice when injected intraperitoneally

and enhance the toxicity of cord factor.[20,24] Sulfatides of MTB may also inhibit the microbicidal activities of monocyte-derived macrophages by inhibiting phagosome–lysosome fusion,[20,25] although the method used in studies of such fusion may influence the results.[26]

Mycosides are species-specific glycolipids and peptidoglycolipids of mycobacteria.[27] The complex chemical structure of many of these compounds has been elucidated by Brennan et al.[28] The surface glycolipids of MTB consist of trehalose-containing lipooligosaccharides. Brennan suggested that the simple acyltrehaloses present in human strains of virulent strains of MTB are incapable of further glycosylation of the core lipooligosaccharides whereas the avirulent Canetti strain of MTB demonstrates extended glycosylation.[28,29] Certain mycosides of mycobacteria induce formation of an electron transparent zone in bacilli phagocytized by macrophages.[14] The role of the electron transparent zone in protection of MTB against intracellular killing has not been determined. The available data, however, suggest that the species-specific surface mycosides may confer some of the resistance to intracellular killing of virulent organisms.

IV. NATIVE RESISTANCE TO *MYCOBACTERIUM TUBERCULOSIS* (MTB)

A. ANIMAL MODELS

In their classic studies, Lurie and Dannenberg followed the course of mycobacteria in alveolar macrophages in lung and other tissues after inhalation of the bacilli by genetically resistant versus susceptible rabbits.[6] In resistant rabbits, alveolar macrophages contained more mycobacteria than susceptible rabbits but the subsequent early forming tubercles within alveolar structures were decreased in size and number. Seven days after inhalation of bacilli (BCG), susceptible rabbits had 20- to 30-fold higher levels of bacilli in the lung than resistant rabbits (reviewed in Reference 30). Resistance of rabbits was attributed to the native resistance of alveolar macrophages, conceivably through increased uptake and killing of mycobacteria.

Collins demonstrated in parabiotic rats that there is an influx of monocytes into alveolar spaces after infection with tubercle bacilli.[31] In Lurie's animal model, more mycobacteria were found in macrophages (recently arrived from the blood) in early granulomata than in alveolar macrophages or in blood-derived macrophages activated in response to cell-mediated immune mechanisms, a finding that is consonant with their importance as effector cells. There was an influx of blood-derived macrophages into alveolar structures and these cells contained high numbers of bacilli. This finding was attributed to efficiency of immature macrophages in phagocytosis and to undeveloped microbicidal mechanisms.[6,30] These immature macrophages also appeared to be relatively unharmed by the bacteria. Thus a state of symbiosis developed in which mycobacteria grew logarithmically within cells but the cells were not lysed.[6,30] At approximately 7 to 21 days after infection of the rabbits with mycobacteria, the rate of multiplication of bacilli in the lungs of resistant and susceptible rabbits was comparable presumably because cell-mediated immunity had not developed yet in either group of rabbits and therefore the recruited monocytes remained inactivated during this period.

In Lurie and Danneberg's rabbit model, at approximately 3 weeks after infection the phase of logarithmic growth of bacilli plateaued in both the resistant and sensitive animals.[6] Histologically, activated macrophages were evident (as demonstrated morphologically and by staining for lysosomal enzymes), epithelioid cells (degenerating macrophages) had appeared, and granulomas were caseating. At this stage, acquired immunity to MTB had likely developed. More bacilli spread to hilar nodes in the resistant animals but growth of the organism in this region appeared to be more inhibited. These findings were ascribed, as in the alveoli, to the native resistance of tissue macrophages to growth of mycobacteria.

In a guinea pig model developed by Smith et al., 3 weeks after infection by the aerosol route, bacilli had disseminated hematogenously back to the lung in large numbers.[32] Previous vaccination with BCG resulted in a decrease in the bacillemia. The mechanisms of protection against dissemination of infection, however, are unclear.

B. MONONUCLEAR PHAGOCYTES
1. Mycobactericidal Mechanisms
There is no evidence that MTB is killed extracellularly. Since cells of the mononuclear phagocyte series phagocytose MTB and the bacilli ultimately are destroyed, mycobactericidal mechanisms of these cells are the key to resistance against infection. Furthermore, it is agreed generally that the degree of virulence of MTB depends on its relative capacity to multiply within host macrophages. There are three general ways that the growth of MTB may be inhibited; each involves mononuclear phagocytes and the latter two require both lymphocytes and mononuclear phagocytes. First, mononuclear phagocytes have a natural armamentarium against the bacillus, that is known as natural resistance, and this will be discussed in this section. Second, mononuclear phagocytes can be activated to kill MTB through cytokines or other mediators and

when such activation is conferred by sensitized T-lymphocytes, acquired resistance has evolved, i.e., the process of cell-mediated immunity in its strictest sense. Third, mononuclear phagocytes containing bacilli may be lysed by cytotoxic T cells but the *in vivo* significance for the containment of MTB by this mechanism is not clear; bacilli released when macrophages are lysed either may disseminate uncontrollably or be taken up by more activated macrophages better able to control their growth. (These latter two mechanisms will be discussed in Sections VII and VIII.)

2. Phagocytosis by Monocytes
Swartz et al. observed that different species of mycobacteria vary in their extent of ingestion by blood monocytes.[33] *M. avium* complex was taken up by many monocytes; whereas, MTB, *M. kansasii*, and other mycobacteria were taken up by fewer monocytes. Serum was found to be important in the uptake of *M. avium* complex and to a lesser extent of MTB. Complement had a major role on this effect of serum.[33] Schlessinger et al. demonstrated that complement receptor 1 (CR1) and CR3 mediate phagocytosis of virulent MTB by blood monocytes and that the C3 component of complement is the bacterial-bound ligand.[34] FcR and the β-glucan inhibitable receptor for zymosan had no role in phagocytosis.

3. Phagocytosis and Growth Inhibition by Alveolar Macrophages
Although alveolar macrophages are believed to be the major defenders of the lung against infectious agents such as MTB, little is known about the effector or immunoregulatory functions of alveolar macrophages in response to MTB. Recently we assessed directly the phagocytosis and growth inhibition of MTB (avirulent strain H37Ra) by human alveolar macrophges. To assess compartmentalization of function, these effector functions of alveolar macrophages were compared to that of blood monocytes from which alveolar macrophages are derived. Alveolar macrophages from healthy subjects phagocytosed and inhibited the growth of this strain of MTB significantly better than blood monocytes.[35a] Phagocytosis by alveolar macrophages was mediated through CR4 to a greater extent than CR1 or CR3. The basis for the improved growth inhibition of MTB by alveolar macrophages was attributed, in part at least, to increased expression of TNF-α by alveolar macrophages after phagocytosis of the organisms. Previously we showed that BCG and PPD stimulate TNF-α production by human alveolar macrophages,[35b] and TNF-α production by alveolar macrophages exceeds that of blood mono-

cytes.[36] Since healthy subjects were the source of alveolar macrophages in these studies, the growth inhibition by these cells is a reflection of the natural resistance of these cells. The role of alveolar macrophages in T-cell-dependent acquired immunity is not known.

4. Role of Lysosomal Enzymes

Myrvik et al. demonstrated the capacity of virulent strains of MTB to disrupt the phagosomal membrane and multiply freely in the cytoplasm of rabbit alveolar macrophages.[37] Armstrong and Hart observed that after phagocytosis of damaged or non-viable MTB by mouse peritoneal macrophages, phagosomes fuse with lysosomes.[38] Phagosomes containing viable MTB, however, did not fuse with lysosomes. Although both normal and immune serum increased phagosome–lysosome fusion (by unknown mechanisms), growth of MTB was unaffected by such pretreatment; MTB survived and multiplied even in phagolysosomes. Thus, the *in vivo* significance of phagosome–lysosome fusion with respect to mycobacterial burden in the host remains to be determined.

Lurie and Dannenberg's histologic studies in rabbits demonstrated an increase in lysosomal enzymes in activated macrophages and that these macrophages appeared to be killing tubercle bacilli.[6,30] Moreover, lysosomes from activated cells contain more cathepsins. Lurie and Dannenberg showed by histochemical techniques that the macrophages in granulomas with less AFB contained high numbers of lysosomal granules.[6,30] Flesch and Kaufmann demonstrated that chloroquine, a compound that increases fusion of phagosomes and lysosomes, increases growth inhibition of *M. bovis* in mouse bone marrow-derived macrophages[39] although this finding may not be relevant to MTB. As described above, however, the serum-induced increase in fusion by mouse peritoneal macrophages did not increase growth inhibition of MTB.[38] Therefore, although intuitively it would appear that digestion of MTB by lysosomal enzymes of macrophages is important in control of growth of the organism, this concept has not been proven formally.

5. Role of Oxygen Radicals

Mitchison et al. found that resistance of MTB to hydrogen peroxide is associated with virulence.[40] Other studies showed, in contrast, that although resistance to peroxide is necessary, it is not sufficient for virulence and differences in susceptibility to peroxidative killing do not correlate with virulence of MTB.[41,42] Furthermore, Douvas et al. showed that the increased growth inhibition of MTB by monocyte-derived macrophages as compared to monocytes was not associated with increased release of reactive oxygen species.[42] Although mycobacteria are sensitive to oxygen radicals, Flesch and Kaufmann demonstrated that scavengers of toxic oxygen metabolites failed to influence the capacity of interferon-γ (IFN-γ)-activated mouse bone marrow macrophages to inhibit growth of *M. bovis*.[39] Thus, at this time there is little convincing evidence that oxygen radicals, so relevant to killing of other microbes, are important as mycobactericidal molecules for mononuclear phagocytes.

C. NEUTROPHILS

MTB persists as a facultative intracellular pathogen within macrophages and chronically produces granulomatous inflammation. Neutrophils are, however, among the first cells to arrive at the site of a tuberculous infection in humans.[43] Moreover, injection of mycobacteria or their products into tissues or the pleural space of animals produces an inflammatory response initally dominated by neutrophils that can persist for up to 48 h.[43-46] Neutrophils stimulated by BCG release chemotaxins for blood monocytes into pleural spaces in rabbits and *in vitro*.[47]

Brown et al. demonstrated first that neutrophils from healthy humans are capable of killing MTB *in vitro*.[48] The mechanism of killing of MTB by neutrophils, however, is not clear. May and Spagnuolo found that MTB induces a respiratory burst in neutrophils.[49] Neutrophils from patients with chronic granulomatous disease kill MTB as do neutrophils from healthy subjects, suggesting nonoxidative mechanisms are involved in the mycobactericidal process.[48] Furthermore, inhibitors of oxygen radical formation do not neutralize killing of MTB by human neutrophils.[50] These data suggest that oxygen radicals are unlikely to be important in the killing of MTB by neutrophils. IFN-γ increases the killing efficiency of *M. fortuitum* by neutrophils.[51] Phorbol myristate acetate enhances killing of MTB by human neutrophils.[48]

In summary, neutrophils are present only early in response to MTB in animals and humans but may, through release of chemotaxins in response to mycobacteria, participate in the initial influx of monocytes from the blood to the infected region (usually the lung). Neutrophils also can kill MTB *in vitro*. The mechanism probably is nonoxidative. Neutrophils, like macrophages, can be activated by products of T-lymphocytes and by external stimuli to kill MTB more efficiently. The precise mechanisms of intracellular and extracellular killing of MTB by neutrophils and the relative capacity of neutrophils and macrophages to inhibit the growth of MTB are, however, not known.

D. GENETIC INFLUENCES ON NATIVE RESISTANCE

1. Animal Models

Genetic resistance in Lurie and Dannenberg's inbred rabbit model was attributed both to better natural resistance of alveolar macrophages and to acquired cell-mediated immunity.[6,30] Variation among mouse strains in resistance to mycobacteria has been demonstrated by many investigators (reviewed in Reference 52). Skamene discovered that susceptibility of mice to tuberculous infection is controlled by a single, dominant, autosomal gene, the *Bcg* gene, located on chromosome 1 within a linkage group showing structural homology with a conserved region of human chromosome 2.[52,53] This genetic locus in mice regulates the natural resistance of macrophages to mycobacteria as well as to other intracellular pathogens such as *Salmonella typhimurium* and *Leishmania donovani*.[52,53] The *Bcg* gene influences the activation of macrophages independent of T-lymphocytes. Macrophages isolated from the peritoneal cavity or from the spleens of uninfected resistant mice are superior to macrophages from susceptible mice in the inhibition of intracellular growth of BCG, and express increased lymphokine-stimulated Ia, accessory function for antigen and mitogen-induced T-cell proliferation, and bactericidal activity against many bacteria. Skamene proposes that macrophages from resistant mice are genetically programmed to be in a primed or more activated state such that on exposure to intracellular pathogens, microbicidal activity is upregulated quickly. The possibility that there is a human equivalent to the *Bcg* gene of mice is being examined by Skamene and others by searching for cosegregation of certain restriction fragment length polymorphisms (RFLPs) with the pattern of resistance to TB in families living in areas with endemic TB (personal communication).

2. Human Observations

The issue of whether humans have genetic resistance and susceptibility to infection with MTB is difficult to address. Stead has shown that blacks are more likely than Caucasians to convert their tuberculin skin test to positive after exposure to a case of TB in an institutional setting.[54] There is clearcut epidemiologic evidence of a genetic predisposition to develop active TB. Identical twins and blood relatives in a household with a case of TB are more likely to be concordant for disease than nonidentical twins and nonblood relatives.[55]

3. HLA Phenotype, Thinness, and Race/Ethnicity

Class I and Class II MHC loci restrict T-cell interactions with macrophages, and peptide antigens bind to Class I and Class II determinants. It therefore is quite conceivable that individuals with certain HLA types would be unable to respond to key MTB constituents, thereby increasing their susceptibility to disease. Also, associations between HLA phenotype and other intracellular pathogens have been demonstrated, for example, with leishmaniasis and *M. leprae*.[56-58] It is of interest that affected sibs (with TB) in India demonstrate excess haplotype sharing.[59] Several efforts have been made to show an association between HLA phenotype and TB and the results are widely divergent. For example, expression of some HLA-B and HLA-DR2 antigens in various populations is associated with development of TB. These antigens include B8, Bw15, Bw35, B27, and DR2.[60-65] Antibody titers to the 38-kDa antigen of *M. tuberculosis* were strongly associated with DR2.[64]

Association of other Class I and Class II MHC phenotypes with TB have been reported in other populations[65-69] but will not be discussed here. Each of these studies was performed in unrelated subjects. Because there was no *a priori* hypothesis that a specific HLA type was associated with TB, the statistical analysis is questionable as it did not correct for the multiple alleles under study. The fact that different phenotypes identified in disparate populations are associated with TB is not discouraging in itself as the HLA genes may be in linkage disequilibrium with one or a few genes that determine susceptibility to TB. Linkage studies of HLA phenotypes among multiple family members with or without TB or tuberculous infection, however, have not been reported. Such studies are required to confirm a genetic paradigm for resistance or susceptibility.

Cox et al. assessed HLA-DR in a group of Mexican Americans with TB.[70] There was no association of a Class II MHC locus with disease or tuberculin skin test reactivity. Of interest, however, was a relationship between HLA-DR and *in vitro* lymphocyte responses to PPD. In fact the haplotype HLA-B14-DR1 was associated with low blastogenic responses. This is of considerable interest since this haplotype is associated with nonclassical adrenal 21-hydroxylase deficiency;[71] the gene for this abnormality maps to chromosome 6, within the Class II MHC, and is a trait that is associated with altered expression of HLA-DR1 such that there is failure to activate alloreactive or Class II-restricted T-cell clones.

Besides the data on HLA type there is some information that body build and race and ethnicity are associated with risk of TB. In a study of naval recruits, the TB case rate in tuberculin reactors was three times higher for men who were 10% or more below ideal body weight than for those who were

10% above ideal body weight.[72] In a study of Norwegians, the relative risk for those with lowest mass index was more than 5-fold that of those with highest mass index.[73] Potential links between thinness and an immunologic or pathogenetic basis for predisposition to TB have not been sought.

An interesting link between genetic and environmental factors in the racial predisposition to TB was noted by Davies in an effort to explain the increased incidence of TB among Asians compared to white people in the United Kingdom.[78] Metabolites of vitamin D activate macrophages for killing of MTB and the food in the United Kingdom is not supplemented with this vitamin. The dark-skinned Asian residents photosynthesize vitamin D less well. Thus lower photosynthesis of vitamin D may be the genetic factor, whereas inadequate sunlight and lack of nutritional sources of vitamin D are environmental factors perhaps together resulting in an increased susceptible to TB among residents of Asiatic origin compared to white residents.

Pathologic studies show that TB is a more aggressive disease in blacks. TB also reportedly is more frequent and more difficult to treat in black than in white people.[74-77] The incidence is higher among people of Asian origin than white people in the United Kingdom.[78] The basis for the epidemiologic and clinical observations of differences in susceptibility to TB among races of people, however, is far from understood. Crowle and Elkins addressed this issue by studying the growth of MTB in monocytes and monocyte-derived macrophages from black and white people.[79] Both monocytes and monocyte-derived macrophages from black people killed MTB better during phagocytosis but significantly less well during culture thereafter, especially in the presence of black donor serum. Furthermore the macrophage activating factor 1,25-(OH)-vitamin D_3 provided less protection against the growth of tubercle bacilli in macrophages from black compared to white donors. Although these data implicate a genetic predisposition to the increase in TB observed among black people, more and larger studies will be required to confirm this observation and to understand more fully the basis for the susceptibility.

V. ACQUIRED RESISTANCE TO MTB

A. DEFINITION OF CELL-MEDIATED IMMUNITY (CMI)

CMI is a consequence of the activation of macrophages by products of sensitized T-lymphocytes such as IFN-γ. In general, cellular immune responses are initiated by exposure to a foreign antigen. The antigen is taken up, processed, and presented on the surface of antigen-presenting cells (accessory cells) such as macrophages and dendritic cells to T-lymphocytes. Subsequent T-cell activation and proliferation in response to the presented antigen occur if such presentation is accompanied by HLA molecules on the surface of antigen-presenting cells as well as by amplifying cytokines such as interleukin-1 (IL-1) and interleukin-6 (IL-6). CD4+ helper T cells react with Class II HLA molecules whereas CD8+ cytotoxic/suppressor T cells react with Class I HLA molecules. The interaction of antigen, T cells, and antigen-presenting cells results not only in immediate proliferation of T cells and cytokine release but also in development of sensitized or memory T cells that will respond to the antigen within 1 or 2 days of subsequent exposure. Cytotoxic effector cells are a second effector arm and may lyse overburdened macrophages.

B. CELL-MEDIATED IMMUNITY TO MTB

Circulating antibodies to mycobacteria are demonstrable in patients with TB.[80] Levels of immunoglobulin G (IgG) generally increase during active disease.[80-82] During treatment for active TB, levels rise for 1 to 2 months, then fall, but remain detectable for one to several years.[83] IgM antibodies are directed at nonspecific polysaccharide antigens and do not correlate with active disease.[81] Serum IgA antibodies are found at low levels in patients with active TB but not in healthy subjects.[81] In spite of the demonstration of humoral responses to MTB, however, the evidence against a protective role of these antibodies is solid. Numerous animal studies have demonstrated that specific antisera do not confer passive protection to mycobacterial antigens whereas protection is conferred by transfer of T cells.[84-87]

Koch reported in 1891 that guinea pigs infected for 4–6 weeks with MTB and then challenged intracutaneously with a small number of virulent bacilli developed a localized area of induration and necrosis at the dermal inoculation site within 48 h.[88] This Koch phenomenon is the classical tuberculin delayed-type hypersensitivity (DTH) reaction. A half-century later, Chase demonstrated that tuberculin DTH was transferred by lymphocytes.[89] Several passive transfer studies in animals now have convincingly demonstrated that both DTH and protective immunity are mediated by T-lymphocytes and not by components of serum.[84-87] Nevertheless a still unresolved and important issue in tuberculoimmunity is whether CMI (protective immunity) and DTH are the same or coincident, separable events. Protection and DTH are linked epidemiologically in that tuberculin skin test positive subjects are relatively resistant to exogenous reinfection.[90] Mackaness discussed the evidence that DTH and antituberculous protective immunity are inexorably linked.[91] Others have argued that DTH and protective immunity are completely separate phenomena (reviewed in Reference 92). The argument that DTH and protective immunity are dissociable stems from studies demonstrating that animals can be desensitized without loss of protection; they can be rendered hypersensitive without causing an increase in protection; and certain fractions of tubercle bacilli incur resistance without producing cutaneous hypersensitivity.[92] Furthermore, Orme and Collins demonstrated that DTH and protective antituberculous immunity are mediated by separate subpopulations of T-lymphoctes in mice (Ly-1 for DTH and Ly-2 for protection).[92a]

Perhaps Rook summarized this issue of the relationship between protective immunity and DTH best by acknowledging the sheer complexity of tuberculoimmunity.[93] Thus, the issue is not resolved but with the insights gained from recent technologic advances, it seems quite certain that DTH and CMI are dissociable yet overlapping and complex events subserved by subpopulations of T-lymphocytes and macrophages and perhaps neutrophils that express and secrete an intricate network of amplifying, suppressive and injurious versus beneficial cytokines and other nonprotein cellular products. This cellular scenario is complicated further by the accumulating evidence that CMI is differentially expressed in various tissues. The following sections seek to summarize the knowledge to date about the functions of each of the major cellular players in response to MTB or its products *in vitro*, and in patients with TB.

C. PROTECTIVE IMMUNITY AND T-LYMPHOCYTE-DEPENDENT MACROPHAGE ACTIVATION

1. Animal Studies

Immunization of mice with BCG results in the acquisition by splenic lymphocytes of the capacity to adoptively transfer protective immunity against an aerogenic challenge with virulent MTB.[92] Furthermore, immunization with live but not heat-killed organisms generates protective immunity in mice.[94] Heat-killed organisms transfer nonspecific resistance and DTH. These data suggest that products of metabolically active mycobacteria may be particularly important in the protective response to MTB.

2. CD4+ AND CD8+ Subsets

During the course of infection with *M. tuberculosis*, protective CD4+ lymphocytes appear early in the spleen, produce large quantities of IFN-γ, and are associated temporally with the onset of bacterial elimination; cytolytic T cells appear later and

have less of a clear role in protective immunity.[95] Depletion experiments using monoclonal antibodies against CD4+ and CD8+ cells in mice indicate that protection against mycobacteria can be conferredboth by CD4+ [95-97] and by CD8+ [97] T-lymphocytes. Recent studies by Bloom et al. indicate that animals unable to express Class I MHC are more susceptible to tuberculosis (Bloom, personal communication).

Studies in murine models have allowed for a subdivision of CD4+ cells based on their patterns of cytokine expression into Th1 (IFN-γ, IL-2, TNF-β, or lymphotoxin) and Th2 (IL-4, IL-5, IL-6, and IL-10).[98] Th1 and Th2 cells function in cellular and humoral immunity, respectively. The Th1 and Th2 populations, however, do not function independently but have cross-modulatory effects.[99,100] For example, IL-10 acts on antigen-presenting cells to suppress the production of cytokines by Th1 cells.[100] Although there are no formal experimental data, it can be assumed based on studies with other infectious agents[101-104] and with human T-cell clones responsive to mycobacterial antigens[105,106] that Th1 cells would be the subpopulation important for protective immunity against MTB. Also, it is important to note that human T-cell clones are not subdivided readily into Th1 and Th2 equivalents.[107]

Although the mechanism by which these subpopulations of T cells protect the animals against subsequent challenge with MTB is difficult to discern directly, *in vitro* studies indicate two potential mechanisms for protection. T-lymphocytes secrete lymphokines such as IFN-γ and granulocyte–macrophage colony-stimulating factor capable of activating the intracellular mycobactericidal mechanisms of macrophages. The protective consequences of activation of killing of mycobacteria are evident. The other mechanism by which T cells may be protective is via cytotoxicity of those T cells for mycobacterial-laden macrophages as discussed below.

3. γδ T-Lymphocytes

The αβ T-cell receptor is expressed on the majority of T-lymphocytes, whereas the γδ T-cell receptor is found on a distinct subset of T cells comprising 5% of T cells in lymphoid organs and 1–5% of circulating blood T cells.[108,109] Since γδ T cells often are found in the lung and in epithelia, it has been suggested that they may act as a first line of defense against foreign antigens.[110] γδ T cells were expanded in lymph nodes and lung following exposure to mycobacterial antigens.[111,112] Most γδ T-cell hybridomas from neonatal murine thymocytes responded to the 65-kDa antigen of MTB.[113] Havlir et al. found that live MTB, but not heat-killed organisms, ingested by monocytes, selectively induce the expansion of human peripheral blood γδ T cells.[114] The ability of other infectious pathogens such as *Salmonella, Listeria monocytogenes,* and *Staphylococcus aureus* to induce γδ T cells further suggests that this subpopulation has a general role in the primary immune response to infectious agents.[115] *In vitro,* γδ T cells express cytotoxic or natural killer cell-like activities.[116-118] γδ T-cell clones are capable of secreting cytokines such as IL-2 and IFN-γ,[116,118] suggesting that these cells may activate macrophages for mycobacterial killing. Whether γδ T cells ultimately will prove to be of major importance in protection against MTB *in vivo,* however, remains to be determined.

4. Pleural Lymphocytes

Although TB is acquired via the inhalation of droplet nuclei containing MTB and the majority of tuberculous patients have pulmonary TB, almost nothing is known about the human immune response in the lung. A few recent studies have begun to address this hole in our knowledge of the pathogenesis of TB by studying pleural fluid cells. Pleural TB generally is a self-limited process and recurrent pleurisy is rare, suggesting that immune responses in this compartment are highly protective. Pleural fluid contains increased numbers of MTB-reactive CD4+ T-lymphocytes as compared with blood[119,120] and these cells are predominantly of the CD4+CDw29+ T-cell phenotype that are thought to represent memory T cells.[120] Approximately 30% of patients with tuberculous pleurisy have decreased blastogenic responses of blood mononuclear cells to PPD and often skin test anergy.[121] Fujiwara and Tsuyuguchi have shown that the frequency of antigen-reactive blood lymphocytes in patients with tuberculous pleurisy is normal, whereas the frequency is increased in pleural fluid.[122] Therefore the increase in pleural fluid antigen-reactive CD4+ T cells may be the result of *in situ* expansion rather than sequestration of such cells from the circulating pool. Despite the adequate numbers of antigen-reactive T cells, it appears that the response of blood mononuclear cells to PPD is depressed relative to healthy tuberculin reactors and relative to the pleural fluid response in the same patients.[123] This finding is due to the presence of suppressive monocytes (see below) in the blood but not the pleural fluid. Pleural fluid also contains several-fold increased levels of IFN-γ and TNF-α relative to serum[124] in keeping with the vigorous and effective local immune response.

Since local protective mechanisms are effective in containing the pleural infection despite the inadequacy of the systemic response, Wallis et al. sought to identify potentially protective antigens using cells from the pleural fluid.[125] B-lymphocytes from the pleural fluid were tranformed with Epstein-Barr virus. Such transformed cells spontaneously elaborate immunoglobulin and can be maintained in culture indefinitely, thus circumventing the lack of a suitable nonsecreting human myeloma fusion partner. The frequency of MTB-reactive clones was 54 and 9% in two subjects. Most (83%) of the clones secreted IgM, and the remainder IgG, antibodies. Western blot analysis of MTB using these antibodies identified several patterns of reactivity. Most of the monoclonal antibodies, however, identified a 31.5-kDa band in culture filtrate identified as the 30-kDa α-antigen (antigen 6) suggesting that secreted mycobacterial proteins in general may be accessible to the human immune response during the course of naturally occurring infection. Recently monoclonal antibody reactivity has been used to identify a gene encoding a 47-kDa protein that appears to be a target of these human monoclonal antibodies.[126]

5. Alveolar Lymphocytes

Bronchoalveolar lavage has allowed access to the immune cells protecting the alveoli. Studies indicate that alveolar cells and their functions reflect the pattern of activity found in the interstitium. A fundamental observation is that the cells from the lung do not reflect the cells from the blood either phenotypically or functionally. To date, however, bronchoalveolar lavage scarcely has been used to study the immunopathogenesis of TB. Lenzini et al. analyzed the cellular pattern in the bronchoalveolar lavage fluid of several patients with various lung diseases.[127] One patient with acute TB had 53% lymphocytes and 45% alveolar macrophages (normal 6–10% lymphocytes, 90–95% macrophages). In another patient with chronic TB there were 20% lymphocytes and 80% macrophages. Other more recent studies also demonstrate a lymphocytic alveolitis.[128-132] Since studies of other lung diseases demonstrate that what we learn from the blood does not reflect necessarily what is happening in the lung, investigators must focus more on the lung in the future to understand the pathogenesis of human TB.

D. ANTIGENIC TARGETS OF THE T-CELL RESPONSE TO MTB

MTB-infected persons are identified on the basis of a positive tuberculin PPD skin test. As such infected individuals are relatively immune to exogenous reinfection, protective T cells are likely to be present in the blood as well as other compartments. Since the blood is the most accessible source in humans, the reactivity of blood T cells to putative protective mycobacterial antigens has been assessed.

The results to date have been somewhat disappointing. Although a number of mycobacterial antigens have been characterized molecularly and stimulate T cells in some tuberculin reactors, there is enormous heterogeneity in the human immune response to MTB and it is not clear that the antigens that have been characterized are the most relevant.

The first major approach to define protective mycobacterial proteins was to generate murine monoclonal antibodies from heat-killed MTB-infected mice.[133] Proteins from these monoclonal antibodies were purified and have molecular weights of 12, 14, 19, 38, 65, and 71 kDa. Some blastogenic responses of human blood T cells to each of these antigens have been reported.[134-136] Nevertheless, these antigens do not appear to be major targets of the T-cell response in infected humans because responsiveness is infrequent. It is of considerable interest, however, that several of these proteins correspond to heat shock proteins found not only in other mycobacteria but also in other prokaryotic and in eukaryotic cells. The 65- and 71-kDa antigens, for example, are heat shock proteins with extensive homology to GroEL and DnaK of *E. coli*.[137-140] Although these heat shock proteins do not elicit responses of T cells from most PPD-positive individuals, they may be involved in autoimmune processes targeted to peptides shared by mycobacteria and humans.

Other antigens of potential importance as targets of the human immune response have been identified and are the subject of a recent review.[141] Secreted mycobacterial proteins are of particular interest since live but not heat-killed mycobacteria and culture filtrates confer protection in animal models.[94] The 85 complex of MTB is a group of three major extracellular antigens of MTB encoded by separate genes and secreted by actively proliferating cultures.[142-146] Each of these three proteins is a major secretory product of growing bacilli. Two of these antigens, 85A and 85B, bind to fibronectin and are of molecular weights 30–32 kDa. 85B is identical to a previously recognized MTB antigen termed antigen 6 or the α-antigen,[147] the gene of which was cloned by Matsuo et al.[148] This protein, which will be designated 30 kDa here, contains specific and cross-reactive determinants and stimulates blastogenesis and IFN-γ production by T cells from healthy donors, and elicits DTH in sensitized guinea pigs. This 30-kDa secreted protein may be a particularly important antigenic target of T cells because live metabolically active mycobacteria but not heat-killed organisms generate protective immunity in mice.[94]

Another approach to define targets of the T-cell response to MTB has been to separate lysates and filtrates of MTB by physicochemical techniques and assess the relative reactivity of T cells to the separated fractions. The most consistent finding has been heterogeneity of the targets of the human T-cell response. For example, we found that T cells from tuberculin-positive healthy donors showed peaks of reactivity to fractions of culture filtrate of MTB H37Rv of 30, 37, 44, 57, 71, and 88 kDa.[149] Western immunoblotting indicated that three of these fractions contained previously defined antigens (30, 64, and 71 kDa). This technique does not allow determination of whether these previously identified proteins account for the activity found in the respective fractions. Schoel et al. found numerous and diverse responses to 400 fractions prepared by 2-D gel electrophoresis of lysates of MTB, underscoring the extensive heterogeneity in the mycobacterial antigen targets of human T cells.[150]

It is possible, if not likely, that the heterogeneity of antigens recognized by T cells at least partly reflects the diversity of T-cell subpopulations and functions. Actually, certain antigens may be dominant in terms of a specific function. For example, the 65-kDa heat shock protein of BCG is a target molecule for CD4+ cytotoxic T cells that in turn lyse human monocytes pulsed with this protein.[135] Only approximately 20% of BCG vaccinees respond, however, to this 65-kDa protein.

VI. TNF-α IN RESISTANCE TO MTB AND GRANULOMA FORMATION

Rook suggested in 1983 that secretory products of mononuclear phagocytes may induce the symptoms and tissue necrosis so characteristic of TB.[151] TNF-α is a likely candidate. This cytokine is produced primarily by mononuclear phagocytes. Some of the functions attributed to TNF-α that might explain some of the symptoms and signs in TB include induction of fever and weight loss, stimulation of collagenase production by fibroblasts, and activation of T cells and endothelial cells.

TNF-α is not necessarily only a detrimental cytokine in TB. The mycobactericidal activity of TNF-α is becoming clear. Denis found that TNF-α inhibits the growth of *M. avium* in human monocytes and monocyte-derived macrophages and that the mechanism involves nitrogen intermediates.[152] Bermudez and Young also demonstrated that TNF-α with or without IL-2 inhibits the growth of *M. avium* complex.[153] The role of TNF-α alone in the killing of MTB by mononuclear phagocytes is not clear. The combination of IFN-γ, calcitriol, and TNF-α, however, decreased the growth of MTB in blood monocytes.[154] Our data indicate that TNF-α is an important mediator of growth inhibition of MTB by human alveolar macrophages.[35a]

Kindler et al. demonstrated that granuloma formation in the liver of mice infected with BCG correlates with local synthesis of TNF-α.[155] Injection of anti-TNF-α decreased the number and size of granulomas and the development of epithelioid cells and allowed for massive replication of BCG. Therefore TNF-α is a major mediator of granuloma formation and such formation is critical to containment of mycobacteria. Toossi has examined the expression of TNF-α and transforming growth factor-β (TGF-β) in granulomas obtained from two patients with untreated TB. TGF-β but not TNF-α was expressed in multinucleated giant cells and to a lesser extent in the epithelioid cells (personal communication). TGF-β pretreatment of blood monocytes increased mycobacterial growth in monocytes whereas TNF-α decreased the growth. Using the polymerase chain reaction to amplify 14 cytokines, Yamamura recently demonstrated that resistance and susceptibility were correlated with distinct patterns of cytokine expression in granulomatous skin lesions of *M. leprae*.[156] The balance of production of deactivating and activating cytokines as well as other products of the cellular constituents of granulomas likely contributes significantly to the fate of infecting mycobacteria within them and ultimately to expression of disease.

Not only does TNF-α mediate both protection and pathology in TB in these *in vitro* studies and animal models, but TNF-α also is produced to an increased extent in human TB. Monocytes from patients with TB produce higher levels of TNF-α when stimulated with lipopolysaccharide than monocytes from healthy subjects.[157,158] BCG, PPD, antigen 5, and lipoarabinomannan of MTB stimulate production of TNF-α by human monocytes.[35,159,160] Barnes et al. showed that pleural fluid from patients with TB contains higher levels of TNF-α and IFN-γ than the blood, and that mycobacterial cell wall components stimulate release of TNF-α by pleural fluid mononuclear cells.[161] Thus, TNF-α produced locally and in response to mycobacteria may induce many of the clinical manifestations of TB and provide protection by enhancing the mycobactericidal activity of mononuclear phagocytes.

VII. MODULATION OF MACROPHAGE EFFECTOR FUNCTIONS BY GROWTH-ENHANCING AND MACROPHAGE-DEACTIVATING CYTOKINES

North demonstrated that acquired nonspecific resistance in mice is reduced greatly in T-cell-deficient mice as a result of their failure to acquire adequate numbers of activated macrophages.[84]

Although multiple lymphokines may activate macrophages, the lymphokine that has been studied the most for its potential as a macrophage-activating factor for growth inhibition of MTB by mononuclear phagocytes is IFN-γ. Murine peritoneal macrophages respond to IFN-γ with increased killing of MTB.[162,163] Murine bone marrow macrophages also are activated by IFN-γ for increased killing of MTB but the response to IFN-γ is specific to the strain of MTB, some being much more affected than others. In contrast to these animal studies, Douvas et al. reported that IFN-γ does not activate killing of MTB in human blood monocyte-derived macrophages and in fact enhances growth.[164] Rook et al., however, found that although IFN-γ has little effect on killing of MTB in human blood monocytes, this lymphokine enhances growth inhibition of MTB by monocyte-derived macrophages.[165] The mechanism by which IFN-γ exerts its macrophage activation was suggested to be through induction of the enzyme necessary for conversion of 25-hydroxyvitamin D_3 to the active metabolite of vitamin D, 1,25-dihydroxyvitamin D_3. This metabolite in turn induces the differentiation of monocytes into macrophages better capable of killing MTB. In summary, the macrophage-activating factor activity of IFN-γ in mononuclear phagocytes from animals is more potent than in monocytes from humans but probably has some activity on monocyte-derived macrophages at least for some strains of MTB.

Surprisingly, little has been done to characterize additional macrophage-activating factors for MTB. The story is more complete, however, for *M. avium*; moreover, these data may have some relevance for MTB. For *M. avium* the macrophage-activating factor activity of IFN-γ is weak and inconstant.[166,167] It appears, however, that these unimpressive results may be due partly to a masking effect. Thus, indomethacin increases the macrophage-activating factor activity of IFN-γ.[167] Bermudez also has shown that TGF-β is produced by monocytes that have ingested *M. avium*, and blocks the activity of IFN-γ.[168] GM-CSF and TNF-α, with and without IL-2, also exhibit macrophage-activating factor activity against *M. avium*.[169-171] IL-6, on the contrary, promotes the intracellular and extracellular growth of *M. avium*[167,172] and appears to down-regulate receptors for TNF-α.[173]

For the case of MTB, we also have found that intracellular growth represents a balance between the monocyte-deactivating effects of TGF-β and the macrophage-activating factor effects of TNF-α. Characteristically, there is little intracellular replication of MTB within the first 4 days of culture; in fresh monocytes, thereafter, the organism begins to replicate at an impressive rate. The phase of intracellular growth corresponds to the delayed induction of TGF-β. Although it is conjectural as to whether the TNF-α/TGF-β ratio and kinetics determine the intracellular growth curve of MTB, it is quite clear that the balance between growth-enhancing and growth-inhibitory influences may determine the outcome of infection in the host.

VIII. CLASS II-RESTRICTED CYOTOXICITY: ROLE IN PROTECTION AND IMMUNOPATHOLOGY

As noted, cytolytic T cells appear during the course of experimental MTB infections.[95] Most of the support for CTL as an effector mechanism in MTB is based on in vitro studies and conjecture. Blood T-lymphocytes from MTB or M. leprae-infected individuals are cytotoxic for monocytes pulsed with mycobacterial antigens.[135] The cytotoxicity was found to be a property of CD4+ T cells. Recently Boom et al. demonstrated further that CD4+ T-cell clones from PPD-reactive individuals were cytotoxic to mycobacterial antigen-pulsed or MTB-infected monocytes.[107] The cytotoxicity was independent of the profile of cytokines released by these clones (IL-2 versus IL-4) and was the property of most of the clones.

Mustafa and Godal demonstrated that CD4+ blood lymphocytes and clones from BCG-vaccinated subjects were cytotoxic to mycobacterial-antigen pulsed monocytes.[174] Interestingly the cytotoxic CD4+ clones also suppressed proliferation of some BCG-specific T-cell clones in response to BCG. Whether the suppression of T-cell responses was a consequence of cytotoxicity for antigen-presenting cells or direct suppression of T-cell responses was not resolved by this study. Macrophages that have ingested MTB or have been pulsed with soluble products such as PPD are targets of the CTL response.[107,135] Some, but not all clones, seem to be targeted on the 65-kDa antigen. In fact, endogenous heat shock proteins produced by monocytes stressed by cytomegalovirus infection or stimulation with IFN-γ may render these cells targets of the CTL response.[175]

What then is the significance of Class II-mediated cytotoxicity? Most investigators speculate that it is a default mechanism by which MTB is released from overburdened and therefore dysfunctional effector cells. Presumably, once the organisms are released they will be ingested and killed by fresh monocytes drawn to the fray. Alternatively, the CTL, by lysing host cells, must be considered a factor in immunopathology. Clearly, additional in vivo studies in experimental animals will be necessary to resolve the relative importance of these two diverse sequelae of CTL.

IX. IMMUNE RESPONSES IN TUBERCULOSIS

A. T-LYMPHOCYTES

T-cell responsiveness to mycobacterial antigens during TB may underlie antigen-specific and/or nonspecific anergy during active disease. From 17 to 25% of patients with active TB are unresponsive to PPD skin tests.[176-178] Moreover, in vitro blastogenic responses of blood T-lymphocytes to PPD are absent in approximately 40% of patients with active TB including most skin test nonreactors and some reactors.[179-186] Hyporesponsiveness to mycobacterial antigens has been described from various geographic areas and therefore seems to be relatively constant regardless of prior immunization with BCG, etc. Several studies have indicated that the responses to nonmycobacterial antigens and mitogens are intact so that depression of tuberculin reactivity is relatively specific.[179,182,183,186] Blood lymphocytes from patients with active TB also show selectively decreased PPD-stimulated expression of IL-2 and expression of IL-2R.[185] In a recent study, both blastogenesis and IFN-γ production by blood mononuclear cells were decreased, whereas TNF-α production (probably monocyte-derived) was increased in newly diagnosed patients with TB.[187] During treatment, blastogenic and IFN-γ responses increased, whereas the TNF-α production decreased.[187] It is important to emphasize that the depressed responses are seen in untreated patients and, where studied, responses to PPD tend to increase during treatment.

Such hyporesponsiveness of circulating T cells in active pulmonary TB may be attributed either to T-cell dysfunction or to direct suppression of T-cell responses by other cells or products of MTB. Exogenous IL-2 did not increase the T-cell response in one study,[185] suggesting T-cell unresponsiveness in TB. In another study, however, IL-2 restored responsiveness.[188] Suppressor cells described in TB include cytotoxic CD4+ lymphocytes,[135] blood monocytes (discussed below),[179] and Fcγ receptor-positive T cells.[182] When monocytes take up MTB in vitro, they release an MTB-derived suppressor cell-activating factor identified as phosphatidylethanolamine and phosphatidylinositol.[189] These products, in turn, activate suppressor T cells.[190] Other MTB constituents that may activate suppressive pathways are lipoarabinomannan[191] and arabinogalactan.[192]

A critical and unanswered question is what is the significance of suppression of T-cell responses to mycobacterial antigens in patients with TB? In the absence of data, divergent possibilities exist. Depressed T-cell responses may be a factor in the pathogenesis of reactivation TB. Alternatively, suppression of the systemic response in a patient with uncontrolled local infection may minimize pathophysiologic sequelae such as septic shock. Another issue to be addressed is the relationship between suppressed responses in the blood and regulation of the immune response locally at the site of infection. It is of interest that TGF-β has both a suppressive activity and may be relevant as a mediator of suppression and a macrophage-deactivating factor activity that may undermine local defenses. In this situation, although it is suppressive activity that is measured, other properties of cytokines produced locally may have greater bearing on the host–parasite balance.

B. BLOOD MONOCYTES

Cunningham et al. first noted in 1925 that patients with TB have a peripheral blood monocytosis.[193] Circulating monocytes are immature based on cytochemical and DNA labeling studies.[194] Patients with TB have a corresponding increase in monocytopoiesis as determined by bone marrow studies. These data may indicate that TB confers a stimulus for bone marrow production and/or there is high monocyte consumption presumably due to influx into granulomatous inflammatory sites in the tissues. The immaturity of monocytes in TB may be a factor in the altered functional activity that has been observed.

The capacity of blood monocytes from patients with TB to function as antigen-presenting cells is unknown. Ellner demonstrated, however, that adherent mononuclear cells (predominantly monocytes) from patients with pulminary TB and skin test anergy were specifically suppressive of lymphocyte blastogenic responses to PPD.[179] This suppressive activity was not affected by depletion of T-lymphocytes from the adherent cell population and has been ascribed to the contained monocytes. Depletion of Fc$_\gamma$ R$^+$ cells from nonadherent blood mononuclear cells resulted in a population uniformly sensitive to suppression by adherent cells in all patients with TB.[182] Yet (and surprisingly) depletion of CD16 positive cells from the lymphocyte population rendered them less sensitive to suppression by monocytes. The selective suppression of PPD-induced blastogenesis by monocytes also extended to production of IL-2.[184]

Several studies have addressed the basis for depression of T-cell responses by monocytes and their apparent antigen specificity. On isolation, monocytes from patients with pulmonary TB show

depressed surface expression of Class II MHC determinants.[186] During culture for 4 h, a sharp increase in HLA-DR is observed. The group with depressed PPD-stimulated blastogenesis had the greatest abnormality in HLA-DR expression. It seems likely that decreased expression of Class II MHC is a marker for a suppressive monocyte rather than the mechanism of suppression; this assumption is based on the finding that depletion of monocytes increased the T-cell response to PPD rather than decreasing it as might be the case if the depressed HLA-DR was limiting the capacity for accessory cell function. IL-1 also is important in the immunoregulatory function of mononuclear phagocytes. Adherent mononuclear cells from patients with TB produce higher levels of IL-1 than healthy controls in response to lipopolysaccharide.[181] In the course of these experiments PPD was shown to be a direct stimulus for monocyte production of IL-1,[195] a signal observation that is discussed below. Also, tuberculosis patients showed increased PPD-stimulated IL-1 production.[181] The apparent paradox between increased production of IL-1 with its key role in immune induction and the suppression by adherent cells may be explained by concurrent production of other suppressive molecules produced by adherent cells.

Some progress has been made concerning the potential mediators of suppression. Adherent cells from patients with TB do not produce higher levels of the immunosuppressive molecule prostaglandin E2 than monocytes from healthy subjects.[180] They do express surface IL-2 receptors and also release IL-2R into medium during culture.[196] In fact, consumption of IL-2 may be relevant to suppression; it appears, however, to be a minor factor, as exogenous IL-2 did not reverse depressed PPD-stimulated blastogenesis.[178] This experiment must be interpreted with care as T cells from patients are known to have decreased IL-2R and therefore may be hyporesponsive to exogenous IL-2 on that basis alone.[185] Recently Toossi and Ellner demonstrated that blood monocytes from tuberculous patients produce increased amounts of TGF-β;[197] as TGF-β is a potent suppressor of PPD-stimulated IL-2 production and blastogenesis, it may be a key factor in suppression. Other suppressive cytokines that deserve further study are IL-10 and IL-1Ra.

C. REGULATION BY MONOCYTE STIMULATORY ANTIGENS

The basis for the antigen specificity of suppression is a matter of great interest. As noted, PPD is a direct stimulus for monocytes to produce IL-1.[195] Subsequently, PPD was shown to stimulate TNF-α production,[35] and IL-2R expression and secretion.[196] Both polysaccharide (lipoarabinomannan) and protein mycobacterial products have the capacity to stimulate cytokine production by monocytes.[198-200] Wallis et al. have demonstrated that most of the monocyte stimulatory activity of mycobacterial culture filtrates resides in a 58-kDa protein.[126] Interestingly, the 30-kDa α-antigen of MTB also has the capacity of stimulating expression of cytokines by monocytes and may do so by binding to surface fibronectin (unpublished observation).

The direct stimulatory properties of mycobacterial proteins for monocytes is of intrinsic interest; it may be relevant to immunity and/or immunopathology as cytokine products such as TNF-α display macrophage-activating factor activity and also may be injurious to host tissues. This property is of particular interest, however, in the context of antigen-specific immunosuppression. It now appears that the basis for the selectivity of suppression by monocytes is the action of PPD not just as a specific antigen for T cells but as a stimulus for monocytes primed during the course of TB to overproduce immunosuppressive factors.

A comparison of the response of tuberculous patients and healthy tuberculin positive controls to purified mycobacterial antigens also may reflect this pathway of immunomodulation. We recently observed that patients with pulmonary TB fail to respond to the 30-kDa α-antigen whereas healthy tuberculin-positive donors and household contacts of patients respond briskly.[149] Seven of eight healthy tuberculin-positive donors and none of six tuberculous patients (treated for 6–20 weeks) showed a blastogenic response to this antigen. These results were confirmed and extended by Sada et al. in studies of 10 households with index cases of active pulmonary TB in Mexico City; despite comparable responses to mycobacterial sonicates, 73% of 21 tuberculin-positive household contacts and none of the TB patients responded to the 30-kDa α-antigen (Sada, personal communication). It is possible that the hyporesponsiveness of the tuberculous patients is due to stimulation of monocyte production of suppressive mediators by the 30-kDa antigen. Regardless of its basis, the failure to respond to this antigen may be a factor in reactivation of TB.

Falla et al. demonstrated that household contacts and tuberculous patients showed similar responses to sonic extracts of MTB H37Rv.[201] Nonetheless, 84% of household contacts and only 48% of newly diagnosed patients responded to MTP40, a 14-kDa antigen; moreover, only 52% of treated patients demonstrated responsiveness.[201] Tuberculous patients also were hyporesponsive to an A60 complex extract.[187] In this case, 60% developed responsiveness with treatment.

X. HIV AND PATHOGENESIS OF TUBERCULOSIS

A. TUBERCULOIMMUNITY IN HIV INFECTION

HIV is the greatest known risk both for reactivation of latent MTB infection[202,203] and for development of primary TB on exposure to infected persons.[204] TB occurs relatively early in HIV infection in 50–67% of the cases in the United States at a mean of 6 to 9 months before an AIDS-defining condition.[205] The mean CD4+ count is approximately 200 cells/μl. This early onset of TB in HIV-infected individuals suggests a strict requirement for a fully competent cell-mediated immune response for protection against MTB. The response to recall antigens, including PPD, is decreased in HIV-infected persons. Generalized anergy was uncommon with a CD4+ count > 500 cells/μl (<10%), but thereafter increased as CD4+ counts dropped (80% for CD4+ < 50 cells/μl).[206] HIV infection also increases the likelihood of a negative tuberculin skin test in MTB-infected people.[207] Although anergy is common in HIV infection, surprisingly HIV-infected patients with TB often have a positive cutaneous DTH response to PPD. In Uganda 68% of patients with TB are HIV infected. Okwera et al. demonstrated that 18% of HIV-infected mothers without TB were positive in a cohort in which 60% of healthy HIV-negative subjects were skin test positive.[207] T-cell proliferation and cytokine production (IFN-γ and TNF-α) by peripheral blood mononuclear cell responses in response to PPD also were increased in the tuberculin skin test-positive HIV-infected patients with TB as compared to HIV-positive, PPD skin test-reactive but asymptomatic women studied in a mother–infant cohort.[208] These data support the concept that immunity to MTB can be boosted by active TB even in the presence of the immunosuppression of HIV. Why such tuberculoimmunity fails to protect against disease, however, is unanswered. Are subtle defects in cell-mediated immunity sufficient for susceptibility to TB or are defects in native resistance operable? The known abnormalities in T-cell and mononuclear phagocyte function in HIV infection may provide clues.

B. T-LYMPHOCYTES IN HIV INFECTION

During infection with HIV, CD4+ T helper cells are progressively depleted and profoundly impaired with respect to proliferation and production of cytokines such as IL-2.[209] B-lymphocyte activity increases during HIV infection with resulting hypergammaglobulinemia. The loss in T helper cell function appears to occur first as unresponsiveness to recall antigens, then to allo-MHC antigens, and finally to the mitogen phytohemagglutinin.[210]

As reviewed by Clerici and Shearer, the mechanisms of such progressive dysfunction include selective loss of memory cells, immunoregulatory dysfunction of mononuclear phagocytes (see below), immunosuppression by products of HIV such as gp120 and tat, induction of suppressor cells and mediators, and production of immunoregulatory cytokines.[210] Each of these mechanisms also may impact on susceptibility to TB in HIV infection. The production of immunoregulatory cytokines in HIV infection may be especially important as regards TB. Daly recently reported that in a cohort of >100 HIV-positive individuals, a selective loss of IL-2 and IFN-γ production in response to recall antigens is correlated with an increase in phytohemagglutinin-stimulated IL-4 and IL-10 production.[204] These data strongly suggest a decline in Th1 function and an increase in Th2 function in HIV infection. Since immunity in TB is associated with Th1 type responses, this switch in the balance toward Th2 function in HIV infection likely contributes to the increased susceptibility to TB in HIV-infected persons.

C. MONONUCLEAR PHAGOCYTES IN HIV INFECTION

Mononuclear phagocytes including blood monocytes and tissue macrophages may be infected with HIV *in vitro* and *in vivo*.[211] Since MTB is an intracellular pathogen, mononuclear phagocytes may be affected particularly by dual infection with HIV and MTB. The properties and functions of mononuclear phagocytes from HIV-infected subjects are not well defined and studies often are contradictory (reviewed in Reference 211). Nevertheless most studies indicate that the number of monocytes, expression of cytokines including IL-1 and TNF-α, production of oxygen radical production, expression of phenotypic markers such as Class II MHC, CR1, and CR3, and microbicidal activity against several pathogens are preserved. Antigen presentation by monocytes, however, is decreased. Neither the microbicidal activity nor the response to macrophage activating factors for MTB by monocytes from HIV-infected subjects is known.

We demonstrated that alveolar macrophages from healthy subjects are more susceptible *in vitro* to productive infection with HIV than are blood monocytes due to the state of differentiation or activation of these cells.[212] Several immunologic and effector functions of alveolar macrophages from HIV-infected subjects are up-regulated including accessory function for T-cell responses to mitogens,[213] expression of markers of activation including HLA-DR and transferrin receptor,[214] and cytokine expression including IL-1,[215] IL-6,[216] and TNF-α.[217] Microbicidal activity of alveolar macrophages from subjects with AIDS is normal for *Toxoplasma gondii* and *Chlamydia psittaci* and killing is up-regulated by IFN-γ.[218]

Whether these findings extend to native and acquired resistance to MTB, however, is not known. Since TNF-α is critical to both granuloma formation and to control of mycobacterial growth, the increased production of TNF-α by alveolar macrophages from HIV-infected patients suggests that these cells may inhibit mycobacterial growth normally or to an increased extent. Because HIV-infected subjects are not protected against MTB, however, other mechanisms of protection by alveolar macrophages may be defective in HIV infection. Another potential consequence of the increased TNF-α expression by alveolar macrophages during HIV infection noted *in vitro* is lung pathology. The increased accessory activity of alveolar macrophages potentially could enhance transmission of HIV from alveolar macrophages to T cells on stimulation by microbial agents such as MTB resulting in further dysfunction or depletion of local T cells important in mycobacterial resistance. The number of cytotoxic alveolar lymphocytes from HIV-infected persons is increased and these cells are of the phenotype CD8+.[219,220] These cytotoxic T cells kill antigen-pulsed alveolar macrophages in a Class I-restricted manner.[221] Should such activity exist for MTB-infected alveolar macrophages, release of tubercle bacilli with dissemination could occur. Alternatively, released bacilli could be phagocytized and killed by other alveolar macrophages or monocyte-derived macrophages in granulomas providing increased protection.

D. IMPACT OF TUBERCULOSIS ON HIV INFECTION

Not only is HIV infection a major risk factor for TB, but the impact of TB on HIV infection also is receiving recognition. For example, in Zaire, HIV-infected child-bearing women with TB had a 2.7-fold higher mortality as compared to those without TB.[222] In Uganda, the mortality of TB in HIV-infected patients is 30%; this finding is thought to be due primarily to progressive HIV disease, and not to the tuberculosis disease.[223] Serum levels of β2-microglobulin, a marker of HIV disease progression, were twofold higher in HIV-infected Ugandan patients with pulmonary TB compared with HIV-infected nontuberculous subjects and HIV-seronegative patients with TB.[208] Recent data from the United States indicate that HIV-infected patients with TB show reduced survival, more opportunistic infections, and a greater decrease in CD4+ counts relative to CD4+-matched controls (C. Whalen, personal communication). Since TB tends to occur early in the course of HIV infection, the interaction of the two diseases may have a pronounced effect on viral burden and may facilitate the progression of HIV disease to advanced stages.

Replication of HIV *in vitro* and presumably *in vivo* both in lymphocytes and monocytes requires activation by various stimuli such as antigens, mitogens, growth factors, and cytokines including TNF-α, IL-1, and IL-6. These stimuli initiate viral replication in part through activation of nuclear factor kB (NFkB) that in turn binds to, the long terminal repeat (LTR) in the promoter region of HIV, thereby stimulating viral transcription. Blood monocytes from patients with TB release increased amounts of TNF-α, IL-1, and IL-6 on stimulation with lipopolysaccharide. Furthermore mycobacteria and protein and polysaccharide constituents of mycobacteria stimulate production of TNF-α by mononuclear phagocytes. These considerations make it likely that TB in HIV-infected persons may result in an increase in HIV replication *in vivo*. In fact, Toossi et al. recently demonstrated that monocytes from patients with pulmonary TB are more susceptible to productive infection with HIV *in vitro* than are monocytes from healthy subjects.[224] The increased production was not attributable to increased viral entry, reverse transcription, or frequency of infected cells, suggesting either that integration or viral transcription was upregulated in these cells. The role of cytokines produced by monocytes from patients with TB in the enhanced replication of HIV is being examined. These data suggest, however, that the cytokines relevant to protection against MTB, such as TNF-α, may be deleterious for persons with HIV infection and that anticytokine therapy may be effective in limiting HIV replication during treatment of active TB in HIV-positive subjects.

REFERENCES

1. Flugge, C., Ueber Luftinfection, *Z. Hyg. Infectionskr.*, 25, 179, 1897.
2. Wells, W. F., Wells, M. W., Wilder, T. S., The environmental control of epidemic contagion. I. An epidemiologic study of radiant disinfection of air in day schools, *Am. J. Hyg.*, 35, 97, 1942.
3. Riley, R. L., Mills, C. C., O'Grady, F., Sultan, L.U., Wittstadt, F., Shivpuri, D. N., Infectiousness of air from a tuberculosis ward. Ultraviolet irradiation of infectiousness of different patients, *Am. Rev. Resp. Dis.*, 85, 511, 1962.
4. Smith, D. W., McMurray, D. N., Wiegeshaus, E. H., Grover, A. A., Harding, G. E., Host-parasite relationships in experimental airborne tuberculosis. IV. Early events in the course of infection in vaccinated and nonvaccinated guinea pigs, *Am. Rev. Resp. Dis.*, 102, 937, 1970.
5. Lurie, M. B., *Resistance to Tuberculosis: Experimental Studies in Native and Acquired Defensive Mechanisms,* Harvard University Press, Cambridge, MA, 1964.
6. Lurie, M. B., Dannenberg, A. M., Jr., Macrophage function in infectious disease with inbred rabbits, *Bacteriol. Rev.*, 29, 466, 1965.
7. Meylan, P. R. A., Richman, D. D., Kornbluth, R. S., Reduced intracellular growth of mycobacteria in human macrophages cultivated at physiologic oxygen pressure, *Am. Rev. Resp. Dis.*, 145, 947, 1992.
8. Dannenberg, A. M., Immune mechanisms in the pathogenesis of pulmonary tuberculosis, *Rev. Infect. Dis.*, 52, 369, 1989.
9. North, R. J., T-cell dependence of macrophage activation and mobilization during infection with *Mycobacterium tuberculosis*, *Infect. Immun.*, 10, 66, 1974.
10. Bates, J. H., Tuberculosis: Susceptibility and resistance, *Am. Rev. Resp. Dis.*, 125, 20, 1982.
11. Medlar, E. M., The behavior of pulmonary tuberculous lesions: a pathological study, *Am. Rev. Tuberc.*, 71, 1, 1955.
12. Yamamura, Y., Ogawa, Y., Maeda, H., Yamamura, Y., Prevention of tuberculous cavity formation by desensitization with tuberculin-active peptide, *Am. Rev. Resp. Dis.*, 109, 594, 1974.
13. Rastogi, N., David H. L., Mechanisms of pathogenicity in mycobacteria, *Biochimie*, 70, 1101, 1988.
14. Rastogi, N., Recent observations concerning structure and function relationships in the mycobacterial cell envelope: elaboration of a model in terms of mycobacterial pathogenicity, virulence and drug-resistance, *Res. Microbiol.*, 142, 464, 1991.
15. Middlebrook, G. Dubos, R., Pierce, G., Virulence and morphological characteristics of mammalian tubercle bacilli, *J. Exp. Med.*, 86, 175, 1947..
16. Bloch, H., Studies on the virulence of tubercle bacilli, *J. Exp. Med.*, 91, 197, 1950.
17. Noll, H., The chemistry of cord factor, a toxic glycolipid of M. tuberculosis, *Adv. Tuberc. Res.*, 7, 149, 1956.
18. Artman, M., Bekierkunst, A., Goldenberg, I., Tissue metabolism in infection: biochemical changes in mice treated with cord factor, *Arch. Biochem. Biophys.*, 105, 80, 1964.
19. Kato, M., Site II-Specific inhibition of mitochondial oxidative phosphorylation by trehalose-6,6'-dimycolate (cord factor) of *Mycobacterium tuberculosis*, *Arch. Biochem. Biophys.*, 140, 379, 1970.

20. Goren, M. B., *Tuberculosis*, Youmans, G. P., Ed., W. B. Saunders, Philadelphia, 1979, 63.

21. Dubos, R., Middlebrook, G., Letters to the editor: cytochemical reaction of virulent tubercle bacilli, *Am. Rev. Tuberc.*, 58, 698, 1948.

22. Goren, M. B., Sulfolipid I of *Mycobacterium tuberculosis* strain H37Rv. I. Purification properties, *Biochim. Biophys. Acta*, 210, 116, 1970.

23. Goren, M. B., Sulfolipid I of *Mycobacterium tuberculosis* strain H37Rv. II. Structural studies, *Biochim. Biophys. Acta,* 210, 127, 1970.

24. Kato, M., Goren, M. B., Synergistic action of cord factor and mycobacterial sulfatides on mitochondria, *Infect. Immun.*, 10, 733, 1974.

25. Goren, M. B., D'Arcy Hart, P., Young, W. R., Armstrong, J. A., Prevention of phagosome-lysosome fusion in cultured macrophages by sulfatides of *Mycobacterium tuberculosis, Proc. Natl. Acad. Sci. U.S.A.,* 73, 2510, 1976.

26. Goren, M. B., Swendsen, C. L., Fiscus, J., Miranti, C., Fluorescent markers for studying phagosome-lysosome fusion, *J. Leukocyte Biol.*, 36, 273, 1984.

27. Smith, D. W., Randall, H. M., Gaastambide-Odier, M. D., and Koevoet, A. L., Mycosides: a new class of type-specific glycolipids of mycobacteria, *Ann. N.Y. Acad. Sci.*, 69, 145, 1960.

28. Brennan, P. J., Hunter, S. W., McNeil, M., Chatterjee, D., Daffe, M., Reappraisal of the chemistry of mycobacterial cell walls, with a view to understanding the roles of individual entities in disease processes, in *Microbial Determinants of Virulence and Host Response*, Ayoub, E. M., Cassell, G. H., Branch, W. C., Jr., Henry, T. J., Eds., American Society for Microbiology, Washington, D.C., 1990, 55.

29. Daffe, M., Lacave, C., Lanelle, M.-A., Gillois, M., Lanelle, G., Polyphythinenacyl trehalose, glycolipids specific for virulent strains of the tubercule bacillus, *Eur. J. Biochem.*, 112, 579, 1988.

30. Dannenberg, A. M., Jr., Review: delayed-type hypersensitivity and cell mediated immunity in the pathogenesis of tuberculosis, *Immunol. Today*, 12, 7, 228, 1991.

31. Collins, F. M., Dynamics of the phgagocytic cell response within the lungs of parabiotic mice infected with mycobacteria with decreasing virulence for mice, *Infect. Immun.*, 58, 2303, 1990.

32. Smith, D. W., McMurray, D. N, Wiegeshaus, E. H., Grover, A. A., Harding, G. E., Host-parasite relationships relationships in experimental airborne tuberculosis. IV. Early events in the course of infection in vaccinated and nonvaccinated guinea pigs, *Am. Rev. Resp. Dis.*, 102, 937, 1970.

33. Swartz, R. P., Naal, D., Vogel, C.-W., Yeager, H., Jr., Differences in uptake of mycobacteria by human monocytes: a role for complement, *Infect. Immun.*, 56, 9, 2223, 1988.

34. Schlessinger, L., Bellinger-Kawahara, C. G., Payne, N. R., Horwitz, M. A., Phagocytosis of *Mycobacterium tuberculosis* is mediated by human monocyte complement receptors and complement component C3, *J. Immunol.*, 144, 7, 2771, 1990.

35a. Hirsch, C. S., Ellner, J. J., Russell, D. G., Rich, E. A., complement receptor-mediated uptake and tumor necrosis factor-α-mediated growth inhibition of *Mycobacterium tuberculosis* by human alveolar macrophages, *J. Immunol.,* 152, 743, 1994.

35b. Valone, S. E., Rich, E. A., Wallis, R. R., Ellner, J. J., Expression of tumor necrosis factor *in vitro* by human mononuclear phagocytes stimulated with BCF and mycobacterial antigens, *Infect. Immun.*, 56, 3313, 1988.

36. Rich, E. A., Panuska, J. R., Wallis, R. S., Wolf, C. B., Ellner, J.J., Dyscoordinate expression of tumor necrosis factor-alpha by human blood monocytes and alveolar macrophages, *Am. Rev. Resp. Dis.,* 139, 1010, 1989.

37. Myrvik, Q. N., Leake, E.E., Wright, M. J., Disruption of phagosomal membranes of normal alveolar macrophages by the H37Rv strain of *Mycobacterium tuberculosis:* a correlate of virulence, *Am. Rev. Resp. Dis.,* 129, 322, 1984.

38. Armstrong, J. A., Hart, P. d'A., Phagosome-lysosome interactions in cultured macrophages infected with virulent turucle bacilli. Reversal of the usual nonfusion pattern and observations on bacterial survival, *J. Exp. Med.,* 142, 1, 1975.

39. Flesch, I. E. A., Kaufmann, S. N. E., Attempts to characterize the mechanisms involved in mycobacterial growth inhibition by gamma-interferon-activated bone marrow macrophages, *Infect. Immun.,* 56, 1464, 1988.

40. Mitchison, D. A., Selkon, J. B., Lloyd, J., Virulence in the guinea-pig, susceptibility to hydrogen peroxide, and catalase activity of isoniazid-sensitive tubercle bacilli from South Indian and British patients, *J. Pathol. Bacteriol.*, 377, 1963.

41. Jackett, P. S., Aber, V. R., Lowrie, D. B., Virulence of *Mycobacterium tuberculosis* and susceptibility of peroxidative killing systems, *J. Gen. Microbiol.*, 106, 273, 1978.

42. Douvas, G. S., Berger, E. M., Repine, J. E., Crowle, A. J., Natural mycobacteriostatic activity in human monocyte-derived adherent cells, *Am. Rev. Resp. Dis.*, 134, 44, 1986.

43. Bloch, H., The relationship between phagocytic cells and human tubercle bacilli, *Am. Rev. Tuberc.*, 58, 662, 1948.

44. Martin, S. P., Pierce, C. H., Middlebrook, G., Dubos, R. J., The effect of tubercle bacilli on the polymorphonuclear leukocytes of normal animals, *J. Exp. Med.*, 91, 381, 1950.

45. Montgomery, L. G., Lemon W. S., The cellular reaction of the pleura to infection with *Mycobacterium tuberculosis*, *J. Thorac. Surg.*, 2, 429, 1933.

46. Vorwald, A. J., The early cellular reactions in the lungs of rabbits infected intravenously with human tubercle bacilli, *Am. Rev. Tuberc.*, 25, 74, 1932.

47. Antony, V. B., Sahn, S. A., Antony, A. C., Repine, J. E., *Bacillus Calmette-Guerin*-stimulated neutrophils release chemotaxins for monocytes in rabbit pleural spaces and *in vitro*, *J. Clin. Invest.*, 76, 1514, 1985.

48. Brown, A. E., Holzer, T. J., Andersen, B. R., Capacity of human neutrophils to kill *Mycobacterium tuberculosis*, *J. Infect. Dis.*, 156, 985, 1987.

49. May, M. E., Spagnuolo, P. J., Evidence for activation of a respiratory burst in the interaction of human neutrophils with *Mycobacterium tuberculosis*, *Infect. Immun.*, 55, 2304, 1987.

50. Jones, G. S., Amirault, H. J., Andersen, B. R., Killing of *Mycobacterium tuberculosis* by neutrophils: a nonoxidative process, *J. Infect. Dis.*, 162, 700, 1990.

51. Geertsma, M. F., Nibbering, P. H., Pos, O., van Furth, R., Interferon-γ-activated human granulocytes kill ingested *Mycobacterium fortuitum* more efficiently than normal granulocytes, *Eur. J. Immunol.*, 20, 869, 1990.

52. Skamene, E., Genetic control of susceptibility to mycobacterial infections, *Rev. Infect. Dis.*, 2(Suppl. 1), S394, 1989.

53. Skamene, E., Genetic regulation of host resistance to bacterial infection, *Rev. Infect. Dis.*, 5, S823, 1983.

54. Stead, W. W., Racial differences in susceptibility to infection by *Mycobacterial tuberculosis*, *N. Engl. J. Med.*, 322, 422, 1990.

55. Comstock, G.W., Tuberculosis in twins: a reanalysis of the prophit survey, *Am. Rev. Resp. Dis.*, 117, 621, 1978.

56. Collins, F. M., Cellular mechanisms of antimycobacterial immunity, in *Host Defenses to Intracellular Pathogens,* Eisenstein, T., Actor, P., Friedman, H., Eds., Plenum Press, New York, 1983, 157.

57. Abel, L., Demenais, F., Detection of major genes for susceptibility to leprosy and its subtypes in a Caribbean island: Desirade Island, *Am. J. Human Genet.*, 42, 256, 1988.

58. van Eden, W., de Bries, R. R. P., Occasional review-HLA and leprosy: a re-evaluation, *Lepr. Rev.*, 55, 89, 1984.

59. Singh, S. P. N., Mehra, N. K., Dingley, H. B., Pande, J. N., Vaidya, M. C., HLA haplotype segregation study in multiple case families of pulmonary tuberculosis, *Tissue Antigens*, 23, 84, 1984.

60. Selby, R., Barnard, J. M., Buehler, S. K., Crumley, J., Larsen, B., Marshall, W. H., Tuberculosis associated with HLA-B8, BfS in a Newfoundland community study, *Tissue Antigens*, 11, 403, 1978.

61. Al-Arif, L. I., Goldstein, R. A., Affronti, L. F., Janicki, J. W., HLA Bw15 and tuberculosis in a North American black population, *Am. Rev. Resp. Dis.*, 120, 1275, 1979.

62. Jian, Z. F., An, J. B., Sun, Y. P, Mittal, K. K., Lee, T. D., Association of HLA-BW35 with tuberculosis in the Chinese, *Tissue Antigen*, 22, 86, 1983.

63. Khomenko, A. G., Litvinov, V. I., Chukanova, V. P., Pospelov, L. E., Tuberculosis in patients with various HLA phenotypes, *Tubercle*, 71, 187, 1990.

64. Bothamley, G.H., Beck, J.S., Schreuder G.M.Th., D'Amaro, J., deVries, R.R.P., Kardjito, T., Ivanyi, J., Association of tuberculosis and *M. tuberculosis*-specific antibody levels with HLA, *J. Infect. Dis.*, 159, 549, 1989.

65. Hwange, C. H., Khan, S., Ende, N., Mangura, B. T., Reichman, L. B., Chou, J., The HLA-A, -B, and -DR phenotypes and tuberculosis, *Am. Rev. Resp. Dis.*, 132, 382, 1985.

66. Hafez, M., El-Salab, S. H., El-Shennawy, F., Bassiony, M. R., HLA-antigens and tuberculosis in the Egyptian population, *Tubercle*, 66, 35, 1985.

67. Zervas, J., Castantopoulos, C, Toubis, M, Anagnostopoulos, D., Cotsovoulou, V., HLA-A and B antigens and pulmonary tuberculosis in Greeks, *Br. J. Dis. Chest*, 81, 147, 1987.

68. Cox, R. A., Arnold, D. R., Cook, D., Lundberg, D. I., HLA phenotypes in Mexican Americans with tuberculosis, *Am. Rev., Resp. Dis.*, 126, 653, 1982.

69. Singh, S. P. N., Mehra, N. K., Dingley, H. B., Pande, J. N., Vaidya, M. C., HLA-A, -B, -C, and -DR antigen profile in pulmonary tuberculosis in North India, *Tissue Antigens*, 21, 380, 1983.

70. Cox, R. A., Downs, M., Neimes, R. E., Ognibene, A. J., Yamashita, T. S., Ellner, J. J., Immunogenetic analysis of human tuberculosis, *J. Infect. Dis.*, 158, 1302, 1988.

71. Davis, J. E., Rich, R. R., Van, M., Le, M. V., Pollach, M. S., Cook, R. G., Defective antigen presentation and novel structural properties of DR1 from an HLA haplotype associated with 21-hydroxylase deficiency, *J. Clin. Invest.*, 80, 898, 1987.

72. Palmer, C. E., Jablon, S., Edwards, P. G., Tuberculosis morbidity of young men in relation to tuberculin sensitivity and body build, *Am. Rev. Tuberc. Pulm. Dis.*, 76, 517, 1967.

73. Tverdal, A., Body mass index and incidence of tuberculosis, *Eur. J. Resp. Dis.*, 69, 355, 1986.

74. Centers for Disease Control, A strategic plan for the elimination of tuberculosis in the United States, *J. Am. Med. Assoc.*, 261, 2929, 1989.

75. Rook, G. A. W., The role of vitamin D in tuberculosis, *Am. Rev. Resp. Dis.*, 138, 768, 1988.

76. Snider, D. E., Reorientation of tuberculosis control programs in the USA, *Bull. Int. Union Tuberc.*, 64, 25, 1989.

77. Snider, D. E., Hutton, M. D., Tuberculosis in correctional institutions, *J. Am. Med. Assoc.*, 261, 436, 1989.

78. Davies, P. D. O., A possible link between vitamin D deficiency and impaired host defence to *Mycbacterium tuberculosis*, *Tubercle*, 66, 301, 1985.

79. Crowle, A., Elkins, N., Relative permissiveness of macrophages from black and white people for virulent tubercle bacilli, *Infect. Immun.*, 58, 632, 1990.

80. Arloing, S., Agglutination ode bacile de la tuberculose vraie, *Compt. Rend. Acad. Sci.*, 126, 1398, 1898.

81. Daniel, T. M., Debanne, S. M., State of the art: The serodiagnosis of tuberculosis and other mycobacterial diseases by enzyme-linked immunosorbent assay, *Am. Rev. Resp. Dis.*, 135, 1137, 1987.

82. Chan, S. L., Reggiardo, Z., Daniel, T. M., Girling, D. J., and Mitchison, D. A., Serodiagnosis of tuberculosis using an enzyme-linked immunosorbent assay (ELISA) with antigen 5 and a hemagglutination assay with glycolipid antigens. Results in patients with newly diagnosed pulmonary tuberculosis ranging in extent of disease from minimal to extensive, *Am. Rev. Resp. Dis.*, 142, 385, 1990.

83. Daniel, T. M., Debanne, S. M., van der Kuyp, F., Enzyme-linked immunoabsorbent assay using *Mycobacterium tuberculosis* antigen 5 and PPD for serodiagnosis of tuberculosis, *Chest*, 88, 388, 1985.

84. North, R. J., Importance of thymus-derived lymphocytes in cell-mediated immunity to infection, *Cell. Immunol.*, 7, 166, 1973.

85. Lefford, M. J., Transfer of adoptive immunity to tuberculosis in mice, *Infect. Immun.*, 11, 1174, 1975.

86. Orme, I. M., Collins, F. M., Passive transfer of tuberculin sensitivity from anergic mice, *Infect. Immun.*, 46, 850, 1984.

87. Orme, I. M., Collins F. M., Protection against *Mycobacterium tuberculosis* infection by adoptive immunotherapy, *J. Exp. Med.*, 158, 74, 1983.

88. Koch, R., Weitere mitteilungen uber ein heilmittel gegen tuberculose, *Dtsch. Med. Wschr.*, 17, 101, 1891.

89. Chase, M. W., The cellular transfer of cutaneous hypersensitivity to tuberculin, *Proc. Soc. Exp. Biol. Med.*, 59, 134, 1945.

90. Stead, W. W., Pathogenesis of the sporadic case of tuberculosis, *N. Engl. J. Med.*, 277, 1008, 1967.

91. Mackaness, G. B., The immunology of antituberculous immunity, *Am. Rev. Resp. Dis.*, 97, 337, 1968.

92. Youmans, G. P., Relation between delayed hypersensitivity and immunity in tuberculosis, *Am. Rev. Resp. Dis.*, 111, 109, 1975.

92a. Orme, I. M., Collins, F. M., Adoptive protection of the *Mycobacterium tuberculosis*-infected lung: dissociation between cells that passively transfer protective immunity and those that transfer delayed-type hypersensitivity to tuberculin, *Cell. Immunol.*, 84, 113, 1984.

93. Rook, G. A. W., Immunity and hypersensitivity, *Practitioner*, 227, 4, 1983.

94. Orme, I. M., Induction of nonspecific acquired resistance and delayed type hypersensitivity, but not specific acquired resistance, in mice inoculated with killed mycobacterial vaccines, *Infect. Immun.*, 56, 3310, 1988.

95. Orme, I. M., Miller, E. S., Roberts, A. D., Furney, S. K., Griffin, J. P., Dobos, E. M., Chi, D., Rivoire, B., Brennan, P. J., T-lymphocytes mediating protection and cellular cytolysis during the course of *Mycobacterium tuberculosis*, *J. Immunol.*, 148, 189, 1992.

96. Orme, I. M., Characteristics and specificity of acquired immunologic memory to *M. tuberculosis* infection, *J. Immunol.*, 140, 3589, 1988.

97. Muller, I. Cobbold, S., Waldmann, H., Kaufmann, S. M. E., Impaired resistance to *M. tuberculosis* after selective *in vivo* depletion of L3T4+ and Lyt-2+ T-cells, *Infect. Immun.*, 55, 2037, 1987.

98. Mosmann, T. R., Coffman, R. L., TH1 and TH2 cells: Different patterns of lymphokine secretion lead to different functional properties, *Annu. Rev. Immunol.*, 7, 145, 1989.

99. Fiorentino, D. F., Bond, M.W., Mosmann, T.R., Two types of mouse T helper cell IV. Th2 clones secrete a factor that inhibits cytokine production by Th1 clones, *J. Exp. Med.*, 170, 2081, 1989.

100. Fiorentino, D. F., Zlotnik, A., Vieira, P., Mosmann, T.R., Howard, M., Moore, K. W., O'Garra, A., IL-10 acts on the antigen-presenting cell to inhibit cytokine production by Th1 cells, *J. Immunol.*, 146, 3444, 1991.

101. Scott, P., Natovitz, P., Coffman, R. L., Pearce, E., Scher, A., Immunoregulation of cutaneous leishmaniasis, *J. Exp. Med.*, 168, 1675, 1988.

102. Heinzel, F. P., Sadick, M.D., Holaday, B. J., Coffman, R. L., Locksley, R. M., Reciprocal expression of interferon-γ or interleukin 4 during the resolution or progression of murine leishmaniasis. Evidence for expansion of distinct helper T-cell subsets, *J. Exp. Med.*, 169, 59, 1989.

103. Romani, L., Menacacci, A., Grohmann, U., Micci, S., Mosci, P., Puccetti, P., and Bistoni, F., Neutralizing antibody to interleukin 4 induces systemic protection and T helper type 1-associated immunity in murine candidiasis, *J. Exp. Med.*, 176, 19, 1992.

104. Pearce, E. J., Caspar, P., Grzych, J. M., Lewis, F. A., Sher, A., Downregulation of Th1 cytokine production accompanies induction of Th2 responses by a parasitic helminth, *Schistosoma mansoni, J. Exp. Med.*, 173, 159, 1991.

105. del Prete, G. F., deCarli, M., Mastromauro, C., Biagiotti, R., Marchia, D., Falagiani, P., Ricci, M., Romagnani, S., Purified protein derivative of *Mycobacterium tuberculosis* and excretory-secretory antigen(s) of *Toxocara canis* expand *in vitro* human T-cells with stable and opposite (Type 1 T helper or Type 2 T helper) profiles of cytokine production, *J. Clin. Invest.*, 88, 346, 1991.

106. Haanen, J. B. A. G., deWaal, M. R., Res, P. C. M., Kraakman, E.M., Ottenhoff, T. H. M., deVries, R. R. P., Spits, H., Selection of a human T helper type 1-like T-cell subset by mycobacteria, *J. Exp. Med.*, 174, 583, 1991.

107. Boom, W. H., Wallis, R. S., Chervenak, K. A., Human *M. tuberculosis*-reactive CD4+ T-cell clones: heterogeneity in antigen recognition, cytokine production, and cytotoxicity for mononuclear phagocytes., *Infect. Immun.*, 59, 2737, 1991.

108. Lanier, L. L., Ruitenberg, J. J., Phillips, J. H., Human CD3+ T-lymphocytes that express neither CD4+ or CD8+ antigens, *J. Exp. Med.*, 164, 339, 1986.

109. Band, H., Hochstenback, I., McLean, J., Hata, S., Krangel, M. S., Brenner, M. B., Immunochemical proof that a novel rearranging gene encodes the T-cell receptor δ subunit, *Science*, 238, 682, 1987.

110. Janeway, C. A., Jones, B., Hayday, A., Specificity and function of T-cells bearing gamma-delta receptors, *Immunol Today*, 9, 73, 1989.

111. Janis, E. M., Kaufmann, S. H. E., Schwartz, R. H., Pardoll, D. M., Activation of γδ T-cells in the primary immune response to *Mycobacterium tuberculosis*, *Science*, 244, 2754, 1989.

112. Augustin, A., Kubo, R. T., Sim, G., Resident pulmonary lymphocytes expressing the γδ T-cell receptor, *Nature(London)*, 340, 239, 1989.

113. O'Brien, R., Happ, M. P., Dallas, A., Palmer, E., Kubo, R., Born, W. K., Stimulation of a major subset of lymphocytes expressing T-cell receptor γδ by an antigen derived from *Mycobacterium tuberculosis*, *Cell*, 57, 667, 1989.

114. Havlir, D. V., Ellner, J. J., Chervenak, K. A., Boom, W. H., Selective expansion of human γδ T-cells by monocytes infected by live *Mycobacterium tuberculosis, J. Clin. Invest.*, 87, 729, 1991.

115. Munk, M. E., Gatrill, A. J., Kaufman, S. H. E., Target cell lysis and IL-2 secretion by γδ T-lymphocytes after activation with bacteria, *J. Immunol.*, 145, 2434, 1990.

116. Patel, S. G., Weicholty, M. C., Duby, A. D., Thiele, D. L., Lipsky, P.E ., Analysis of the functional capabilities of the CD3+, CD4−, CD8− and CD3−, CD4+, CD8+ human T-cell clones, *J. Immunol*, 143, 1108, 1989.

117. Rivas, A., Koide, J., Cleary, M. L., Engleman, E. G., Evidence for involvement of the γ,δ T-cell antigen receptor in cytotoxicity mediated by human alloantigen-specific T-cell clones, *J. Immunol.*, 142, 1840, 1989.

118. Raulet, A. H., The structure-function and molecular genetics of the γ/δ T-cell receptor, *Annu. Rev. Immunol.*, 7, 175, 1989.

119. Fujiwara, H., Okuda Y., Fukukawa T., Tsuyuguchi I., *in vitro* tuberculin reactivity of lymphocytes from patients with tuberculous pleurisy, *Infect. Immun.*, 35, 402, 1982.

120. Barnes, P. F., Mistry, S. D., Cooper, C. L., Pirmez, C., Rea, T. H., Modlin, R. L., Compartmentalization of a CD4+ T-lymphocyte subpopulation in tuberculous pleuritis, *J. Immunol.*, 142, 1114, 1989.

121. Berger, H. W., Mejia, E., Tuberculous pleurisy, *Chest,* 63, 88, 1973.

122. Fujiwara, H., Tsuyuguchi, I., Frequency of tuberculin-reactive T-lymphocytes in pleural fluid and blood from patients with tuberculous pleurisy, *Chest,* 89, 530, 1984.

123. Ellner, J. J., Pleural fluid and peripheral blood lymphocyte function in tuberculosis, *Ann. Intern. Med.,* 89, 932, 1978.

124. Barnes, P. F., Fong, S. J., Brennan, P. J., Twomey, P. E., Mazumder, A., Modlin, R. L., Local production of tumor necrosis factor and interferon-γ in tuberculous pleuritis, *J. Immunol.,* 145, 149, 1990.

125. Wallis, R. S., Alde, S. L., Havlir, D. V., Amir-Tahmasseb, H., Daniel, T. M., Ellner, J.J., Identification of antigens of *Mycobacterium tuberculosis* using human monoclonal antibodies, *J. Clin Invest.,* 84, 214, 1989.

126. Wallis, R. S., Raranjape, R., Phillips, M., Identification of 2-D gel electrophonesis of a 58 kD TNF-reducing protein of *M. tuberculosis, J. Immun.,* 61, 627, 1993.

127. Lenzini, L., Heather, C. J., Rottoli, L., Rottoli, P., Studies on bronchoalveolar cells in humans. I. Preliminary morphological studies in various respiratory diseases, *Respiration,* 36, 145, 1978.

128. Venet, A., Niaudet, P., Bach, J. F., Even, P., Study of alveolar lymphocytes obtained by bronchoalveolar lavage, *Ann. Anest. Franc.,* 6, 634, 1980.

129. Sharma, S. K., Pande, J. N., Verma, K., Bronchoalveolar lavage (BAL) in miliary tuberculosis, *Tubercle,* 69, 175, 1988.

130. Dhank, R., De, A., Ganguly, N. K., Gupta, N., Jaswal, S., Malik, S. K., Kohli, K. K., Factors influencing the cellular response in bronchoalveolar lavage and peripheral blood of patients with pulmonary tuberculosis, *Tubercle,* 69, 161, 1988.

131. Baughman, R. P., Dohn, M. N., Loudon, R. G., Trame, P. T., Bronchoscopy with bronchoalveolar lavage in tuberculosis and fungal infections, *Chest,* 99, 92, 1991.

132. Ozaki, T., Nakahira, S., Tani, K., Ogushi, F., Yasuoka, S., Ogura, T., Differential cell analysis in bronchoalveolar lavage fluid from pulmonary lesions of patients with tuberculosis, *Chest,* 102, 54, 1992.

133. Husson, R. W., Young, R. A., Genes for the major protein antigens of *M. tuberculosis*: The etiologic agents of tuberculosis and leprosy share an immunodominant antigen, *Proc. Natl. Acad. Sci. U.S.A.,* 84, 1679, 1987.

134. Emmrich, F., Thole, J., Van Embden, J., Kaufmann, S. H. E., A recombinant 64 kD protein of *Mycobacterium bacillus calmette guerin* specifically stimulates human T4 clones reactive to mycbacterial antigens, *J. Exp. Med.,* 163, 1024, 1986.

135. Ottenhoff, T. H. M., Kale, B., van Embden, J. D. A., Thole, J. E. R., Kiessling, R., The recombinant 65 kD heat shock protein of *Mycobacterium bovis bacillus calmette guerin*/*M. tuberculosis* is a target molecule for CD4+ cytotoxic T-lymphocytes that lyse human monocytes, *J. Exp. Med.,* 168, 1947, 1988.

136. Munk, M.E., Schoel, B., Kaufmann, S. H. E., T cell responses of normal individuals towards recombinant protein antigens of *M. tuberculosis, Eur. J. Immunol.,* 18, 1835, 1988.

137. Shinnick, T. M., Vodkin, M. N., Williams, J. C., The *M. tuberculosis* 65 kilodalton antigen is a heat shock protein which corresponds to common antigen and to the *Escherichia coli* GroEL protein, *Infect. Immun.,* 56, 446, 1988.

138. Garsia, R. J., Hellquist, L., Booth, R. J., Redford, A. J., Britton, W. J., Astbury, L., Trent, R. J., Basten, A., Homology of the 70-kilodalton antigens from *M. leprae* and *M. bovis* with *M. tuberculosis* 71-kilodalton antigen and with the conserved heat shock protein 70 of eucaryotes, *Infect. Immun.,* 56, 204, 1989.

139. Lathigra, R. B., Young, D. B., Sweetser, D., Young, R. A., A gene from *Mycobacterium tuberculosis* which is homologous to the DnaJ heat shock protein of *E. coli, Nucl. Acids Res.,* 16, 1636, 1639, 1988.

140. Young, D., Lathigra, R., Sweetser, D., Young, R. A., Stress proteins are immune targets in leprosy and tuberculosis, *Proc. Natl. Acad. Sci. U.S.A.,* 4267, 1988.

141. Young, D. B., Kaufmann, S. H. E., Hermans, P. W. M., Thole, J. E. R., Mycobacterial proteins, a compilation, *Mol. Micro.,* 6, 133, 1992.

142. Wiker, H. G., Sletten, K., Nagai, S., Harboe, M., Evidence for three separate genes encoding the proteins of the mycobacterial antigen 85 complex, *Infect. Immun.,* 58, 272, 1990.

143. Rambukkhan, A., Das, P. K., Chand, A., Baas, J. G., Grothuis, D. G., Kold, A. H. J., Subcellular distribution of monoclonal antibody-defined epitopes on immuno dominant 33-kilodalton proteins of *M. tuberculosis*: identification and localization of 29/33 kilodalton doublet proteins in mycobacterial cell walls, *Scand. J. Immunol.,* 33, 763, 1991.

144. Abou-Zeid, C., Ratliff, T. L., Wiker, H. G., Harboe, M., Bennedsen, J., Rook, G. A. W., Characterization of fibronectin-binding antigens released by *M. tuberculosis* and *M. bovis* BCG, *Infect. Immun.*, 56, 3046, 1988.

145. Abou-Zeid, C., Smith, I., Grange, J. M., Ratliff, T. L., Steele, J., Rook, G. A. W., The secreted antigens of *M. tuberculosis* and their relationship to those recognized by the available antibodies, *J. Gen. Microbiol.*, 134, 531, 1988.

146. Wiker, H. G., Harboe, M., Lea, T. E., Purification and characterization of two protein antigens from the heterogenous BCG85 complex in *M. bovis* BCG, *Int. Arch. Allergy Appl. Immunol.*, 81, 298, 1986.

147. Salata, R. A., Sanson, A. J., Malhotra, I. J., Wiker, H. G., Harboe, H. G., Phillips, N. B., Daniel, T. M., Purification and characterization of the 30,000 dalton native antigen of *Mycobacterium tuberculosis* and characterization of six monoclonal antibodies reactive with a major epitope of this antigen, *J. Lab. Clin. Med.*, 118, 589, 1991.

148. Matsuo, K., Yamaguchi, R., Yamakazi, A., Tasaka, H., Yamada, T., Cloning and expression of the *M. bovis* BCG gene for extracellular alpha antigen, *J. Bacteriol.*, 160, 3847, 1988.

149. Havlir, D. V., Wallis, R. S., Boom, W. H., Daniel, T. M., Chervenak, K., Ellner, J. J., Human immune response to *M. tuberculosis* antigens, *Infect. Immun.*, 59, 665, 1991.

150. Schoel, B., Gulle, M., Kaufmann, S. H. E., Heterogeneity of the repertoire of T-cells of tuberculosis patients and healthy contacts to *M. tuberculosis* antigens separated by high resolution techniques, *Infect. Immun.*, 60, 1717, 1992.

151. Rook, G. A. W., Importance of recent advances in our understanding of antimicrobial cell-mediated immunity to the International Union for the Prevention of Tuberculosis, *Bull. Int. Union Tuberc.*, 58, 60, 1983.

152. Denis, M., Tumor necrosis factor and granulocyte macrophage-colony stimulating factor stimulates human macrophages to restrict growth of virulent *Mycobacterium avium* and to kill avirulent *M. avium*. Killing effector mechanism depends on the generation of reactive nitrogen intermediates, *J. Leukocyte Biol.*, 49, 380, 1991.

153. Bermudez, L. E. M., Young, L. S., Tumor necrosis factor alone or in combination with IL-2 but not IFN-γ, is associated with macrophage killing of *Mycobacterium avium* complex, *J. Immunol.*, 140, 3006, 1988.

154. Rook, G. A. W., Steele, J., Fraber, L., Barker, S., Karmali, R., O'Riordan, J., Standford, J., Vitamin D3, gamma interferon and control of proliferation of *Mycobacterium tuberculosis* by human monocytes, *Immunology*, 56, 159, 1986.

155. Kindler, V., Sappino, A.P., Grau, G.E, Piquet, P.I., Vassali, P., The reducing role of tumor necrosis factor in the development of bactericidal granulomas during BCG infection, *Cell*, 56, 731, 1989.

156. Yamamura, M., Oyemura, K., Keans, R. J., Weinberg, K., Rea, T. H., Bloom, B. R., Modlin, R. L., Defining protective responses to pathogens: cytokine profiles in leprosy lesions, *Science*, 254, 277, 1991.

157. Ogawa, T., Uchida, H., Kusumoto, Y., Mori, Y., Yamamura, Y., Hamada, S., Increase in tumor necrosis factor alpha and interleukin 6-secreting cells in peripheral blood mononuclear cells from subjects infected with *Mycobacterium tuberculosis*, *Infect. Immun.*, 59, 3021, 1991.

158. Takashima, T., Ueta, C., Tsuyuguchi, I., Kishimoto, S., Production of tumor necrosis factor alpha by moncytes from patients with pulmonary tuberculosis, *Infect. Immun.*, 58, 3286, 1990.

159. Moreno, C., Taverne, J., Mehlert, A., Bate, C. A. W., Brealey, R. J., Meager, A., Rook, G. A. W., Playfair, J. H. J., Lipoarabinomannan from *Mycobacterium tuberculosis* induces the production of tumor necrosis factor from human and murine macrophages, *Clin. Exp. Immunol.*, 76, 240, 1989.

160. Barnes, P. F., Chatterjee, D., Abrams, J. S., Lu, S., Wang, E., Yamamura, M., Brennan, P. J., Modlin, R. L., Cytokine production induced by *Mycobacterium tuberculosis* lipoarabinomannan, *J. Immunol.*, 149, 541, 1992.

161. Barnes, P. F., Fong, S. J., Brennan, P. J., Twomey, P. E., Mazumder, A., Modlein, R. L., Local production of tumor necrosis factor and interferon-γ in tuberculous pleuritis, *J. Immunol.*, 145, 149, 1990.

162. Flesch, I., Kaufmann, S. H. E., Mycobacterial growth inhibition by interferon-γ activated bone marrow macrophages and differential susceptibility among strains of *M. tuberculosis*, *J. Immunol.*, 138, 4408, 1987.

163. Flesch, I. E., Kaufmann, S. H. E., Mechanisms involved in mycobacterial growth inhibition by gamma interferon-activated bone marrow macrophages: role of reactive nitrogen intermediates, *Infect. Immun.*, 59, 3213, 1991.

164. Douvas, G. S., Looker, D. L., Vatter, A. E., Crowle, A. J., Gamma interferon activates human macrophages to become tumoricidal and leishmanicidal but enhances replication of macrophage-associated mycobacteria, *Infect. Immun.*, 50, 1, 1985.

165. Rook, G. A. W., Steele, J., Fraher, L., Barker, S., Karmali, R., O'Riordan, J., Stanfor, J., Vitamin D3, gamma interferon, and control of proliferation of *Mycobacterium tuberculosis* by human monocytes, *Immunology*, 57, 159, 1986.

166. Toba, H., Crawford, J. T., Ellner, J. J., Pathogenicity of *Mycobacterium avium* for human monocytes: absence of macrophage activating factor activity of gamma interferon, *Infect. Immun.*, 56, 239, 1989.

167. Shiratsuchi, M., Johnson, J. L., Ellner, J. J., Bidirectional effects of cytokines on the growth of *Mycobacterium avium* within human monocytes, *J. Immunol.*, 146, 3165, 1991.

168. Bermudez, L. E., Production of transforming growth factor-β by *Mycobacterim avium*-infected human macrophages is associated with unresponsiveness to IFN-γ, *J. Immunol.*, 150, 1838, 1993.

169. Blanchard, D. K., Michelini-Norris, M. B., Pearson, C. A., McMillen, S., Djeu, J. Y., Production of granulocyte-macrophage colony stimulating factor (GM-CSF) by monocytes and large granular lymphocytes stimulated by *Mycobacterim avium-M. intracellulare*: activation of bactericidal activity by GM-CSF, *Infect. Immun.*, 59, 2396, 1991.

170. Bermudez, L. E., Young, L. S., Tumor necrosis factor, alone or in combination with IL-2 but not interferon-gamma is associated with macrophage killing of *Mycobacterium avium* complex, *J. Immunol.*, 140, 3006, 1988.

171. Orme, I., Furney, S. K., Skinner, P. S., Roberts, A. B., Brennan, P. J., Russell, D. G., Shiratsuchi, H., Ellner, J. J., Wiser, W. Y., Inhibition of growth of *Mycobacterium avium* in murine and human mononuclear phagocytes by migration inhibitory factor, *Infect. Immun.*, 61, 338, 1993.

172. Denis, M., Gregg, E. O., Recombinant tumor necrosis factor-alpha decreases, whereas recombinant interleukin-6 increases growth of a virulent strain of *Mycobacterium avium* in human monocytes, *Immunology*, 71, 139, 1990.

173. Bermudez, L. E., Petrofsky, M., Young, L. S., Interleukin-6 antagonizes tumor necrosis factor-mediated mycobacteriostatic and mycobactericidal activities in macrophages, *Infect. Immun.*, 60, 4245, 1992.

174. Mustafa, A. S., Godal, T., BCG-induced CD4+ cytotoxic T-cells from BCG vaccinated healthy subjects: relation between cytotoxicity and suppression *in vitro*, *Clin. Exp. Immunol.*, 69, 255, 1987.

175. Koga, T., Wand-Wurttenberger, A., Debruyn, J., Munk, M. E., Schoel, B., Kaufmann, S. H. E., T-cells against a bacterial heat shock protein recognize stressed macrophages, *Science*, 1112, 1989.

176. Daniel, T. M., Oxtoby, M. J., Pinto, E., Moreno, E., The immune spectrum in patients with pulmonary tuberculosis, *Am. Rev. Resp. Dis.*, 123, 556, 1981.

177. Nash, D.R., Douglass, J.E., Anergy in pulmonary tuberculosis. Comparison between positive and negative reactors and an evaluation of 5TU and 250 TU skin test doses, *Chest*, 77, 32, 1980.

178. Rooney, J. J., Crocco, J. A., Kramer, S., Lyons, H. A., Further observations on tuberculin reactions in tuberculosis, *Am. J. Med.*, 60, 517, 1976.

179. Ellner, J. J., Suppressor adherent cells in human tuberculosis, *J. Immunol.*, 121, 2573, 1978.

180. Ellner, J. J., Spagnuolo, P. J., Schacter, B. Z., Augmentation of selective monocyte functions in tuberculosis, *J. Infect. Dis.*, 144, 391, 1981.

181. Fujiwara, H., Kleinhenz, M. E., Wallis, R. S., Ellner, J. J., Increased interleukin-1 production and monocyte suppressor cell activity associated with human tuberculosis, *Am. Rev. Resp. Dis.*, 133, 73, 1986.

182. Kleinhenz, M. E., Ellner, J. J., Antigen responsiveness during tuberculosis: regulatory interaction of T-cell subpopulations and adherent cells, *J. Lab. Clin. Med.*, 110, 31, 1987.

183. Kleinhenz, M. E., Ellner, J. J., Immunoregulatory adherent cells in human tuberculosis: radiation-sensitive antigen-specific suppression by monocytes, *J. Infect. Dis.*, 152, 171, 1985.

184. Toossi, Z., Edmonds, K. L., Tomford, W. J., Ellner, J. J., Suppression of PPD-induced interleukin-2 production by interaction of Leu-22 (CD16) lymphocytes and adherent mononuclear cells in tuberculosis, *J. Infect. Dis*, 159, 352, 1989.

185. Toossi, Z., Kleinhenz, M. E., Ellner, J. J., Defective interleukin-2 production and responsiveness in human pulmonary tuberculosis, *J. Exp. Med.*, 163, 1162, 1986.

186. Tweardy, D. J., Schacter, B. Z., Ellner, J. J., Association of altered dynamics of monocyte surface expression of human leukocyte antigen-DR with immunosuppression in tuberculosis, *J. Infect. Dis.*, 149, 31, 1984.

187. Carlucci, S., Beschin, A., Tuosto, L., Ameglio, F., Gandolfo, G., Cocito, C., Fiorucci, F., Saltini, C., Piccolella, E., Mycobacterial antigen complex A60-specific T-cell repertoire during the course of pulmonary tuberculosis, *Infect. Immmun.*, 61(2), 439, 1993.

188. Shiratsuchi, H., Okuda, Y., Tsuyuguchi, I., Recombinant human interleukin-2 reverses *in vitro*-deficient cell-mediated immune responses to tuberculin purified protein derivative by lymphocytes of tuberculous patients, *Infect. Immun.*, 55, 2126, 1987.

189. Wadee, A. A., Mendelsohn, D., Rabson, A. R., Characterization of a suppressor cell-activating factor (SCAF) released by adherent cells trated with *M. tuberculosis*, *J. Immunol.*, 130, 5, 2266, 1983.

190. Wadee, A. A., Rabson, A. R., Binding of phosphatidylethanolamine and phosphatidylinositol to OKT8+ lymphocytes activates suppressor cell activity, *J. Immunol.*, 130, 2271, 1983.

191. Ellner, J. J., Daniel, T. M., Immunosuppression by mycobacterial arabinomannan, *Clin. Exp. Immunol.*, 35, 250, 1979.

192. Kleinhenz, M. E., Ellner, J. J., Spagnulo, P. J., Daniel, T. M., Suppression of lymphocyte response by tuberculous plasma and mycobacterial arabinogalactan: monocyte dependence and indomethacin reversibility, *J. Clin. Invest.*, 68, 153, 1981.

193. Cunningham, R. S., Sabin, F. R., Sugiyama, S., Kindwall, J. A., The role of the monocyte in tuberculosis, *Bull. Johns Hopkins Hosp.*, 37, 231, 1925.

194. Schmitt, E., Meuret, G., Stix, L., Monocyte recruitment in tuberculosis and sarcoidosis, *Br. J. Hematol.*, 35, 11, 1977.

195. Wallis, R. S., Fujiwara, H., Ellner, J. J., Direct stimulation of monocyte release of interleukin-1 by mycobacterial protein antigens, *J. Immunol.*, 136, 193, 1986.

196. Toossi, Z., Lapurga, J. P., Ondash, R. J., Sedor, J. R., Ellner, J. J., Expression of functional IL-2 receptors by peripheral blood monocytes from patients with active pulmonary tuberculosis, *J. Clin. Invest.*, 1777, 1990.

197. Toossi, Z., Ellner, J. J., The potential role of transforming growth factor-beta in monocyte-dependent suppression of PPD-induced T-cell responses in tuberculosis. Twenty-fifth Joint Research Conference on Tuberculosis: U.S.-Japan Cooperative Medical Science Program, Sapporo, Japan, 1990, 1223.

198. Moreno, C., Taverne, J., Mehlert, A., Bate, C. A. W., Brealey, R. J., Meager, A., Rook, G. A. W., Playfair, J. H. L., Lipoarabinomannan from *Mycobacterium tuberculosis* induces the production of tumor necrosis factor from human and murine macrophages, *Clin. Exp. Immunol.*, 76, 240, 1989.

199. Brennan, P. J., Hunter, S. W., McNeil, M., Chatterjee, D., Daffe, M., Reappraisal of the chemistry of mycobacterial cell walls, with a view to understanding the roles of individual entities in disease processes, in *Microbial Determinants of Virulence and Host Response*, Ayoub, E. M., Cassell, G. H., Branche, W. C., Henry, T. J., Eds., American Society for Microbiology, Washington, D.C., 1990, 55.

200. Wallis, R. S., Amir-Tahmasseb, M., Ellner, J. J., Induction of interleukin-1 and tumor necrosis factor by mycobacterial proteins: the monocyte Western blot, *Proc. Natl. Acad. Sci. U.S.A.*, 87, 3348, 1990.

201. Falla, J. C., Parra, C. A., Mendoz, M., Franco, L. C., Guzman, F., Forero, J., Orozco, O., Patarroyo, M.E., Identification of B- and T-cell epitopes within the MTP40 protein of *M. tuberculosis* and their correlation with the disease course, *Infect. Immun.*, 59, 2265, 1991.

202. Pitchenik, A. E., Cole, C., Russel, B. W., Fischl, M. A., Spira, T. J., Snider, D. E., Tuberculosis, atypical mycobacterioses, and AIDS among Haitians and non-Haitians in south Florida, *Ann. Intern Med.*, 101, 641, 1984.

203. Reider, H. L., Cauthen, G. M., Bloch, A. B., Cole, C. H., Holtzman, D., Snider D. E., Bigler, W. J., Witte, J. J., Tuberculosis and AIDS Florida, *Arch. Intern. Med.*, 149, 1268, 1989.

204. Daley, C. L., Small, G. F., Schecter, G. K., Schoolnik, G. K., McAdam, R. A., Jacobs, W. R., Hopewell, P.C., An outbreak of tuberculosis with accelerated progression among persons infected with HIV, *N. Engl. J. Med.*, 326, 2131, 1992.

205. Ellner, J. J., Tuberculosis in the time of AIDS. The facts and the message [editorial], *Chest*, 98, 1051, 1990.

206. Daniel, T. M., Recent advances in alternate methods for the rapid diagnosis of mycobacterial diseases. Presented at Clinical Research for the 90s (workshop sponsored by the Division of Tuberculosis Control, Centers for Disease Control), Atlanta, GA, 1990.

207. Okwera, A., Eriki, P.P., Guay, L.A., Ball, P., Daniel, T.M., Tuberculin reactions in HIV-seropositive and HIV-seronegative healthy women in Uganda, *MMWR*, 39, 638, 1990.

208. Wallis, R. S., Vjecha, M., Amir-Tahmasseb, M. Okwera, A., Byekwaso, F., Nyole, J., Kabengera, J., Mugerwa, R.D., Ellner, J. J., Influence of tuberculosis on HIV: enhanced cytokine expression and elevated B2 microglobulin in HIV-1 associated tuberculosis, *J. Infect. Dis.*, 167, 43, 1992.

209. Fauci, A.S., The human immunodeficiency virus: infectivity and mechanisms of pathogenesis, *Science,* 239, 617, 1988.

210. Clerici, M., Shearer, G. M., A TH1→TH2 switch is a critical step in the etiology of HIV infection, *Immunol. Today,* 14, 107, 1993.

211. Meltzer, M. S., Skillman, D. R., Gomatos, P. J., Kalter, D. C., Gendelman, H. E., Role of mononuclear phagocytes in the pathogenesis of human immunodeficiency virus infection, *Annu. Rev. Immunol.,* 8, 169, 1990.

212. Rich, E.A., Chen, I.S.Y., Zack, J.A., Leonard, M.L., O'Brien, W.A., Increased susceptibility of differentiated mononuclear phagocytes to productive infection with human immunodeficiency virus-1 (HIV-1), *J. Clin. Invest.,* 89, 176, 1992.

213. Twigg, H. L., Lipscomb, M. F., Yoffe, B., Barbaro, D. J., Weissler, J. C., Enhanced accessory cell function by alveolar macrophages from patients infected with the human immunodeficiency virus: potential role for depletion of CD4+ cells in the lung, *Am. J. Resp. Cell Mol. Biol.,* 1, 391, 1989.

214. Buhl, R., Jaffe, H. A., Holroyd, K. J., Borok, Z., Roum, J. H., Mastrangeli, A., Wells, F. B., Kirby, M., Saltini, C., Crystal, R. G., Activation of alveolar macrophages in asymptomatic HIV-infected individuals, *J. Immunol.,* 150, 1019, 1993.

215. Twigg, H. L., Iwamoto, G. K., Soliman, D. M., Role of cytokines in alveolar macrophage accessory cell function in HIV-infected individuals, *J. Immunol.,* 149, 1462, 1992.

216. Trentin, L., Barbisa, S., Zambello, R., Agostini, C., Caenazzo, C., di Francesco, C., Cipriani, A., Francavalla, E., Semenzato, G., Spontaneous production of IL-6 by alveolar macrophages form human immunodeficiency virus type 1-infected patients, *J. Infect. Dis.,* 166, 731, 1992.

217. Agostini, C., Zambello, R., Trentin, L., Garbisa, S., DiCelle, P. F., Bulian, P., Onisto, M., Poletti, V., Spiga, L., Raise, E., Foa, R., Semenzato, G., Alveolar macrophages from patients with AIDS and AIDS-related complex constitutively synthesize and release tumor necrosis factor alpha, *Am. Rev. Resp. Dis.,* 144, 195, 1991.

218. Murray, H. W., Gellene, R. A., Libby, D. M., Roth, E., Armmel, C. D., Rubin, B. Y., Activation of tissue macrophages from AIDS patients: *in vitro* responses of AIDS alveolar macrophages to lymphokines and interferon-γ, *J. Immunol.,* 135, 2374, 1985.

219. Young, K. R., Rankin, J. A., Naegel, G. P., Paul, E. S., Reynolds, H. Y., Bronchoalveolar lavage cells and proteins in patients with the acquired immunodeficiency syndrome: an immunological analysis, *Ann. Intern. Med.,* 103, 522, 1985.

220. Agostini, C., Poletti, V., Zambello, R., Trentin, L., Siviero, F., Spiga, L., Gritti, F., Semenzato, G., Phenotypical and functional analysis of bronchoalveolar lavage lymphocytes in patients with HIV infection, *Am. Rev. Resp. Dis.,* 138, 1609, 1988.

221. Plata, F., Autran, B., Pedroza Martins, L., Wain-Hobson, S., Raphael, M., Mayaud, C., Denis, M., Guillon, J. M., Debre, P., AIDS virus-specific cytotoxic T-lymphocytes in lung disorders, *Nature(London),* 328, 348, 1987.

222. Braun, M. M., Nsanga B., Ryder, R. W., A retrospective cohort study of the risks of tuberculosis among women of childbearing age with HIV infection in Zaire, *Am. Rev. Resp. Dis.,* 143, 501, 1991.

223. Vjecha, M., Okwera, A., Byekwaso, F., Nakibali, J., Nyole, F., Okot-nwang, M., Aisu, T., Eriki, P., Mugerwa, R., Daniel, T., Heubner, R., Ellner, J., Predictors of mortality and drug toxicity in HIV-infected patients from Uganda treated for pulmonary tuberculosis, VIIIth International Conference on AIDS/IIIrd STD World Congress, Amsterdam, Netherlands, July 1992.

224. Toossi, Z., Sierra-Madero, J.G., Blinkhorn, R.A., Mettler, M.A., Rich, E.A., Enhanced susceptibility of blood monocytes from patients with pulmonary tuberculosis to productive infection with human immunodeficiency virus-1 (HIV-1), *J. Exp.Med.,* 177, 1511, 1993.

Chapter 3

Transmission and Safety Issues

Edward A. Nardell, M.D.

CONTENTS

I. INTRODUCTION

In the early part of this century when tuberculosis was the major cause of death and misery in the United States and Europe, control of airborne spread, then a theory of growing popularity, became an important component of evolving scientific strategies to combat the disease. Isolation of contagious patients was in part the rationale for sanatorium treatment, although at times only early cases were admitted in hope of cure while ad-vanced, more infectious cases were sent home to die, thereby undoing the benefits of isolation.[1] In 1934 William Firth Wells proposed a clear distinction between true airborne infections (e.g., TB, measles) transmitted by droplet nuclei, the buoyant, dried residua of aerosolized respiratory droplets, and infections spread by the larger respiratory droplets themselves (e.g., staphylococci, streptococci).[2] Unlike droplet nuclei that disperse widely, large respiratory droplets remain within

0-8493-4825-0/94/$0.00+$.50
© 1994 by CRC Press, Inc.

the immediate vicinity of their source, carrying infection as an extension of direct person to person contact. During the next four decades airborne infection was the subject of intensive research, with the ultimate goal of better environmental control — a strategy analogous to the hygienic control of waterborne infections such as cholera.[3] Unlike the disinfection of public water supplies, however, disinfection of air in the many environments where TB transmission occurs was not a feasible goal. Moreover, with the accelerated decline in tuberculosis in developed countries after the introduction of chemotherapy, and the prospect of immunizations against many of the common respiratory viruses, research on airborne infection and environmental control all but ended. Transmission has continued since the advent of chemotherapy, of course, before the diagnosis is made and in cases where therapy fails, increasingly facilitated in tightly constructed buildings by central heating, ventilating, and air conditioning (HVAC) systems, and by the growing pool of previously uninfected, fully susceptible persons. With the rise both of homelessness and HIV infection since the mid-1980s, and the progressive erosion of the public health system's ability to ensure the completion of tuberculosis treatment, outbreaks of widespread, accelerated tuberculosis transmission have been reported in health care facilities and long-term residential centers such as shelters, prisons, and drug treatment centers, and air disinfection has once again become an important adjunct to diagnosis and effective treatment.[4,5]

Although tuberculosis infection for an individual is considered an all or nothing event, the probability of infection resulting from a given exposure depends on the interaction of a limited number of host and environmental factors, the relative importance of which have been examined epidemiologically, experimentally, and theoretically.[6] However, recent discussions of tuberculosis transmission and its control often have ignored important quantitative concepts and the substantial experimental data on which they are based. Instead, environmental control recommendations have been based largely on tradition, intuition, and strategies used to control such indoor air pollutants as odors or industrial toxins. The premise of this discussion is that a quantitative approach to understanding tuberculosis transmission leads to emphasis on control strategies somewhat different than have been recommended currently.[4] Important differences between factories and health care facilities that limit the application of industrial respirators as personal protection against TB will also be emphasized.

II. EXPERIMENTAL BASIS FOR UNDERSTANDING TB TRANSMISSION

A. EXPERIMENTAL TRANSMISSION TO ANIMALS

Although decades of careful clinical and epidemiologic observations had provided important insights into TB transmission and pathogenesis, early experiments in which rabbits were infected with bovine tuberculosis or guinea pigs with human tuberculosis, organisms to which each species is exquisitely susceptible, provided the foundation for a new level of understanding, much of which remains valid today. Inhalation experiments using dilute aerosols where droplets contained mostly single organisms, for example, resulted in infection in a predictable percentage of exposed animals, depending on the airborne concentration and the volume of air breathed.[7-9] Infections were detected several weeks after inhalation by tuberculin skin test conversion, and this correlated with the finding of single, discrete tubercles visible in the lungs of animals sacrificed 5 to 6 weeks after inhalation.

As noted already, the size of airborne particles is a critical determinant of infection. In experiments using concentrated aerosols of cultured organisms, Wells et al. found 16 times as many tubercles in the lungs of rabbits breathing equal numbers of fine (2-μm) droplets compared to coarse aerosol suspensions (12–15 μm).[7] Fine droplets (droplet nuclei) were dragged with air into the vulnerable alveoli, whereas larger droplets were much more likely to impact on the upper airways, which are highly resistant to infection. Such quantitative inhalation experiments in animals established the fundamental principle that the probability of infection is proportional to the concentration of infectious droplet nuclei in air, and the volume of air breathed over the exposure time.[8] Within the limits of the experimental methods, complete parity was established between the number of bacilli aerosolized into air as determined by colony counts on air centrifuge culture tubes, and the numbers of tubercles in the lungs of exposed animals. The minimum infective dose for highly susceptible experimental animals was a single droplet nucleus containing one or at most several tubercle bacilli. Rabbits and guinea pigs, therefore, have been used as nearly ideal quantitative samplers for infectious droplet nuclei in air.

B. TRANSMISSION FROM HUMANS

The ultimate use of animals as samplers of airborne tubercle bacilli was a remarkable experiment conceived by Wells to demonstrate convincingly that airborne contagion was sufficient to transmit human tuberculosis, and to quantify the infectiousness of patients under hospital conditions. The experiment was carried out between 1956 and 1961 by Riley and colleagues with the cooperation of the Baltimore Veterans Administration Hospital.[10-12] A unique six-bed experimental ward for tuberculosis patients was constructed so that all exhaust air passed through a chamber designed by Wells to expose uniformly more than 100 guinea pigs simultaneously. The six rooms were occupied continuously by newly diagnosed patients about to begin chemotherapy, and by chronic tuberculosis patients, many with drug-resistant disease. During the first 2 years 71 of an average 156 exposed animals were infected, having breathed approximately 1 million cubic feet (cf) of ward air, yielding a calculated average concentration of 1 infectious unit in 14,000 cf of air.[11] During the second 2 years, under slightly modified conditions (to be discussed), 63 of an average 120 exposed animals were infected, for an average concentration of 1 infectious unit in 11,000 cf of ward air.[12] Careful correlation of the presence of individual patients on the ward, guinea pig conversions, and drug resistance patterns of organisms recovered from the animals permitted further analysis of factors associated with infectiousness.[13]

C. SOURCE FACTORS

Clinical, epidemiologic, and experimental observations indicate that some patients with tuberculosis are much more contagious than others. Factors generally associated with greater contagiousness include more extensive lung involvement, especially lung cavitation, laryngeal or endobronchial disease, more frequent cough, greater numbers of tubercle bacilli in sputum, less viscous sputum, and an indolent rather than a fulminant clinical course, allowing more time for transmission.[6,14] In contrast, noncavitary pulmonary tuberculosis generally has been less contagious. However, cases of pulmonary tuberculosis associated with HIV infection have been infectious in the absence of lung cavitation, presumably because lung tissues contain unusually large numbers of organisms.[15] Although extrapulmonary tuberculosis usually is not very contagious, a hip abscess containing large numbers of tubercle bacilli was responsible for extensive transmission in a hospital, in part because high-pressure wound irrigation generated infectious droplet nuclei.[16] In the Baltimore VA Hospital Study, great variability in infectivity of cases was observed, with 35 of 48 bacteriologically traceable guinea pig infections caused by just 3 of 77 patients on the ward during the initial 2 years.[13] Effective disseminators were noted to have had more violent coughing, to have been less likely to have covered their mouths while coughing, and were more likely to have had drug-resistant

tuberculosis, thereby not receiving effective treatment as did the drug-susceptible cases. In recent outbreaks of multidrug-resistant TB in institutions, some of the same transmission factors have been identified, most notably, unrecognized drug resistance.[17]

D. MECHANICAL AIR SAMPLING

Although the lungs of highly susceptible animals proved to be nearly ideal selective air samplers for tuberculosis, their use under clinical conditions was cumbersome to say the least. Mechanical air sampling methods using culture techniques are simpler to use by comparison, and have been used to detect and quantify a variety of airborne microorganisms. Unfortunately, technical limitations prevent the application of mechanical air sampling for tubercle bacilli in clinical settings. At the very low average concentrations of tubercle bacilli found in the air of Riley's experimental TB ward, detection would require prolonged sampling time (5–10 h) at extremely high sampling rates (1000 LPM), whereas the concentration of background environmental microorganisms likely would exceed 1000/liter.[18] Moreover, the slow growth rate of tubercle bacilli compared to most other microorganisms makes their detection doubly difficult. Using the Wells air centrifuge for sampling, First was unable to detect airborne tubercle bacilli during bronchoscopies performed at a Detroit tuberculosis hospital in the prechemotherapeutic era.[19] Polymerase chain reaction (PCR) techniques that selectively amplify identifying segments of mycobacterial nucleic acids amid a soup of other organisms might eventually permit detection of even rare airborne tubercle bacilli, living or dead, but this application of PCR has yet to be reported.

E. TRANSMISSION TO HUMANS

The infecting dose for humans is harder to estimate than for inbred rabbits and guinea pigs. Tubercles in peripheral lung tissue comparable to those found in experimental animals are seen in humans, suggesting that single droplet nuclei also are sufficient to infect.[20] However, while the number of inhalations of viable tubercle bacilli required before infection occurs in humans is uncertain, the very low average concentrations of droplet nuclei estimated under clinical conditions makes multiple inhalations statistically unlikely under most circumstances. Assuming susceptibility to one to three inhalations, the estimated concentrations of infectious droplet nuclei in the air of Riley's experimental tuberculosis ward (1 in 11,000 to 14,000 cf) was sufficient to explain the rate of skin test conversions of student nurses (6 to 18 months) working 40 h per week on general medical wards in the prechemotherapy era.[21]

Not knowing how many droplet nuclei were required to infect humans, Wells coined the term "quanta" to represent an infectious unit of droplet nuclei, whatever the number.[2,22] Quanta, symbolized by q will appear in the mathematical analysis of TB transmission, representing an infecting dose of one or at most a few droplet nuclei — containing one or at most a few viable tubercle bacilli.

Recent epidemiologic data suggest that there may be as much as a twofold difference in the initial rate of tuberculosis infection between blacks and whites under conditions of approximately equal exposure, a finding attributed to greater inherited resistance among whites, resulting from generations of selective genetic pressure, whereas blacks in central Africa historically had been geographically isolated from the disease.[23,24] Individual variation in susceptibility based on innate resistance and concomitant medical conditions is also likely.

Under low prevalence conditions among otherwise healthy persons, previous infection with tuberculosis appears to convey almost complete immunity to exogenous reinfection. Under conditions of repeated exposure and decreased host immunity, however, true exogenous reinfection occurs, and although often difficult to prove, may be an important pathogenic pathway in high prevalence countries and among high-risk persons in congregate settings.[25,26] Furthermore, HIV immunosuppression clearly predisposes persons with new TB infection to progress rapidly to active disease, and persons with old foci of infection to reactivate. There also is a strong suggestion, but as yet no proof, that HIV infection predisposes individuals to acquire TB infection, an event believed to be determined locally by the innate microbicidal capacity of resident alveolar macrophages, not by cell-mediated immunity (CMI).[15,27] However, restriction fragment-length polymorphism (RFLP), a technique for genetic fingerprinting of tubercle bacilli, has shown exogenous reinfection with tuberculosis to be prevalent among persons with advanced HIV immunosuppression, strongly suggesting impairment of innate macrophage killing, as well as of CMI.[26] Increased susceptibility to new infection together with rapid progression to active, communicable disease probably explains the accelerated rate of propagation observed among HIV-infected persons in congregate settings.[25]

Whether the infecting dose is one or several droplet nuclei for a given individual, clearly there is no safe level of exposure for tuberculosis comparable to a threshold limit value (TLV) for chemical and physical agents. When concentrations are extremely low, infection remains possible, but statistically unlikely. The absence of a TLV distinguishes tuberculosis and certain other infectious agents from indoor air pollutants where exposure concentration more often correlates with symptoms or disease, rather than the probability of an all or nothing event.

F. MICROBIAL FACTORS

Tuberculosis is transmitted from person to person with no important intermediary hosts or reservoirs in nature. Whereas buildings can contribute substantially to TB transmission, unlike true building-associated infections like legionellosis, buildings are never the source of infection, and cannot harbor the organism in an infectious state for very long after the source case leaves. Although the half-life of airborne tubercle bacilli of the H37Rv strain was about 6 h under controlled conditions of temperature and humidity, dilution with infection-free air through ventilation limits the long-term potential for infection far more than does viability.[28] Only 1% of airborne droplet nuclei persist for an hour in a room with five air changes (AC) per hour (infection-free air), assuming complete mixing. If droplet nuclei were not being produced continuously by an active case, even relatively poor ventilation would be expected to greatly reduce their concentration (and the probability of infection) within several hours. Although a large fraction of tubercle bacilli in larger respiratory droplets settles onto surfaces, becoming part of room dust, residual viable bacilli pose no threat of infection unless they are resuspended as airborne particles of a respirable size (1–5 μm).[6] Aerosolization from the surface of the respiratory tract requires a thin fluid layer and the high velocity air flow rates generated by coughs and other respiratory maneuvers — conditions not easily reproduced in the environment. The possibility of an environmental source was examined in the Byrd study of shipboard transmission, but no convincing evidence was found.[29] Tuberculosis transmission, therefore, depends heavily on the simultaneous presence both of a contagious source and a potential victim under conditions supportive of transmission.

Virulence of human tubercle bacilli appears to vary somewhat around the world, based on experimental and epidemiologic evidence.[30] The basis for increased virulence appears to be ill-defined microbial factors that allow the organisms to evade macrophage-mediated host defenses. Clinically, virulence is manifest as a relatively high rate of clinical disease for a given level of infection. Experimentally, pathogenicity for guinea pigs has been used to distinguish fully virulent strains from strains of less virulence. Reduced virulence may be a microbial accommodation ("balanced pathogenicity") to endemic infection among highly susceptible persons, a situation where full virulence eventually might adversely affect microbial propagation and survival.[31] Although it is harder to infect guinea pigs with drug-resistant tuberculosis, a large number of outbreaks with such organisms has discredited the notion that drug resistance correlates with decreased virulence for humans.[32] In fact, there is a popular misconception that the multidrug-resistant (MDR) tuberculosis responsible for recent outbreaks in congregate settings must be a supervirulent strain. Although there is no standard biological assay for increased virulence, there is no reason to believe that MDR TB is more virulent than susceptible strains. The accelerated propagation and high fatality rate among HIV-infected persons appear to be explained by rapid progression from infection to active disease, by environmental factors favoring wide transmission, and by a high rate of dissemination outside the lungs.[33]

G. ENVIRONMENTAL FACTORS

In low prevalence countries, tuberculosis spreads almost exclusively within buildings because droplet nuclei are diluted outside to concentrations so low that transmission becomes statistically unlikely. The hostility of outdoor environments for tubercle bacilli, including the germicidal effects of the ultraviolet irradiation in sunlight, may be another, less important factor. Within buildings, droplet nuclei become less concentrated as they disperse from the source, diffusing within the available space, moved by convection currents and forced air movement. Mechanical ventilation redistributes droplet nuclei within buildings, lowering their local concentration by dilution within a larger volume of air, and by dilution with a variable fraction of infection-free, outside air. Outside air replaces a normally small, but variable, volume of mixed air exhausted to the outside, and it is the exhaust air together with air leakage from buildings that actually removes droplet nuclei.

In small, poorly ventilated indoor spaces, droplet nuclei reach relatively high concentrations quickly compared to larger, well-ventilated spaces. If small spaces are crowded, a common condition for the economically disadvantaged, the potential for TB transmission is increased, accounting in part for the high prevalence of TB among the poor.

H. PATTERNS OF TB OUTBREAKS WITHIN BUILDINGS

TB outbreaks within buildings occur in two general patterns, convection and recirculation, and in combinations of the two. In some outbreaks, those in unventilated spaces, for example, transmission occurs predominantly by convection, with greater infection rates closer to the source case, and lower rates at greater distances, presumably the result of the dilution of droplet nuclei as they disperse.[16,34] In other outbreaks, infections occur throughout buildings, not centered around the source case or specific high-risk activities, suggesting the recirculation of droplet nuclei through the ventilation system.[25,29,35] Recirculation mixes, dilutes, and distributes droplet nuclei, producing a relatively uniform exposure within the entire ventilation circuit, as if exposures occurred in one common breathing space. Mobility of the source case and susceptible persons within buildings also contribute to the equalization of exposure. The ultimate indoor exposure was the shipboard epidemic of tuberculosis on the SS Byrd where the source resided in one of two separate living compartments.[29] The infection rate was high in the compartment where the source case resided and worked, where the air largely was recirculated. Infections in the other compartment were proportional to the percentage of air mixing between the two compartments.

III. A MATHEMATICAL MODEL OF AIRBORNE INFECTION

A. THE WELLS–RILEY MODEL OF AIRBORNE INFECTION

While it is not possible to consider all of the transmission factors involved in a given TB exposure, a mathematical model has been developed that accounts for the major determinants, including the statistical probability of escaping infection.[36] The model assumes steady-state conditions, complete air mixing, equal susceptibility to a quanta of infection (assumed to be a single droplet nucleus — as discussed in Section II.E), and other conditions that may not be entirely valid for each exposure, but that have permitted insights not otherwise possible into the relative importance of ventilation and various other factors.[12,25,34]

If infectious droplet nuclei suspended in air were distributed evenly, the number of quanta inhaled by susceptibles, N, would be equal to the concentration of quanta in the air times the volume of air breathed. In the steady state, the concentration of quanta would equal Iq/Q: the number of infectors, I, times the rate of production of quanta per infector, q, divided by the volume of infection-free air (i.e., ventilation) into which the quanta are distributed, Q. The volume of air breathed by susceptibles would equal Stp: the number of susceptibles, S, times the pulmonary ventilation per susceptible, p, times the duration of exposure, t.

$$
\begin{aligned}
N &= \text{concentration} \times \text{volume} \\
&= Iq/Q \times Stp \\
&= S(Iqpt/Q) \quad \textbf{(1)}
\end{aligned}
$$

For simplicity in developing this mathematical model further, consider a hypothetical, high-exposure situation where the combination of transmission factors $(Iqpt/Q) = 1$, in which case $N = S$, that is, all susceptibles would become infected. Cases this infectious occur rarely, although the situation was approximated during a bronchoscopy and intubation in which 10 of 13 exposed persons were infected.[34] Under more commonly encountered conditions, droplet nuclei appear to be separated by large volumes of infection-free air, an average of 10,000 to 14,000 cf of air in the experimental TB ward already discussed, and the distribution of droplet nuclei tends to be random rather than even.[21]

Under random conditions, if $(Iqpt/Q) = 1$ and $N = S$, some susceptibles would, by chance, escape infection, while others would inhale more than one quantum. According to Poisson's law of small chances, the probability of escaping infection under the hypothetical circumstance where $(Iqpt/Q) = 1$ would be approximately e^{-1}, or 0.37, where e is the base of natural logarithms, with a value of approximately 2.7. The probability of infection under the above circumstances would be $S(1 - e^{-1})$, or 63%. Thus, in the hypothetical case where $(Iqpt/Q) = 1$, and the distribution of droplet nuclei is random, 63% of susceptible persons would be infected compared to 100% with even distribution. The general mathematical expression, referred to as the "Wells–Riley Model for Airborne Infection," describing the interaction of transmission factors, therefore, is

$$C = S\left(1 - e^{-Iqpt/Q}\right) \qquad (2)$$

where C = the number of new infections. This modified form of Eq. (1) was derived by E. C. Riley for use in airborne infection.[36] The relationship has been used to analyze measles as well as TB transmission, and a similar mass balance equation has been successfully used to predict the effects of ventilation and filtration on the concentration of aeroallergens in animal quarters.[25,36,37]

B. APPLICATION OF THE WELLS–RILEY MODEL

The model has been applied to TB transmission under circumstances where the quantifiable transmission factors have been known or could be estimated. Knowing all other factors, q, the generation rate of quanta, the infecting dose of droplet nuclei, has been calculated for several TB cases. Estimates for q range from about 1 quanta per hour (qph) for the treated patients transmitting TB to guinea pigs on the Baltimore experimental ward, to 13 qph for a highly infectious office worker, to 60 qph for a case of laryngeal TB on the experimental ward, to

about 250 qph for the bronchoscopy case mentioned already.[12,13,25,34] Even the highest reported level for TB infectivity pales in comparison to a highly infectious measles case where, from the first generation of secondary cases, q was estimated to be more than 5000 qph.[36] The calculated q value should be considered a crude index of infectivity, recognizing that patients probably generate droplet nuclei sporadically, in bursts related to coughing, sneezing, and other respiratory maneuvers, not continuously as the average figures would suggest. Local air concentrations of droplet nuclei presumably vary greatly, depending on production rate, dilution rate, and the other transmission factors. However, air recirculation and personal mobility tend to dampen exposure fluctuations over time. Over a period of years, the true exposure for health care workers serving high-risk populations probably is a mixture of rare, brief exposures to relatively high concentrations, and longer exposures to much lower concentrations. For most individuals, infection ordinarily is a low probability, random event. Table 3-1 lists the transmission factors for several exposures where the Wells–Riley model has been applied.

C. THE LIMITED PROTECTION OF BUILDING VENTILATION

In an office outbreak, 27 of 67 (40%) workers became infected during a 4-week exposure to a co-worker with active TB.[25] The office building had been the subject of chronic air quality complaints, and the Wells–Riley model was applied to assess the importance of outdoor air ventilation as a transmission factor. Infections occurred throughout both floors of the office building, and a case-control analysis failed to reveal risk factors other than being in the building during the 4-week exposure. For analytical purposes, therefore, the office building was considered a single exposure chamber with an average outdoor air ventilation (Q) of approximately 15 cubic feet per minute per person (cfm/person), or a total of 1395 cfm based on air quality measurements made before and after the exposure. Knowing all other transmission factors, q was calculated at 13 qph (see Table 3-1). It was then possible to estimate the infection rate at ventilation rates greater and less than that actually determined for the building, assuming other factors remained unchanged. The results of that analysis are represented in Figure 3-1 (curve marked "Nardell") where infection rate is plotted as a function of ventilation. For comparison, a similar analysis was plotted for the bronchoscopy case where 10 of 13 exposed persons were infected during a 150-min exposure (curve marked "Catanzaro" — see also Table 3-1).[34] In both cases poor outside air ventilation had

Table 3-1 Airborne transmission factors[a] — three different exposures

Factors	VA Hospital[12]	Office Building[25]	Bronchoscopy[34]
Source (I)	6 pts.	1 pt.	1 pt.
Exposure time (t)	730 days	6.7 days	150 min.
Susceptibles (S)	120 guinea pigs	67 people	13 people
Air sampled (Spt)	693,000 cf	230,000 cf	688 cf
Infected (C)	63/120 (52%)	27/67 (40%)	10/13 (77%)
Ventilation (Q)	38 cfm/person	15 cfm/person	11.5 cfm/person
Infectivity (q)	1.25 qph	13 qph	249 qph
Concentration	1/11,000 cf	1/8,500 cf	1/70 cf

[a] See text for further discussion of transmission factors and exposure conditions.

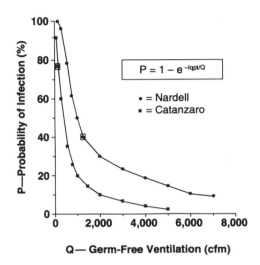

Figure 3-1 Probability of infection (P) as a function of germfree ventilation (Q), based on actual outbreaks published by Cantanzaro[34] and Nardell et al.[25] using the equation of airborne infection shown, where I is the number of infectors, p is the ventilation rate of those exposed, and t is the exposure time. (From Riley, R. L., Nardell, E. A., Controlling transmission of tuberculosis in health care facilities: ventilation, filtration, and ultraviolet air disinfection. Plant, Technology and Safety Management Series, Joint Commission on Accreditation of Healthcare Organizations, Number 1, PTSM Series, 1993, with permission.)

contributed to the extent of transmission observed, and in both cases increased ventilation was predicted to reduce greatly, but not eliminate transmission. The curves show that increasing ventilation of an area that is below the level recommended for comfort achieves the greatest increment in protection. Similar increases when ventilation already meets comfort levels is predicted to result in much smaller improvements in protection. In the office exposure, going from 15 cfm to a generous 35 cfm

of outside air per occupant (3255 cfm total outside air) would be expected to reduce the infection rate by only half, with 13 infections still predicted.

The logarithmic curve of infection and ventilation can be understood better if one considers the low concentrations of infectious quanta calculated for the office exposure, or measured on the Baltimore VA Hospital experimental TB ward: 1 in 8500 to 1 in 11,000 cf of air, respectively (Table 3-1). Under either conditions, approximately 10,000 cf of air would need to be exhausted, on average, to remove a single droplet nucleus. If ventilation were to successfully remove droplet nuclei faster than they were being added by the source case, reducing their concentration, for example, by half, then 20,000 cf of air would have to be vented to remove a single droplet nucleus. Ventilation becomes less and less efficient at removing droplet nuclei as their concentration falls. When the concentration of airborne droplet nuclei is much higher, as in the bronchoscopy case (Table 3-1, Figure 3-1), each cubic foot of air exhausted removes many more droplet nuclei, but unfortunately, many more remain behind, and occupants remain at higher risk than under dilute conditions. Ventilation, indeed all air moving approaches to air disinfection, are inherently limited in their ability to protect occupants from airborne infection, especially when concentrations of infectious droplet nuclei are low, when exposures are potentially long, and where a single inhaled droplet nucleus may be all that is required for infection.

The Wells–Riley model, and other calculation of clearance rates for building contaminants, assume complete air mixing, a condition rarely achieved in reality. Air supply diffusers, for example, often are located too close to exhaust grills, allowing air to enter and leave the room with little effect on air composition. Ideally, when the volume of infection-free air entering a room and the volume of well-mixed air leaving a room equal the volume of the room, one air change (AC) is said to have occurred, and approximately 63% of airborne organisms are flushed out. After five ideal room air changes, approximately 1% of the original airborne organisms remain. Such calculations, presumably, are the basis for recommending six room air changes per hour for isolation rooms, although such simple clearance calculations do not account for incomplete air mixing, and the ongoing generation of droplet nuclei. There are no clinical trials demonstrating protection from airborne infection with six room air changes, or any other ventilation rate.

IV. PRACTICAL APPROACHES TO CONTROLLING TB TRANSMISSION IN BUILDINGS

A. SURVEILLANCE, TREATMENT, PREVENTION, AND ADMINISTRATIVE APPROACHES

1. Patient Isolation Procedures

As stated earlier, because the most important factor in TB transmission is the prolonged presence of the infectious case in the same indoor space with susceptible persons, detection of cases, isolation, and effective therapy are the most important control strategies.[5] This often is far easier said than done. Despite growing awareness of tuberculosis, infectious cases will continue to be missed, or the diagnosis delayed, because of health care access problems, nonspecific symptoms, inadequate tests, and human error.[38] After diagnosis, prompt, continuous, and effective treatment is the single best way to reduce the chance of transmission.[5] With less effective, older treatment regimens, epidemiologic observations suggested that patients started on effective therapy became rapidly noninfectious, even though tubercle bacilli persisted on sputum smear.[39] With recent, more potent, multidrug regimens it has been assumed that noninfectiousness is achieved earlier, but there are few recent data.[40] However, the rising prevalence of drug-resistant tuberculosis in some regions of the country now requires that the infectiousness of TB cases be assessed individually. Parameters for estimating infectiousness include the transmission factors already discussed: cough frequency, cavitation, sputum smear, and culture results, as well as the history of past compliance with therapy, and the probability of drug-resistant organisms.[5,14] Patients who are clinically responding to therapy, as evidenced by decreasing cough, diminished fever, and fewer organisms in sputum, are less likely to be infectious. In a setting where there is the potential for transmission to highly susceptible persons, such as on a hospital floor with HIV-infected patients, evidence of response to therapy should be compelling before the patient is permitted out of isolation. Under these high-risk conditions, there should be a clear and consistent clinical response to therapy, and at least three separate sputum specimens should be negative for AFB on smear. Negative cultures constitute even stronger evidence against infectiousness, but the time required for culture results usually is too long to be of practical use in the day-to-day decisions on isolation in acute care hospitals. Because most newly diagnosed TB patients in developed countries are not hospitalized now, it follows that patients need not be considered noninfectious before discharge, depending on who would be exposed when they do leave the hospital. Of greatest concern are young children at home, and persons sharing congregate living space such as shelters, prisons, and residential care facilities, especially those with HIV infection. Before a patient is released to a high-risk setting, a high degree of certainty is required that the patient is noninfectious, and that effective therapy will continue to be supervised fully after discharge. Because of the serious consequences of transmission of multidrug-resistant tuberculosis, it is essential that such cases be rendered noninfectious before isolation is broken in hospitals, and before discharge, especially to congregate settings. The potential for transmission of multidrug-resistant tuberculosis among HIV-infected persons in congregate living situations is a powerful argument for the necessity of long-term treatment facilities for selected cases.[41]

2. Facemasks on Patients

The subject of particulate respirators for health care workers is discussed in a later section, but the use of face masks for patients deserves mention here, where the subject of patient isolation is discussed. The use of surgical masks on TB patients is more widespread than reason would dictate. No surgical mask or particulate respirator can contain the volume and force of air expelled by vigorous coughing, and leakage must occur around the mask. Surgical masks are designed to keep large respiratory droplets from falling onto surgical fields — not to contain droplet nuclei. The problem is not the pore size, although droplet nuclei can pass through as well as around most surgical masks. Surgical masks serve to stop many large particles that would become droplet nuclei, thereby reducing their number. However, a hand or a tissue held over the mouth serves the same purpose and is far less stigmatizing. If a patient can and will cooperate with this simple hygienic practice, the use of a facemask is unnecessary and undesirable both for social reasons and because a wet facemask may itself become an effective atomizer of droplet nuclei when the patient coughs vigorously. Although they offer some protection, there are few circumstances where even the short-term use of masks on patients is warranted, for example, in transporting infectious patients who cannot or will not cooperate with instructions, or infectious prisoners whose hands are restrained.

3. Administrative Controls

In addition to policies for patient isolation, administrative policies and procedures for surveillance, triage of potentially infectious cases, preventive therapy, and the logistics of patient flow and scheduling may help prevent transmission as much or more than engineering controls. For example, potential transmission may be avoided by scheduling a TB clinic, an HIV clinic, and a high-risk neonatal clinic in separate clinic locations, or at different times. Another policy decision is the administration of pentamidine aerosol treatments or sputum inductions only in booths designed for those purposes, in areas and at times that expose as few others as possible.

In the outpatient setting, administrative controls deserve further consideration, especially the subject of the waiting room. In primary care clinics and emergency waiting rooms, patients with chronic coughs of unknown cause sit together for hours with other patients, some with increased susceptibility to tuberculosis. Pediatricians recognized the problem of airborne infection in common waiting rooms many years ago, and many private offices and clinics have separate sick and well child waiting areas. Although that strategy might protect some otherwise healthy adults from airborne infection, it still leaves the sick with the sick, the potential infector with the vulnerable patient. For control of tuberculosis and other airborne infections, it is the patient with a cough of several weeks duration who should be identified promptly, asked to wait in a separate, environmentally controlled area, or escorted to a special examination room for prompt evaluation. For the reasons mentioned above, masking coughing patients in a waiting area is not a satisfactory alternative solution. Simple triage questions need to be developed and tested to allow a trained desk clerk to identify and separate certain patients with unexplained, chronic cough within minutes of arrival — not 45 min later when interviewed by the triage nurse. Most patients with coughing of 2 or more weeks duration will have chronic bronchitis, asthma, viral infections, or lung cancer — not tuberculosis. However, influenza transmission in waiting rooms also is a serious health risk for the elderly and the infirm, and the triaging of chronically coughing patients may add to the protection afforded by influenza immunization and treatment.

4. Surveillance and Prevention

Early detection of potentially infectious tuberculosis through vigilance and appropriate screening procedures is a highly desirable goal in theory, but often is difficult to achieve in practice. Symptoms and signs of tuberculosis are nonspecific, and tests are neither uniformly sensitive nor rapid. Acute, more critical medical problems often predominate, delaying consideration of chronic problems like tuberculosis.[38] Among immunocompromised patients, respiratory infections are common, and active tuberculosis may present with skin test anergy, nonspecific symptoms, and atypical radiographic findings. Skin testing protocols can often detect TB infection, but positive tuberculin tests rarely are the first clue to active disease. Ideally, positive skin tests lead to INH preventive therapy and fewer future active tuberculosis cases in some long-term facilities, but routine testing of patients is likely to have little effect on TB transmission in acute care settings. Baseline and periodic skin testing of employees potentially exposed to patients with tuberculosis should help detect recent transmission and lead to preventive therapy, and is an important epidemiologic tool for institutions serving high-risk populations.

B. ENVIRONMENTAL CONTROL MEASURES
1. Source Control — Negative Pressure Isolation Rooms

Given the inherent difficulty of removing infectious droplet nuclei from the air once they are dispersed, control at the source is an important preventive strategy. As discussed, effective treatment is the best form of source control. However, for suspected and newly diagnosed cases in institutions, physical isolation is necessary until patients become noninfectious. Source control also makes sense for high-risk procedures such as pentamidine aerosol treatments and sputum inductions, and isolation booths are available to protect the therapist and other building occupants.

The 1990 CDC Guidelines to reduce the risk of TB transmission in health care facilities emphasizes the importance of negative pressure isolation as an environmental strategy.[4] Revisions of that document likely will maintain that priority. However, while isolation is necessary, it assumes that all or most source cases of tuberculosis transmission are known or suspected, whereas it is the undiagnosed case that often is the most dangerous in the health care setting.

The four walls of the isolation room or sputum induction booth are its most important feature, physically limiting dispersion of droplet nuclei. To prevent the egress of contaminated air through the door, however, it is recommended that room exhaust rate exceed intake by approximately 15%, the difference being drawn into the room from the corridor.[42] The isolation room then is under slightly negative pressure relative to adjacent areas, but the pressure difference is so small that it is difficult to measure. It is the direction of airflow into the isolation room, not the pressure difference, that is important, and direction is determined readily by holding a wisp of cotton or a special smoke stick near the bottom of the door.[4]

Directional airflow into isolation rooms can be difficult to achieve if sufficient exhaust capacity is not available. Adding exhaust capacity may require extensive renovations to the central HVAC system and to the building. Operating costs also are high because air must be exhausted directly outside, and not recirculated elsewhere in the building.[4,42] Moreover, once established, directional airflow readily changes as ventilation systems become unbalanced over time, and as airflow in adjacent areas changes due to opening and closing of doors and windows, and countless other variables.[43] In some areas of the country, fire codes require that patient rooms be neutral, or be under positive pressure relative to corridors, to avoid drawing smoke into the room in case of fire elsewhere in the vicinity.

2. Ventilation — Numbers of Room Air Changes — Outside Air Mix

Four walls and directional airflow into isolation rooms protect other building occupants from airborne tuberculosis. Within an isolation room the probability of infection for health care workers depends on the transmission factors already discussed, most importantly, the volume of infection-free air diluting, removing, or inactivating the infectious droplet nuclei generated by the patient. Six room air changes per hour are recommended for isolation rooms, at least two of which are outside air.[4] Using the Wells–Riley model already discussed, it is possible to estimate the infection risk for hypothetical exposures of various durations.

A large isolation room, 10×20 ft with an 8 ft ceiling, contains 1600 cf of air, and six room air changes per hour is a ventilation rate of 9600 cf per hour or 160 cfm, assuming that all supply air is infection free (Table 3-2). The risks of infection have been calculated for cumulative exposures of 1 and 8 h, assuming the patient in the room is as infectious as the case in the office building discussed earlier (13 qph on average), about 10 times more infectious than the 6 treated patients on Riley's experimental ward, but much less infectious than the most infectious recorded TB cases (Table 3-1).[25,34] This moderately infectious case was chosen because such infectious patients probably are

not unusual, and because such cases present a substantial risk of transmission — one that any environmental intervention must address.

These infection risks seem somewhat high compared to the anecdotal experience of most hospitals, although very little broad-based data on hospital worker conversions is available. The relatively high predicted infection rates may indicate that cases as infectious as that of the office building exposure are not really common, that droplet nuclei actually are generated in bursts, episodically, not continuously as the model assumes, and that some innately resistant persons may inhale more than one droplet of nucleus without infection. The point of the calculation is to illustrate that, in theory at least, six room air changes would not be expected to protect fully a health care worker in an isolation room with an active case of tuberculosis. The calculation favors maximum benefit by assuming that all six air changes are nonrecirculated, infection-free air, and that there is complete mixing within the room. Current recommendations are for two outside air changes per hour and four recirculated, presumably from low-risk areas.[4]

3. High-Efficiency Particle Air (HEPA) Filtration

HEPA filters remove 99.97% of airborne particles over 0.3 μm in diameter and have long been used to remove airborne microorganisms in laboratory, pharmaceutical, and medical settings. A number of devices are being marketed in which a fan or blower is combined with an HEPA filter in a portable air filtration machine designed to supplement the air disinfection provided by ventilation. Given the cost of ventilation renovations, the ability to disinfect air with portable filtration units is attractive. Moreover, there are large potential cost savings in recirculating air within an isolation room rather than exhausting six room changes per hour of conditioned air to the outside as is recommended currently. Depending on the region of the country, the annual energy savings from heating or cooling for one isolation room ranges from about 1000 to 7000 dollars, using standard engineering energy consumption formulas.[44] HEPA filtration also is being used in central ventilation ducts to remove droplet nuclei from recirculated air, and to disinfect air being exhausted to the outside in congested areas. Unfortunately, there are a number of problems, both practical and theoretical, with this otherwise attractive approach to air disinfection.

The fundamental problem with HEPA filtration is the potential for a single droplet nucleus to cause infection, the enormous dilution of droplet nuclei in air, already discussed, and the necessity to move large volumes of air to remove or further dilute

Table 3-2 Risk of infection in an isolation room with variable ventilation[a]

Air Changes (AC/h)	Ventilation (CFM)	Cumulative Exposure	
		1 h	8 h
6	160	2.8 %	20 %
10	267	1.7 %	13 %
15	400	1.1 %	9 %
25	667	0.7 %	5 %

[a] Assumptions: room volume, 1600 cf; all infection-free supply air; infectivity of hypothetical source case (q), 13 qph. See text for additional details.

droplet nuclei. The relationship between ventilation and risk of infection in Figure 3-1 and in Table 3-2 applies as well to HEPA-filtered air. Mathematical modeling indicates that it is extremely difficult to move enough air through a filter to reduce the risk of infection substantially unless ambient ventilation is grossly inadequate, and the task gets progressively harder as the concentration of droplet nuclei falls. Because HEPA filters offer considerable resistance to airflow, larger, noisier blowers are required to move large volumes of air compared to ordinary HVAC specifications. Air mixing within the room is another problem, especially when air supply and exhaust ducts are located in close proximity, as in most portable fan-filter units. A variable portion of the air that was just filtered is likely to be entrained again by the intake (i.e., "short-circuiting"), whereas other air in the room may not be filtered at all. Room furnishings and other obstructions may preclude optimal air circulation patterns. Effective room air changes may be far fewer than the advertised high flow rates through the machine would suggest. Leakage around filters is an inherent problem with HEPA filtration, requiring that great care be given to seal filters within their housings, and that filter systems be tested for leaks, both at the manufacturing stage and periodically after delivery, since any movement of the device may break seals. Filter seals must also be retested whenever filters are replaced. Leakage around HEPA filters in duct installations is harder to detect. In-place filter testing routines should precisely follow the procedures established for biological safely cabinets (available from NSF International, P.O. Box 130140, Ann Arbor, MI 48113).

Ultimately, the efficacy of all HEPA filtration devices (and ventilation) should be tested in room experiments in which airborne particulates of a respirable size are removed. Air should be sampled in various room locations over time to produce clearance curves under controlled conditions

designed to approximate the conditions in which the devices will be used. Although it is difficult to recommend any of the available fan-HEPA filter devices without independent test data, there may be high-risk situations not suitable for other interventions where any improvement would be welcome. There is no doubt that HEPA filters can remove droplet nuclei; the issue is effectiveness and efficiency compared to the alternative methods of air disinfection.

A unique fan-filter device has been marketed to retrofit hospital rooms as negative pressure isolation rooms for infectious patients. Room air is drawn into a fan-filter unit located near the head of the bed, and filtered air is exhausted through a duct above the ceiling to the corridor, or anteroom. Air flow is, therefore, from the corridor into the isolation room, and away from health care workers entering the room. Filtered air is recirculated for substantial energy savings. The effectiveness of the system in lowering concentrations of respirable airborne particulates needs to be evaluated carefully under a variety of conditions that approximate those found in hospitals.

4. Ultraviolet Germicidal Irradiation (UVGI)

William Firth Wells not only pioneered the scientific study of droplet nuclei transmission, he also explored the use of UVGI to halt transmission of tuberculosis and the common epidemic respiratory viral infections, such as measles.[45] More than 40 years after the publication of his landmark monograph on air hygiene, however, the full potential of upper room UVGI in halting airborne transmission has yet to be realized.[3] The advent of effective treatment for tuberculosis and of immunizations for some of the epidemic viral infections accounts in part for the decline in interest in UVGI. However, disillusionment also followed the failure of UVGI to prevent common colds in offices, and measles in several clinical trials where infections occurred outside of irradiated classrooms, on school buses, and in crowded urban tenements.[46-48] Wells had raised expectations by demonstrating UVGI efficacy in halting measles transmission in a carefully conducted field trial in suburban Philadelphia schools under conditions where infection outside of school was unlikely.[3] McLean later used the same technology effectively to prevent influenza transmission on a ward for respiratory patients.[49] Through these and other successes and failures it is now understood that air disinfection can work only for infections that are spread predominantly as droplet nuclei — not by direct contact or as larger respiratory droplets — and where the site of air disinfection is the principal site of transmission, thereby excluding some common infections even though the pathogenic agents are highly susceptible to UVGI. The use of UVGI to reduce tuberculosis transmission in a number of high-risk areas should be effective, but wide application remains hampered by several longstanding obstacles: (1) general misconceptions about the application of UVGI, (2) specific concerns about radiation injury, (3) the lack of technical expertise to plan UV installations, and (4) the absence of controlled clinical trials to support its use for tuberculosis. The general lack of information about UVGI and the personal interest of the author are the reasons for its disproportionate discussion in this chapter.

a. UV Misconceptions

The most common misconceptions regarding UVGI are that it is dangerous and of unproven efficacy, requiring extensive maintenance, i.e., regular cleaning. Although there is some basis for each of these concerns, in the aggregate they reflect widespread unfamiliarity with the technology and its application. These concerns are discussed below.

b. UVGI Safety

UVGI utilizes a narrow-band (95% output at 253.7 nm wavelength) of the ultraviolet portion of the electromagnetic spectrum (200–400 nm) to inactivate airborne pathogens. Short wavelength UV irradiation (253.7 nm, UV-C) is rapidly lethal for airborne bacteria at intensity levels achieved easily in the upper room, above people's heads, but it is safe for occupants at the much lower intensity levels permitted in the occupied part of the room.[50] Longer wavelength UV-B has a much greater penetrating capacity than does UV-C, and chronic exposure to the intensive UV-B in sunlight has been associated with skin cancer and cataracts. UV-C has more energy than UV-B, and might be more damaging to tissues than UV-B were it not almost completely (95%) absorbed by the outer, dead layer of the stratum corneum.[51] Accidental direct exposure to high intensity UV-C can cause temporary, painful, but superficial irritation of eyes (photokeratoconjunctivitis) or skin erythema. Eye irritation is transient due to the normally rapid turnover of the corneal epithelium. Painters and maintenance personnel have experienced photokeratoconjuctivitis due to accidental direct UV-C exposure after working in the upper room without first turning off UV fixtures. Because UV-C does not penetrate the cornea, it does not reach the lens to cause cataracts.[51] Intensive, direct skin exposure can cause erythema, and could cause a mild to moderate "sunburn" in sensitive individuals. Prolonged high-intensity irradiation of hairless mice with UV-C has produced skin cancers, but at the low level exposures permitted for people in the lower room

(6 mJ/cm^2), Urbach has estimated that human skin cancer would require more than 300 years of exposure![53-56]

Although systemic immunosuppression has been induced by UV-B irradiation of mice, the UV dosage required was relatively large compared to potential UVGI exposures in the lower room.[57] Moreover, the immunosuppressive effect presumably requires UV penetration to the cellular level — readily achieved with more penetrating UV-B in mice due to their relatively thin epidermis, but unlikely in thicker skinned humans with low-level, low-penetrating UV-C exposure. There is no evidence of systemic immunosuppression in humans from UV-C exposure. Activation of HIV virus in cell cultures exposed to UV-B or UV-C has been reported, and concerns have been raised that PUVA therapy and sunbathing could be an important activation factor for HIV-infected persons.[58] If true, the effect should be discernible epidemiologically given the numbers of HIV-infected persons under observation, and the wide range of sun exposure, geographically, and among individuals. By comparison to ordinary outdoor exposures to the more intense and penetrating UV-B in sunlight, the low levels of UV-C permitted in the lower room should pose no significant added risk, while it should offer substantial protection from TB infection, a much more established hazard for HIV-infected persons.

Current exposure safety guidelines for UV-C are based on a combination of animal data and voluntary human exposures using eye irritation as the end-point.[59] The exposure limit for 254 nm UV of 0.2 μW/cm^2 over 8 h already incorporates a margin of safety, and furthermore assumes continuous eye exposure at the maximum level detected by a meter aimed at the fixture (i.e., stare time). Movement within rooms, angles of incidence of UV rays reflected from ceilings, and shielding by brows and eyelids all greatly reduce true UV exposure to the cornea — the same factors that ordinarily prevent photokeratoconjunctivitis outside from exposure to UV-B in sunlight.

For over 50 years, upper room UVGI has been used safely in hospitals, clinics, jails, and shelters around the country without injuries more serious than an occasional, transient photokeratoconjunctivitis from accidental direct exposure.[60] Until recently, however, little attention has been paid to the measurement of UV in the lower room, and to the design of fixtures intended for upper room UV air disinfection. In rooms equipped with some common UVGI fixtures of older design, UV intensity at eye level has been measured at well over the 0.2 μW/cm^2, as high as 6.0 μW/cm^2 in one installation. Fortunately, such fixtures have been used for years without photokeratitis, a fact attributable to the safety margin built into the exposure standard, which, as noted, was based on "stare time" rather than the relatively brief, indirect exposures common in real life. The safety margin should be much greater for newer fixtures designed to effectively confine irradiation to the space above peoples heads.[61] Common sense dictates that UV-C exposure in occupied spaces should be as low as possible while allowing for effective upper room air disinfection.

c. Technical Expertise

The application of UVGI in health care facilities falls into no established area of technical expertise. While building engineers are expert at HVAC systems, most are unfamiliar with the use of UVGI, and often are biased in their views on UVGI by rumors of health hazards, unproven efficacy, and high maintenance requirements. Manufacturers have traditionally sold fixtures, but neither have planned installations nor checked UV fixtures postinstallation with a sensitive UV meter before use. Federal agencies have offered little guidance, and often have contributed some of the misconceptions, lumping UVGI (UV-C) together with more hazardous forms of UV (UV-B) found in the workplace.[62] As demand for practical environmental interventions rises, however, engineers and other technically qualified consultants undoubtedly will acquire the skills needed to assist institutions wanting to apply UVGI and other environmental interventions safely and effectively.

d. The Absence of Clinical Trials

Although a large body of credible basic research supports the use of UVGI, and the lethal UV dose for various airborne pathogens has been established, there are no clinical field trials demonstrating UVGI efficacy in protecting workers from nosocomial tuberculosis.[50] The major problem preventing clinical trials is the highly variable nature of TB transmission, as demonstrated by Sultan and colleagues.[13] Infection rates among hospital staff, for example, are heavily influenced by the number and infectiousness of TB patients who happen to be under their care, the duration of exposure before effective treatment, environmental conditions, and the variable susceptibility to infection of those exposed. One highly infectious undiagnosed TB patient could badly skew even a large clinical trial. The lack of clinical trials applies as well to isolation policies, isolation rooms, ventilation, HEPA filtration, and the use of particulate respirators to prevent TB transmission. However, there is less reluctance to question the protection attributed to negative pressure isolation rooms and respirators, both time-honored and relatively risk-free methods of infection control, the underlying principles of which seem intuitive.

e. Upper Room UVGI — Theory and Experimental Basis

Using culture techniques to determine viability, the relative and absolute susceptibility of a variety of airborne microbes, including both virulent tuberculosis and avirulent BCG strains, has been determined under controlled experimental conditions.[50,63,64] Mycobacteria were approximately seven times harder to kill than aerosolized *E. coli* or *S. marcescens*, but easier to kill than common fungal spores. For virulent tubercle bacilli and for BCG, exposure to 10 μW/cm^2 for 60 s or 50 μW/cm^2 for 12 s killed 90% of airborne organisms. That a powerfully germicidal dose was achievable within ventilation ducts under hospital conditions was convincingly demonstrated on Riley's experimental tuberculosis ward where UVGI completely protected an average of 120 guinea pigs exposed to patient-generated contagion over a 2-year period.[12] An equal number of guinea pigs breathing nonirradiated air from the same ward became infected at approximately the same rate as during the first 2 years of the experiment, already discussed. Drug-resistant organisms infected many of the control animals breathing nonirradiated air, demonstrating that organisms resistant to chemotherapy were quite susceptible to UVGI. Despite this highly successful demonstration of efficacy when UVGI is used between the infectious source and the susceptibles, the main limitation to using UVGI in ventilation ducts remains exactly that described for HEPA filters, and that of outdoor air ventilation itself — the need to move large volumes of air to substantially reduce the risk of infection for occupants of the same room as an infectious case. Compared to HEPA filters, UVGI in ducts requires less maintenance and offers less airflow resistance, permitting the use of smaller, quieter blowers to achieve a given air flow. According to Riley, there was no routine maintenance of the duct UV lamps during the guinea pig experiments, yet they performed flawlessly for 2 years. While dust accumulation can diminish UV output, within ducts it is possible to overcome any anticipated fall-off with higher initial UV intensity. Despite the theoretical limitations of duct irradiation, the National Jewish Center for Immunology and Respiratory Medicine in Denver has long used UVGI within air-recirculating units, mounted above the ceiling, in isolation rooms on the inpatient unit for drug-resistant tuberculosis.[65] Air flow through the units is said to be equivalent to 12 to 15 room air changes per hour. Although there had been several infections among staff before the room units were installed, there have been only two infections over the last 10 years. The air-moving UVGI units are more costly than upper room UV fixtures, which have produced the equivalent of 20 added room air changes under experimental conditions, as described below, and which are more suitable for larger spaces such as waiting areas, emergency rooms, and shelters for the homeless.

Room air disinfection through upper air UVGI is achieved through the surprisingly rapid, but imperceptible dilution of contaminated lower room air with germ-free, irradiated upper room air.[66-69] Effective mixing within the room is due to natural convection currents, mechanical ventilation, radiant heat, agitation of air due to the opening of doors, and the movement of occupants within the room. Rather than forcing room air rapidly through a relatively small duct for disinfection, upper room UVGI uses the entire cross-sectional area of a room as the duct and irradiation chamber, permitting high-volume, low-velocity mixing of disinfected upper with contaminated lower room air. Although the susceptibility of tubercle bacilli is known, given the many variables within a room, it was not possible to predict the air disinfection achievable in the lower room by upper room UV without actual room experiments. Riley and colleagues aerosolized test organisms into sealed rooms, mixed and distributed airborne droplet nuclei with a fan, then sampled and cultured lower room air quantitatively over time, with and without upper room irradiation.[64]

Because of the health risk of aerosolizing virulent tubercle bacilli into a room it was necessary to perform room experiments using safer surrogate organisms, the UV susceptibility of which had been established relative to virulent TB by previous controlled experiments, as noted above. The results of one experiment using aerosolized BCG are shown in Figure 3-2. A single 17-W UV tube irradiating the upper 2 feet of a 200 ft² room inactivated airborne organisms at a rate equivalent to adding 10 air changes to the existing 2 air changes of the room. Many more room experiments were performed using aerosolized *S. marcescens* under a variety of conditions intended to increase mixing between the upper and lower room, thereby increasing air disinfection in the lower room. Results in an unventilated room using *Serratia* confirmed the findings of the BCG experiments, allowing for the sevenfold difference in susceptibility to UV light.[66-69]

f. The Application of UVGI — Practical Considerations

Based on the above room experiments, and on the remarkable ability of UVGI in ducts to protect guinea pigs from patient-generated droplet nuclei, upper room UVGI has long been used in a variety of indoor environments where TB transmission has been a problem. The criteria for applying UVGI are

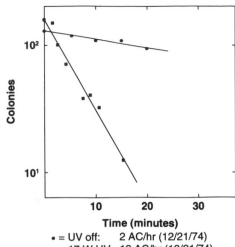

Figure 3-2 Disappearance of bacillus Calmette–Guérin (BCG) from a naturally ventilated, sealed room, with and without upper room ultraviolet air disinfection, using one 17-W tube; AC/h = air changes per hour. (From Riley et al.,[64] reprinted with permission.)

(1) a demonstrably high-risk indoor environment for TB transmission, (2) a comparatively low risk of infection outside of the proposed area, (3) sufficient unobstructed ceiling height (i.e., 8 ft or more) to install fixtures at 7 ft (to avoid direct or reflected eye overexposure), with at least one additional foot for air disinfection, and (4) understanding and acceptance by room occupants, or those responsible for their well being.

Although the planning of an upper room UV installation is not difficult, some experience, and access to a 254-nm wavelength UV radiometer, sensitive down to 0.1 µW/cm², are required. The objective is to flood the upper room (7.5 ft) with UV irradiation at the highest intensity possible (at least 50 µW/cm² at a distance of 3 ft from the fixture, 10 to 15 µW/cm² at 10 ft) while maintaining safe exposure levels in the lower room (< 0.2 µW/cm², at eye level — 5.5 ft high), depending on the estimated true duration of exposure. New, multilouvered fixture designs have made safe upper room UV installations possible in rooms with ceilings as low as 8 ft.[61] One or two 15-W wall fixtures (Riley design) are generally used for an average size (150–200 ft²) single hospital room, depending on its configuration. Air disinfection equivalent to about 10 to 20 room air changes is anticipated, without noise, drafts, reconstruction, and energy costs. The placement of UVGI in corridors as well as rooms has been shown to prevent transfer of airborne test organisms, and has been suggested as an alternative to negative pressure isolation when the latter cannot be achieved.[69,70]

The estimated protection predicted for 25 room air changes, 20 equivalent air changes added by UVGI, plus 5 produced by mechanical ventilation, is listed in Table 3-2. Compared to major ventilation renovations, high-volume ventilation, and self-contained air disinfecting units (HEPA filter or UV), upper room UVGI is likely to be more effective, much less costly to install and operate, and more applicable to shelters, emergency rooms, waiting rooms, and other large spaces. Operating rooms have high levels of ventilation, but are under positive pressure by design in order to prevent wound infections. TB transmission has been associated with operating room procedures, and rooms used for necessary procedures on patients known or suspected of having TB, including certain cases of extrapulmonary TB, should be equipped with upper room germicidal UV.

Ideally, an engineering consultant or industrial hygienist thoroughly familiar with ventilation, filtration, UV air disinfection, and personal respirators should evaluate buildings in consultation with infection control staff and recommend the appropriate environmental control interventions for each potential exposure situation.

g. Air Recirculation

As noted, outbreaks of tuberculosis have been documented in which recirculation of infectious droplet nuclei were thought to have played an important role.[25,29,35] Under those circumstances, air disinfection centrally, through HEPA filtration or UVGI, should be highly effective. However, central air disinfection does little to protect the health worker in the same room with an infectious case, whereas room by room air disinfection does reduce the chance that droplet nuclei will be recirculated. Under most circumstances, therefore, central air disinfection should be a second tier defense against transmission, to be employed after source control and room control measures are in place.

5. Personal Respirators

In the traditional hierarchy of controls for environmental hazards, source control, environmental controls, and administrative controls all precede the use of personal protective devices, in this case, personal respirators (PRs) to prevent the inhalation of droplet nuclei. In the current terminology, "masks" refer to mouth and nose covers designed to protect the patient from the wearer's large respiratory droplets (e.g., surgical masks). PRs can appear similar to masks, but are designed to protect the wearer from a variety of hazards, depending on the design. Personal respiratory protection is employed when control by the other three tiers is considered inadequate. Although it is unlikely that 100% protection from TB infection can be achieved in health care settings, PRs, however technically sophisticated, may not play a major role for the following reasons: (1) except in unusual circumstances, PRs are applicable for health care workers only, whereas patients and their visitors also must be protected. This is different from industrial applications where everyone in a high-risk area can be required to comply; (2) cooperation and training are required for the proper use of PRs, and failures through lapses in technique are inevitable; (3) simple, inexpensive masks are least intrusive, most acceptable to workers, but offer the least protection because of leaks between the face and the PR; (4) sophisticated PRs designed to prevent leaks are expensive, cumbersome, impair verbal communication, and are least acceptable to workers, and their patients. However, there are high risk settings, bronchoscopies and autopsies, for example, where some form of effective PR is warranted; and (5) a PR strategy assumes that most potential transmitters are identified, whereas unsuspected cases in emergency rooms, intensive care units, and other clinical settings are important. Health care workers cannot function wearing respirators all day.

Despite these considerations, OSHA now requires the use of HEPA respirators to prevent TB transmission in three settings: TB isolation rooms, high-risk procedures, and transporting patients known or suspected to have TB. The efficacy of this requirement remains to be demonstrated.[71]

REFERENCES

1. Bates, B., *Bargaining for Life: A Social History of Tuberculosis, 1876–1938,* University of Pennsylvania Press, Philadelphia, 1992, 16.
2. Wells, W. F., On airborne infection: Study II. Droplet and droplet nuclei, *Am. J. Hyg., 20,* 611, 1934.
3. Wells, W. F., *Airborne Contagion and Air Hygiene,* Harvard University, Cambridge, MA, 1955.
4. Centers for Disease Control, Guidelines for preventing transmission of tuberculosis in health-care settings, with special focus on HIV-related issues, *MMWR,* 39(no. RR-17), 1, 1990.
5. American Thoracic Society, Control of tuberculosis in the United States, *Am. Rev. Resp. Dis.,* 146, 1623, 1992.
6. Riley, R. L., O'Grady, F., *Airborne Infection,* Macmillan, New York, 1961.
7. Wells, W. F., Ratcliff, H. L., Crumb, C., On the mechanism of droplet nuclei infection II: Quantitative experimental airborne infection in rabbits, *Am. J. Hyg.,* 47, 11, 1948.

8. Lurie, M. B., Heppleston, A. G., Abramson, S., Swartz, I. B., An evaluation of the method of quantitative airborne infection and its use in the study of the pathogenesis of tuberculosis, *Am. Rev. Tuberc.*, 61, 765, 1950.

9. Ratcliff, H. L., Tuberculosis induced by droplet nuclei infection: pulmonary tuberculosis of predetermined initial intensity in mammals, *Am. J. Hyg.*, 55, 36, 1952.

10. Riley, R. L., Wells, W. F., Mills, C. C., Nyka, W., McLean, R., Air hygiene in tuberculosis: quantitative studies of infectivity and control in a pilot ward, *Am. Rev. Tuberc. Pulm. Dis.*, 75, 420, 1957.

11. Riley, R. L., Mills, C.C., Nyka, W., Weinstock, N., Storey, P. B., Sultan, L. U., Riley, M. C., Wells, W. F., Aerial dissemination of pulmonary tuberculosis — a two year study of contagion in a tuberculosis ward, *Am. J. Hyg.*, 70, 185, 1959.

12. Riley, R.L., Mills, C.C., O'Grady, F., Sultan, L. U., Wittstadt, F., Shivpuri, D. N., Infectiousness of air from a tuberculosis ward — ultraviolet irradiation of infected air: comparative infectiousness of different patients, *Am. Rev. Resp. Dis.*, 84, 511, 1962.

13. Sultan, L., Nyka, C., Mills, C., O'Grady, W., Riley, R. L., Tuberculosis disseminators — a study of the variability of aerial infectivity of tuberculosis patients, *Am. Rev. Resp. Dis.*, 82, 358, 1960.

14. Loudon, R. G., Spohn, S. K., Cough frequency and infectivity in patients with pulmonary tuberculosis, *Am. Rev. Resp. Dis.*, 99, 109, 1969.

15. Barnes, P. F., Bloch, A. B., Davidson, P. T., Snider, D. E., Tuberculosis in patients with human immunodeficiency virus infection, *N. Engl. J. Med.*, 324, 1644, 1991.

16. Hutton, M. D., Stead, W. W., Cauthen, G. M., Bloch, A. B., Ewing W. M., Nosocomial transmission of tuberculosis associated with a draining abscess, *J. Infect. Dis.*, 161, 286, 1990.

17. Edlin, B. R., Torkars, J. I., Grieco, M. H., Crawford, J. T., Williams, J., Sordillo, E. M., Ong, K., Kilburn, J. O., Dooley, S. W., Castro, K. G., Jarvis, W. R., Holmberg, S. D., An outbreak of multi-drug resistant tuberculosis among hospitalized patients with the acquired immunodeficiency syndrome, *N. Engl. J. Med.*, 326, 1514, 1992.

18. American Conference of Governmental and Industrial Hygienists, *Guidelines for the Assessment of Bioaerosols in the Indoor Environment*, Cincinnati, Ohio, 1989.

19. First, M., personal communication, 1993.

20. Dannenberg, A. M., Delayed-type hypersensitivity and cell-mediated immunity in the pathogenesis of tuberculosis, *Immunol. Today*, 12, 228, 1991.

21. Riley, R. L., Aerial dissemination of tuberculosis, *Am. Rev. Tuberc. Pulm. Dis.*, 76, 931, 1957.

22. Wells, W. F., Response and reaction to inhaled droplet nuclei, in *Airborne Contagion and Air Hygiene*, Harvard University, Cambridge, MA, 1955, 123.

23. Stead, W. W., Senner, J. W., Reddick, W. T., Lofgren, J. P., Racial differences in susceptibility to infection by *Mycobacterium tuberculosis*, *N. Engl. J. Med.*, 322, 422, 1990.

24. Stead, W. W., Genetics and resistance to tuberculosis: could resistance be enhanced by genetic engineering? *Ann. Intern. Med.*, 116, 937, 1992.

25. Nardell, E. A., Keegan, J., Cheney, S.A., Etkind, S. C., Airborne infection: theoretical limits of protection achievable by building ventilation, *Am. Rev. Resp. Dis.*, 144, 302, 1991.

26. Small, P. M., Shafer, R. W., Hopewell, P. C., Singh, S. P., Murphy, M. J., Desmond, E., Sierra, M. F., Schoolnik, G. K., Exogenous reinfection with multidrug-resistant M. Tuberculosis in patients with advanced HIV infection, *N. Engl. J. Med.*, 328, 1137, 1993.

27. Nardell, E., Pathogenesis of tuberculosis, in *Tuberculosis*, Reichman, L. B., Hershfield, E., Eds., Marcel Dekker, New York, 1993, chap. 5.

28. Loudon, R. G., Bumbarner, L. R., Lacy, J., Coffman, G. K., Aerial transmission of mycobacteria, *Am. Rev. Resp. Dis.*, 100, 165, 1969.

29. Houk, V. N., Baker, J. H., Sorensen, K., Kent, D. C., The epidemiology of tuberculosis infection in a closed environment, *Arch. Environ. Health*, 16, 26, 1968.

30. Myrvik, Q. N., Leake, E. S., Goren, M. B., Mechanisms of toxicity of tubercle bacilli for macrophages, in *Mycobacterium Tuberculosis: Interactions with the Immune System*, Bendinelli, M., Friedman, H., Eds. Plenum Press, New York, 1988, chap. 14.

31. Mims, C. A., *The Pathogenesis of Infectious Disease*, 3rd ed., Academic Press, London, 1987, chap. 1.

32. Dooley, S. W., Jarvis, W. R., Martone, W. J., Snider, D. E., Multidrug resistant tuberculosis, *Ann. Intern. Med.*, 117, 257, 1992.

33. Daley, C. L., Small, P. M., Schecter, G. F., Schoolnik, G. K., McAdam, R. A., Jacobs, W. R., Hopewell, P. C., An outbreak of tuberculosis with accelerated progression among persons infected with the human immunodeficiency virus, *N. Engl. J. Med.*, 326, 231, 1992.

34. Catanzaro, A., Nosocomial tuberculosis, *Am. Rev. Resp. Dis.,* 125, 559, 1982.

35. Centers for Disease Control, *Mycobacterium tuberculosis* transmission in a health clinic — Florida, *MMWR,* 38, 256, 1989.

36. Riley, E. C., Murphy, G., Riley, R. L., Airborne spread of measles in a suburban elementary school, *Am. J. Epidemiol.,* 107, 421, 1978.

37. Swanson, M. C., Campbell, A. R., O'Hollaren, M. T., Reed, C. E., Role of ventilation, air filtration, and allergen production rate in determining concentrations of rat allergens in the air of animal quarters, *Am. Rev. Resp. Dis.,* 141, 1578, 1990.

38. Lin-Greenberg, A., Anez, T., Delay in respiratory isolation of patients with pulmonary tuberculosis and human immunodeficiency virus infection, *Am. J. Infect. Control,* 20, 16, 1992.

39. Gunnels, J. J., Bates, J. H., Swindoll, H., Infectivity of sputum-positive tuberculosis patients on chemotherapy, *Am. Rev. Resp. Dis.,* 109, 323, 1974.

40. Noble, R. C., Infectiousness of pulmonary tuberculosis after starting chemotherapy: review of available data on an unresolved question, *Am. J. Infect. Control,* 9, 6, 1981.

41. Etkind, S., Boutotte, J., Ford, J., Singleton, L., Nardell, E. A., Treating hard-to-treat tuberculosis patients in Massachusetts, *Sem. Resp. Infect.,* 6, 273, 1991.

42. Lindberg, P. R., Improving hospital ventilation systems for tuberculosis infection control, *Joint Commission: 1993 Plant, Technology and Safety Management (PTSM) Series,* Number 1, 19, 1993.

43. Keene, J. H., Sansone, E. B., Airborne transfer of contaminants in ventilated spaces, *Lab. Anim. Sci.,* 34, 453, 1984.

44. Nelson, T., Recirculating air from respiratory isolation rooms: evaluation of energy loss due to exterior venting, unpublished promotional information distributed by Component Systems, Inc., Cleveland, Ohio, 1992.

45. Wells, W. F., Wells, M. W., Wilder, T. S., The environmental control of epidemic contagion I — An epidemiologic study of radiant disinfection of air in day schools, *Am. J. Hyg.,* 35, 97, 1942.

46. *Medical Research Council Special Report Series No. 283,* Disinfection with ultra-violet irradiation of classrooms — its effects on illness in school-children, London, 1954.

47. Kingston, D., Lidwell, O. M., Williams, R. E. O., The epidemiology of the common cold — III, The effects of ventilation, air disinfection and room size, *J. Hyg. London,* 60, 341, 1962.

48. Perkins, J. E., Bahlke, A. M., Silverman, H. F., Effects of ultraviolet irradiation of classrooms on the spread of measles in large rural central schools, *Am. J. Public Health,* 37, 529, 1947.

49. McLean, R., The effect of ultraviolet radiation upon the transmission of epidemic influenza in long-term hospital patients, International Conference on Asian Influenza, Feb. 17–19, 1960, Bethesda, Discussion, *Am. Rev. Resp. Dis.,* 83(Suppl.), 36, 1961.

50. Riley, R. L., Nardell, E. A., Clearing the air — The theory and application of ultraviolet air disinfection, *Am. Rev. Resp. Dis.,* 139, 1286, 1989.

51. Bruls, W. A. G., Transmission of human epidermis and stratum corneum as a function of thickness in the ultraviolet and visible wavelengths, *Photochem. Photobiol.,* 40, 485, 1984.

52. Sliney, D. H., Ultraviolet radiation and the eye, in *Light Lasers and Synchroton Radiation,* Grandolfo, M., Ed., Plenum, New York, 1990, 237.

53. Blum, H. F., Lippincott, S. W., Carcinogenic effectiveness of ultraviolet radiation of wavelength 2537 A, *J. Natl. Cancer Inst.,* 1, 211, 1942.

54. Forbes, P. D., Urbach, F., Experimental modification of carcinogenesis I. Fluorescent whitening agents and shortwave ultraviolet radiation, *Food Cosmet. Toxicol.,* 13, 335, 1974.

55. Urbach, F., Unpublished presentation, Potential carcinogenic effects for human skin of ultraviolet radiation of 253.7 nm wavelength, Centers for Disease Control, Consultant Meeting on Ultraviolet Germicidal Irradiation, Atlanta, December 10–11, 1991.

56. Sterenborg, H. J. C. M., The dose-response relationship of tumorigenesis by ultraviolet radiation of 254 nm, *Photechem. Photobiol.,* 47, 245, 1988.

57. Jeevan, A., Kripke, M., Alteration of the immune response to M. bovis BCG in mice exposed chronically to low dose of UV irradiation, *Cell. Immunol.,* 130, 32, 1990.

58. Zmudzka, B. Z., Beer, J., Activation of human immunodeficiency virus by ultraviolet radiation, *Photochem. Photobiol.,* 52, 1153, 1990.

59. National Institute for Occupational Safety and Health, Criteria for a recommended standard for occupational exposure to ultraviolet radiation, NIOSH, Cincinnati, OH, 1972.

60. Rose, R. C., Parker, R. L., Erythema and conjunctivitis. Outbreak caused by inadvertent exposure to ultraviolet light, *J. Am. Med. Assoc.,* 242, 1155, 1979.

61. Nardell, E. A., Riley, R. L., A new ultraviolet germicidal irradiation (UVGI) fixture design for upper room air disinfection with low ceilings, in *Program and Abstracts of the World Congress on Tuberculosis,* Bethesda, 1992, 38.

62. Moss, C. E., Seitz, T. A., Case studies — Ultraviolet radiation exposure to health care workers from germicidal lamps, *Appl. Occup. Environ. Hyg.,* 6, 168, 1991.

63. Riley, R. L., Kaufman, J. E., Effect of relative humidity on the inactivation of airborne *Serratia marcescens* by ultraviolet radiation, *Appl. Microbiol.,* 23, 1113, 1972.

64. Riley, R. L., Knight, M., Middlebrook, G., Ultraviolet susceptibility of BCG and virulent tubercle bacilli, *Am. Rev. Resp. Dis.,* 113, 413, 1976.

65. Iseman, M. D., A leap of faith — What can we do to curtail intrainstitutional transmission of tuberculosis? (editorial), *Ann. Intern. Med.,* 117, 251, 1992.

66. Riley, R. L., Permutt, S., Kaufman, J. E., Convection, air mixing and ultraviolet air disinfection in rooms, *Arch. Environ. Health,* 22, 200, 1971.

67. Riley, R. L., Permutt, S., Room air disinfection by ultraviolet irradiation of upper air — air mixing and germicidal effectiveness, *Arch. Environ. Health,* 22, 208, 1971.

68. Riley, R. L., Permutt, S., Kaufman, J. E., Room air disinfection by ultraviolet irradiation of upper room air, *Arch. Environ. Health,* 23, 35, 1971.

68a. Kundsin, R. B., Ed., Airborne contagion, *Ann. N. Y. Acad. Sci.,* 353, 1, 1980.

69. Riley, R. L., Kaufman, J. E., Air disinfection in corridors by upper air irradiation with ultraviolet, *Arch. Environ. Health,* 22, 551, 1971.

70. Nardell, E. A., Iseman, M. D., Kubica, G., Riley, R. L., Stead, W. W., Urbach, F., Multidrug-resistant tuberculosis, (letter), *N. Engl. J. Med.,* 327, 1173, 1992.

71. Clark, R. A., OSHA enforcement policy and procedures for occupational exposure to tuberculosis, *Infect. Contr. Hosp. Epidemiol.,* 14, 694, 1993.

Chapter 4

The Working Mycobacteriology Laboratory

Ronald W. Smithwick, M.S.

CONTENTS

I. INTRODUCTION

Mycobacteriology is the field of science dedicated to the study of the group of microorganisms in the genus *Mycobacterium*, which includes the species *tuberculosis* and more than 50 other described species. These microorganisms have features similar to both fungi and bacteria, thus the genus name *Mycobacterium*.

The role of the mycobacteriology laboratory is to confirm the physician's diagnosis of tuberculosis and other mycobacterioses, to test mycobacterial isolates for susceptibility to antimicrobial drugs, to monitor therapy with bacteriologic tests, to support epidemiologic investigations, and to identify isolates from mycobacterioses.

Microscopically, mycobacteria vary in appearance from spherical to short filaments, which may be branched. Although *M. tuberculosis* (*M. tb.*, tubercle bacilli) from clinical specimens usually appear as short to moderately long rods, they can be curved and are seen frequently in a closely bound mass or clump. Individual bacilli are generally 0.5–1.0 μm in diameter and 1.5–10 μm long.[1,2]

One of the distinguishing characteristics of mycobacteria is the ability to retain dyes that are removed easily from other microorganisms by alcohols and dilute solutions of strong mineral acids like hydrochloric acid. Consequently, mycobacteria are termed acid-fast and are called acid-fast bacilli or just AFB. This ability to resist destaining by acids and alcohols has been attributed to a wax-like layer composed of long-chain fatty acids, the mycolic acids, in their cell wall.[1]

The detection of tubercle bacilli in specimens from tuberculosis patients begins with specimen collection. Both the quality of the specimen and the conditions for transport to the laboratory can affect how accurately the laboratory report reflects the status of the patient. Good quality laboratory work cannot compensate for a poor quality specimen.

Acid-fast microscopy usually is the first and most rapid diagnostic test done on a specimen. Subsequently, the specimen is processed in an attempt to grow the AFB on artificial media. This growth is used to do tests for drug susceptibility, species identification, and any other required testing.

II. LABORATORY SAFETY

Since tuberculosis is transmitted by the airborne route, protecting the laboratory worker against infection should be the first consideration in mycobacteriology. The recent increase in multidrug-resistant tuberculosis has made safety even more critical to laboratory operation.

Most laboratory manipulations of clinical specimens and cultures of microorganisms create aerosols. Since breaking the surface tension of a liquid almost always creates an aerosol, in the laboratory, these aerosols are created by bursting bubbles, by removing an instrument from a liquid or moist surface, or by a drop leaving a pipet or landing on a medium surface. These aerosols then dry to form droplet nuclei, which remain suspended in the air and may contain infectious microorganisms, including tubercle bacilli. Although it is impossible to prevent aerosol production and the resultant droplet nuclei, aerosol formation can be minimized, and those aerosols that are produced can be contained. Procedures that avoid both bubble production and agitation of liquids or moist materials help minimize aerosol production. The control of airflow, such as one-pass air conditioning with negative

0-8493-4825-0/94/$0.00+$.50
© 1994 by CRC Press, Inc.

71

pressure containment laboratories and biological safety cabinets, helps isolate and eliminate any droplet nuclei created from laboratory-generated aerosols. Protective clothing, autoclave sterilization, ultraviolet light, and disinfectants all contribute to protecting laboratory workers and others from infection in the laboratory.

III. SPECIMEN COLLECTION

Proper specimen collection and transport are critical to producing a laboratory report that reflects the microbiological condition of the patient. To ensure the best sputum for mycobacteriology, the specimen collector must be trained properly, the patient must be given instructions and must understand them, and the patient must be supervised during sputum collection. Frequently, collecting a good sputum specimen is not easy. Collectors must manage some patients who are uncooperative, very young, very old, or debilitated. They must attempt to collect sputum only. Saliva and nasopharyngeal discharges are not acceptable.

Three single specimens should be collected on different days within one week, usually on three consecutive days. Because a tuberculous lesion may drain intermittently into the bronchial tree, it is possible for a specimen taken one day to be AFB negative and a specimen taken the next day to be positive. Pooled specimens should not be collected because AFB isolations frequently are lost due to overgrowth by contaminating microorganisms that multiply in the specimen during the extended collection period.[3]

Unsupervised sputum collection should be avoided. Sputum collection by unsupervised patients allows not only for the submission of unacceptable sputum but for substitution as well.

Since coughing, sneezing, and talking all create aerosols, precautions must be taken to protect workers and patients from infection. Transmission of tuberculosis in the sputum collection area can be prevented by efficient directional airflow exhausted to the outside and away from public areas, by using sputum collection booths, and by proper use of particulate respirator masks or other respiratory protection devices by the sputum collection staff.

The sputum collection area should be well organized to have a smooth flow of patients who are supervised by the sputum collectors. There should be a waiting area with sufficient seating. All materials should be prepared beforehand with adequate supplies to last throughout the collection period. Sputum collection containers must be clean, sterile, preferably new, with a 2- to 5-cm opening, and with a tight-fitting lid. The lid should seal well enough to prevent leaks and, for transported specimens, should be strong enough to withstand air pressure changes during air transport. Fifty-milliliter, screw-capped, plastic centrifuge tubes frequently are recommended for sputum collection and subsequent processing in the laboratory. There must be a label on the *side* of the container with the patient's name and/or identification number.

The sputum collector should not collect sputum from more patients than can be effectively supervised at one time; usually no more than three and frequently only one. The immediate area of sputum collection should be free of onlookers. Easily read instructions, illustrated with photos or drawings, should be posted to reinforce the sputum collector's verbal instructions.

Before collecting a sputum it is advisable to have the patient rinse food particles and unwanted bacteria from the mouth with water and also clear the throat of postnasal discharge. Although water can contain saprophytic mycobacteria, these organisms rarely are isolated and present less of a problem for the laboratory than the food and other material that may be collected.

To collect sputum, the patient should be instructed to take four deep breaths: the first two times to inhale deeply, hold the breath for a few seconds, then exhale slowly; the third time, to forcefully blow the air out; and the fourth time, to inhale deeply and cough. The patient may have to cough several times before producing sputum. The patient should rest after coughing three or four times or when appearing stressed. The sputum collector may need to use back-percussion to supplement the patient's efforts.

The patient should hold the sputum container to the lower lip and gently release the specimen into the container. An adequate specimen is 5 to 10 ml of sputum. More than 10 ml may be too much for laboratory processing. If attempts to collect the minimum of 5 ml are unsuccessful, the specimen should be submitted to the laboratory with an explanation for the small amount.

A nebulizer may be used for sputum induction but should not be considered the method of choice. Naturally produced sputa are preferred to the thin watery ones obtained by nebulizer induction. Also, nebulizer sputum induction may cause a patient unnecessary respiratory distress for several hours after use. Nebulizer maintenance and parts replacement create an additional expense.

A throat swab should be done only if sputum cannot be collected because of the patient's inability to cooperate or if it is impractical or impossible to collect a specimen by other means.

Some other specimens that may be submitted to the laboratory for mycobacteria isolation are specimens collected during bronchoscopy, gastric washings, body fluids, tissue, urine, and feces.[4]

Collecting feces to isolate mycobacteria should be limited to immunocompromised patients.

Instructions for storing and transporting specimens must be obtained from the receiving laboratory; specimens can become useless when improperly stored or transported. Some general rules are (1) always use sterile collection containers, even for feces, (2) use aseptic collection techniques if possible, (3) do not freeze specimens, (4) refrigerate specimens when possible, and (5) obtain and follow all regulations for mailing and other transport.

IV. ACID-FAST MICROSCOPY

Acid-fast microscopy is a rapid and easy laboratory test for the presence of mycobacteria in a clinical specimen. It usually is the first bacteriologic test to confirm the clinical diagnosis of tuberculosis. Microscopy also identifies potentially infectious patients, helps to monitor the effects of therapy, and helps the laboratory staff to determine inoculum adjustments for tests. However, the method has limitations. *Mycobacterium* species cannot be identified by acid-fast microscopy. It is relatively insensitive compared with isolation by culture. Because only a small portion of sputum is used to prepare a smear and only a portion of the smear is examined by microscopy, it has been estimated that 1 ml of sputum must contain approximately 6000 AFB to have a 50% chance of finding 3 AFB and reporting the smear as positive for AFB.[5] Another estimate indicates that at least 10,000 AFB must be present in 1 ml of sputum to find consistently 3 AFB by microscopy.[1] This means that a smear could be reported as negative for AFB even though as many as 600 colonies could grow if 0.1 ml of this material was used to inoculate a tube of isolation medium. This assumes that all AFB in this theoretical specimen would be viable; usually, they are not. Because aerosols are generated during smear preparation, the smears must be prepared in a biological safety cabinet.

A smear is prepared by spreading approximately 0.01 ml of specimen or specimen concentrate over an area approximately 1×2 cm on a new, labeled, glass microscope slide. Smears are then dried at ambient temperature and heat-fixed at approximately 75°C for 2 h or over a flame for 2–3 s. It then is stained with specific dyes and searched by microscopy to find AFB. Heat-fixing kills many but not all AFB in a smear. The infection hazard from any tubercle bacilli that remain viable in a smear is very small because the bacilli would have to be either rubbed off the slide in particles smaller than 5 μm and be inhaled or they would have to enter the skin by puncture from a broken slide.

Phenol in acid-fast staining solutions will kill any AFB on the slide, so staining smears soon after preparation is best.[6]

Considerable experience is required to maintain proficiency in acid-fast microscopy. The usual rate for AFB-positive smears is about 5% of submitted specimens. An AFB-positive control smear should be stained with each day's group of smears. The quality of stain solutions and the reagents for their preparation decrease with time. For these reasons, laboratories that do acid-fast microscopy on fewer than 15 or 20 specimens per week probably will have trouble maintaining proficiency. Such laboratories should have all acid-fast microscopy results confirmed by a laboratory that processes a higher number of specimens per week.

A smear, prepared from a specimen without initial processing, usually is referred to as a direct smear.

Concentrated specimen smears usually are prepared from the sediments of specimens centrifuged for isolating AFB by culture. A concentrate smear also can be made by mixing sputum with an equal volume of approximately 5% sodium hypochlorite (household bleach), waiting for 10 min, centrifuging at 3000× g for 15 min, and then preparing a smear from the sediment.

There are a number of acid-fast staining techniques. The standard technique is the 1883 Neelsen modification of the 1882 Ziehl method.[5] The Ziehl–Neelsen method requires moderate heat for optimum AFB staining. The Kinyoun cold staining method has a higher concentration of dye, and stains AFB just as well as the Ziehl–Neelsen method. The dye used in these staining solutions is the phenyl methane dye, basic fuchsin, also known as magenta, which stains AFB red. The background tissue debris may be lightly stained a contrasting blue, green, or yellow through which the microscopist searches to find the red-stained AFB.

For fluorescence acid-fast microscopy, the fluorescent dye auramine or a combination of auramine and rhodamine is used. The staining process is the same as for the Ziehl–Neelsen method and is not a fluorescent antibody technique. When stained with auramine alone and observed with a fluorescence microscope, AFB appear as white to yellow-green fluorescing bacilli. They fluoresce pink or orange when stained with the auramine and rhodamine combination.

Phenol is a primary ingredient in acid-fast staining solutions. Its function is to accelerate dye penetration of the mycolic acid portion of the AFB cell wall. The phenol used to prepare acid-fast stain solutions must be pure colorless crystals. Any yellow or brown discoloration indicates deterioration of the phenol, which must not be used.

After the initial specific staining, the smear is destained with an acid and alcohol solution leaving only the AFB stained. Then a counterstain of a contrasting color is applied.

Smears are scanned in an orderly fashion, usually in successive horizontal sweeps across the smear. A magnification of 800× to 1000× is used to scan Ziehl–Neelsen-stained smears. Fluorescing AFB appear as bright points of light in a dark background; therefore, they are more easily detected than the red, fuchsin-stained bacilli seen by standard transmitted light microscopy. For fluorescence microscopy, a lower magnification of 200× to 250× is used to observe smears, and AFB morphology is then confirmed at 400× to 600×. The area of a 250× field is usually more than 10 times larger than a field at 1000×. It is recommended that 300 fuchsin-stained microscope fields of view be observed before reporting a smear negative for AFB whereas observing only 30 fields at 200–250× is required for fluorescence microscopy. This saving in work time usually justifies the additional cost of a fluorescence microscope.[5] Fluorescence acid-fast microscopy is considered the method of choice because the shorter observation time allows for earlier reporting of results.

There are several methods for reporting the results of acid-fast microscopy. Table 4-1 displays the currently recommended method.[5,7]

The tenfold increments for reporting microscopy results help the physician follow the effect of

TABLE 4-1 Recommended method for reporting acid-fast microscopy results on smears scanned at 1000×[a]

Number of AFB Seen	Preferred Report	Alternate Report
0	Negative for AFB	–
1–2/300 fields	Number/smear	+/–
1–9/100 fields	Number/100 fields	1+
1–9/10 fields	Number/10 fields	2+
1–9/field	Number/field	3+
>9/field	>9/field	4+

[a] Reports for Ziehl–Neelsen-stained smears are usually based on magnifications of approximately 1000×, for fluorochrome stained smears, 600× to 400×. The area of a 600× field is approximately twice that of 1000×, and that of 400× is approximately four times the area at 1000×. These area differences must be considered when comparing results of the two methods of acid-fast microscopy. A report of one or two AFB per smear is not considered positive because of a possible observation error or contamination with AFB from the environment. The microscopist should review the results of companion specimens or request a replacement specimen.

patient therapy and give laboratory workers the information needed to prepare inocula for direct drug susceptibility tests.

Distinctive cell morphology and staining characteristics have been described for some species of mycobacteria but are not seen consistently and are shared by more than one species. Although these clues are helpful for species identification, *Mycobacterium* species cannot be identified by microscopy alone.

Although AFB are considered Gram-stain positive, this test has no real meaning in defining mycobacteria and therefore has no useful purpose in mycobacteriology.

Several reports on fluorescent antibody (FA) tests for mycobacteria have been published. However, reliable commercial FA conjugates for mycobacteria have not been produced, and the test is not available for general use.[8]

V. ISOLATION BY CULTURE

Sputa contain many different non-acid-fast microorganisms, which reproduce much faster than tubercle bacilli. The goal in the laboratory is to kill or inhibit the growth of these unwanted microorganisms while promoting the growth of AFB. Sodium hydroxide has been the most widely used substance to decontaminate sputa and other clinical specimens for isolating mycobacteria. Trisodium phosphate is another strong base often used. Acids such as sulfuric and oxalic are used for special specimen decontamination applications.[7]

Mycobacteria are resistant to many of the quaternary ammonium detergents. Benzalkonium chloride and cetylpyridinium chloride are two of these compounds used to decontaminate specimens to isolate mycobacteria.[9,10]

The ideal decontaminant works rapidly, is inexpensive, eliminates all unwanted microorganisms, and does not kill any mycobacteria present in the specimen. Unfortunately no decontaminant is ideal, and most will kill or inhibit some mycobacteria in the specimen.

Since mycobacteria are resistant to many of the common antimicrobial drugs, several have been incorporated into media to inhibit contaminant growth and still allow mycobacterial growth. Some of the penicillin derivatives, cycloheximide, trimethoprim, amphotericin B, and nalidixic acid, have been used.[11,12]

The mucus in sputum must be liquefied for effective decontamination to take place. This liquefaction process is called digestion. The entire process is often referred to as "digestion and decontamination." Four percent sodium hydroxide will both digest and decontaminate sputa. If mucolytic substances such as

N-acetyl-L-cysteine or dithiothreitol are used, the concentration of sodium hydroxide can be lowered and still obtain good decontamination with more surviving mycobacteria.[13]

Immediately after decontamination, sterile buffer or distilled water is added to the specimen either to neutralize or dilute the decontaminant and to balance the centrifuge load. Solid material and any AFB are concentrated at the bottom of the tube by centrifugation at a relative centrifugal force (RCF) of 3000× g. The supernatant is decanted into a pan of disinfectant, and the sediment is resuspended in 1 or 2 ml of sterile, buffer solution, distilled water, or bovine serum albumin solution. Media are then inoculated and smears are prepared from this suspension.

An RCF of 3000× g is necessary to attain adequate sedimentation of tubercle bacilli during centrifugation.[14] Although a higher RCF would be more efficient, some plastic centrifuge tubes may fail and additional frictional heat could kill tubercle bacilli.[7] Using a refrigerated centrifuge is advisable since frictional heating can reduce the number of viable tubercle bacilli in centrifuged specimens.[7]

There are many formulations of growth media for mycobacteria; they can be characterized by three basic types. The first is coagulated egg represented by the well-known Lowenstein–Jensen (L-J) medium. It is composed of whole eggs, potato starch, glycerol, other nutrients, and trace elements plus a dye, usually malachite green, which inhibits contaminant growth. This medium is prepared as a liquid; after being dispensed in screw-capped glass containers and placed in the desired position, it is solidified by coagulation at 85°C for 45 min. Several other egg-based media, such as American Trudeau Society (ATS) medium, frequently are used for mycobacteriology.

The second type of medium also is solid and is composed of soluble nutrients and trace elements, with agar as a solidifier. The most common of this type are Middlebrook 7H10 and 7H11. These media have several advantages over the egg-based media. Colonies are more distinct on the transparent agar than on the opaque egg media, some tubercle bacilli prefer it to other media, and drugs for susceptibility testing tend to be more stable in it than in egg media.[15] Two disadvantages are that exposure to heat and light cause formaldehyde production, which inhibits mycobacterial growth,[16] and growth of tubercle bacilli from specimens requires an atmosphere containing 5–10% carbon dioxide.[17]

The third type of medium is a clear liquid and is egg free; the most common one is Middlebrook 7H9. This medium is used primarily to produce cultures consisting of single cells and very small clumps. These easily diluted cultures are used to prepare inocula to produce isolated colonies on solid media for drug susceptibility and identification tests. Modifications of Middlebrook 7H9 are used as isolation media in the BACTEC method (Beckton Dickinson Diagnostic Instrument Systems, Sparks, MD) and the Septi-Chek method (Beckton Dickinson). When used to isolate tubercle bacilli from specimens, Middlebrook 7H9 and its modifications also require a 5–10% carbon dioxide atmosphere.

Compared with other microorganisms, tubercle bacilli grow very slowly. Cell doubling time is 15 to 24 h, depending on growth conditions,[2] compared with 20 min for some of the common bacteria. Colonies can be seen on solid media in 2 to 3 weeks for some strains, but visible growth can take as long as 8 weeks for other strains. This slow growth has been a perpetual problem in laboratory confirmation of tuberculosis and the timely reporting of drug susceptibility test results. Tubercle bacilli from specimens usually do not produce visible colonies on solid media until about 3 weeks after inoculation and may take 6 weeks or more if only a few colonies are present. Growth can be detected earlier by the BACTEC and the Septi-Chek methods, especially if the specimen contains a relatively large number of viable AFB.[18-20]

In the BACTEC system, growth of the mycobacteria is detected radiometrically. The modified 7H9 liquid medium (BACTEC 12B) contains palmitic acid with ^{14}C as a component. Radioactive carbon dioxide is a metabolic byproduct of this palmitic acid. The air in the 12B vial is sampled and evaluated by the BACTEC 460 instrument. Any sampled radioactive carbon dioxide produced is evaluated, and a relative value is printed as the growth index, which indicates the level of metabolism in each vial. When growth is detected, a smear of the medium is prepared to confirm the presence of AFB. Drug susceptibility tests are done after the presence of $M.$ $tb.$ is indicated by the growth rate and the NAP test, described later.

The BACTEC 12B medium was developed for use with all specimens except blood. A slightly different modified 7H9 medium, BACTEC 13A, with a greater volume in a larger vial is used for blood specimens. BACTEC 13A medium also is recommended for bone marrow aspirates.

The Septi-Chek system is a biphasic medium system using both solid and liquid media. The liquid medium is a modified 7H9. The Septi-Chek System uses three kinds of solid media: egg-based, 7H11, and chocolate agar. During media production, carbon dioxide is added to the bottle containing the modified 7H9. After the bottle containing the modified 7H9 is inoculated with the decontaminated specimen, it is mated with another bottle containing a paddle supporting the three solid media. The sealed bottles are inverted to inoculate the solid media from the 7H9, and then are incubated at 37°C. The mated bottles are observed daily for colony growth on the solid media for the first week, then weekly for an additional 7 weeks before discarding and reporting as negative for growth of a culture. At each observation, the mated bottles are inverted to reinoculate the solid media if no growth was observed.

Growth of contaminants is restricted by adding a solution of inhibitory drugs to both the BACTEC and Septi-Chek bottles before they are inoculated with a decontaminated specimen.

The primary advantages of the BACTEC system over the use of solid medium alone is the earlier detection of a very small amount of mycobacterial growth and the ability to complete drug susceptibility tests on the primary antituberculosis drugs within 5 days. Using L-J and 7H10 or 7H11 in conjunction with BACTEC improves the isolation rate of tubercle bacilli.[18] In the Septi-Chek system, several types of solid media are combined with a liquid medium to provide optimal opportunity for an isolation. Although detection of growth is not as rapid as with BACTEC, growth is seen earlier than when a solid medium alone is used.[20]

Occasionally isolation by culture fails with a patient whose symptoms, medical history, X-ray findings, or acid-fast bacilli positive smears indicate tuberculosis or other mycobacterioses. This can occur for many reasons, including poor specimen collection, specimen mixup, overheating or freezing specimens during storage or shipment, misdiagnosis, overdecontamination, effective therapy, collecting specimens shortly after administering drugs, toxic substances in specimens, and improper specimen processing. Unusual growth requirements also are an infrequent cause. Some rare strains of *M. tb* are carbon dioxide dependent. *M. bovis* may not grow in the presence of glycerol. *M. africanum* prefers a medium supplemented with pyruvic acid or its salt. Mycobacteria other than tubercle bacilli may prefer temperatures higher or lower than 37°C or, in the case of *M. haemophilum*, require a medium rich in iron. It is important that the physician give the laboratory staff all information about the source and any conditions concerning a specimen to help to determine if any unusual processing or growth conditions are needed.

False-positive reports frequently are caused by a mixup in specimens during collection or processing; this is avoided best by good organization and careful attention to detail. However, other factors can cause misleading AFB-positive reports. Mycobacteria other than tubercle bacilli are present in most water supplies, even in nonsterile distilled water.[21,22] These potential troublemakers can be introduced into the specimen during collection or during processing in the laboratory. They must be recognized as contaminants. As a rule, when five or less colonies of AFB not appearing to be tubercle bacilli are isolated from only one specimen, all testing should stop unless the physician is convinced the isolate is causing disease. The expensive identification of AFB contaminants seldom serves any useful medical purpose. Such isolates from immunocompromised patients should be considered as an exception to the rule.

VI. DRUG SUSCEPTIBILITY TESTING

Drug-resistant mutants are produced spontaneously in actively growing populations of tubercle bacilli. For any one drug, the proportion of spontaneous mutations that occurs in a population is relatively constant, but the proportion varies from drug to drug. The number of drug-resistant mutants in a susceptible population may range between one per 100,000 to one per several million bacilli, depending on the drug and its concentration.[23,24] Since the mutations are spontaneous and not induced, the drug need not be present for the mutations to occur. The presence of only a single drug then can select for those mutants resistant to that drug, and they will become the replacement population of tubercle bacilli.

In the past it was considered impractical to test initial *M. tb.* isolates for drug susceptibility unless the patient was from a population in which drug-resistant tuberculosis was common. Because of the recent emergence of multidrug-resistant *M. tb.*, this policy has changed. All initial isolates of tubercle bacilli are to be tested for drug susceptibility. As in the past, susceptibility testing is indicated for apparent drug treatment failures, retreatment cases, and isolates from close contacts of patients with known drug-resistant tuberculosis.[4] Also, drug susceptibility test investigations are done on isolates from patients not previously treated for tuberculosis to determine the level of primary drug resistance in specified populations.

Drug susceptibility tests detect selective growth of drug-resistant tubercle bacilli on drug-containing media. Of the several methods for determining drug resistance, the proportion method is the most widely accepted and is recommended for use in the United States. Colonies are counted on the drug-containing medium and compared with the number of colonies on the control medium without drugs. Growth in the presence of drugs is reported as a percent of the growth on the control, i.e., the proportion of drug resistance compared to control growth.

The critical concentration of each drug must be determined for each medium before routine use because drugs are affected differently by each type of medium used for testing. Critical concentration has been defined as "the weakest concentration at which susceptible bacilli are unable to grow in the presence of the drug."[25] This definition is based on the average results of tests of many different strains. Middlebrook 7H10 has been used extensively in the United States and will be the example medium used in this discussion.

Minimal inhibitory concentration (MIC) is not quite the same as critical concentration. The MIC is based on the test results of a single strain with a drug.

The inoculum for testing must contain a selection of bacilli that represents the population in the patient, it must contain only single cells or only very small clumps of bacilli, and it must contain the appropriate number of colony-forming units to achieve valid test results.

For the direct drug-susceptibility test the microbiologist first must observe an acid-fast-stained smear prepared from the decontaminated specimen concentrate. If the smear is positive for AFB, the bacilli are enumerated for a report to the physician, and centrifuge-concentrate dilutions are calculated for the drug-testing inoculum. The inoculum theoretically contains a representative sample of the patient's *M. tb* population. The dilutions are prepared and the susceptibility test media are inoculated.

Direct drug-susceptibility tests can be done only on AFB smear-positive specimens because it is wasteful to test specimens containing no tubercle bacilli and it is necessary to know the approximate number of AFB in the inoculum to ensure useful numbers of colonies on the drug-test control medium.

Indirect susceptibility tests are done on isolated cultures of *M. tb*. The inoculum is prepared by scraping or rubbing the medium surface to dislodge portions of all of the colonies to obtain a representative sample of the patient's *M. tb*. population. These clumps of colonies are used either to inoculate a tube of liquid medium or placed in a sterile glass tube containing glass beads and a buffer solution, which is vortex-mixed to produce a fine suspension of single cells and very small clumps.

Drug-susceptibility test medium plates are inoculated with appropriate dilutions of the resuspended specimen sediment, the ground culture, or the liquid medium culture grown for 1 week at 37°C. The plates are sealed in carbon dioxide-permeable plastic bags and incubated at 37°C. An atmosphere of 5–10% carbon dioxide is required for the direct-susceptibility tests but not for the indirect tests. After 3 weeks, colonies are counted on the controls and the percent of resistance is calculated for any growth seen on the drug-containing medium. Microcolonies seen on drug-susceptibility test media also are considered evidence of drug resistance. Therefore, the surfaces of the media are scanned at 10× to 20× with a stereomicroscope to ensure all colonies are counted.

A calculated resistance of 1% or greater at the critical concentration is considered to be significant resistance, and it is likely that the tested drug no longer will be effective for antituberculosis therapy.

As mentioned, drug-susceptibility testing may be completed within 5 days using the BACTEC system. The inoculum is prepared from an *M. tb*-positive BACTEC isolation vial or from other culture media as for the solid media susceptibility tests. The control vial is inoculated with a 100-fold dilution of the inoculum used for the tests to demonstrate growth at less than or greater than 1% in the test medium compared to the control. Growth of 1% or more in a test vial would indicate that the drug probably would not be effective, just as in the results from solid media.

Most of the slowly growing species of mycobacteria other than tubercle bacilli are resistant to the antituberculosis drugs, and testing them for drug susceptibility has not been practical. The exception is *M. kansasii*, which usually is susceptible to some of the antituberculosis drugs.

A drug susceptibility-testing procedure has been developed for the rapidly growing mycobacteria, and several laboratories offer this service.

VII. IDENTIFICATION TESTS

Species identification refers to the act of differentiating a particular life form, or a pure culture in the field of microbiology, from others to determine its species name among the classified species. The term speciation refers to the evolutionary production of new species. Speciation or speciate are not used in the context of species identification in this text.

From the 1950s until the late 1980s, a series of tests using growth characteristics, specific enzyme activity, and growth inhibition were used to identify *M. tb*. and differentiate the other *Mycobacterium* species. Although these tests remain valid, they can take several weeks to complete and require a large number of test media and reagents. Newer methods are making many of those older tests all but obsolete.

In the early 1980s *p*-nitro-1-acetylamino-2-hydroxypropiophenone (NAP) was introduced in conjunction with the BACTEC system to differentiate *M. tb.* complex from the other species of mycobacteria. Tubercle bacilli rarely grew at the recommended concentration of NAP, and the other mycobacteria were rarely inhibited by it. This enabled an early presumptive diagnosis of tuberculosis.[26]

Later, in the mid-1980s, genetic probes were introduced to identify *M. tb.*, *M. avium*, and *M. intracellulare*, species that cause pulmonary mycobacterioses most often. Since then, genetic probes have been developed for *M. gordonae*, a frequent contaminant from the environment, and *M. kansasii*, which also causes pulmonary mycobacterioses (Gen-Probe, Inc., San Diego, CA).[27]

Deoxyribonucleic acid (DNA) is most stable in its double-stranded configuration and, under favorable conditions, matching single strands unite to form a double strand by the bonding of matching nucleotide base pairs. The function of genetic probes depends on this affinity of the base pairs of nucleotides on matching single chromosome strands. If two single-strand chromosomes are not a matched pair, the small amount of bonding that takes place between a few nucleotides will be too unstable for complete double-strand chromosome formation. Since closely related species have some portions of chromosomes that match, it is necessary to choose only portions of chromosomes that are species specific to produce a probe that does not cross-react with other species. For the genetic probes, the species-specific portions of single strands of DNA are labeled with a detectable substance such as radioisotopes, fluorescents, enzymes, or enzyme substrates.

The target for the probe can be either strands of DNA or ribonucleic acid (RNA). Ribosomal RNA (rRNA) is the target for the probes developed for *Mycobacterium* species because there are many more rRNA strands per cell than chromosomes. There are a number of possible methods to use probes. The basic steps are (1) place cells for testing in a container and then rupture them to release the DNA or rRNA, (2) react the DNA or rRNA with the probe, hybridization, (3) remove the unhybridized probe or inactivate the label on the unhybridized probe, and (4) use a detection system to determine positive or negative reactions for identification reports (see Chapter 5, this volume).

A method to identify *Mycobacterium* species using high-performance liquid chromatography (HPLC) also was introduced in the mid-1980s.[28] As mentioned earlier, mycobacteria and related genera produce long-chain fatty acids, the mycolic acids, that compose a waxy portion of the cell wall. Mycolic acids are 60 to 90 carbons long in mycobacteria. The amount of each chain length produced varies from one species to another. HPLC determines the amount of each of the mycolic acids produced by a culture. The relative amounts of each mycolic acid then are displayed as a pattern on a chart. This culture then is identified to *Mycobacterium* species by matching its HPLC pattern to a standard species pattern.

Gas chromatography (GC) is used in another identification system for mycobacteria (MIDI, 115 Barksdale Prof. Center, Newark, DE). In this system, patterns of shorter chained fatty acids are produced to identify *Mycobacterium* species[29] (see Chapter 5, this volume).

Restriction fragment-length polymorphism (RFLP) is a method of determining strain relatedness within a species. This method compares patterns of different sized segments of DNA. These segments of DNA are produced by enzymatically breaking chromosomes at specific sites, separating them in sequence by electrophoresis within a thin, flat, moist matrix, and then using labeled genetic probes to produce a pattern of specific segment bands in the matrix. Patterns then are compared to demonstrate strain relatedness. This method, whimsically called DNA fingerprinting, is used in epidemiologic studies and is expected to replaced phage typing in tuberculosis epidemiology and cross-contamination investigations in mycobacteriology (see Chapter 5, this volume).

VIII. LABORATORY OPERATION

The function of a clinical laboratory is to receive clinical specimens, evaluate the information provided with the specimens, perform appropriate specimen tests, and provide understandable and accurate reports in a timely manner. Reports should give the physician the necessary specimen information to help provide effective health care.

Specimens sent to the laboratory for diagnostic evaluation should be the best possible specimen for the required testing. Specimens and requested tests should be only those necessary to provide good quality patient care. Specimens should be transported from the collection site to the testing laboratory in a manner sufficient to maintain specimen quality and to ensure the safety of the general population and laboratory staff. The testing laboratory staff should be given enough information about the patient and the specimen to ensure that all appropriate testing methods are used.

Quality assurance is an essential part of the operation of a clinical laboratory. Quality control is the use of known positive and negative controls for tests to ensure that the testing system is functioning properly. This part of laboratory testing is essential to quality assurance, but quality assurance has other aspects.

Clinical laboratories usually are required to participate in proficiency testing programs. Central laboratories or outside agencies send "unknown" samples to the tested clinical laboratory for evaluation. The tested laboratory is graded on its ability to evaluate the samples properly and return a report within a reasonable time. This system provides an unbiased evaluation of the tested laboratory's ability to give an accurate and timely report.

On-site evaluations by licensing agencies also are part of the quality assurance process. Some examples of evaluated items are effective safety programs and equipment, personnel qualifications, equipment maintenance, reagent quality, testing controls, recordkeeping, and reports. These evaluations ensure safe, correct, and efficient laboratory operation.

Internal quality control measures, proficiency testing, and on-site evaluations all are part of the laboratory quality assurance process.

In conclusion, to provide first quality health care it is important that good quality specimens and information be provided to the laboratory and that the laboratory provide easily understood, accurate reports. At times the quality of submitted specimens or this exchange of information has been less than ideal. Too often the response to a breakdown in communication has been negative rather than there being an attempt to enhance the lines of communication. Unfortunately everyone loses when this happens: the patient, the physician, the laboratory staff, and the health care system. The physician must give adequate specimen information and request clarification of unfamiliar test reports. The testing laboratory should specify the characteristics of a good quality specimen to be submitted for evaluation. Laboratory staff should be free to request additional specimen information to avoid improper or inadequate testing, or to request replacements for unsatisfactory specimens. Laboratory reports should provide information about normal parameters, cut-off levels, and avoid or define such ambiguous terms as 2+ or few.

Open, clear communication between the health care providers and clinical laboratory staff is both a responsibility of and a benefit to everyone.

REFERENCES

1. Barksdale, L., Kim, K. S., *Mycobacterium*, *Bacteriol. Rev.*, 41, 217, 1977.
2. Darzins, E., *The Bacteriology of Tuberculosis*, University of Minnesota Press, Minneapolis, 1958.
3. Kestle, D. G., Kubica, G. P., Sputum collection for cultivation of mycobacteria — An early morning specimen or the 24- to 72-hour pool?, *Tech. Bull. Reg. Med. Tech.*, 37, 347, 1967.
4. Bass, J. B., Farer, L. S., Hopewell, P. C., Jacobs, R. F., Snider, D. E., Diagnostic standards and classification of tuberculosis, *Am. Rev. Resp. Dis.*, 142, 725, 1990.
5. Smithwick, R. W., *Laboratory Manual for Acid-Fast Microscopy*, Department of Health and Human Services, Public Health Service, Center for Disease Control, Atlanta, GA, 1976.
6. Allen, B. W., Survival of tubercle bacilli in heat-fixed sputum smears, *J. Clin. Pathol.*, 34, 719, 1981.
7. Kent, P. T., Kubica, G. P., *Public Health Mycobacteriology — A Guide for the Level III Laboratory*, U.S. Department of Health and Human Services, Public Health Service, Centers for Disease Control, Atlanta, GA, 1985.
8. Nassau, E., Parsons, E. R., Johnson, G. D., Detection of antibodies to *Mycobacterium tuberculosis* by solid phase radioimmunoassay, *J. Immunol. Methods*, 6, 261, 1975.
9. Wayne, L. G., Krasnow, I., Kidd, G., Finding the "hidden positive" in tuberculosis eradication programs. The role of the sensitive trisodium phosphate-benzalkonium (Zephiran) culture techniques, *Am. Rev. Resp. Dis.*, 86, 537, 1962
10. Smithwick, R. W., Stratigos, C. B., David, H. L., Use of cetylpyridinium chloride and sodium chloride for decontamination of sputum specimens that are transported to the laboratory for the isolation of *Mycobacterium tuberculosis*, *J. Clin. Microbiol.*, 1, 411, 1975.
11. Gruft, H., Isolation of acid-fast bacilli from contaminated specimens, *Health Lab. Sci.*, 8, 79, 1971.
12. Mitchison, D. A., Allen, B. W., Carrol, L., Dickinson, J. M., Aber, V. R., A selective oleic acid albumin agar medium for tubercle bacilli, *J. Med. Microbiol.*, 5, 165, 1972.
13. Kubica, G.P., Dye, W. E., Cohn, M. L., and Middlebrook, G., Sputum digestion and decontamination with N-acetyl-L-cysteine-sodium hydroxide for culture of mycobacteria, *Am. Rev. Resp. Dis.*, 87, 775, 1963.
14. Rickman, T. W., Moyer, N. P., Increased sensitivity of acid-fast smears, *J. Clin. Microbiol.*, 11, 618, 1980.
15. Kubica, G. P., Dye, W. E., *Laboratory Methods for Clinical and Public Health Mycobacteriology*, Public Health Service Publication No. 1547, United States Government Printing Office, Washington, D.C., 1967.
16. Miliner, R. A., Stottmeier, K. D., Kubica, G. P., Formaldehyde: a photothermal activated toxic substance produced in Middlebrook 7H10 medium, *Am. Rev. Resp. Dis.*, 99, 603, 1969.
17. Beam, R. E., Kubica, G. P., Stimulatory effect of carbon dioxide on the primary isolation of tubercle bacilli on agar-containing medium, *Am. J. Clin. Pathol.*, 50, 395, 1968.

18. Stager, C. E., Libonati, J. P., Siddiqi, S. H., Davis, J. R., Hooper, N. M., Baker, J. F., Carter, M. E., Role of solid media when used in conjunction with the BACTEC system for mycobacterial isolation and identification, *J. Clin. Microbiol.*, 29, 154, 1991.

19. Abe, C., Hosojima, S., Fukasawa, Y., Kazumi, Y., Takahashi, M., Hirano, K., Mori, T., Comparison of MB-Check, BACTEC, and egg-based media for recovery of mycobacteria, *J. Clin. Microbiol.*, 30, 878, 1992.

20. Isenberg, H. D., D'Amato, R. F., Heifets, L., Murray, P. R., Scardamaglia, M., Jacobs, M. C., Aperstein, P., Niles, A., Collaborative feasibility study of a biphasic system (Roche Septi-Chek AFB) for rapid detection and isolation of mycobacteria, *J. Clin. Microbiol.*, 29, 1719, 1991.

21. Wright, E. P., Collins, C. H., Yates, M. D., *Mycobacterium xenopi* and *Mycobacterium kansasii* in a hospital water supply. *J. Hosp. Infect.*, 6, 175, 1985.

22. Wenger, J. D., Spika, J. S., Smithwick, R. W., Pryor, V., Dodson, D. W., Carden, G. A., Klontz, K. C., Outbreak of *Mycobacterium chelonae* infection associated with use of jet injectors, *J. Am. Med. Assoc.*, 264, 373, 1990.

23. David, H. L. Probability distribution of drug-resistant mutants in unselected populations of *Mycobacterium tuberculosis*, *Appl. Microbiol.*, 20, 810, 1970.

24. Canetti, G., Present aspects of bacterial resistance in tuberculosis, *Am. Rev. Resp. Dis.*, 92, 687, 1965.

25. Canetti, G., Froman, S., Grosset, J., Hauduroy, P., Langerova, M., Mahler H. T., Meissner, G., Mitchison, D. A., Sula, L., Mycobacteria: laboratory methods for testing drug sensitivity and resistance, *Bull. WHO.*, 29, 565, 1963.

26. Morgan, M. A., Horstmeier, C. D., DeYoung, D. R., Roberts G. D., Comparison of a radiometric method (BACTEC) and conventional culture media for recovery of mycobacteria from smear-negative specimens, *J. Clin. Microbiol.*, 18, 384, 1983.

27. Lebrun, L., Espinasse, F., Poveda, J. D., Vincent-Levy-Frebault, V., Evaluation of nonradioactive DNA probes for identification of mycobacteria, *J. Clin. Microbiol.*, 30, 2476, 1992.

28. Butler, W. R., Ahern, D. G., Kilburn, J. O., High-performance liquid chromatography of mycolic acids as a tool in the identification of *Corynebacterium, Nocardia, Rhodococcus,* and *Mycobacterium* species, *J. Clin. Microbiol.*, 23, 182, 1986.

29. Lambert, M. A., Moss, C. W., Silcox, V. A., Good, R. C., Analysis of mycolic acid cleavage products and cellular fatty acids of *Mycobacterium* species by capillary gas chromatography, *J. Clin. Microbiol.*, 23, 731, 1986.

Chapter 5

New Diagnostic Methods

Joseph H. Bates, M.D.

CONTENTS

I. INTRODUCTION

The laboratory techniques most commonly employed in the United States and around the world for the diagnosis of tuberculosis were developed in the last century and have been modified only slightly over the past decades. The tubercle bacillus replicates slowly, dividing only once every 18–21 h, and efforts to reduce the time required for its division have been unsuccessful. This has meant that reports of positive culture growth from clinical specimens have required several weeks and sometimes up to 2 months. In addition, dependence on the stained smear of sputum or other clinical specimens has marked limitations. Although the smear report can be returned quickly from the laboratory, the sensitivity is poor because many thousands of organisms per milliliter must be present in the sample for the microscopist to detect their presence. Thus the laboratory diagnosis of tuberculosis has remained little changed and rather unsatisfactory by modern-medicine standards for many years. Now there is promise for improvement. New laboratory techniques using advances in immunology, molecular biology, and instrumentation provide a framework for significant change. This chapter will review recent developments in this regard.

II. SEROLOGICAL METHODS

A. IMMUNOASSAYS FOR MYCOBACTERIAL ANTIBODIES

Serological methods have been applied widely for the diagnosis of a variety of infectious diseases and it was only in 1898, a few years after Koch's identification of the tubercle bacillus, that Arloing published the first report of the value of a serological method for the diagnosis of tuberculosis.[1] He developed an agglutination test and noted that 57% of sera from tuberculosis patients showed an agglutinating antibody; healthy controls and persons ill with other diseases showed positive reactions in 11%. Over the years since that time many serological tests have been put forward as showing promise, but each failed to find wide acceptance. When Engvall and Perlmann described the sensitive and relatively simple enzyme-linked immunosorbent assay (ELISA) in 1972 it opened the way for a new approach to the serodiagnosis of tuberculosis and since that time many different antigens and antibodies have been studied.[2]

The largest single problem in the serodiagnosis of tuberculosis has turned on the antigen employed. A detailed description of more than 50 of these antigens has been published by Young et al.[3] Many workers have referred to mycobacterial antigens on the basis of approximate subunit molecular weights as judged by sodium dodecyl sulfate–polyacrylamide gel electrophoresis. The development of mycobacterial genes in *Escherichia coli* allowed the demonstration of immunological activity associated with a particular polypeptide, and sequence analysis gave insights to the biochemical function of the native protein. As this methodology improves, the ultimate mycobacterial antigens used for serodiagnosis will be cloned and sequenced and the events regarding expression of its gene will be understood. Currently, knowledge of this type is very fragmentary for all mycobacterial antigens.

0-8493-4825-0/94/$0.00+$.50
© 1994 by CRC Press, Inc.

At present most mycobacterial antigens are nonspecific because these proteins are widely shared among species and genera.[4] Since humans and most animals have repeated contacts with environmental mycobacteria that may have little or no capacity to cause disease but do provoke an antibody response; a test subject infected or diseased by *M. tuberculosis* may demonstrate antibody production that is a combination of both present and past antigenic stimuli. The development of a simple and rapid test to sort out this complex immunological pattern has proven to be a demanding task with great potential for error.

Nassau et al. were the first to use ELISA techniques for the diagnosis of tuberculosis.[5] They used as antigen a filtrate of *M. tuberculosis* H37Rv and studied healthy controls together with diseased subjects and reported a sensitivity of 56% and a specificity of 98%. Few workers have been able to improve on these initial results. Grange and Kardijito published a series of studies with ELISA assays using sonicates of *M. bovis* BCG as the antigen.[6] They measured IgG, IgM, and IgA antibody levels and obtained the best results with IgG antibody. Tuberculin status did not influence the IgM and IgA antibody levels. Their best sensitivity was 68% and their best specificity was 98%. Other reports using unheated culture filtrates of *M. tuberculosis* H37Ra, as well as saline extracts and sonicates, have failed to improve on these initial reports.

The use of tuberculin purified protein derivative (PPD) as an antigen has been studied extensively in ELISA serodiagnostic tests. The most complete report using PPD is that of Kalish et al. who found a sensitivity of 67% and a specificity of only 79%, with IgG antibody providing the best results, although IgA antibody also correlated with the diagnosis of tuberculosis.[7] Daniel and his co-workers have published several reports testing PPD as the antigen with the ELISA technique. PPD was found to rank below antigen 5, but ahead of antigen 6 and crude filtrates in terms of sensitivity and specificity.[8-10]

False-positive results with ELISA probably result from antibodies induced by mycobacteria that come from the environment or from normal flora that share common antigens with *M. tuberculosis*. To avoid these nonspecific results, efforts have been made to use purified or semipurified antigens that might be unique to the tubercle bacillus. The most commonly used protein for this purpose has been designated by Daniel and Anderson as antigen 5, but this antigen also contains nonspecific epitopes found in other mycobacteria.[11] In a study of South American and North American patients, antigen 5 gave a sensitivity of 84% for serum obtained from bacteriologically positive patients in

Bolivia and a sensitivity of 68% for patients in Ohio.[12] About one-third of the patients with atypical mycobacterial infections also were positive.

A significant disadvantage of antigen 5 is its instability under conditions of storage and shipping, whereas antigen 6 can be lyophilized without loss of activity.[13] In general antigen 6 has been found to be a less satisfactory antigen for ELISA serodiagnosis than either antigen 5 or PPD.[14]

Reggiardo and Vazques described three serologically active mycobacterial glycolipids and tested their value in the serodiagnosis of tuberculosis.[15] These antigens when compared with antigen 5 give the same efficiency of prediction for disease.[16]

Lipoarabinomannan (LAM) is a component of the cell wall of many, if not all, mycobacteria including *M. leprae*. Hunter et al. purified it in its native acylated state and this product has been tested for use as an antigen in the serodiagnosis of tuberculosis.[17] Sada et al. evaluated sera from 66 patients with pulmonary or extrapulmonary tuberculosis using LAM with an ELISA technique and found 91% specificity and 72% sensitivity.[18] Subsequently they tested the serum of patients with tuberculosis for the presence of LAM antigenemia.[19] The antigen was detected using a coagglutination method and the test was able to detect as little as 50 ng/ml of LAM in a test sample. The sensitivity for patients having pulmonary tuberculosis who had no acid-fast bacilli present on stained sputum smears was 67%, the specificity was 100%.

Charpin et al. evaluated an ELISA method using an antigen designated as A60 obtained from *M. bovis* BCG.[20] The patients studied were suspected of having pulmonary tuberculosis, but had negative sputum stains. Both IgM and IgG antibody activity were measured and, combining the results of IgG and IgM, the sensitivity was 68%, the specificity was 100%, and the positive predictive value was 100%.

In an effort to simplify the technical aspects of ELISA serodiagnosis, McDonough et al. evaluated a dot enzyme immunoassay using nitrocellulose strips to which had been added a *M. tuberculosis* antigen of 30,000 Da molecular weight.[21] This method was compared using an ELISA procedure for measuring IgG antibody. The dot assay results were less satisfactory than the ELISA, but it was suggested that this simple technique might be useful as a screening test in areas having limited technical support.

The role of ELISA serodiagnosis of extrapulmonary tuberculosis was reported by Wilkins and Ivanyi who evaluated 64 patients with involvement of lymph nodes in 31, pleura and/or pericardium in 14, bones and joints in 10, meninges in 4, genitourinary tract in 3, soft tissue in 3, gastrointestinal tract in 2, and skin disease in 2.[22] Ten patients had disease in multiple extrapulmonary sites. Antibodies were detected in 73% of these patients and in 5% of uninfected controls. Mathai et al. studied the cerebrospinal fluid of patients having suspected tuberculous meningitis using a dot immunoassay to detect antibody to antigen 5 among 40 such patients.[23] The specificity of this assay was 100% and this technology is simpler than ELISA.

The value of ELISA serodiagnosis for tuberculosis patients who also have AIDS has not been studied extensively. Theuer et al. and Eriki et al. observed that similar levels of IgG antibody to purified protein derivative were present in tuberculosis patients with and without AIDS.[24,25] Subsequently Daniel reviewed more complete studies from his laboratory and found that about 10% of patients with AIDS and tuberculosis in Uganda demonstrated antibody detectable by the ELISA method.[26]

Thus there is a large body of literature regarding ELISA serodiagnosis of tuberculosis and a comprehensive review has been published by Daniel and Debanne.[16] ELISA is well suited for use in developing countries where tuberculosis is common, and it gives information comparable to that of a direct sputum smear, and may be very useful for those patients from whom a sputum sample cannot be obtained and for patients with extrapulmonary tuberculosis. A major drawback has been the instability of antigen 5; thus more stable antigens are being evaluated. It is not clear which of the many variations of the serodiagnostic tests will prove to be the best.

B. IMMUNOASSAYS FOR MYCOBACTERIAL ANTIGENS

The detection of mycobacterial antigens in clinical specimens to provide a laboratory diagnosis of tuberculosis has been reported by several groups of investigators, many of whom concentrated on its value in tuberculous meningitis. Sada et al. were the first to use ELISA for the detection of *M. tuberculosis* antigen in cerebrospinal fluid. Since this report, a number of assay techniques for this purpose have been reported using competitive inhibition ELISA, latex agglutination, hemagglutination, and double antibody sandwich ELISA.[27,28] Radhakrishnan and Mathai studied cerebrospinal fluid from 40 patients having a clinical diagnosis of tuberculous meningitis using an inhibition ELISA technique to detect the presence of antigen 5.[29] Antigen 5 was detected in all 10 culture-positive specimens, in 21 of 30 culture-negative specimens, in none of the 40 control specimens. Krambovitis et al. assayed sera from patients with pulmonary and extrapulmonary tuberculosis for plasma

membrane antigens and reported 45% sensitivity.[30] Wadee et al. detected *M. tuberculosis* antigens by a sandwich assay using two purified *M. tuberculosis* antibodies.[31] They studied 63 cerebrospinal fluid specimens from patients with tuberculous meningitis. A total of 253 cerebrospinal fluids specimens were studied and there were 4.3% false positives, but no false negatives. Radhakrishnan and Mathai developed an assay for detection of antigen 5 using an inhibition ELISA and found 85% sensitivity with 100% specificity.[32] A preliminary report by Sada et al. described the measure of lipoarabinomannan in the serum of patients who had tuberculosis with and without AIDS.[33] The test in persons with tuberculosis alone was 90% sensitive, with both diseases was 85% sensitive, and, overall, the test was 93% specific.

Thus the detection of mycobacterial antigens in cerebrospinal fluid may prove to be a significant laboratory advance for the diagnosis of tuberculous meningitis, especially in countries where this diagnosis is relatively common. Its value for the study of chronic meningitis in countries where tuberculous meningitis is rare has not been studied sufficiently.

III. NUCLEIC ACID PROBES

DNA is composed of four repeating nucleotides — adenine, guanine, cytosine, and thymine — that are joined together in a coiled, double helix, double-stranded DNA (dsDNA). The two strands are held together by hydrogen bonds that can be broken by heat or high pH. Single strands of DNA (ssDNA) are very stable and on removal of the heat source or correction of the pH, the DNA molecule will reform (reanneal) into the double-stranded configuration. When the ssDNA molecules are from different sources, the reannealing is called hybridization. Reannealing comes about because the hydrogen bonds reform only with specific complementary bases; adenine pairs only with thymine and cytosine only with guanine. It is the same for RNA except uracil replaces thymine and pairs only with adenine. The stability of hybridization depends on the nucleotide sequence of both strands; a perfect match in the sequence of nucleotides produces a very stable dsDNA, but if there are mismatches there will be increasing instability of the molecule that leads to progressive weakening of the hybridization.

A nucleic acid probe is usually a short sequence of nucleotide bases that will bind or hybridize to highly specific regions of a target sequence of nucleotides. To develop a specific probe, a sequence of nucleotides must be found that is highly specific for the organism in question, then the probe must be reproduced in large quantity and tagged with a label that can be detected. An ideal probe usually consists of a short piece of single-stranded nucleic acid composed of 15 to 30 nucleotides. It can be composed of either DNA or RNA, but DNA probes are more common. For statistical uniqueness a minimum of 20 nucleotides is needed for a probe. Short probes hybridize at very high rates (in minutes) whereas long probes may require hours to achieve stable hybridization. Longer probes are more specific and hybridize at higher temperatures. The base sequence of the probe and the conditions under which the probe is used determine its specificity. It is not necessary to know the function of the target nucleic acid before a probe can be used. The only requirements are that the probe hybridize specifically to the target nucleic acids and that the target nucleic acids be unique to the cell or organism in question.

Most probes are labeled so that they can be detected after they hybridize. Isotopes such as ^{32}P, ^{35}S, and ^{125}I can be incorporated into the structure of the molecule. Enzymes such as alkaline phosphatase can be covalently linked to the probe or biotin can be incorporated into the probe and then the biotin can be detected by enzyme-labeled avidin molecules. Probes can be designed to detect genera, species, or even strains of various organisms. Targets in RNA are used because there are so many more copies per cell of RNA than DNA; this increases sensitivity of detection. Ribosomal RNA is the most useful target in a screening assay. The 16 S and 23 S ribosomal units are very useful for detecting taxonomic groups because these genes are highly conserved. There may be 10,000 ribosomes per cell compared with only a few or one copy of a DNA target per cell. Plasmid DNA (i.e., extrachromosomal circular DNA) may serve as a target for some organisms, but plasmids may not be present in many strains and for *M. tuberculosis*, plasmids have never been described.

DNA and RNA probes have proven very useful to detect mycobacteria in a specimen if the number of organisms present is large. Two probe systems are available commercially. The Gen-Probe system (Gen-Probe, San Diego, CA) uses a labeled DNA probe complementary to the ribosomal RNA in *M. tuberculosis*. Another available probe is designated SNAP (Syngene, San Diego, CA) and it utilizes a probe labeled with alkaline phosphatase that is directed against ribosomal RNA. These probes are used after the specimen to be tested has been processed and cultured long enough for the organism to have multiplied to a large number, perhaps 1×10^5 organisms per sample. The probe can be used to identify organism in a liquid or solid medium and are 99–100% specific.[34-37]

Another probe developed by Gen-Probe is labeled with an acridinium ester and this allows target detection using chemiluminescence. Experience indicates that this probe also is highly specific.[38] This assay is nonradioactive, rapid, and simple to carry out. Probes also are available for *Mycobacterium avium*, *M. intracellulare*, *M. avium* complex, *M. gordonae*, and *M. kansasii*.[39] When probes are combined with the BACTEC system, two-thirds of clinical specimens can be processed and the mycobacteria can be detected and identified to species within 2 weeks of inoculation. However, a standard procedure to combine BACTEC culture methods with DNA probes has yet to be established. With this system, if the number of organism present in the initial test sample is small, sensitivity may suffer if the probe is used after only 2 weeks incubation. This deficiency can be overcome by allowing the broth culture to reach a higher growth index before probe testing.[40]

Thus probes are used widely in the clinical mycobacteriology laboratory to speciate mycobacteria that have been grown in large number, either in broth or on a solid medium. These probes are highly specific, but are not sensitive. The probes do not help in detecting drug resistance, but this may be possible in the future. The probes serve as a substitute for biochemical testing to speciate mycobacteria and are more accurate than biochemical methods (see Chapter 4, this volume).

IV. PHAGE TYPING FOR *M. TUBERCULOSIS*

The first phages lytic for mycobacteria were reported by Gardner and Weiser in 1947 and their report was followed by studies done by Hnatko who used a number of phages isolated from soil to type a variety of strains of rapidly growing mycobacteria.[41,42] These phages failed to infect *M. tuberculosis* or *M. bovis* and it was not until Froman et al. reported the isolation of phages D28, D29, D32, and D34 in 1954 that there were any known phages that were lytic for virulent mycobacteria.[43] They tested a large number of strains of tubercle bacilli with various phages and no clear pattern of phage susceptibility was found. Although their work suggested that some phages might be useful for speciating mycobacteria, their technique of spotting large concentrations of phage particles onto the bacterial lawn resulted in nonspecific lysis or lysis from without. This form of lysis is highly nonspecific since the disruption of the bacterial cell wall is a result of many phages attaching to the cell wall causing cell lysis without any phage DNA penetrating the cell wall and inserting into the bacterial chromosome. Thus there would be no phage replication. It was only after the adoption of a "routine test dilution" as proposed by Ward and Redmond that true phage infection of *M. tuberculosis* could be detected using a spotting technique on a bacterial lawn.[44] With this technique, reproducible results were obtained and low concentrations of phage particles were shown to infect and lyse certain highly susceptible strains.

Redmond and Cater were the first to use phages isolated from soil to differentiate with great accuracy strains of *M. tuberculosis* and *M. bovis* from other virulent and avirulent mycobacteria.[45] Very significant results were obtained with phages designated DS6A and GS4E. Phage DS6A, isolated from soil, was specific for *M. tuberculosis* and *M. bovis* and would lyse no other species. Phage GS4E would lyse *M. tuberculosis* but not *M. bovis*. This work was confirmed by Murohashi et al. who studied 163 strains of *M. tuberculosis* and found all to be sensitive to phage DS6A, but noted some differences in sensitivity to phage GS4E.[46]

The first report of subdividing the species *M. tuberculosis* by phage typing was published by Bates and Fitzhugh in 1967.[47] Using 14 phages, 92 strains of *M. tuberculosis* were subdivided into 3 types on the basis of sensitivity to the phages DS6A, BG1, GS4E, and D34. Type A strains (76%) were sensitive to DS6A only, type B strains (14%) were sensitive to DS6A, BG1, and GS4E, and type C strains (10%) were sensitive to all four phages. This nomenclature was the first system adopted for phage typing mycobacteria. No correlation was found between phage type and either the geographic location of the patient or the drug sensitivity of the strains.

Later additional studies of tubercle bacilli isolated from Europe, Africa, and Asia were reported by Bates and Mitchison.[48] A study of 255 pretreatment isolates showed that a number of strains did not give uniform results and could not be classified as type A or B, and striking differences in geographic distribution by phage type were noted. In Hong Kong, type A predominated, while in Great Britain many of the strains were type B. The strains that could not be uniformly designated type A or B all were from southern India. A number of patients were observed to relapse after treatment and the pretreatment phage type was the same as the post-treatment phage type and there was no correlation between phage type and drug sensitivity.

These studies and others laid the groundwork for the development of a reliable phage typing scheme for *M. tuberculosis*. An international working group was formed by the World Health Organization to standardize procedures and nomenclature. This formed the foundation for the methods in general use today.[49] The phages were designated Mycobacterial Typing Phage Human and numbered (MTPH) 1–14. With this system most strains of *M. tuberculosis* can be reliably subdivided into phage types, although there is some variability inherent in the system. It is clear that phage type is a constant feature of the strain and does not change while the strain replicates in the host or after extensive subculturing in the laboratory. A detailed description of the technique for phage typing of *M. tuberculosis* has been published by Crawford and Bates.[50]

After the standard methods were confirmed, phage typing was carried out by the Centers for Disease Control, U.S. Public Health Service as a service to individuals and organizations, and for its own use to study the epidemiology of selected tuberculosis outbreaks. Phage typing was used to determine whether clusters of cases of tuberculosis were epidemiologically related and it was used as an aid to study the transmission of tubercle bacilli within a closed population unit such as a hospital or prison. The data obtained by phage typing are useful, but there are marked limitations. Since such a large percentage of all strains are included within a few phage types, the sensitivity of the test is markedly limited. Thus, when two or more subjects are infected with the same phage type, it could be explained by chance alone or by direct transmission of the same phage type from subject A to subject B. The phage typing data are of greater use when the phage types of isolates from a small epidemic are not all the same. Such information will indicate that the outbreak is due neither to a single source nor to a single strain passing progressively through a susceptible population group.

Phage typing has not been adopted for routine use in service laboratories because of its expense and technical difficulty. It never has been used for laboratory identification of unknown mycobacterial species, although this is a theoretical possibility. Again the expense and technical difficulty preclude such use. In recent years phage typing for epidemiological purposes has been replaced in many laboratories by a much more sensitive technique, restriction fragment-length polymorphism.

V. RESTRICTION FRAGMENT LENGTH POLYMORPHISM

The use of laboratory techniques to support studies of the epidemiology of tuberculosis have been few because of the limited ability of the laboratory to differentiate between specific strains of *M. tuberculosis*. In the past, investigators were forced to depend first on comparisons of drug resistance patterns and later on phage typing data. These methods provided only limited assistance since most strains showed identical drug susceptibility patterns and only a few phage types were known — thus most strains showed the same phage type. This meant that there were no highly specific laboratory tools available to help the epidemiologist study the movement of strains of *M. tuberculosis* through a community or other defined host group.

This deficiency was completely eliminated with the advent of a much more sophisticated technique employing restriction fragment-length polymorphism (RFLP) that detects genotypic variations among members of the species *M. tuberculosis*. These studies have shown that RFLP analysis can be used to obtain a "fingerprint" for each isolate of *M. tuberculosis*. Thus far, it appears that each tubercle bacillus shows a unique fingerprint clearly different from all other isolates. The exception to this rule will be found only when strains are obtained from persons infected by a common source or where persons are tested who have experienced the spread of a particular strain from person to person in a small epidemic. Thus the epidemiologist now has the ultimately sensitive laboratory test to study the epidemiology of tuberculosis.

The most common fingerprinting process depends on the putative insertion sequence IS6110, present in the genome of all *M. tuberculosis* and *M. bovis* strains, and not found in any other mycobacterial species. As a general rule, strains of *M. tuberculosis* contain multiple copies of IS6110, while strains of *M. bovis* contain only a few, although there are a few exceptions.[51,52] This DNA fragment moves about within the chromosome in an almost random manner, but movement is an infrequent event. For each unrelated wild isolate, copies of IS6110 vary in number and location within the chromosome. A restriction enzyme is used that cleaves multiple areas of the chromosome, but cleaves IS6110 at a single site only. It is thus possible to obtain DNA fragments of varying length with which a specific probe, representing a partial sequence of IS6110, will hybridize. The number of fragments produced that will react with the probe will depend on the number of copies of IS6110 in the chromosome. The fingerprint is produced by gel electrophoresis of the digested DNA, which is then transferred to a nylon membrane where the fragments are hybridized with an IS6110-labeled probe. The banding pattern of the DNA fragments of specific sizes constitutes a "fingerprint" unique to each strain.

The IS6110 fingerprinting method has been a very useful tool to study tuberculosis outbreaks. It has been used to study transmission within households, communities, and hospitals.[53-58] Data from these outbreaks (see Figure 5-1) have shown that epidemiologically related groups share organisms

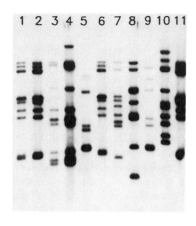

Figure 5-1 Shown above are 11 DNA fingerprints of *M. tuberculosis* isolated from 10 different HIV positive patients. Note that the fingerprints in lanes 1, 2, 6, and 11 are identical although each of these strains was isolated from a different patient. The identity of the fingerprint suggests epidemiologic relatedness. The isolates in lanes 3 and 4 came from the same patient, and are identical as expected. The fingerprints in the other lanes are unique, each representing an isolate from a different patient, each with a distinct fingerprint pattern.

having identical or nearly identical fingerprints, while unrelated isolates have totally different patterns. These outbreaks have demonstrated person-to-person spread that never would have been suspected based on the epidemiological data alone. In some cases the fingerprinting demonstrated that the outbreak had spread to adjacent communities even though the traditional methods of outbreak analysis had failed to reveal any links between the two communities.

Both animal models and *in vitro* studies demonstrate that the fingerprint pattern is very stable, remaining unchanged after passage of *M. tuberculosis* strains through a guinea pig for 2 months and after passage in cultured macrophages for 4 weeks.[54-59] The fingerprints of BCG strains grown in broth cultures for 6 months remain unchanged. Differences in the fingerprint may be limited to only a few bands. That is, the majority of the bands are identical except for one or two that differ in size. The fingerprints of two different cultures of the standard laboratory strain of *M. tuberculosis* designated H37Rv differ in the size of a single band.

The full impact of DNA fingerprinting on the epidemiological study of tuberculosis is yet to unfold. In the future one can expect an increasing fraction of new isolates of *M. tuberculosis* to be fingerprinted as a result of this service being offered by the Mycobacteriology Laboratory at the Centers for Disease Control in Atlanta, Georgia. Of special importance will be the fingerprinting of outbreak strains, of strains isolated from persons having to do with prisons, of strains obtained from health care workers, and of strains obtained from persons who live or are associated with others who are living or working in shelters for the homeless. It is expected that new and unsuspected epidemiological links among many of these persons will be found, and this observation will lead to improved methods of infection control. In some countries such as the Netherlands, all isolates from newly diagnosed patients are being fingerprinted and the fingerprint profile included in a computer-generated data bank. This approach will provide abundant new information regarding the epidemiology of tuberculosis for an entire country.

VI. POLYMERASE CHAIN REACTION

Since its introduction in 1985, the polymerase chain reaction (PCR) has transformed the way DNA analysis is performed.[60] This process involves the *in vitro* synthesis of millions of copies of a specific DNA segment and is based on the annealing and extension of two oligonucleotide primers that flank the target area in the DNA. First the DNA is denatured and then each primer hybridizes to one of the two separated strands so that extension from each 3′ hydroxyl end is directed toward the other. The annealed primers are extended on the template strand with a DNA polymerase. These three steps (denaturation, primer binding, and DNA synthesis) represent a single PCR cycle. Repeated cycles of denaturation, primer annealing, and extension produce an exponential accumulation of a discrete fragment (target). PCR can amplify single- or double-stranded DNA and RNA can serve as a target if reverse transcription is used to make a DNA copy. This technology permits one to amplify a highly specific DNA segment to millions or billions of copies in only a few hours. Thus when once it would have been almost impossible to find a single DNA segment in a sample, PCR permits the amplification of this DNA to such a quantity that it can be detected by simple laboratory means. This technology has made possible new methods for the diagnosis of many infectious diseases including tuberculosis.

To use PCR for detecting *M. tuberculosis* in clinical samples, it first was necessary to identify and characterize a DNA segment within the *M. tuberculosis* chromosome specific and unique for this organism. Hance et al. reported the detection of mycobacteria by PCR using a segment of DNA that codes for the 65-kDa antigen (the gro EL heat shock protein) as the target, however, this DNA segment is present in all mycobacterial species and is not specific for *M. tuberculosis*.[61] Also, PCR using this target technique has not been shown to be sensitive enough for use in clinical samples and it is unlikely to be adopted for widespread clinical use. Manjunath identified a target segment of DNA specific for *M. tuberculosis* and additional PCR methods for diagnosis of tuberculosis have been reported by Pao et al., by Shanker et al., by Sjobring et al., and by Plikaytis et al.[62-66] Boddinghaus et al. used the 16 S ribosomal gene as a PCR target, a segment that is conserved in all mycobacterial species. This target offers the advantage of a high copy number of rRNA sequences, but despite this apparent advantage the reported sensitivity is no higher than that obtained with single-target DNA sequences.[67]

The most attractive target specific for *M. tuberculosis* and *M. bovis* is that described by Eisenach et al.[68] The target sequence is repeated within the *M. tuberculosis* chromosome up to 20 or more times and each individual copy can be amplified using the same primers. This duplication increases the sensitivity by a factor of up to 20 or more compared to those methods that utilize a chromosomal target that occurs only once per chromosome. The target sequence is part of a larger repeated segment that is most probably an insertion sequence that has been designated IS6110.[69] An example of PCR analysis of several clinical sputum samples is shown in Figure 5-2.

In a clinical trial of 314 sputum samples, 93% of the patients with tuberculosis were PCR positive.[70] Among the 104 PCR-positive patients, 83 were smear and culture positive, 2 were smear negative and culture positive, 16 were smear positive and culture negative, and 4 were smear and culture negative. Four patients who had completed or partially completed chemotherapy had PCR positive specimens. Of the 136 specimens obtained from patients who did not have tuberculosis (72 had nontuberculous mycobacterial infection and 64 had no known mycobacterial infection) there were 4 specimens found to be PCR positive. This study demonstrated the utility of the IS6110 PCR assay and it is expected that this assay will be adapted for use to detect *M. tuberculosis* in clinical samples of cerebrospinal fluid, pleural fluid, blood, and tissue. This test will detect low numbers of organisms in a sample, perhaps as few as 10 under ideal circumstances, and it will detect nonviable organisms as well. The problems with any PCR method for the diagnosis of tuberculosis will include the risk of obtaining false-positive results due to contamination of clinical specimens with *M. tuberculosis* DNA product from the PCR laboratory, the inability of the PCR method to detect a difference between viable and nonviable organisms, and the inability of the PCR

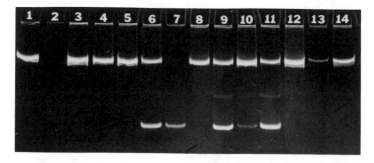

Figure 5-2 Shown above are examples of electrophoretic separation of mycobacterial DNA (amplified by PCR) from clinical sputum samples. Control DNA that produces a 600-base pair PCR product with the same set of primers is included in each test as an internal control. Lanes 1, 3, 4, 5, 8, 12, 13, and 14 show samples from patients without tuberculosis. Lanes 6, 7, 9, 10, and 11 show samples from patients with tuberculosis. The sample fragment migrating more rapidly is the specific amplified target (123 base pairs). The larger fragment, migrating more slowly, is the internal control. Note that lane 2 shows no amplification of control DNA meaning that the reaction was inhibited and the test on this sample must be repeated. Note that in lane 7 control DNA did not amplify, but the tuberculosis specific fragment is amplified. This is because the specific tuberculosis segment combined with all available primers so that no primer was available for annealing with the control DNA.

method to determine drug susceptibility. For the future it should be possible to use PCR methodology to detect drug susceptibility as the genetic mechanisms for drug resistance of *M. tuberculosis* become understood. For those drugs whose resistance mechanism depends on chromosomal mutations, it should be possible to detect these target changes using PCR amplification of the gene in question followed by base analysis of the segment.

VII. TUBERCULOSTEARIC ACID

Tuberculostearic acid (TBSA) is a structural component found in all mycobacterial species and in other members of the *Actinomycetales* such as diptheroids, actinomyces, and nocardia, but not in normal human tissues.[71] It is reasoned that detection of TBSA in body fluids such as sputum, gastric aspirates, urine, cerebrospinal fluid, pleural fluid, ascitic fluid, and tissue extracts would indicate the likely presence of *M. tuberculosis*. A number of studies to evaluate the value of TBSA detection in clinical samples have been reported with mixed results. The expensive technology required and the highly developed skills required of the laboratory worker have limited the availability of testing to a few research laboratories only.

Frequency-pulsed electron-capture gas–liquid chromatography has been used to detect femtomole quantities of TBSA in samples.[72-73] In some situations it would seem possible to diagnose tuberculous meningitis within 3 h. In a study of 40 patients suspected of having active pulmonary tuberculosis who could not produce sputum or whose sputum smears were negative for acid-fast bacilli, 29 were found to have tuberculosis and 23 of these showed positive TBSA tests; there were 2 false positives.[74] Brooks et al. studied clinical cases of tuberculous meningitis with gas–liquid chromatography and reported the specificity to be 91% and the sensitivity to be 95%.[75]

At present this technology should be used to evaluate the cerebrospinal fluid of patients who are suspected of having tuberculous meningitis. The fluid should be sent to the Centers for Disease Control where this test is readily available. Its use to diagnose tuberculosis at other sites is of less value, particularly for pulmonary disease where other mycobacteria may be found as saprophytes or as pathogens and where other actinomycetes may be present as part of the "normal flora." In all these instances one would encounter false positives (see Chapter 4, this volume).

VIII. ADENOSINE DEAMINASE

Adenosine deaminase (ADA) catalyzes the conversion of adenosine to inosine and is released by lymphocytes and macrophages during the cellular immune response. Increased ADA levels have been used to aid in the diagnosis of tuberculous pleural effusions, but this enzyme also is found in inflammatory fluids associated with rheumatoid arthritis, lymphoma, empyema, parapneumonic effusions, and mesothelioma.[76-79] Banales et al. studied 218 consecutive patients with exudative pleural effusions hospitalized in Mexico City.[80] In this population with a relatively high prevalence of tuberculosis, the ADA analysis was a very useful marker for tuberculosis since the determination can be made quickly and at low cost. There were 2.7% false-positive reports for patients who had cancer with pleural effusions and there was one patient with tuberculosis that gave a false-negative ADA value. They reviewed results from 10 other studies and combined these reports with their own and found a sensitivity of 99% and a specificity of 89% for the diagnosis of tuberculosis.

Additional studies have evaluated ADA levels in tuberculous peritonitis and tuberculous meningitis. In those areas where tuberculosis is very prevalent, the test may be very useful. Voigt et al. working in Cape Town, South Africa studied 41 patients with microbiologically confirmed tuberculous peritonitis together with 41 control patients having ascites from other causes such as cirrhosis, tumor, and pancreatitis.[81] They found a sensitivity of 95% and a specificity of 98% in distinguishing between the two groups. However, in geographic regions where exudative reactions of serosal surfaces are not often a result of tuberculosis, the false-positive rate of elevated ADA levels in these fluids is too frequent for the test to be applied broadly.[82]

REFERENCES

1. Arloing, S., Agglutination de becille de la tuberculose vraie, *Compt. Rend. Acad. Sci.*, 136, 1398, 1898.
2. Engvall, E., Perlmann, P., Enzyme-linked immunosorbent assay, ELISA III. Quantation of specific antibodies by enzyme-labeled anti-immunoglobulin in antigen-coated tubes, *J. Immunol.*, 109, 129, 1972.
3. Young, D. B., Kaufmann, S. H. E., Hermans, P. W. M., Thole, J. E. R., Mycobacterial protein antigens: a compliation, *Mol. Microbiol.*, 6, 133, 1992.
4. Daniel, T. M., Janicki, B. W., Mycobacterial antigens: a review of their isolation, chemistry and immunological properties, *Microbiol. Rev.*, 42, 84, 1978.
5. Nassau, E., Parsons, E. R., Johnson, G. D., The detection of antibodies to Mycobacterium tuberculosis by microplate enzyme-linked immunosorbent assay (ELISA), *Tubercle*, 57, 67, 1976.
6. Grange, J. M., Kardijito, T., Serological tests for tuberculosis: can the problem of low specificity be overcome?, *Indian J. Chest Dis.*, 24, 108, 1982.
7. Kalish, S. B., Radin, R. C., Phair, J. P., Levitz, D., Zeiss, C. R., Metzger, E., Use of an enzyme-linked immunosorbent assay technique in the differential diagnosis of active pulmonary tuberculosis in humans, *J. Infect. Dis.*, 147, 523, 1983.
8. Daniel, T. M., Debanne, S. M., van der Kuyp, F., Enzyme-linked immunosorbent assay using *Mycobacterium tuberculosis* antigen 5 and PPD for the serodiagnosis of tuberculosis, *Chest*, 88, 388, 1985.
9. Benjamin, R. G., Debanne, S. M., Ma, Y., Daniel, T. M., Evaluation of mycobacterial antigens in an enzyme-linked immunosorbent assay (ELISA) for the serodiagnosis of tuberculosis, *J. Med. Microbiol.*, 18, 309, 1984.
10. Balestrino, E. A., Daniel, T. M., de Latini, M. D. S., Latini, O. A., Ma, Y., Scocozza, J. B., Serodiagnosis of pulmonary tuberculosis in Argentina by enzyme-linked immunosorbent assay (ELISA) of IgG antibody to *Mycobacterium tuberculosis* antigen 5 and tuberculin purified protein derivative, *Bull. WHO*, 62, 755, 1984.
11. Daniel, T. M., Anderson, P. A., The isolation by immunosorbent affinity chromatography and physiochemical characterization of *Mycobacterium tuberculosis* antigen 5, *Am. Rev. Resp. Dis.*, 117, 533, 1978.
12. Benjamin, R. G., Daniel, T. M., Serodiagnosis of tuberculosis using the enzyme-linked immunosorbent assay (ELISA) of antibody to *Mycobacterium tuberculosis* antigen 5, *Am. Rev. Resp. Dis.*, 126, 1013, 1982.
13. Lau, J. H. K., Long, J. C. Y., Stroebel, A. B., A longitudinal study of antibody titers to antigen 6 in patients with bone and joint tuberculosis, *Int. Orthop.*, 7, 205, 1983.
14. Kiran, U., Shriniwas, K. R., Sharma, A., Efficacy of three mycobacterial antigens in the serodiagnosis of tuberculosis, *Eur. J. Resp. Dis.*, 66, 187, 1985.
15. Reggiardo, Z., Vazquez, E., Comparison of enzyme-linked immunosorbent assay and hemogglutination test using mycobacterial glycolipids, *J. Clin. Microbiol.*, 13, 1007, 1981.
16. Daniel, T. M., Debanne, S. M., The serodiagnosis of tuberculosis and other mycobacterial diseases by enzyme-linked in immunosorbent assay (ELISA), *Am. Rev. Resp. Dis.*, 135, 1137, 1987.
17. Hunter, S. W., Gaylord, H., Brennan, P. J., Structure and antigenicity of the phosphorylated lipopolysaccharide antigens from the leprosy and tubercle bacilli, *J. Biol. Chem.*, 261, 12345, 1986.
18. Sada, E., Brennan, P. J., Herrera, T., Torres, M., Evaluation of lipoarabinommana for the serological diagnosis of tuberculosis, *J. Clin. Microbiol.*, 28, 2587, 1990.
19. Sada, E., Aguilar, D., Torres, M., Herrera, T., Detection of lipoarabinomannan as a diagnostic test for tuberculosis, *J. Clin. Microbiol.*, 30, 2415, 1992.

20. Charpin, D., Herbault, H., Gevaudan, M. J., Saadjian, M., De Micco, P., Arnaud, A., Vervloet, D., Charpin, J., Value of ELISA using A60 antigen in the diagnosis of active pulmonary tuberculosis, *Am. Rev. Resp. Dis.*, 142, 380, 1990.

21. McDonough, J. A., Sada, E., Sippola, A. A., Ferguson, L. E., Daniel, T. M., Microplate and dot immunoassays for the serodiagnosis of tuberculosis, *J. Lab. Clin. Med.*, 120, 318, 1992.

22. Wilkins, E. G. L., Ivanyi, J., Potential value of serology for diagnosis of extrapulmonary tuberculosis, *Lancet*, 336, 641, 1990.

23. Mathai, A., Radhakrishnan, V. V., Thomas, M., Rapid diagnosis of tuberculous meningitis with a dot enzyme immunoassay to detect antibody in cerebrospinal fluid, *Eur. J. Clin. Microbiol. Infect. Dis.*, 10, 440, 1992.

24. Theuer, C. P., Chaisson, R. E., Elias, D., Schecter, G. L., Glassroth, J., Zeiss. C. R., Phair, J. P., Hopewell, P. C., Detection of circulating antibodies to purified protein derivative in tuberculous patients with and without human immunodeficiency virus infection, *Am. Rev. Resp. Dis.*, 139, (Part 2) A395, 1987.

25. Eriki, P. P., Kataaha, P. K., Daniel, T. M., The detection of IgG antibody to a 30,000 dalton antigen of *Mycobacterium tuberculosis* in the serum of HIV-positive and HIV-negative patients in Uganda (abstract), IVth International Conference on AIDS and Associated Cancers in Africa, Marseilles, France, 1989.

26. Daniel, T. M., The rapid diagnosis of tuberculosis: a selective review, *J. Clin. Lab. Med.*, 116, 277, 1990.

27. Sada, E., Ruiz-Palacios, G.M., Lopez-Vidal, Y., Ponce de Leon, S., Detection of mycobacterial antigens in the cerebrospinal fluid of patients with tuberculous meningitis by enzyme-linked immunosorbent assay (ELISA), *Lancet*, 2, 651, 1983.

28. Jacobs, R. F., Eisenach, K. D., Childhood tuberculosis, *Ad. Ped. Infect. Dis.*, 8, 23, 1993.

29. Radhakrishnan, V. V., Mathai, A., Detection of *Mycobacterium tuberculosis* antigen 5 in cerebrospinal fluid by inhibition ELISA and its diagnostic potential in tuberculous meningitis, *J. Infect. Dis.*, 163, 650, 1991.

30. Krambovitis, E., Harris, M., Hughes, D. T. D., Improved serodiagnosis of tuberculosis using two assay test, *J. Clin. Pathol.*, 39, 779, 1986.

31. Wadee, A. A., Boting, L., Reedy, S. G., Antigen capture assay for detection of a 43-kilodalton *Mycobacterium tuberculosis* antigen, *J. Clin. Microbiol.*, 28, 2786, 1990.

32. Radhakrishnan, V. V., Mathai, A., Enzyme-linked immunosorbent assay to detect *Mycobacterium tuberculosis* antigen 5 and antimycobacterial antibody in cerebrospinal fluid of patients with tuberculous meningitis, *J. Clin. Lab. Anal.*, 5, 233, 1991.

33. Sada, E., Anguilar, D., Torres, M., Lipoarabinomannan antigenemia in patients with AIDS and tuberculosis. Presented at the 31st Interscience Conference on Antimicrobial Agents and Chemotherapy, Chicago, September 1991.

34. Lim, S. D., Todd, J., Lopez, J., Ford, E., Janda, J. M., Genotypic identification of pathogenic mycobacterium species by using a non-radioactive oligonucleotide probe, *J. Clin. Microbiol.*, 29, 1276, 1991.

35. Gonalez, R., Hanna, B. A., Evaluation of Gen-Probe DNA hybridization systems for the identification of *Mycobacterium tuberculosis* and *Mycobacterium avium-intracellulare*, *Diagn. Microbiol. Infect. Dis.*, 8, 69, 1980.

36. Musial, C. E., Tice, L. S., Stockman, L., Roberts, G. D., Identification of mycobacteria from culture by using the Gen-Probe rapid diagnostic system for *Mycobacterium avium* complex and *Mycobacterium tuberculosis* complex, *J. Clin. Microbiol.*, 26, 2120, 1988.

37. Sderman, I., Sherman, I., Harrington, N., Rothrock, A., George, H., Use of a cutoff range in identifying mycobacteria by the Gen-Probe rapid diagnostic system, *J. Clin. Microbiol.*, 27, 241, 1989.

38. Goto, M., Oka, S., Okuzumi, K., Kimura, S., Shimada, K., Evaluation of acridinium-ester labeled DNA probes for identification of *Mycobacterium tuberculosis* and *Mycobacterium avium* — *Mycobacterium intracellulare* complex in culture, *J. Clin. Microbiol.*, 29, 2473, 1991.

39. Jacobs, R. E., Eisenach, K. D., Childhood tuberculosis, *Ad. Ped. Infect. Dis.*, 8, 23, 1993.

40. Body, B., Warren, N. G., Spicer, A., Henderson, D., Chery, M., Use of Gen-Probe and BACTEC for rapid isolation and identification of mycobacteria correlation of probe results with growth index, *Am. J. Clin. Pathol.*, 93, 415, 1990.

41. Gardner, G. M., Weiser, R. S., A bacteriophage for *Mycobacterium smegmates*, *Proc. Soc. Exp. Biol. Med.*, 66, 205, 1947.

42. Hnatko, S. I., The isolation of bacteriophages for mycobacteria with reference to phage typing of the genus, *Can. J. Med. Sci.*, 31, 462, 1953.

43. Froman, S., Will, D. W., Bogen, E., Bacteriophage active against virulent *Mycobacterium tuberculosis*, *Am. J. Public Health*, 44, 1326, 1954.

44. Ward, D. M., Redmond, W. B., Spotting method of phage typing of mycobacteria, *Am. Rev. Resp. Dis.*, 85, 883, 1962.

45. Redmond, W. B., Cater, J. D., A bacteriophage specific for *Mycobacterium tuberculosis*, varieties hominis and bovis, *Am. Rev. Resp. Dis.*, 82, 781, 1960.

46. Murohashi, T., Tokunago, T., Mizuguchi, Y., Maruyama, Y., Phage typing of slow-growing mycobacteria, *Am. Rev. Resp. Dis.*, 88, 664, 1963.

47. Bates, J. H., Fitzhugh, J. K., Subdivision of the species *M. tuberculosis* by mycobacteriophage typing, *Am. Rev. Resp. Dis.*, 96, 7, 1967.

48. Bates, J. H., Mitchison, D. A., Geographic distribution of bacteriophage types of *Mycobacterium tuberculosis*, *Am. Rev. Resp. Dis.*, 100, 189, 1969.

49. Rado, T. A., Bates, J. H., Engel, H. W. B., Mankiewicz, E., Murohashi, T., Mizuguchi, Y., Sula, L., World Health Organization studies on bacteriophage typing of mycobacteria. Subdivision of the species *Mycobacterium tuberculosis*, *Am. Rev. Resp. Dis.*, 111, 459, 1975.

50. Crawford, J., Bates, J. H., Phage typing of mycobacteria, in *The Mycobacteria,* Part A, Kubica, G., Wayne, L. G., Eds., Marcel Dekker, New York, 1984, 123.

51. Cave, M. D., Eisenach, K. D., McDermott, P. F., Bates, J. H., Crawford, J. T., IS6110: conservation of sequence in the *Mycobacterium tuberculosis* complex and its utilization in DNA fingerprinting, *Mol. Cell Probes* 5, 73, 1991.

52. van Soollingen, D., Hermans, P. W. M., Haas, P. E., Soll, D. R., van Embden, J. D. A., Occurrence and stability of insertion sequences in *Mycobacterium tuberculosis* complex strains: evaluation of an insertion sequence-dependent DNA polymorphism as a tool in the epidemiology of tuberculosis, *J. Clin. Microbiol.*, 4, 2578, 1991.

53. Mazurek, G. H., Cave, M. D., Eisenach, K. D., Wallace, R. J., Bates, J. H., Crawford, J. T., Chromosomal DNA fingerprint patterns produced with IS6110 as strain-specific markers for epidemiologic study of tuberculosis, *J. Clin. Microbiol.*, 29, 2030, 1991.

54. van Soolingen, D., Herman, P. W. M., Haas, P. E., Soll, D. R., van Embden, J. D. A., Occurrence and stability of insertion sequence-dependent DNA polymorphism as a tool in the epidemiology of tuberculosis, *J. Clin. Microbiol.*, 4, 2578, 1991.

55. Daley, C. L., Small, P. M., Schechter, G. S., Schoolnik, G. K., McAdam, R. A., Jacobs, W. R., Hopewell, P. C., An outbreak of tuberculosis with accelerated progression among persons infected with human immunodeficiency virus, *N. Engl. J. Med.*, 326, 231, 1992.

56. Pearson, M., Jereb, J. A., Frieden, T. R., Crawford, J. T., Davis, B. J., Dooley, S. W., Jarvis, W. R., Nosocomial transmission of multidrug-resistant *Mycobacterium tuberculosis*, *Ann. Intern. Med.*, 117, 191, 1992.

57. Edlin, B. R., Tokars, J. I., Grieco, M. H., Crawford, J. T., Williams, J., Sordillo, E. M., Ong, K. R., Kilburn, J. O., Dooley, S. W., Castro, K. G., Jarvis, W. R., Holmberg, S. D., An outbreak of multidrug-resistant tuberculosis among hospitalized patients with acquired immunodeficiency syndrome, *N. Engl. J. Med.*, 326, 1514, 1992.

58. Beck-Sague, C., Dooley, S. W., Hutton, M. D., Otten, J., Bruden, A., Crawford, J. T., Pitchenik, A. E., Woodley, C., Cauthen, G., Jarvis, W., Hospital outbreak of multidrug-resistant Mycobacterium tuberculosis infections, *J. Am. Med. Assoc.*, 268, 1280, 1992.

59. Hermans, P. W. M., van Soolingen, D., Dale, J. W., Schuikema, A. R. J., McAdams, R. A., Catty, D., van Embden, J. D. A., Insertion element IS986 from *Mycobacterium tuberculosis*: a useful tool for diagnosis and epidemiology of tuberculosis, *J. Clin. Microbiol.*, 28, 2051, 1990.

60. Mullis, K. B., Faloona, F., Specific synthesis of DNA in vitro via a polymerase catalyzed chain reaction, *Methods Enzymol.*, 155, 335, 1987.

61. Hance, A. J., Grandchamp, B., Lavy-Frebault, V., Lecossier, D., Rauzier, J., Bocart, D., Gicqual, B., Detection of mycobacteria by amplification of mycobacterial DNA, *Mol. Microbiol.*, 3, 843, 1989.

62. Manjunath, N., Evaluation of a polymerase chain reaction for the diagnosis of tuberculosis, *Tubercle,* 72, 21, 1991.

63. Pao, C. C., Yen, T. S. B., You, J. B., Maa, J. S., Fiss, E. H., Chang, C. H., Detection and identification of *Mycobacterium tuberculosis* by DNA amplification, *J. Clin. Microbiol.*, 28, 1877, 1990.

64. Shankar, P., Manjunath, N., Lakshmi, R., Aditi, B., Seth, P., Shriniwas, K., Identification of *Mycobacterium tuberculosis* by polymerase chain reaction, *Lancet,* 355, 423, 1990.

65. Sjobring, U., Mecklenburg, M., Anderson, A. B., Miorner, M., Polymerase chain reaction for detection of *Mycobacterium tuberculosis*, *J. Clin. Microbiol.*, 28, 2200, 1990.

66. Plikaytis, B. B., Eisenach, K. D., Crawford, J. T., Shinnick, T. M., Differentiation of *Mycobacterium tuberculosis* and *Mycobacterium bovis* by a polymerase chain reaction assay, *Mol. Cell Probes,* 5, 215, 1991.

67. Boddinghaus, B., Rogall, T., Flohr, T., Blocker, H., Bottger, E. C., Detection and identification of mycobacteria by amplification of r RNA, *J. Clin. Microbiol.,* 28, 1751, 1990.

68. Eisenach, K. D., Cave, M. D., Bates, J. H., Crawford, J. T., Polymerase chain reaction amplification of a repetitive DNA sequence specific for *Mycobacterium tuberculosis, J. Infect. Dis.,* 161, 977, 1990.

69. Thierry, D., Cave, M. D., Eisenach, K. D., Crawford, J. T., Bates, J. H., Gicqual, B., Guesdon, T. L., IS6110, and IS-like element of *Mycobacterium tuberculosis* complex, *Nucl. Acids Res.,* 18, 188, 1990.

70. Eisenach, K. D., Sifford, M. D., Cave, M. D., Bates, J. H., Crawford, J. T., Detection of *Mycobacterium tuberculosis* in sputum samples using a polymerase chain reaction, *Am. Rev. Resp. Dis.,* 144, 1160, 1991.

71. Anderson, R. J., Chargaff, E., The chemistry of the lipids of tubercle bacilli. VI. Concerning tuberculostearic acid and phthioic acid from the acetone-soluble fat, *J. Biol. Chem.,* 85, 77, 1929.

72. Brooks, J. B., Craven, R. B., Schlossberg, D., Alley, C. C., Pritts, F. M., Possible use of frequency-pulse-modulated electron capture gas-liquid etromalography to identify septic and aseptic causes of pleural effusions, *J. Clin. Microbiol.,* 8, 203, 1978.

73. Brooks, J. B., Daneshvar, M. I., Fast, D. M., Good, R. C., Selective procedures for detecting femtomole quantities of tuberculostearic acid in serum and cerebrospinal fluid by frequency-pulsed electron-capture gas-liquid chromatography, *J. Clin. Microbiol.,* 25, 1201, 1987.

74. Pang, J. A., Chan, H. S., Chan, C. Y., Cheung, S. W., French, G. L., A tuberculostearic acid assay in the diagnosis of sputum smear-negative pulmonary tuberculosis, *Ann. Intern. Med.,* 111, 650, 1989.

75. Brooks, J. B., Daneshvar, M. I., Haberberger, R. L., Mikhail, I. A., Rapid diagnosis of tuberculous meningitis by frequency-pulsed electron-capture gas-liquid chromatography detection of carboxylic acids in cerebrospinal fluid, *J. Clin. Microbiol.,* 28, 989, 1990.

76. Petterson, T., Osala, K., Weber, T. H., Adenosine deaminase in the diagnosis of pleural effusions, *Acta Med. Scand.,* 215, 299, 1984.

77. Ocana, I., Martinez-Vazquez, J. M., Segura, R. M., Fernandez de Sevilla, T., Capdevila, J. A., Adenosine deaminase in pleural fluid. Test for diagnosis of tuberculous pleural effusion, *Chest,* 84, 51, 1983.

78. Maritz, F. J., Malan, C., le Roux, I., ADA estimations in the differentiation of pleural effusions, *S. Afr. Med. J.,* 62, 556, 1982.

79. Strankinga, W. F., Navta, J. J., Straub, J. P., Stam, J., Adenosine deaminase activity in tuberculous pleural effusions: a diagnostic test, *Tubercle,* 68, 137, 1987.

80. Banales, J. L., Pineda, P. R., Fitzgerald, J. M., Rubio, H., Selman, M., Salazar-Legama, M., Adenosine deaminase in the diagnosis of tuberculous pleural effusions, *Chest,* 99, 355, 1991.

81. Voigt, M. D., Kalvaria, I., Trey, C., Berman, P., Lombard, C., Kirsch, R. E., Diagnostic value of ascites adenosine deaminase in tuberculous peritonitis, *Lancet,* 1, 751, 1989.

82. Van Keimpema, A. R., Sloats, E. H., Wagenaar, J. P., Adenosine deaminase activity, not diagnostic for tuberculous pleurisy, *Eur. J. Resp. Dis.,* 71, 15, 1987.

Chapter 6

Pulmonary Tuberculosis: Primary, Reactivation, HIV Related, and Non-HIV Related

Lloyd N. Friedman, M.D. and Peter A. Selwyn, M.D., M.P.H.

CONTENTS

I. PRIMARY PULMONARY TUBERCULOSIS

Historically, primary pulmonary tuberculosis has been a childhood infection (see Chapter 10, this volume). However, the frequency of infection has declined markedly, and many uninfected persons now are susceptible to infection. Myers et al. showed the prevalence of tuberculous infection in Minnesota schoolchildren to be 47.3% in 1926, 18.9% in 1936, and only 3.9% in 1954.[1] Although rates may be higher in other parts of the country, it would not be unusual today for an elderly person to be newly exposed to tuberculosis and to develop primary disease.

Although the majority of air is drawn into the lower lobes, it has been shown in autopsy studies by Ghon that the primary focus of tuberculosis is equally distributed between the upper and lower lobes, with a slight predilection for the right lung.[2] Palmer stated that primary pulmonary tuberculosis is more common in the upper lobes.[3] On chest radiographic readings, Poulsen showed a predilection for disease in the mid-lung fields with an equal distribution of the remainder between upper and lower zones.[4] Segmental atelectasis was much more common in the upper lobes in studies by Frostad[5] and Weber et al.[6] and similar but less pronounced differences were found by Daly.[7] In most studies, even the anterior segment of the upper lobes have a substantial number of primary complexes and atelectatic segments. Thus, an upper lobe infiltrate may represent either primary or reactivated disease.

Lymphadenopathy is common in primary tuberculosis and may exceed by far the size of the original parenchymal focus.[8] Lymphadenopathy plays a major role in the pathogenesis of atelectasis, sometimes referred to as epituberculosis,[2] and also plays a major role in the obstructive emphysema seen in children in as many as 34% of cases of primary tuberculosis.[5-9] The long-term sequelae of lymphadenopathy with airway involvement may be bronchostenosis, bronchiectasis, or both.

In an important study by Poulsen[4,10] of 517 Faroe Islanders, an attempt was made to document the initial time and subsequent sequelae of tuberculous infection. The Pirquet test, a scarification procedure utilizing old tuberculin, was used to document conversion. Although it is a less sensitive test than the Mantoux test, it is not clear whether this biased the findings once the group of convertors was assembled.

Initial fever was reported in 430 (83%) of the 517 known convertors. The temperature was as high as 40.5°C with more than 30% of persons having temperatures above 39.5°C. In many cases, the patients were completely unaware of the presence of fever. Although today, most patients with primary infection are thought to be asymptomatic, 117 (27%) of 430 persons in Poulsen's study with initial fever had subjective symptoms that most commonly included retrosternal and side pain, and rarely, cough, fatigue, sore throat, and joint pain. The retrosternal pain began with the onset of fever, lasted a week or two, and usually was exacerbated by swallowing. The duration of fever most commonly was 2 weeks, and was less than 6 weeks in more than 90% of persons.

Erythema nodosum occurred in 78 (15%) of cases, predominantly on the shins of women and children, and appeared to coincide with the onset of delayed hypersensitivity. In five instances it involved the arms.

There were 139 (27%) of 517 convertors with parenchymal infiltrates consistent with primary tuberculosis, 44% of which were demonstrated in the first month after conversion. Hilar adenitis, more often right sided and often bilateral, occurred with or without infiltrates in 333 (64%) of cases and was more common in children. The incidence of radiographic abnormalities was even higher, i.e., 86%, in persons studied during the initial fever.

Much of this study was similar to the work of Gedde-Dahl, who studied 272 tuberculin convertors (Pirquet test) and found that 41% had a primary lesion on chest radiograph and 35% had hilar adenitis. He also found erythema nodosum to be more common in women and children, and stated that its presence indicated a less favorable prognosis.[11]

Lincoln and Sewell stated that the primary presentation of tuberculosis may mimic a typical bacterial pneumonia with fever, chills, and a lobar infiltrate.[12] Any process that causes air space consolidation cannot be distinguished from primary pulmonary tuberculosis. In addition, diseases that cause lymph node enlargement such as sarcoidosis and lymphoma may mimic primary disease.

Often the only residua of a primary tuberculous infection are a positive skin test and the Ranke complex. The Ranke complex comprises the small fibrotic parenchymal Ghon focus with an associated calcified lymph node.[13] Although the complex often is called the Ghon complex, the association of the parenchymal infiltrate and lymph node originally was made by Parrot in 1876, the significance of the association first was made clear by Kuss,[14] and the term "primary complex" was coined by Ranke.[15]

Progressive primary pulmonary tuberculosis is a condition where the primary parenchymal disease progresses either at the site of the Ghon focus, or elsewhere, usually in the upper lobes.[13] It had been reported up to 10 years after the onset of primary disease in untreated individuals,[4,11] but many of these individuals initially had normal chest radiographs and today probably would have been classified as having reactivation tuberculosis. In Gedde-Dahl's study of tuberculin convertors, 33 (12.1%) of 272 convertors developed "progressive primary tuberculosis," with 20 (7.4%) progressing in the first year, but these were not separated by initial radiographic findings. In Poulsen's study, 20 (3.9%) of 517 infected persons with an initial parenchymal infiltrate developed progressive primary pulmonary disease with 3 (0.6%) progressing in the first year. However, today, with modern screening and therapy, it would be very unusual to see progressive primary tuberculosis ensue after initial presentation and treatment, unless the disease was unresponsive to therapy.

Cavitation was described as a sequela of this process in 8 (11%) of 78 persons with primary parenchymal infiltrates in Gedde-Dahl's group and 4 (3%) of 139 persons with primary parenchymal infiltrates in Poulsen's group.

Lincoln and Sewell stated that calcifications may occur within 6 months in infants, require at least 1 year in children, and take longer to appear in adults. In 964 children who survived primary pulmonary tuberculosis, 90% had definite calcifications on chest radiograph.[12]

Patients with primary tuberculosis often have a cough, but rarely produce adequate sputum. Gastric aspiration sometimes is successful in obtaining organisms, but as a rule, the diagnosis is based most often on the clinical findings, exposure history, radiographic findings, and skin test status. Bronchoscopy may be useful because of the high incidence of endobronchial lesions, i.e., 28%, in Weber's study.[6]

A. LOWER LOBE TUBERCULOSIS IN ADULTS

Lower lobe tuberculosis is becoming more prevalent in adults, with involvement in as many as 7%

of pulmonary tuberculosis cases.[16] It has been described recently in several studies and is thought to be more prevalent in AIDS, diabetes, pregnancy, the elderly, and persons on steroid therapy.[16-19] It may reflect partially an increasing incidence of primary disease in older persons.

II. REACTIVATION PULMONARY TUBERCULOSIS

Reactivation, or postprimary, pulmonary tuberculosis (see Chapter 10, this volume), refers to tuberculous disease that occurs after the primary infection has resolved. When an apical calcified focus (Simon focus) or a granuloma or caseous node with dormant tuberculous organisms reactivates, the delayed hypersensitivity response may lead to massive inflammation, necrosis, liquefaction, and cavitation. The infection may involve the airways and spread to other parts of the lung, and uncommonly involves the lymph nodes. The reactivation focus usually was seeded in the well-oxygenated upper lobes during the primary lymphohematogenous dissemination, and reactivation occurs most often within 10 years after the primary infection. Adler found that 85% of the dominant tuberculous lesions in adults were in the apical or posterior segment of an upper lobe, and that an additional 9.5% were in the superior segment of a lower lobe.[20] Although it has been stated that reactivation tuberculosis almost never occurs solely in the anterior segment of an upper lobe, Spencer et al. recently described 9 adult patients with predominantly or solely anterior segment tuberculosis,[21] and Adler showed that 3% of dominant lesions occurred in the anterior segment with an additional 36% of secondary lesions in that segment.[20] Tuberculosis of the basilar segments was described as a dominant lesion in 1.9% of patients, and as a secondary lesion in 23.2% of patients in Adler's study.

Contrary to popular opinion, the presence of intrathoracic lymphadenopathy does not rule out reactivation tuberculosis. Woodring et al. found that 5% of definite cases of reactivation tuberculosis were associated with lymphadenopathy.[22]

There are numerous radiographic findings in tuberculosis. Fraser et al.[13] define "local exudative tuberculosis" as a patchy or confluent air-space consolidation, sometimes with cavitation, and "local fibrocaseous or fibrocalcific tuberculosis" as a finding where "the relatively poor definition of the exudative lesion is replaced by a more sharply defined shadow, usually somewhat irregular and angular in contour." Bronchogenic spread refers to a picture of bronchopneumonia where the contents of a cavity have spilled into the airways and have been aspirated into an entire segment, lobe, or lung.

It has the features of a typical bacterial pneumonia, with lower lobe involvement in 19% of cases,[23] and a toxic appearing patient.

A. CAVITATION

Vascular involvement is common in the area of active infection, and vessels may show both vasculitis and thrombosis. Endarteritis obliterans may occur and lead to necrosis and cavitation, frequent findings in advanced reactivation tuberculosis.[24] Hadlock et al.[23] found cavitation in 51% of cases of reactivation disease, Woodring et al.[25] found cavitation in 45% of cases, and Choyke et al.[26] found cavitation in 7.7% of cases. The cavitation may be solitary or multiple, may vary in size and shape, may have a variable thick or thin wall, and may be internally nodular.[13,27] An air fluid level may be present and, in one study, was demonstrated in 20% of cases.[25] Changes in the cavity size or tension in the cavity may develop due to impaired drainage.[27] The cavity may rupture into the pleural space and cause an empyema. Cavities also may be a source of bleeding. A locally dilated artery in the wall of a cavity (Rasmussen's aneurysm) may cause exsanguination or, more commonly, asphyxia.[28,29] Such hemoptysis may require management with angiographic embolization.[30] As the process resolves, the natural course of the cavity is to diminish gradually in size. However, it may persist and lead to further complications such as the development of an aspergilloma.

III. ASPERGILLOMA

The Research Committee of the British Thoracic and Tuberculosis Association studied 544 treated tuberculosis patients with cavities greater than 2.5 cm in diameter who had been culture negative for at least 1 year and found 61 (12%) to have an aspergilloma.[31] The most likely time for development of the aspergilloma in that study was within 7 to 11 years after the diagnosis of cavitary tuberculosis.[32] Another study found the average latency period to be 8.5 years.[33] Hemoptysis is common, and may be massive, but rarely leads to exsanguination. Asphyxia is the major risk. Most of the patients in a study by Tomlinson and Sahn presented with varying degrees of hemoptysis, and 10 patients underwent surgical resection for massive or recurrent hemoptysis. Recommendations for management varied from watchful waiting to arterial embolization to surgical resection.[33]

IV. ENDOBRONCHIAL TUBERCULOSIS

Endobronchial involvement was described previously as a complication of advanced cavitary tuberculosis where the airway becomes infected and tracheobronchitis ensues.[34] However, it has been described with and without parenchymal involvement in adults and the elderly,[35] and may be due to lymph node erosion.[36] There often is peripheral collapse of the involved segment or lobe, and bronchostenosis is a common sequela.[36] The sputum is not necessarily smear positive, and in one study, 85% of cases with demonstrated endobronchial involvement were sputum smear negative.[37] In three patients with endobronchial tuberculosis and AIDS, tumor like masses were seen, and even so, spontaneously induced sputum smears were negative.[38]

Bronchostenosis may occur due to inflammation and scarring of the bronchus, and bronchiectasis may result from bronchostenosis and obstructive pneumonitis with distal bronchiectasis, or it may occur from chronic scarring of the parenchyma with traction on the bronchus. Broncholithiasis also has been reported, usually as a complication of old inactive disease.[13]

V. TUBERCULOMA

A tuberculoma may occur during primary or reactivation tuberculosis. It is a smooth, round, or ovoid lesion ranging in size from 0.5 to 4.0 cm in diameter.[39,40] Satellite lesions may be identified nearby in 80% of cases.[40] Tuberculomas may be multiple and are mistaken easily for coin lesions or metastatic disease.[18] The lesions may or may not be active, and may or may not be calcified, but activity has been reported to correlate directly with size. Cavitation may occur in 10–50% of tuberculomas but lymphadenopathy is a very rare association.[3]

VI. PNEUMOTHORAX AND BRONCHOPLEURAL FISTULA

A pneumothorax or pneumomediastinum may occur at any time during the disease process, even with miliary tuberculosis,[41] and probably is due to subpleural disease with formation of a cyst and subsequent rupture.

A bronchopleural fistula usually is due to rupture of a tuberculous cavity. It is a feared complication, for if the cavity is active, an empyema will result. The tear may be 1 mm to 4 cm in size,[42] and cure often requires a definitive surgical procedure.[43]

VII. ENDOCRINOLOGIC MANIFESTATIONS

Hyponatremia commonly is associated with tuberculosis and was present in 56 (10.7%) of 522 new consecutively diagnosed cases in one study.[44] The mechanism has been shown to involve the inappropriate secretion of antidiuretic hormone.[45] The syndrome resolves after several weeks of antituberculous therapy.

Hypercalcemia also is commonly associated with tuberculosis, and was present in a study by Abassi et al. in 22 (28%) of 79 patients with tuberculosis.[46] However, 95% of the patients were receiving supplemental vitamin D. Interestingly, all patients were normocalcemic on admission, and the onset of hypercalcemia occurred within 4 to 16 weeks after therapy was started. Calcium levels returned to normal over a period of 1 to 7 months, despite the continuation of vitamin D supplementation. Resolution of the hypercalcemia appeared to correlate with the conversion to a negative sputum. Candranel et al. recently confirmed the participation of the pulmonary macrophage by showing that conversion of 25-hydroxyvitamin D to 1,25-dihydroxyvitamin D was performed *in vitro* by pulmonary macrophages from a patient with pulmonary tuberculosis, but stated that the participation of macrophages was not enough to explain entirely the hypercalcemia associated with tuberculosis.[47]

VIII. RADIOLOGIC DIFFERENTIAL

Radiologic findings of other diseases may mimic tuberculosis (see Chapter 10, this volume). Upper lobe infiltrates and cavitation with or without fibrosis may be seen with atypical mycobacteria, sarcoidosis, ankylosing spondylitis, aspiration pneumonia, silicosis, Wegener's granulomatosis and other collagen vascular diseases, adenosquamous cancer, lymphomas (especially Hodgkins), infarcts, and actinomycosis.[48] Upper lobe bullous disease may be seen in emphysema and neurofibromatosis, and may mimic cavitary disease, especially where there is a periemphysematous infection.

In the setting of HIV infection, pulmonary tuberculosis often must be distinguished radiologically from bacterial pneumonia, upper lobe *Pneumocystis carinii* pneumonia, which may occur in the setting of chronic aerosolized pentamidine administration, and, less commonly, nocardia and rhodococcus infections.[49,50]

IX. DIAGNOSIS OF TUBERCULOSIS
A. HISTORY AND PHYSICAL
In pursuit of the diagnosis of tuberculosis, the history and physical examination are notoriously misleading. Reactivation tuberculosis develops insidiously and may exist for months with few symptoms. The classic symptoms of cough, hemoptysis, fever, night sweats, and weight loss rarely are seen concurrently except in advanced disease. The patient may present acutely during an upper respiratory

viral infection or a superinfecting bacterial pneumonia, and it may appear that the tuberculous condition is causing the acute presentation, but often the tuberculous process has been present for months. In a study of preemployment screening where 9 (0.9%) of 970 adults had active tuberculosis, the only sensitive indicator was the presence of a cough. Other symptoms were present variably, and none of the subjects felt ill enough to seek medical attention independently, despite the presence, in some, of far advanced disease.[51]

Even when symptoms and signs are present they are not specific for tuberculosis. Weight loss is seen in many diseases. Night sweats are reported in persons with nontuberculous infections, cancer, and even heavy alcohol or drug use. The physical exam sometimes adds little to the evaluation, and the classic posttussive rales often are absent in the area of involvement. Although choroidal tubercles were shown in one study[52] to be present in 30% of patients with pulmonary tuberculosis and were thought to be a specific finding, this has not been tested widely. Therefore, the appropriate use of the history and physical examination is to prompt the physician to order a chest radiograph, sputum analysis, or both where the suspicion of tuberculosis is present.

The PPD has little use in the evaluation of reactivation tuberculosis. A positive test does not indicate that an infiltrate is tubercular in nature, and a negative test that shows less than 5 mm of induration to 5 TU of PPD has been reported in 17.4 to 21.0% of cases of active tuberculosis (see Chapter 13, this volume).[53-55]

B. SMEAR, CULTURE, AND BRONCHOSCOPY

The diagnosis of tuberculosis hinges on the procurement of several adequate sputum samples for analysis and culture. Sputum AFB smears are estimated to be positive in 65–75% of patients who have had multiple specimens, and 30–40% of those with a single specimen.[56] In 1991, there were 22,829 reported cases in which pulmonary tuberculosis was a major or additional site of disease.[56a] Of these, 17,671 (77%) were documented by culture of any lung specimen,[56a] 14,859 (65%) were sputum-culture-positive, and 8576 (38%) were both sputum-smear- and culture-positive (Centers for Disease Control and Prevention, unpublished data).

The early morning sputum is the best specimen for the diagnosis of pulmonary tuberculosis. Pooled specimens are not advised because of problems with contamination.[57] It is recommended that if acid-fast bacilli are present on two of three morning specimens, it is unnecessary to continue collections. However, if no acid-fast bacilli are seen, and if tuberculosis is suspected strongly, it is recommended that sputum collection continue, although there is little advantage to collecting more than five sputa per patient.[57] If the patient is unable to produce sputum, then sputum induction with normal or hypertonic saline should be attempted. The specimen should be labeled clearly as an induced specimen because its watery nature may cause the laboratory to mistake the sample for saliva and discard it. Another effective technique is the early morning gastric aspiration of 50 ml of fluid after an 8 to 10 h fast. This modality is especially useful in children or patients who do not produce sputum. Gastric aspirates should be processed within 4 h or else be neutralized to a pH of 7.0 and stored under refrigeration. Gastric smears are not thought to be reliable due to the possibility of atypical mycobacterial contaminants in food. However, in a small study in Louisiana, Klotz and Penn showed that where AFBs were identified on smear, they always were associated with true typical or atypical mycobacterial disease.[58] Urine may be collected and, in one study, was reported positive in 4.7% of cases of pulmonary tuberculosis without evidence of renal disease by history, physical, or urinalysis.[59] The author stated that asymptomatic tubercle bacilluria, even without pyuria or IVP abnormalities, always represents genitourinary tuberculosis. This assumption has not been proven. It certainly is possible that bacilluria can occur during bacteremia without infecting the kidneys. If the patient is very sick and the process is thought to be disseminated, blood cultures also may be drawn. They are very useful in HIV-related tuberculosis, and have been shown to be positive in as many as 38% of such cases.[60]

If sputum cannot be obtained, or if it is imperative to make an immediate diagnosis, bronchoscopy is the next best course of action.[61] Bronchoscopy has been shown clearly to aid in the immediate diagnosis of tuberculosis. Danek and Bower obtained 34% positive smear and 95% positive culture results with brushings, washings, and biopsies in 41 sputum smear-negative patients.[62] De Gracia et al. obtained 18% positive smear and 88% positive culture results with lavage in 17 patients with smear-negative tuberculosis.[63] Wallace et al. analyzed 22 patients with documented smear-negative pulmonary tuberculosis and found that, for a single procedure, the best yield for an immediate diagnosis was 30% with a transbronchial biopsy procedure that included histology and AFB stains.[64] The biopsy was exclusively positive in 26% of patients and had a far better yield than brushings or washings. Postbronchoscopy smears were considered part of the bronchoscopy procedure and added an additional 9%. However, the prebronchoscopy sputa proved to be a more sensitive test for culture diagnosis than bronchoscopic cultures, 67 versus 44%, although the bronchoscopy cultures occasionally were positive where the sputum culture was negative. Stenson et al. also obtained their highest yield (75%) by prebronchoscopy sputa.[65] The lower yield on bronchoscopy has been thought to be due in part to the mycobacterial inhibitory effects of the lidocaine employed as an anesthetic during the bronchoscopic procedure.[66,67] Based on these studies, one may conclude that it is important to perform a complete bronchoscopic procedure where indicated, including biopsy and lavage, and that all specimens should be stained and cultured. It also is important to collect postbronchoscopy sputa. For information on diagnostic modalities in HIV-related tuberculosis, see Section X.

Careful cleaning of the bronchoscope is essential to reduce the risk of cross-contamination of specimens,[68] and the risk of actual transmission of tuberculosis to the next patient in whom bronchoscopy is performed.[69] Various cleaning regimens and solutions have been recommended, and glutaraldehyde, phenol, or ethylene oxide are effective agents.[70-72]

Rapid diagnostic methods are discussed in Chapter 5 (this volume).

X. HIV INFECTION AND PULMONARY TUBERCULOSIS

The presentation of pulmonary tuberculosis in patients early in the course of HIV disease may not be different from the presentation in the normal host. Tuberculosis early in the course of HIV disease tends to occur at a CD4 count of 300 cells per mm^3 or less.[49,50,73,74] The skin test may be less reactive, but otherwise the body still is capable of responding to and controlling tuberculosis in the usual way.[49,75] However, as noted earlier, the development of tuberculosis in HIV-positive patients often indicates that other AIDS-related illnesses will follow soon.[76-78] Where tuberculosis develops in persons with preexisting AIDS, the T helper cell count usually is low,[79] and both cell-mediated immunity and delayed-type hypersensitivity are depressed. The body is less able to fight the infection, but also is less able to respond with destructive processes such as caseation, liquefaction, and cavitation.[19,80] Tuberculous pneumonia may present typically, and has been associated with cavitation, or it may present atypically with a diffuse or miliary pattern, a mid or lower lung field infiltrate, and, frequently, hilar adenopathy.[19,49,81] In fact, AIDS patients occasionally may present with pulmonary tuberculosis and a normal chest radiograph. It is not clear what proportion of tuberculosis in AIDS patients represents primary versus reactivation tuberculosis, and, indeed, there is evidence for both mechanisms.

Data from early in the AIDS epidemic, and especially among HIV-infected patients who did not have AIDS at the time they were diagnosed with tuberculosis, suggested that reactivation of latent infection was the main mechanism to explain the increased risk of tuberculosis in AIDS.[49,50,82-84] Data from Selwyn et al.[85] indicated that HIV-infected drug users with previously positive skin tests developed active tuberculosis at a rate 20 times greater than that among HIV-infected drug users without previously positive skin tests. No cases of active tuberculosis developed in HIV-seronegative drug users in the same patient population, even in those with prior positive tuberculin tests. However, recent data, especially those obtained through investigations of nosocomial outbreaks of tuberculosis among HIV-infected patients, have indicated that primary infection with *M. tuberculosis* and rapid disease progression also may be an important mechanism for the increased risk of tuberculosis in this population, especially in late-stage AIDS patients.[86-90] Studies by Di Perri et al. and Daley et al. documented high tuberculosis attack rates and rapid disease progression within weeks to months in HIV-infected patients exposed to an active tuberculosis index case in a residential or hospital setting.[87,88] Some of these investigations have been carried out through the use of restriction fragment-length polymorphisms and other molecular genetic techniques that enable investigators to link cases epidemiologically and to document person-to-person transmission.[86,87,90] These data strongly suggest that highly immunosuppressed patients may be at risk not only for acquiring tuberculosis but also for developing symptomatic disease in the short-term. In contrast to presumed reactivation tuberculosis occurring earlier in the course of HIV infection, which for pulmonary disease tends to occur at CD4$^+$ T-lymphocyte counts of approximately 300 cells per mm^3, late-stage tuberculosis tends to occur at CD4$^+$ counts of 200 cells per mm^3 or lower.[73,74,79] Extrapulmonary tuberculosis also becomes increasingly more likely as CD4$^+$ counts decline, as described below.

Several studies have examined the yield and sensitivity of sputum examination in diagnosing tuberculosis in HIV-infected patients. Although some have found sputum analysis to be extremely sensitive, i.e., 61–83% smear positive and 88–100% culture positive, in four studies of HIV-positive patients,[81,83,91,92] others have postulated that the lower incidence of cavitary disease and necrosis makes it less likely that sputum examination will yield positive results. Klein et al. showed that only 11 (29%) of 38 AIDS/ARC patients had an initial positive smear compared with 35 (61%) of 57 controls.[93] Five smears increased the yield to 40% as opposed to 87.1% of the control group. Another study found that the failure to diagnose tuberculosis promptly in HIV-infected patients was not due to decreased sensitivity of sputum smear examination, but rather to a failure to obtain the recommended minimum number of sputum smears from patients suspected of having tuberculosis.[60] Long et al.[94] addressed this issue more definitively in 289 Haitian patients with culture proven pulmonary mycobacterial disease (tuberculous and nontuberculous). He found the sensitivity of AFB smears in culture-positive pulmonary tuberculosis in 55 HIV-positive patients and 181 HIV-negative patients to be 67.3 versus 79.0%, respectively. In analysis of the entire cohort of 289 patients, the positive predictive accuracy of a positive smear in diagnosing pulmonary tuberculosis in HIV-positive versus HIV-negative patients was 80 versus 90%, respectively. The authors concluded that although tuberculous smear positivity was slightly reduced in HIV-positive disease, it was still a sensitive and accurate means of diagnosis in the right epidemiologic setting.

Bronchoscopy data also vary widely. Smear positivity in three studies ranged from 10 to 47%, while culture positivity ranged from 43 to 89%.[60,91,92] Granulomas were present in 19% of biopsies in one study[60] and thus support the use of biopsy. Salzman et al.[95] agree with the use of the transbronchial biopsy in HIV-related pulmonary tuberculosis. Their study showed that an immediate diagnosis by smear or histology was made in 12 (39%) of 31 patients; and in 7 it was the sole means of an immediate diagnosis. Miro et al.[96] did not support the use of the transbronchial biopsy, although their data did show an increase in yield with brushings and biopsy. The lack of significance in their study may be due to a type 2 error.

Pulmonary tuberculosis in HIV-positive patients often coexists with extrapulmonary disease. Extrapulmonary disease occurs commonly in as much as 20% of most series of tuberculosis cases without HIV infection, but may occur in over 50% of cases of HIV-related tuberculosis at advanced stages of immunosuppression.[73,74,97,98] De Cock et al., in a recent review on tuberculosis and AIDS, determined that the median CD4+ count at the time of diagnosis of localized extrapulmonary tuberculosis was approximately 240 cells per mm³, compared to 140 cells per mm³ for meningeal tuberculosis, and less than 100 cells per mm³ for disseminated tuberculosis.[73] Small et al. showed that 42 (32%) of 132 patients with HIV-related tuberculosis had coexistent pulmonary and extrapulmonary disease.[92] Therefore, in addition to the lungs, other sites such as urine, stool, blood, lymph nodes, bone marrow, and cerebrospinal fluid may yield a diagnosis. Further discussion on this matter may be found in Chapter 7 (this volume).

The acuity of the process and the atypical presentation often lead the practitioner to pursue other diagnoses, and unsuspected tuberculosis is found on autopsy in a substantial number of cases.[60,99] Also, HIV-infected patients may be more likely colonized with atypical mycobacteria and may be more susceptible to symptomatic disease with organisms such as *M. kansasii* and *M. avium*.[100,101] Thus, in individuals who harbor both tuberculous and nontuberculous mycobacteria, overgrowth with atypical organisms may in some cases obscure the tuberculous disease.[102] Thus, when tuberculosis is suspected in an HIV-positive person, it is important to pursue the diagnosis aggressively at multiple sites.

XI. DIAGNOSTIC CLASSIFICATION OF TUBERCULOSIS

All tuberculosis cases must be categorized and reported to the Centers for Disease Control according to the standards set forth in the "Official Statement of the American Thoracic Society" in June 1989.[103] They are found in Table 6-1.

XII. TREATMENT OF DISEASE

The goal of therapy is to eradicate the tuberculous organisms in the various environments within the host, and to prevent the emergence of drug resistant strains. Accordingly, Mitchison described four basic environments, three of which are targeted for attack.[104,105] First are the extracellular organisms that grow most rapidly along cavity walls and in a liquid necrotic medium, and represent the largest load of bacilli. These are killed most effectively by isoniazid. Second are the slower growing semidormant extracellular organisms sometimes found in caseous material that may have only spurts of activity. These are killed most effectively by rifampin because it has the fastest onset of action (15–20 min) and is the drug most capable of killing the organism during one of the growth spurts. Third are the slowly growing or semidormant bacilli found intracellularly in the acidic environment (pH 5.5) of macrophages. These are attacked most effectively by pyrazinamide, which works best at an acid pH. The fourth environment contains the dormant organisms that cannot be killed until they begin to grow. Although isoniazid and rifampin work best in the environments described, they are each effective in all but the fourth environment. It should be noted that the concept of the acidic internal milieu of the macrophage has been challenged recently, and some feel that the pH actually may be neutral.[106]

These mechanisms in part explain the philosophy of utilizing three of the currently prescribed

Table 6-1 **Diagnostic classification of tuberculosis**[a]

Class	Diagnosis
0	No tuberculosis exposure, not infected
1	Tuberculosis exposure, no evidence of disease, i.e., a negative skin test
2	Tuberculous infection, no disease, i.e., a positive skin test and no disease
3	Tuberculosis, clinically active. The location of the disease should be listed as pulmonary, pleural, lymphatic, bone and/or joint, genitourinary, disseminated (miliary), meningeal, peritoneal, and/or other. The predominant site should be listed and the bacteriologic status, chemotherapy status, chest radiograph findings, and tuberculosis skin test reaction should be recorded
4	Tuberculosis, not clinically active. The diagnosis is made either by history or by a positive skin test with a stable radiograph consistent with tuberculosis. The past or present chemotherapy status should be recorded
5	Tuberculosis suspect (diagnosis pending). Persons may only remain in this category for 3 months. After that time they should be placed in one of the other categories. The chemotherapy status should be recorded

[a] Adapted from American Thoracic Society/Center for Disease Control.[103]

drugs, i.e., isoniazid, rifampin, and pyrazinamide, in the initial phase of short-course therapy. Other reasons for using multidrug chemotherapy include the rapid decrease of the burden of organisms, and a decreased chance for the emergence of resistant strains. According to David, the highest proportions of resistant organisms that were found in unselected populations in 1970 were 3.5×10^{-6} for isoniazid, 3.1×10^{-8} for rifampin, 3.8×10^{-6} for streptomycin, and 5×10^{-5} for ethambutol.[107] These *in vitro* studies indicate that there might be a significant number of resistant organisms found in cavities, which may harbor as many as 10^9 organisms, and explain why more than one drug must be used to treat active tuberculosis. The chance occurrence of an organism that is resistant to more than one drug is equal to the product of the resistance rates for each drug. Therefore, the use of three bactericidal drugs makes it very unlikely that a resistant organism will emerge. Furthermore, the actual mutation rate per generation is approximately 100 times less frequent than the above rates, and explains why 2-drug maintenance therapy is adequate once the initial burden of organisms is reduced and the initially resistant strains largely are eliminated. The low burden of organisms in tuberculous infection without disease explains why isoniazid may be used alone in chemoprophylaxis without leading to the development of resistance, and why less rigorous therapy may be used in smear-negative disease.

Because of the slow replication time, as long as the bacillus is exposed to adequate antimicrobial levels at some period of time over several divisions (i.e., several days) therapy will be effective. This allows for daily, twice, or thrice weekly therapy even if blood levels are inadequate for a portion of the day or week.

A. CURRENT DRUGS

First line drug therapy is shown in Table 6-2 and second line drug therapy in Table 6-3. For further descriptions of these drugs, refer to Chapter 11 (this volume).

B. CURRENT THERAPY

Since 1970, therapy has been shortened from 18 to 9 and then to 6 months. This has been made possible by the use of rifampin with isoniazid, and then by the addition of pyrazinamide. The basis for adopting any new short course regimen may be found in the statement by the Centers for Disease Control that "an acceptable short course chemotherapy regimen should allow reduction in the duration of therapy while resulting in a rate of relapse not greater than 5%."[108] Pyrazinamide seems to be the key additional drug in 6-month regimens.[109] At least one other drug must be used where isoniazid resistance is possible. The ability to use twice weekly or thrice weekly therapy allows easier monitoring by public health officers.

The current therapy recommendations for new cases of tuberculosis are displayed in Table 6-4 and are based on the official American Thoracic Society (ATS)/Centers for Disease Control (CDC) recommendations from 1993[109] and the CDC recommendations from 1992.[110] The dosages of the first and second line drugs are displayed in Tables 6-2 and 6-3, respectively. It is recommended that drug susceptibility studies be performed on all initial isolates from patients with newly diagnosed tuberculosis.[109] Furthermore, as noted in Table 6-4, it is essential to begin therapy with four drugs in areas where the prevalence of primary isoniazid resistance has not been demonstrated to be less than 4%.

The basis for the 6-month treatment regimen defined in Table 6-4, option 1, rests partly on a study

Table 6-2 **Dosage recommendation for the initial treatment of tuberculosis in children[a] and adults[b]**

Drugs	Daily Dose		Twice Weekly Dose		Thrice Weekly Dose	
	Children	Adults	Children	Adults	Children	Adults
Isoniazid (mg/kg)	10–20	5	20–40	15	20–40	15
maximum (mg)	300	300	900	900	900	900
Rifampin (mg/kg)	10–20	10	10–20	10	10–20	10
maximum (mg)	600	600	600	600	600	600
Pyrazinamide (mg/kg)	15–30	15–30	50–70	50–70	50–70	50–70
maximum (g)	2	2	4	4	3	3
Ethambutol[c] (mg/kg)	15–25	15–25	50	50	25–30	25–30
Streptomycin (mg/kg)	20–40	15	25–30	25–30	25–30	25–30

[a] Children ≤12 years of age.

[b] From American Thoracic Society/Centers for Disease Control.[109]

[c] Ethambutol is generally not recommended for children whose visual acuity cannot be monitored (<8 years of age). However, ethambutol should be considered for all children with organisms resistant to other drugs, when susceptibility to ethambutol has been demonstrated, or susceptibility is likely.

Table 6-3 **Second line antituberculosis drugs[a,b]**

Drug	Dosage Forms	Daily Dose in Children and Adults[c] (mg/kg)	Maximal Daily Dose in Children and Adults (g)	Major Adverse Reactions	Recommended Regular Monitoring
Capreomycin	Vials: 1 g	15 to 30 im	1	Auditory, vestibular, and renal toxicity	Vestibular function audiometry, blood urea nitrogen, and creatinine
Kanamycin	Vials: 75 mg, 500 mg, 1 g	15 to 30 im	1	Auditory and renal toxicity, rare vestibular toxicity	Vestibular function, audiometry, blood urea nitrogen, and creatinine
Ethionamide	Tablets: 250 mg	15 to 20 p.o.	1	Gastrointestinal disturbance, hepatotoxicity, hypersensitivity	Hepatic enzymes
p-Aminosalicylic acid	Tablets: 500 mg, 1 g; Bulk powder	150 p.o.	12	Gastrointestinal disturbance, hypersensitivity, hepatotoxicity, sodium load	
Cycloserine	Capsules: 250 mg	15 to 20 p.o.	1	Psychosis, convulsions, rash	Assessment of mental status

[a] From American Thoracic Society/Centers for Disease Control.[109]

[b] These drugs are more difficult to use than drugs listed in Table 6-2. They should be used only when necessary and should be given and monitored by health providers experienced in their use.

[c] Doses based on weight should be adjusted as weight changes.

Table 6-4 **Current recommendations for therapy of actual or probable drug sensitive tuberculosis[a,b]**

6-Month Therapy

Option 1

Eight weeks of daily isoniazid, rifampin, and pyrazinamide, followed by 16 weeks of isoniazid and rifampin, daily or 2 to 3 times per week. In areas where the isoniazid resistance rate is not documented to be less than 4%, ethambutol or streptomycin should be added to the initial regimen until susceptibility to isoniazid and rifampin is demonstrated. If the results of susceptibility studies are not available at 8 weeks, and the rate of isoniazid resistance is not documented to be less than 4%, then pyrazinamide may be discontinued, but the fourth drug (i.e., either ethambutol or streptomycin) must be continued until the isolate is shown to be drug susceptible. The treatment duration should total at least 6 months and 3 months beyond culture conversion. All regimens administered twice or thrice weekly should by monitored by directly observed therapy. A tuberculosis medical expert should be consulted if the patient is symptomatic or smear or culture positive after 3 months.

Option 2

Two weeks of daily isoniazid, rifampin, pyrazinamide, and streptomycin or ethambutol followed by 6 weeks of the same drugs, twice weekly, administered by directly observed therapy, followed by 16 weeks of isoniazid and rifampin administered twice weekly by directly observed therapy in cases where the organsim is shown to be drug susceptible. A tuberculosis medical expert should be consulted if the patient is symptomatic or smear or culture positive after 3 months.

Option 3

Thrice weekly isoniazid, rifampin, pyrazinamide, and ethambutol or streptomycin for 6 months, administered by directly observed therapy. (The strongest evidence from clinical trials shows the effectiveness of all four drugs administered for the full 6 months.) There is weaker evidence that streptomycin can be discontinued after 4 months if the isolate is susceptible to all drugs. The evidence for stopping pyrazinamide before the end of 6 months is equivocal for the thrice weekly regimen, and there is no evidence for the effectiveness of this regimen with ethambutol for less than the full 6 months. A tuberculosis medical expert should be consulted if the patient is symptomatic or smear or culture positive after 3 months.

HIV-Related Tuberculosis

Option 1, 2, or 3 under 6-month therapy can be used, but patients should be followed much more closely. If there is any problem with response to treatment, the usual evaluation should ensue, and therapy may be prolonged.

9-Month Therapy

Nine months of daily isoniazid and rifampin, or 1 to 2 months of daily isoniazid and rifampin followed by 7 to 8 months of daily or twice weekly isoniazid and rifampin for a total of 9 months of therapy. Directly observed therapy should be used for twice weekly administration. Ethambutol or streptomycin should be added for the first 2 months in areas where the isoniazid resistance rate is not documented to be less than 4%.

4-Month Therapy

Treat as per options 1, 2, or 3 under 6-Month Therapy, truncated after 4 months in patients who are not at high risk and have smear-negative, culture-negative pulmonary tuberculosis.

[a] Adapted from American Thoracic Society/Centers for Disease Control.[109]

[b] For cases where isoniazid, rifampin, or pyrazinamide cannot be used, please see the text for therapy modifications.

in Poland by Snider et al. that compared 56 patients who received isoniazid, rifampin, pyrazinamide, and streptomycin for 2 months followed by isoniazid and rifampin for 4 months with 116 patients who received the same regimen without streptomycin.[111] The entrants were all new cases of smear-positive pulmonary tuberculosis. The numbers analyzed in the study and presented here are those who completed therapy. In the group receiving initial streptomycin, there was only one (1.8%) relapse, whereas in the group not receiving initial streptomycin, there were two (1.7%) treatment failures that developed isoniazid-resistant strains while on therapy, and there were four (3.4%) relapses for a total of six (5.2%) overall failures. Although these differences were not found to be significant, the sample size was not large enough for reassurance that the treatment outcomes were equivalent.

However, further study showed improved efficacy of the new 3-drug 6-month regimen in the USPHS Short Course Chemotherapy Trial 21 which analyzed 1062 eligible study entrants and compared 617 on the currently accepted 6-month regimen with 445 on the previous 9-month standard therapy.[112] In light of the fact that only 15% of the 6 month treatment group had greater than 50 colonies on culture, one must assume that most of the study entrants were smear negative. Thus, this group represents cases with a lower bacillary load than the study from Poland. In comparison with the 9-month regimen, those in the 6-month regimen converted their sputa more rapidly at 16 weeks (94.6 versus 89.9%), had lower noncompliance rates (16.8 versus 29.2%), and had similar relapse rates 96 weeks after completing therapy (3.5 versus 2.8%). Approximately 25% of each group initially also received ethambutol because of suspected resistance, and this was positively associated with early sputum conversion. There were no significant differences in adverse drug reactions. These data showed the efficacy of 6 month therapy in this population. Cohn et al. studied 108 patients with pulmonary tuberculosis (7 of whom also had extrapulmonary tuberculosis) on a 6-month largely intermittent regimen.[112a] Of these patients, 80 (74%) were smear-positive and 100% of patients converted their sputa by 20 weeks of therapy. There were no treatment failures and there were 2 relapses. The study excluded 4 patients who died soon after beginning therapy because of overwhelming tuberculosis. Further confirmation of the efficacy of the standard 6 month initial 3-drug regimen in smear-positive patients may be found in the British Medical Research Council Study in Singapore,[113] as well as a more recent Singapore study.[114] However, a recent Hong Kong study suggests that the initial addition of a fourth drug, i.e., streptomycin, in smear-positive disease is superior to the 3-drug regimen.[115]

Pyrazinamide is the best third drug to add to isoniazid and rifampin for short course therapy,[109] and, for patients receiving the regimen outlined in Table 6-4, option 1, there is no advantage to the use of pyrazinamide after the first 2 months of therapy of drug-susceptible tuberculosis.[116] However, if the organism is resistant to isoniazid, isoniazid may be discontinued, but pyrazinamide should be continued for the entire 6-month duration of treatment, as noted below.

The course of therapy outlined in Table 6-4, option 3, i.e., thrice-weekly 4-drug therapy for 6 months, is based on a study performed in Hong Kong where five different 6-month regimens were compared, two of which were 4-drug thrice weekly regimens using isoniazid, rifampin, pyrazinamide, and either ethambutol or streptomycin.[117] In drug-susceptible patients who were followed over a 5-year period, there were 2 (1.3%) relapses in 151 patients who were taking the regimen containing streptomycin, and there were 7 (4.4%) relapses in 160 patients who were taking the regimen containing ethambutol. Overall, the rate of relapse in the regimens containing pyrazinamide versus the regimen that did not contain pyrazinamide was 3.4 versus 10.3%, respectively. Therefore, it was suggested that for thrice weekly therapy, pyrazinamide was beneficial where used for the entire 6-month period,[109] although the Hong Kong study did not address this issue specifically because there was no comparison with a 6-month regimen that used initial pyrazinamide for 2 months only. Analysis of a small group of 131 patients who were resistant to isoniazid, streptomycin, or both, showed that those who took pyrazinamide fared much better than those who did not; there were 4 (3.8%) relapses in 104 patients in the pyrazinamide series versus 6 (22.2%) in 27 patients in the nonpyrazinamide series. Therefore, in all treatment options in Table 6-4 where isoniazid cannot be used due to resistance or toxicity, pyrazinamide should be continued for the entire 6-month duration of therapy.[109]

In cases where both isoniazid and pyrazinamide cannot be used, ethambutol and rifampin have been recommended for 12 months.[109] This is based largely on a study by the National Research Institute for Tuberculosis, Poland, where a regimen of 12 weeks of daily therapy [rifampin (600 mg) and ethambutol (25 mg/kg)] followed by twice-weekly rifampin (600 mg) and ethambutol (50 mg/kg) for a total of 12 months of therapy, was used in the retreatment of 40 patients with isoniazid-resistant pulmonary tuberculosis.[117a,118] There was a 10% overall failure rate (5% treatment failures plus 5% relapses). The results from a similar Hong Kong study were even less favorable.[118a] Better results were obtained by Lees et al. and Nitti et al.[118b,118c] Nevertheless, it might be advisable to add a third drug to such a regimen.

In cases where rifampin alone cannot be used, isoniazid, pyrazinamide, and streptomycin may be used daily for 9 months,[118d] or isoniazid and ethambutol may be used daily or twice weekly for 18 months.[118e,118f] Ethambutol always should be started at 25 mg/kg/day for the first 2 months.

In cases where both isoniazid and rifampin cannot be used because of toxicity, it would be wise to apply the principles of treatment for multidrug-resistant tuberculosis (see Chapter 12, this volume). In these instances, it is preferable to use at least three new drugs and continue until culture conversion is documented, followed by at least 12 months of 2-drug therapy. Often, a total of 24 months is administered empirically.[109]

The previous standard of 9-month therapy was established in 1980[108] and has been shown to be very effective in most forms of tuberculosis.[119-125] In fact, there are still those who prefer to use this regimen. In view of the rising problems with isoniazid resistance, it is prudent in most cases to add ethambutol during the initial phase until culture sensitivity reports are available, and recommended strongly where the incidence of primary isoniazid resistance is not documented to be less than 4%.

In general, it appears that the smaller the bacillary load in pulmonary tuberculosis, the less vigorous the therapy. Dutt and Snead have shown success in smear-negative culture-positive pulmonary tuberculosis with 6 months of isoniazid and rifampin,[126] and have shown further success in smear-negative culture-negative pulmonary tuberculosis with 4 months of isoniazid and rifampin.[127] Furthermore, there is evidence that smear-negative pulmonary tuberculosis, with or without positive cultures, responds well to 4 months of either daily or thrice weekly 4-drug therapy.[128] Therefore, in smear-negative culture-negative tuberculosis, the American Thoracic Society and Centers for Disease Control recommend that it is acceptable to reduce the basic 6-month regimen to 4 months.[109] Recommendations for treatment of tuberculosis in the pregnant woman, the child, and the neonate may be found in Chapter 8, this volume.

C. MONITORING FOR ADVERSE REACTIONS

Baseline evaluation for one of the standard regimens should include a complete blood count with platelets, liver function tests, blood urea nitrogen, creatinine, and calcium. If pyrazinamide is used, uric acid should be obtained, and if ethambutol is used, uric acid, visual acuity, and red/green color perception should be assessed. Isoniazid toxicity should be monitored as described in Chapter 13 (this volume) except that in persons with normal baseline liver function tests and in the absence of symptoms, routine monitoring of liver function tests is not necessary. Patients should be instructed about the complications of therapy and the natural course of the disease. If symptoms develop that suggest drug toxicity, a full evaluation should ensue.[109] For techniques on reintroducing drugs

after an adverse reaction, please see Chapter 12 (this volume).

D. MONITORING RESPONSE TO THERAPY

Patients should be seen every month to monitor response to treatment and encourage adherence, and directly observed therapy is recommended unless there is evidence that the patient will adhere to therapy. In sputum smear-positive patients, weekly sputum smears with quantitation is encouraged strongly.[109] Otherwise, sputum should be obtained each month until culture conversion is documented. After 2 months of therapy with a standard regimen containing both isoniazid and rifampin, more than 85% of positive sputum cultures should have converted to negative.[109] If the sputum has not converted by that time, the patient should be evaluated carefully and drug susceptibility tests should be repeated. The patient also should be started on directly observed therapy. Treatment should be continued with an emphasis on adherence and, where necessary, supervised therapy.

Fever may be present for prolonged periods. In one study, 34% of patients treated with isoniazid and PAS with or without streptomycin were still febrile at 2 weeks.[129] In another study with more effective therapy (i.e., isoniazid, rifampin, and ethambutol) only 10% were still febrile at 2 weeks.[130] The duration of fever was longer than 100 days in rare cases and correlated with the extent of disease. The presence of fever during the first few weeks should not be of great concern if the patient is improving clinically. A chest radiograph should be performed 2 or 3 months into therapy to assess the radiographic resolution of the disease. If the sputum culture converts within 2 months, the chest radiograph improves, and the patient improves clinically, then a final sputum and chest radiograph should be performed at the completion of therapy. Further follow-up is not necessary. Monitoring and follow-up of high-risk patients should be more intensive and individualized. Patients who have been slow to respond, have significant residual radiographic findings upon completion of treatment, or who are immunosuppressed should be reevaluated 6 months after the completion of treatment, or earlier if symptoms occur.[109] For patients with negative pretreatment sputa, the course of therapy should be followed clinically and by chest radiograph.

Patients whose sputum cultures do not convert after 5 or 6 months are considered treatment failures. Therapy may be continued pending drug susceptibility tests, or the patient may be started immediately on at least three new drugs while continuing the previous regimen, pending the susceptibility report. Direct supervision of therapy should be implemented.

Patients who relapse after completing a regimen containing both isoniazid and rifampin may be restarted on their original therapy as the organisms usually are still susceptible to the original drugs.[109,131] Patients who relapse after a regimen that did not contain both isoniazid and rifampin should be treated as if they are resistant to all previous drugs (see Chapter 12, this volume).

E. ACQUIRED IMMUNODEFICIENCY SYNDROME

Persons with AIDS and tuberculosis often respond well to antituberculous chemotherapy and, once effectively treated, do not usually die from tuberculosis. Small studied 125 persons with advanced HIV infection and tuberculosis who received either 6 or 9 months of short course therapy.[92] The population appeared to be distributed equally among persons with pulmonary disease alone (50 persons), those with extrapulmonary disease alone (40 persons), and those with both (42 persons). There were 52 deaths during therapy, 8 (6.4%) of which were due to tuberculosis. There was 1 additional treatment failure due to resistant organisms. In general, sputa were cleared of acid-fast organisms after a median of 10 weeks of therapy. There were only 3 (5%) relapses in 58 patients who completed therapy, and these were due to poor compliance. Thus, if the tuberculous disease was not overwhelming, it responded well to chemotherapy. The incidence of adverse reactions necessitating a change in therapy was 18%, and was due to rashes, hepatitis, gastrointestinal distress, and anaphylaxis.

The Advisory Committee for the Elimination of Tuberculosis recommended that antituberculous therapy be started as soon as acid-fast bacilli are seen in a specimen from the respiratory tract of a person with known or suspected HIV infection, even if AIDS has not developed yet.[132] Therapy should be the same as for normal hosts (see Table 6-4), but patients should be followed much more closely. This may shorten the previously recommended 9-month regimen.[110] If there is any problem with response to treatment, the usual evaluation should ensue, and therapy may be prolonged.[109]

In most reports, patients with HIV infection treated for tuberculosis have tolerated therapy well.[49,50,92] However, one report found that HIV-infected patients had a higher than expected incidence of allergic reactions to rifampin, which occurred in approximately 20% of patients in that series.[92] It is known that HIV-infected patients do have a higher incidence of hypersensitivity reactions to sulfonamides and thiacetazone,[133,134] and clinicians may choose to monitor patients closely

while on rifampin as well. It should be stressed, however, that a substantial majority of tuberculosis cases with HIV infection can be treated quite successfully with standard tuberculosis regimens, modified only modestly from standard therapy in non-HIV-infected patients, as outlined above. While there are some data from Africa indicating an unacceptably high relapse rate in HIV-infected patients treated with what is considered standard therapy in such settings (i.e., isoniazid, streptomycin, and thiacetazone),[134] there are no data as yet to indicate a significant risk of relapse among HIV-infected patients treated for tuberculosis with regimens containing both isoniazid and rifampin. Additional study is required to determine the optimal duration of treatment for tuberculosis in the setting of HIV infection, including the question of whether continuing prophylaxis with isoniazid after the completion of therapy for active disease is advisable.

F. IMMUNOCOMPROMISED HOSTS

Non-HIV immunocompromised patients respond well to chemotherapy unless they have extensive tuberculous disease. In one study, tuberculosis in patients immunocompromised by cancer, cancer chemotherapy, transplant therapy, hemopathy, or steroid therapy responded well to a regimen of isoniazid, rifampin, and ethambutol for 3 months followed by isoniazid and rifampin for 9 to 12 months.[135] However 2 of 30 patients died, 1 before therapy and 1 just after it began. All others did well. Bobrowitz et al.[136] and Fulkerson et al.[137] noted that persons with coexistent tuberculosis and lung cancer could be irradiated successfully with full doses as long as adequate antituberculous chemotherapy was administered. Therefore, it would seem reasonable for all significantly immunocompromised hosts to follow the same guidelines set forth for the treatment of tuberculosis in HIV infection, but it might be wise to prolong therapy in this group to at least 9 months, since the rapid response to treatment has not been documented as well as it has in HIV-related tuberculosis.

G. SILICOTUBERCULOSIS

As noted earlier, tuberculosis is particularly difficult to treat in the setting of silicosis, and relapses are common, presumably due to the cytotoxicity of silica for alveolar macrophages.[138] Some have recommended indefinite therapy once silicotuberculosis has been diagnosed.[139]

Dubois et al.[140] had success with initial therapy of tuberculosis in 27 silicotic individuals with a regimen of three to four drugs (including rifampin and ethambutol) given until sputum conversion occurred, followed by two drugs for 6 months, and then by isoniazid for 1 year. Sputum conversion occurred in all persons by 5 months, and there was one relapse during a 2- to 6-year period. Escreet et al.[141] claimed success in 36 patients with a 9-month regimen that included thiacetazone. However, their relapse rate was 9%. Lin et al.[142] studied a regimen of 2 months of isoniazid, rifampin, pyrazinamide, and streptomycin, followed by 7 months of isoniazid and rifampin. They had 5% treatment failures and 5% relapses. Cowie et al.[143] treated 1,085 cases with 4.5 months of a weekday regimen of isoniazid, rifampin, pyrazinamide, and streptomycin with no treatment failures and a gross relapse rate of 3.8% after 36 months of follow-up. It was estimated that 14% of the assembled group had atypical mycobacteria. Neither the MOTT cases nor the initial resistance patterns appeared to affect the rate of relapse. Other regimens in the same study with a less intensive initial phase and without rifampin during the maintenance phase were much less successful. The Hong Kong Chest Service compared 6 months versus 8 months of a thrice weekly 4-drug regimen of isoniazid, rifampin, pyrazinamide, and streptomycin, supplemented by ethambutol if the patient had been treated previously. Sputum conversion occurred in 98% of patients at 3 months, but the relapse rate was 7% in the 8-month group, and 22% in the 6-month group.[144]

The official recommendation of the American Thoracic Society and the Centers for Disease Control is that in cases of culture-positive silicotuberculosis, the usual therapy must be extended by at least 2 months.[109] As noted above, 8 months of a thrice weekly 4-drug regimen might be effective.

H. SURGERY

Surgery for pulmonary tuberculosis rarely is performed today. Before the chemotherapy era, it was an important adjunct for "resting" the lung, for resection of cavities and progressive local disease, and for managing empyemas and fibrothoraces. Operations such as the artificial pneumothorax, artificial pneumoperitoneum, artificial phrenic nerve paralysis, plombage, thoracoplasty, pulmonary resection, cavity drainage, Eloesser flap, and decortication had been performed.[145,146] Currently, the indications for surgery are few. They include active localized disease unresponsive to adequate chemotherapy (e.g., a multidrug-resistant strain), empyema or bronchopleural fistula unresponsive to closed pleural space evacuation, and life-threatening hemoptysis unresponsive to arteriographic embolization.[147]

Iseman et al. have studied surgical resection as adjunctive therapy for multidrug-resistant cases in 29 patients. Of 27 survivors (there were two unrelated deaths), 25 (93%) remained sputum culture negative at 36 months postresection.[148]

If drug resistance continues to be a major problem, surgery again may become important in the management of tuberculosis (see Chapter 12, this volume).

I. CORTICOSTEROIDS

Corticosteroids do not play a role in the management of typical pulmonary tuberculosis, unless it is associated with fulminant miliary disease[149] or severe obstructive intrathoracic lymphadenopathy in primary disease.[150] Signs and symptoms may resolve sooner in typical pulmonary and pleural disease, but a long-term benefit has not been demonstrated.

REFERENCES

1. Myers, J. A., Gunlaugson, F. G., Meyerding E. A., et al., Importance of tuberculin testing of school children — a twenty-eight year study, *J. Am. Med. Assoc.*, 159, 185, 1955.
2. Caffey, J., Ed., *Caffey's Pediatric X-ray Diagnosis,* 7th ed., Year Book Medical Publishers, Chicago, 1985.
3. Palmer, P. E. S., Pulmonary tuberculosis — usual and unusual radiographic presentations, *Sem. Roentgenol.*, 14, 204, 1979.
4. Poulsen, A., Some clinical features of tuberculosis. II. Initial fever. III. *Erythema nodosum.* IV. Tuberculosis of lungs and pleura in primary infection. V. Extrapulmonary tuberculosis. VI. Spread of infection. VII. Sequelae of primary tuberculous infection, *Acta Tuberc. Scand.*, 33, 37, 1951.
5. Frostad, S., Segmental atelectasis in children with primary tuberculosis, *Am. Rev. Tuberc.*, 79, 597, 1959.
6. Weber, A. L., Bird, K. T., Janower, M. L., Primary tuberculosis in childhood with particular emphasis on changes affecting the tracheobronchial tree, *Am. J. Roentgenol.*, 103, 123, 1968.
7. Daly, J. F., Endoscopic aspects of primary tuberculosis in children, *Ann. Otol. Rhinol. Laryngol.*, 67, 1089, 1958.
8. Smith, M. H. D., Starke, J. R., Marquis, J. R., Tuberculosis and other opportunistic mycobacterial infections, in *Textbook of Pediatric Infectious Diseases,* 3rd ed., Feigin, R. D., Cherry, J. D., Eds., W. B. Saunders, Philadelphia, 1993, 1321.
9. Singh, D., Richards, W. F., Obstructive emphysema in primary pulmonary tuberculosis, *Tubercle*, 38, 397, 1957.
10. Poulsen, A., Some clinical features of tuberculosis. I. Incubation period, *Acta Tuberc. Scand.*, 24, 311, 1950.
11. Gedde-Dahl, T., Tuberculous infection in the light of tuberculin matriculation, *Am. J. Hyg.*, 56, 139, 1952.

12. Lincoln, E. M., Sewell, E. M., *Tuberculosis in Children,* McGraw-Hill, New York, 1963.
13. Fraser, R. G., Pare, J. A. P., Pare, P. D., et al., Eds., *Diagnosis of Diseases of the Chest,* 3rd ed., W. B. Saunders, Philadelphia, 1989.
14. Fried, B. M., The primary complex (initial anatomic lesion in childhood type of tuberculosis), *Arch. Pathol.*, 22, 829, 1936.
15. Pinner, M., *Pulmonary Tuberculosis in the Adult: Its Fundamental Aspects,* Charles C Thomas, Springfield, IL, 1945.
16. Chang, S. C., Lee, P. Y., Perng, R. P., Lower lung field tuberculosis, *Chest*, 91, 230, 1987.
17. Berger, H. W., Granada M. G., Lower lung field tuberculosis, *Chest*, 65, 522, 1974.
18. Khan, M. A., Kovnat, D. M., Bachus, B., et al., Clinical and roentgenographic spectrum of pulmonary tuberculosis in the adult, *Am. J. Med.*, 62, 31, 1977.
19. Pitchenik, A. E., Rubinson, H. A., The radiographic appearance of tuberculosis in patients with the acquired immune deficiency syndrome and pre-AIDS, *Am. Rev. Resp. Dis.*, 131, 393, 1985.
20. Adler, H., Phthisiogenetic studies by means of tomography in cases of localized pulmonary tuberculosis in adults, *Acta Tuberc. Scand.*, 47, 13, 1959.
21. Spencer, D., Yagan, R., Blinkhorn, R., et al., Anterior segment upper lobe tuberculosis in the adult: occurrence in primary and reactivation disease, *Chest*, 97, 384, 1990.
22. Woodring, J. H., Vandiviere, H. M., Lee, C., Intrathoracic lymphadenopathy in postprimary tuberculosis, *South. Med. J.*, 81, 992, 1988.
23. Hadlock, F. P., Park, S. K., Awe, R. J., et al., Unusual radiographic findings in adult pulmonary tuberculosis, *Am. J. Radiol.,* 134, 1015, 1980.
24. Cudkowicz, L., The blood supply of the lung in pulmonary tuberculosis, *Thorax*, 7, 270, 1952.
25. Woodring, J. H., Vandiviere, H. M., Fried, A. M., et al., Update: the radiographic features of pulmonary tuberculosis, *Am. J. Radiol.*, 146, 497, 1986.
26. Choyke, P. L., Sostman, H. D., Curtis, A. M., et al., Adult-onset pulmonary tuberculosis, *Radiology*, 148, 357, 1983.
27. Jacobson, H. G., Shapiro, J. H., Pulmonary tuberculosis, *Radiol. Clin. North Am.*, 1, 411, 1963.
28. Auerbach, O., Pathology and pathogenesis of pulmonary arterial aneurysm in tuberculous cavities, *Am. Rev. Tuberc.*, 39, 99, 1939.
29. Plessinger, V. A., Jolly, P. N., Rasmussen's aneurysms and fatal hemorrhage in pulmonary tuberculosis, *Am. Rev. Tuberc.*, 60, 589, 1949.
30. Muthuswamy, P. P., Akbik, F., Franklin, C., et al., Management of major or massive hemoptysis in active pulmonary tuberculosis by bronchial arterial embolization, *Chest*, 92, 77, 1987.
31. British Thoracic Association, Aspergilloma and residual tuberculous cavities — the results of a resurvey, *Tubercle*, 51, 227, 1970.
32. British Thoracic Association, Aspergillus in persistent lung cavities after tuberculosis, *Tubercle*, 49, 1, 1968.
33. Tomlinson, J. R., Sahn, S. A, Aspergilloma in sarcoid and tuberculosis, *Chest*, 92, 505, 1987.
34. Auerbach, O., Tuberculosis of the trachea and major bronchi, *Am. Rev. Tuberc.*, 60, 604, 1949.
35. Van den Brande, P. M., Van de Mierop, F., Verbeken, E. K., et al., Clinical spectrum of endobronchial tuberculosis in elderly patients, *Arch. Intern. Med.*, 150, 2105, 1990.
36. Chang, S. C., Lee, P. Y., Perng, R. P., Clinical role of bronchoscopy in adults with intrathoracic tuberculous lymphadenopathy, *Chest*, 93, 314, 1988.
37. Ip, M. S. M., Lam, W. K., Endobronchial tuberculosis revisited, *Chest*, 89, 727, 1986.
38. Wasser, L. S., Shaw, G. W., Talavera, W., Endobronchial tuberculosis in the acquired immunodeficiency syndrome, *Chest*, 94, 1240, 1988.
39. Bleyer, J. M., Marks, J. H., Tuberculomas and hamartomas of the lung: comparative study of 66 proved cases, *Am. J. Radiol.*, 77, 1013, 1957.
40. Sochocky, S., Tuberculoma of the lung, *Am. Rev. Tuberc.*, 78, 403, 1958.
41. Narang, R. K., Kumar, S., Gupta, A., Pneumothorax and pneumomediastinum complicating acute miliary tuberculosis, *Tubercle*, 58, 79, 1977.
42. Johnson, T. M., McCann, W., Davey, W. N., Tuberculous bronchopleural fistula, *Am. Rev. Resp. Dis.*, 107, 30, 1973.
43. Light, R. W., *Pleural Diseases,* 2nd ed., Lea and Febiger, Philadelphia, 1990.
44. Chung, D. K., Hubbard, W. W., Hyponatremia in untreated active pulmonary tuberculosis, *Am. Rev. Resp. Dis.*, 99, 595, 1969.
45. Hill, A. R., Uribarri, J., Mann, J., et al., Altered water metabolism in tuberculosis: role of vasopressin, *Am. J. Med.*, 88, 357, 1990.
46. Abbasi, A. A., Chemplavil, J. K., Farah, S., et al., Hypercalcemia in active pulmonary tuberculosis, *Ann. Intern. Med.*, 90, 324, 1979.
47. Cadranel, J., Hance, A. J., Milleron, B., et al., Vitamin D metabolism in tuberculosis: Production of $1,25(OH)_2D_3$ by cells recovered by bronchoalveolar lavage and the role of this metabolite in calcium homeostasis, *Am. Rev. Resp. Dis.*, 138, 984, 1988.

48. Laforet, E. G., Laforet, M. T., Non-tuberculous cavitary disease of the lungs, *Dis. Chest*, 31, 665, 1957.

49. Barnes, P. F., Bloch, A. B., Davidson, P. T., Snider, D. E., Tuberculosis in patients with human immunodeficiency virus infection, *N. Engl. J. Med.*, 324, 1644, 1991.

50. Hopewell, P. C., Impact of human immunodeficiency virus infection on the epidemiology, clinical features, management, and control of tuberculosis, *Clin. Infect. Dis.*, 15, 540, 1992.

51. Friedman, L. N., Sullivan, G. M., Bevilaqua, R. P., et al., Tuberculosis screening in alcoholics and drug addicts, *Am. Rev. Resp. Dis.*, 136, 1188, 1987.

52. Massaro, D., Katz, S., Sachs, M., Choroidal tubercles: a clue to hematogenous tuberculosis, *Ann. Intern. Med.*, 60, 231, 1964.

53. Holden, M., Dubin, M. R., Diamond, P. H., Frequency of negative intermediate-strength tuberculin sensitivity in patients with active tuberculosis, *N. Engl. J. Med.*, 285, 1507, 1971.

54. McMurray, D. N., Echeverri, A., Cell-mediated immunity in anergic patients with pulmonary tuberculosis, *Am. Rev. Resp. Dis.*, 118, 827, 1978.

55. Rooney, J. J., Crocco, J. A., Kramer S., et al., Further observations on tuberculin reactions in active tuberculosis, *Am. J. Med.*, 60, 517, 1976.

56. Daniel, T. M., Rapid diagnosis of tuberculosis: laboratory techniques applicable in developing countries, *Rev. Infect. Dis.*, 11 (Suppl. 2), S471, 1989.

56a. Centers for Disease Control and Prevention, *1991 Tuberculosis Statistics in the United States,* U.S. Department of Health and Human Services, Atlanta, GA, 1993.

57. Kubica, G. P., Gross, W. M., Hawkins, J. E., et al., Laboratory services for mycobacterial diseases, *Am. Rev. Resp. Dis.*, 112, 773, 1975.

58. Klotz, S. A., Penn, R. L., Acid-fast staining of urine and gastric contents is an excellent indicator of mycobacterial disease, *Am. Rev. Resp. Dis.*, 136, 1197, 1987.

59. Bentz, R. R., Dimcheff, D. G., Neimiroff, M. J., et al., The incidence of urine cultures positive for mycobacterium tuberculosis in a general tuberculosis patient population, *Am. Rev. Resp. Dis.*, 111, 647, 1975.

60. Kramer, F., Modilevsky, T., Waliany, A. R., Leedom, J. M., Barnes, P. F., Delayed diagnosis of tuberculosis in patients with human immunodeficiency virus infection, *Am. J. Med.,* 89, 451, 1990.

61. Fulkerson, W. J., Fiberoptic bronchoscopy, *N. Engl. J. Med.*, 311, 511, 1984.

62. Danek, S. J., Bower, J. S., Diagnosis of pulmonary tuberculosis by flexible fiberoptic bronchoscopy, *Am. Rev. Resp. Dis.*, 119, 677, 1979.

63. De Gracia, J., Curull, V., Vidal, R., et al., Diagnostic value of bronchoalveolar lavage in suspected pulmonary tuberculosis, *Chest*, 93, 329, 1988.

64. Wallace, J. M., Deutsch, A. L., Harrall, J. H., et al., Bronchoscopy and transbronchial biopsy in evaluation of patients with suspected active tuberculosis, *Am. J. Med.*, 78, 1189, 1981.

65. Stenson, W., Aranda, C., Bevelaqua, F. A., Transbronchial biopsy culture in pulmonary tuberculosis, *Chest*, 83, 883, 1983.

66. Conte, B. A., Laforet, E. G., The role of the topical anesthetic agent in modifying bacteriologic data obtained by bronchoscopy, *N. Engl. J. Med.*, 267, 957, 1962.

67. Schmidt, R. M., Rosenkranz, H. S., Antimicrobial activity of local anesthetics: lidocaine and procaine, *J. Infect. Dis.*, 121, 597, 1970.

68. Dawson, D. J., Armstrong, J. G., Blacklock, Z. M., Mycobacterial cross-contamination of bronchoscopy specimens, *Am. Rev. Resp. Dis.*, 126, 1095, 1982.

69. Nelson, K. E., Larson, P. A., Schraufnagel, D. E., et al., Transmission of tuberculosis by flexible fiberbronchoscopes, *Am. Rev. Resp. Dis.*, 127, 97, 1983.

70. Best, M., Sattar, A., Springthorpe, V. S., et al., Efficacies of selected disinfectants against *Mycobacterium tuberculosis, J. Clin. Microbiol.*, 28, 2234, 1990.

71. Davis, D., Bonekat, H. W., Andrews, D., et al., Disinfection of the flexible fibreoptic bronchoscope against *Mycobacterium tuberculosis* and *M. gordonae, Thorax*, 39, 785, 1984.

72. Leers, W. D., Disinfecting endoscopes: How not to transmit *Mycobacterium tuberculosis* by bronchoscopy, *Can. Med. Assoc. J.*, 123, 275, 1980.

73. De Cock, K. M., Soro, B., Lucas, S. B., Coulibaly, I. M., Tuberculosis and HIV infection in Sub-Saharan Africa, *J. Am. Med. Assoc.*, 268, 1581, 1992.

74. Shafer, R. W., Chirgwin, K. D., Glatt, A. E., Dahdouh, M. A., Landesman, S. H., Suster, B., HIV prevalence, immunosuppression, and drug resistance in patients with tuberculosis in an area endemic for AIDS, *AIDS*, 5, 399, 1991.

75. Chaisson, R. E., Slutkin, G., Tuberculosis and human immunodeficiency virus infection, *J. Infect. Dis.*, 159, 96, 1989.

76. Centers for Disease Control, Tuberculosis and AIDS — Connecticut, *MMWR,* 36, 133, 1987.

77. Centers for Disease Control, Tuberculosis and acquired immunodeficiency syndrome — Florida, *MMWR,* 35, 587, 1986.

78. Centers for Disease Control, Tuberculosis and acquired immunodeficiency syndrome — New York City, *MMWR,* 36, 785, 1987.

79. Theuer, C. P., Hopewell, P. C., Elias, D., et al., Human immunodeficiency virus infection in tuberculosis patients, *J. Infect. Dis.*, 162, 8, 1990.

80. Fournier, A. M., Dickinson, G. M., Erdfrocht, I. R., et al., Tuberculosis and nontuberculous mycobacteriosis in patients with AIDS, *Chest,* 93, 772, 1988.

81. Long, R., Maycher, B., Scalcini, M., et al., The chest roentgenogram in pulmonary tuberculosis patients seropositive for human immunodeficiency virus type 1, *Chest,* 99, 123, 1991.

82. Centers for Disease Control, Tuberculosis — United States, 1985 — and the possible impact of human T-lymphotropic virus type III/lymphadenopathy-associated virus infection, *MMWR,* 35, 74, 1986.

83. Chaisson, R. E., Slutkin, G., Tuberculosis and human immunodeficiency virus infection, *J. Infect. Dis.,* 159, 96, 1989.

84. Centers for Disease Control, Tuberculosis and HIV infection: recommendations of the advisory committee for the elimination of tuberculosis (ACET), *MMWR,* 38, 236, 1989.

85. Selwyn, P. A., Hartel, D., Lewis, V. A., et al., A prospective study of the risk of tuberculosis among intravenous drug users with human immunodeficiency virus infection, *N. Engl. J. Med.*, 320, 545, 1989.

86. Beck-Sague, C., Dooley, S. W., Hutton, M. D., et al., Hospital outbreak of multidrug-resistant *Mycobacterium tuberculosis* infections, *J. Am. Med. Assoc.,* 268, 1280, 1992.

87. Di Perri, G., Cruciani, M., Danzi, M. C., et al., Nosocomial epidemic of active tuberculosis among HIV-infected patients, *Lancet,* 2, 1502, 1989.

88. Daley, C. L., Small, P. M., Schecter, G. F., et al., An outbreak of tuberculosis with accelerated progression among persons infected with the human immunodeficiency virus: an analysis using restriction-fragment-length-polymorphisms, *N. Engl. J. Med.*, 26, 231, 1992.

89. Fischl, M. A., Uttamchandani, R. B., Daikos, G. L., et al., An outbreak of tuberculosis caused by multiple-drug-resistant tubercle bacilli among patients with HIV infection, *Ann. Intern. Med.,* 117, 177, 1992.

90. Pearson, M. L., Jereb, J. A., Frieden, T. R., et al., Nosocomial transmission of multidrug-resistant *Mycobacterium tuberculosis, Ann. Intern. Med.,* 117, 191, 1992.

91. Modilevsky, T., Sattler, F. R., Barnes, P. F., Mycobacterial disease in patients with human immunodeficiency virus infection, *Arch. Intern. Med.,* 149, 2201, 1989.

92. Small, P. M., Schecter, G. F., Goodman, P. C., et al., Treatment of tuberculosis in patients with advanced human immunodeficiency virus infection, *N. Engl. J. Med.*, 324, 289, 1991.

93. Klein, N. C., Duncanson, F. P., Lenox, T. H., et al., Use of mycobacterial smears in the diagnosis of pulmonary tuberculosis in AIDS/ARC patients, *Chest,* 95, 1190, 1989.

94. Long, R., Scalcini, S., Manfreda, J., Jean-Baptiste, M., Hershfield, E., The impact of HIV on the usefulness of sputum smears for the diagnosis of tuberculosis, *Am. J. Public Health,* 81, 1326, 1991.

95. Salzman, S. H., Schindel, M. L., Aranda, C. P., Smith, R. L., Lewis, M. L., The role of bronchoscopy in the diagnosis of pulmonary tuberculosis in patients at risk for HIV infection, *Chest,* 102, 143, 1992.

96. Miro, A. M., Gibilara E., Powell S., Kamholz, S. L., The role of fiberoptic bronchoscopy for diagnosis of pulmonary tuberculosis in patients at risk for AIDS, *Chest,* 101, 1211, 1992.

97. Elder, N. C., Extrapulmonary tuberculosis, *Arch. Fam. Med.,* 1, 91, 1992.

98. Braun, M. M., Byers, R. H., Heyward, W. L., Ciesielski, C. A., Bloch, A. B., et al., Acquired immunodeficiency syndrome and extrapulmonary tuberculosis in the United States, *Arch. Intern. Med.,* 150, 1913, 1990.

99. Flora, G. S., Modilevsky, T., Antoniskis, D., et al., Undiagnosed tuberculosis in patients with human immunodeficiency virus infection, *Chest,* 98, 1056, 1990.

100. Levine, B., Chaisson, R. E., *Mycobacterium kansasii*: A cause of treatable pulmonary disease associated with advanced human immunodeficiency virus (HIV) infection, *Ann. Intern. Med.,* 114, 861, 1991.

101. Horsburgh, C. R., *Mycobacterium avium* complex infection in the acquired immunodeficiency syndrome, *N. Engl. J. Med.,* 324, 1332, 1991.

102. Burnens, A. P., Vurma-Rapp, U., Mixed mycobacterial cultures — occurrence in the clinical laboratory, *Zentralbl. Bacteriol. Mikrobiol.,* 271, 85, 1989.

103. American Thoracic Society/Centers for Disease Control, Diagnostic standards and classification of tuberculosis, *Am. Rev. Resp. Dis.,* 142, 725, 1990.

104. Mitchison, D. A., The action of antituberculosis drugs in short-course chemotherapy, *Tubercle*, 66, 219, 1985.

105. Mitchison, D. A., Basic mechanisms of chemotherapy, *Chest*, 76 (Suppl.), 771, 1979.

106. Crowle, A. J., Dahl, R., Ross, E., et al., Evidence that vesicles containing living, virulent *Mycobacterium tuberculosis* or *Mycobacterium avium* in cultured human macrophages are not acidic, *Infect. Immun.*, 59, 1823, 1991.

107. David, H. L., Probability distribution of drug-resistant mutants in unselected population of *Mycobacterium tuberculosis, Appl. Microbiol.*, 20, 810, 1970.

108. Centers for Disease Control, Guidelines for short-course tuberculosis chemotherapy, *MMWR*, 29, 97, 1980.

109. American Thoracic Society/Centers for Disease Control, Treatment of tuberculosis and tuberculosis infection in adults and children, *Am. J. Respir. Crit. Care Med.*, Vol. 149, 1994, in press.

110. Centers for Disease Control, Initial therapy for tuberculosis in the era of multidrug resistance: recommendations of the advisory council for the elimination of tuberculosis, *MMWR*, 42 (No. RR-7), 1, 1992.

111. Snider, D. E., Graczyk, J., Bek, E., et al., Supervised six-months treatment of newly diagnosed pulmonary tuberculosis using isoniazid, rifampin, and pyrazinamide with and without streptomycin, *Am. Rev. Resp. Dis.*, 130, 1091, 1984.

112. Combs, D. L., O'Brien, J., Geiter, L. J., USPHS tuberculosis short-course chemotherapy trial 21: effectiveness, toxicity, and acceptability: the report of final results, *Ann. Intern. Med.*, 112, 397, 1990.

112a. Cohn, D. L., Catlin, B. J., Peterson, K. L., et al., A 62-dose, 6-month therapy for pulmonary and extrapulmonary tuberculosis: a twice-weekly, directly observed, and cost-effective regimen, *Ann. Intern. Med.*, 112, 407, 1990.

113. Singapore Tuberculosis Service/British Medical Research Council, Five-year follow-up of a clinical trial of three 6 months regimens of chemotherapy given intermittently in the continuation phase in the treatment of pulmonary tuberculosis, *Am. Rev. Resp. Dis.*, 137, 1147, 1988.

114. Singapore Tuberculosis Service/British Medical Research Council, Assessment of a daily combined preparation of isoniazid, rifampin, and pyrazinamide in a controlled trial of 3 6-month regimens for smear-positive pulmonary tuberculosis, *Am. Rev. Resp. Dis.*, 143, 707, 1991.

115. Hong Kong Chest Service/British Medical Research Council, Controlled trial of 2, 4, and 6 months of pyrazinamide in 6-month, three-times-weekly regimens for smear-positive pulmonary tuberculosis, including an assessment of a combined preparation of isoniazid, rifampin, and pyrazinamide: results at 30 months, *Am. Rev. Resp. Dis.*, 143, 700, 1991.

116. Singapore Tuberculosis Service/British Medical Research Council, Long-term follow-up of a clinical trial of six-month and four-month regimens of chemotherapy in the treatment of pulmonary tuberculosis, *Am. Rev. Resp. Dis.*, 133, 779, 1986.

117. Hong Kong Chest Service/British Medical Research Council, Five-year follow-up of a controlled trial of five 6-month regimens of chemotherapy for pulmonary tuberculosis, *Am. Rev. Resp. Dis.*, 136, 1339, 1987.

117a. National Research Institute for Tuberculosis, Poland, a comparative study of daily followed by twice- or once-weekly regimens of ethambutol and rifampicin in the retreatment of patients with pulmonary tuberculosis: second report, *Tubercle,* 57, 105, 1976.

118. Zierski, M., Prospects of retreatment of chronic resistant pulmonary tuberculosis patients: a critical review, *Lung*, 154, 91, 1977.

118a. Hong Kong Tuberculosis Treatment Services/Brompton Hospital/British Medical Research Council, A controlled trial of daily and intermittent rifampicin plus ethambutol in the retreatment of patients with pulmonary tuberculosis: results up to 30 months, *Tubercle* 56, 179, 1975.

118b. Lees, A. W., Allan, G. W., Smith, J., et al., Rifampin plus isoniazid in initial therapy of pulmonary tuberculosis and rifampin and ethambutol in retreatment cases. *Chest*, 61, 579, 1972.

118c. Nitti, V., Catena, E., Veneri, F. D., et al., Rifampin in association with isoniazid, streptomycin, and ethambutol, respectively, in the initial treatment of pulmonary tuberculosis, *Am. Rev. Respir. Dis.*, 103, 329, 1971.

118d. Hong Kong Chest Service/British Medical Research Council, Controlled trial of 6-month and 9-month regimens of daily and intermittent streptomycin plus isoniazid plus pyrazinamide for pulmonary tuberculosis in Hong Kong: the results up to 30 months, *Am. Rev. Respir. Dis.*, 115, 727, 1977.

118e. American Thoracic Society, Treatment of mycobacterial disease, *Am. Rev. Respir. Dis.*, 115, 185, 1977.

118f. American Thoracic Society, Intermittent chemotherapy for adults with tuberculosis, *Am. Rev. Resp. Dis.,* 110, 374, 1974.

119. British Thoracic Association, A controlled trial of six months chemotherapy in pulmonary tuberculosis: first report: results during chemotherapy, *Br. J. Dis. Chest*, 75, 141, 1981.

120. Combs, D. L., O'Brien, J., Geiter, L. J., USPHS tuberculosis short-course chemotherapy trial 21: effectiveness, toxicity, and acceptability: the report of final results, *Ann. Intern. Med.*, 112, 397, 1990.

121. Dutt, A. K., Moers, D., Stead, W. W., Short-course chemotherapy for tuberculosis with mainly twice-weekly isoniazid and rifampin: community physicians' seven-year experience with mainly outpatients, *Am. J. Med.*, 77, 233, 1984.

122. Dutt, A. K., Jones, L., Stead, W. W., Short-course chemotherapy for tuberculosis with largely twice-weekly isoniazid-rifampin, *Chest*, 75, 441, 1979.

123. Dutt, A. K., Stead, W. W., Chemotherapy of tuberculosis for the 1980's, *Clin. Chest Med.*, 1, 243, 1980.

124. Dutt, A. K., Moers, D., Stead, W. W., Short-course chemotherapy for extrapulmonary tuberculosis: nine years' experience, *Ann. Intern. Med.*, 104, 7, 1986.

125. Slutkin, G., Schecter, G. F., Hopewell, P. C., The results of 9-month isoniazid-rifampin therapy for pulmonary tuberculosis under program conditions in San Francisco, *Am. Rev. Resp. Dis.*, 138, 1622, 1988.

126. Dutt, A. K., Stead, W. W., Smear-negative, culture-positive pulmonary tuberculosis: six-month chemotherapy with isoniazid and rifampin, *Am. Rev. Resp. Dis.*, 141, 1232, 1990.

127. Dutt, A. K., Stead, W. W., Smear- and culture-negative pulmonary tuberculosis: four-month short-course chemotherapy, *Am. Rev. Resp. Dis.*, 139, 867, 1989.

128. Hong Kong Chest Service/Tuberculosis Research Centre, Madras/British Medical Research Council, A controlled trial of 3-month, 4-month, and 6-month regimens of chemotherapy for sputum-smear-negative pulmonary tuberculosis: results at 5 years, *Am. Rev. Resp. Dis.,* 139, 871, 1989.

129. Berger, H. W., Prolonged fever in patients treated for tuberculosis, *Am. Rev. Resp. Dis.*, 97, 140, 1968.

130. Kiblawi, S. S. O., Jay, S. J., Stonehill, R. B., Norton, J., Fever response of patients on therapy for pulmonary tuberculosis, *Am. Rev. Resp. Dis.*, 123, 20, 1981.

131. Costello, H. D., Caras, G. J., Snider, D. E., Drug resistance among previously treated tuberculosis patients, a brief report, *Am. Rev. Resp. Dis.*, 121, 313, 1980.

132. Centers for Disease Control, Tuberculosis and human immunodeficiency virus infection: recommendations of the Advisory Committee for the Elimination of Tuberculosis, *MMWR,* 38, 236, 1989.

133. Sattler, F. R., Cowan, R., Nielsen, D. M., Ruskin, J., Trimethoprim-sulfamethoxazole compared with pentamidine for treatment of *Pneumocystis carinii* pneumonia in the acquired immunodeficiency syndrome. A prospective, non-crossover study, *Ann. Intern. Med.*, 109, 280, 1988.

134. Perriens, J. H., Colebunders, R. L., Karahunga, C., et al., Increased mortality and tuberculosis treatment failure rate among human immunodeficiency virus (HIV) seropositive compared with HIV seronegative patients with pulmonary tuberculosis treated with "standard" chemotherapy in Kinshasa, Zaire, *Am. Rev. Resp. Dis.,* 144, 750, 1991.

135. Dautzenberg, B., Grosset, J., Fechner, J., et al., The management of thirty immunocompromised patients with tuberculosis, *Am. Rev. Resp. Dis.,* 129, 494, 1984.

136. Bobrowitz, I. D., Elkin, M., Evans, J. C., et al., Effect of direct irradiation on the course of pulmonary tuberculosis (using cancerocidal doses), *Dis. Chest*, 40, 397, 1961.

137. Fulkerson, L. L., Perlmutter, G. S., Zack, M. B., et al., Radiotherapy in chest malignant tumors associated with pulmonary tuberculosis, *Radiology*, 106, 645, 1973.

138. Allison, A. C., Hart, P. D., Potentiation by silica of the growth of *Mycobacterium tuberculosis* in macrophage cultures, *Br. J. Exp. Pathol.*, 49, 465, 1968.

139. Morgan, E. J., Silicosis and tuberculosis, *Chest*, 75, 202, 1979.

140. Dubois, P., Gyselen G., Prignot, J., Rifampin-combined chemotherapy in coal worker's pneumoconio-tuberculosis, *Am. Rev. Resp. Dis.*, 115, 221, 1977.

141. Escreet, B. C., Langton, M. E., Cowie, R. L., Short-course chemotherapy for silicotuberculosis, *S. Afr. Med. J.*, 66, 327, 1984.

142. Lin, T. P., Suo, J., Lee, J. J., et al., Short-course chemotherapy of pulmonary tuberculosis in pneumoconiotic patients, *Am. Rev. Resp. Dis.*, 136, 808, 1987.

143. Cowie, R. L., Langton, M. E., Becklake, M. R., Pulmonary tuberculosis in South African gold miners, *Am. Rev. Resp. Dis.*, 139, 1086, 1989.

144. Hong Kong Chest Service/British Medical Research Council, A controlled clinical comparison of 6 and 8 months of antituberculous chemotherapy in the treatment of patients with silicotuberculosis in Hong Kong, *Am. Rev. Resp. Dis.*, 143, 262, 1991.
145. Gaensler, E. A., The surgery for pulmonary tuberculosis, *Am. Rev. Resp. Dis.*, 125 (3 part 2), 73, 1982.
146. Newman, M. M., The olden days of surgery for tuberculosis, *Ann. Thorac. Surg.*, 48, 161, 1989.
147. Harrison, L. H., Current aspects of the surgical management of tuberculosis, *Surg. Clin. North Am.*, 60, 883, 1980.
148. Iseman, M. D., Madsen, L., Goble, M., et al., Surgical intervention in the treatment of pulmonary disease caused by drug-resistant mycobacterium tuberculosis, *Am. Rev. Resp. Dis.*, 141, 623, 1990.
149. Harris, H. W., Menitove, S., Miliary tuberculosis, in *Tuberculosis,* 3rd ed., Schlossberg, D., Ed., Springer-Verlag, New York, 1993, 233.
150. Nemir, R. L., Cardona, J., Vaziri, F., et al., Prednisone as an adjunct in the chemotherapy of lymph node-bronchial tuberculosis in childhood: a double-blind study. II. Further term observation, *Am. Rev. Resp. Dis.*, 95, 402, 1967.

Chapter 7

Extrapulmonary Tuberculosis

Wilfredo Talavera, M.D., Klaus-Dieter K. L. Lessnau, M.D., and Sandra Handwerger, M.D.

CONTENTS

0-8493-4825-0/94/$0.00+$.50
© 1994 by CRC Press, Inc.

I. INTRODUCTION

Tuberculosis (TB) in organs other than the lung had been observed for many centuries but was not recognized as such. Skeletal TB was present in Egypt in 3500 B.C.[1] Ancient physicians divided phthisis (consumption) into many supposedly distinct diseases. Throughout history, extrapulmonary tuberculosis was referred to by many names (Table 7-1) such as Pott's disease of the spine, lupus vulgaris of the skin, and scrofula of the cervical lymph nodes. It was described as an "evil omen" and a disease that "carried men off after their candle had flickered but a short time." The discovery of the tubercle bacillus in 1882 by Robert Koch advanced the understanding of TB as a systemic infection with varying clinical manifestations.

The classic definition of extrapulmonary TB is the tuberculous involvement of an organ outside of the lung. It includes disseminated disease and bacteremia, pleural disease, and intrathoracic lymphatic disease. It may occur in the presence or absence of pulmonary involvement. The course of extrapulmonary TB can be acute and overwhelming, or chronic and slowly progressive over many years, and any organ may be involved. The spectrum of clinical presentations may mimic other systemic diseases and is partly responsible for misdiagnosis and diagnostic delay.

About 10 million of the 250 million people who live in the United States are infected with the tubercle bacillus.[2] Each year from 1964 to 1989 there were approximately 20,000 reported new cases of TB of which approximately 20% resulted in extrapulmonary involvement.[3-5] In 1991 there were 26,283 cases of TB reported in the United States (CDC, Atlanta, unpublished data), of which 4887 cases were predominately extrapulmonary. Of those

Table 7-1 **Historical terminology**

Bouchut's tubercles	Choroidal tubercles in miliary MTB
Eales' disease	Retinal periphlebitis, retinal vasculitis, retinal hemorrhage with possible retinal detachment and neovascularization
Empyema necessitatis	Empyema with invasion of chest wall or lung
Ghon complex	Calcified area in the chest X-ray due to healed primary tuberculosis
Gibbus	Anterior erosion of vertebral bone leads to collapse and sharp kyphosis (Victor Hugo's Quasimodo; latin for hump, convex, protuberant, humpbacked)
Lupus vulgaris	Cutaneous tuberculosis
Phthisis	Wasting syndrome, "consumption"
Poncet's disease	Polyarthritis, hypersensitivity induced
Pott's disease	Vertebral tuberculosis, tuberculous spondylitis, spinal caries
Scrofula	Cervical lymph nodes (king's evil); latin for "glandular swelling"
Spina ventosa	Tuberculous osteitis of the phalanges in children; "ballooned-out" appearance (ventosa)
Tabes mesenterica	Mesenteric tuberculous lymphadenitis

cases that were predominately extrapulmonary 23.5% were pleural, 30.2% were lymphatic, 8.7% were urogenital, 10.6% involved bones or joints, 7.6% were miliary, 5.4% were meningeal, 4% were peritoneal, and 9.9% involved other sites. At this rate there is an annual risk for extrapulmonary disease of over 1:2500 in tuberculin-positive individuals. In developing countries, there are approximately 7 million new cases of active tuberculosis per year of which 5–10% are extrapulmonary.[6] This apparent underestimation may be due to the difficulty in diagnosis, particularly with the unavailability of advanced technology in some third-world countries.[7,8] Between 20 and 50% of cases of extrapulmonary TB are diagnosed at autopsy only.[3,8,9]

Historically, extrapulmonary TB has afflicted children, decreased in incidence with age, and then peaked in the elderly population.[3] In the post-AIDS era in this country, 1008 patients (22%) with extrapulmonary tuberculosis were over 65 years of age.[10] However, meningitis, lymphadenopathy (scrofula), and miliary disease are more common among children less than 5 years of age.[11] Extrapulmonary disease is more common in Hispanics (4-fold), blacks (6-fold), Asians (11-fold), foreign born, and native Americans.[3,8]

Specific medical risk factors for extrapulmonary TB include HIV infection with low CD4+ cell counts, immunosuppression, chronic renal disease and hemodialysis,[12,13] bone marrow transplantation,[14] and jejunoileal bypass.[15,16] A questionable risk factor is pregnancy.[17]

Low CD4+ cell counts are associated with a greater probability of extrapulmonary disease in patients with AIDS. For example, mean CD4+ cell counts of 350 have been reported with pulmonary disease, 250 with localized extrapulmonary TB

(lymph nodes or effusion), 140 with meningitis, and 70 with bacteremia.[18,19]

It has been estimated that more than 4 million persons worldwide have been infected with both HIV and TB. Two-thirds of these patients potentially have extrapulmonary involvement.[20] Extrapulmonary disease appears to be common among patients infected with HIV in this country. Of 292 HIV-positive patients with TB compiled from several retrospective studies, 181 patients (62%) had extrapulmonary TB (with or without pulmonary disease), 216 patients (74%) had pulmonary TB (with or without extrapulmonary disease), and 36% had both.[21] In the United States during the period of October 1987 through March 1989 48,712 persons with AIDS were reported to the CDC. Of these, 1239 patients (2.5%) were diagnosed with extrapulmonary tuberculosis.[22]

In patients with AIDS multiple sites of infection are common. The bacilli may be found in lymph nodes, blood, bone marrow, urinary tract, liver, gastrointestinal tract, central nervous system, cardiovascular system, skin, and soft tissues.[23-25]

In a study of 44 patients with AIDS or ARC and tuberculosis published by one of these authors (S.H.), 13 patients (29.5%) had extrapulmonary disease alone.[26] In another study of 35 patients with both AIDS and TB, 9 patients (26%) had extrapulmonary disease alone.[27] Both reports were published before the AIDS case definition included extrapulmonary tuberculosis. In 1991, Shafer et al. reported 199 patients with AIDS and extrapulmonary TB at a major New York City hospital; 76 patients (38%) had extrapulmonary involvement alone.[28] More unusual presentations have been seen in HIV-positive patients,[29] such as skeletal disease, scrotal disease, and bacteremia.[30] Miliary and lymphatic disease are observed often, and unusual presentations such as spinal and breast abscesses, and esophagobronchial fistulas have been described.[31] Extrapulmonary TB has become a significant cause of morbidity and mortality in HIV-infected patients in the 1990s.

The diagnosis of extrapulmonary TB often is difficult. The shortest delay in diagnosis is in pleural disease, and the longest is in skeletal disease, probably because tissue is less accessible and symptoms are more subtle.[32] Twenty to fifty percent of extrapulmonary TB is discovered at autopsy, in contrast to 5% of pulmonary TB. Those numbers may be increased in the elderly and in HIV patients.[3,33] Unfortunately there is no inexpensive, rapid, and noninvasive screening test, and a high degree of clinical suspicion is a prerequisite for a timely diagnosis.

Although 9 months of treatment for pulmonary tuberculosis is well established, there are few data available on the use of short-course chemotherapy in extrapulmonary tuberculosis. The extrapulmonary site of disease probably is less consequential since the mycobacterial population is smaller in extrapulmonary versus cavitary pulmonary disease. Dutt et al. [34] reported their experience with short-course chemotherapy in 350 patients with extrapulmonary tuberculosis. Nine-month therapy with isoniazid and rifampin was successful in 95% of patients.[34,35] Cohn et al.[36] reported success with a 62-dose, largely twice-weekly, 6-month tuberculosis treatment regimen in 7 patients with both pulmonary and extrapulmonary disease and 17 patients with extrapulmonary tuberculosis alone who had directly observed therapy. Although it appears that a 6-month short course of therapy may be adequate in selected patients with extrapulmonary tuberculosis, caution must be taken when extrapolating from small series of patients. Specific treatment for each extrapulmonary site will be considered in each section below.

II. PLEURA

A. EPIDEMIOLOGY

Worldwide, tuberculosis is still a significant cause of pleural effusions. In some parts of the world (e.g., Spain) tuberculosis remains the most frequent cause of pleural effusion, in the absence of an obvious pulmonary lesion.[37] In the United States, tuberculosis is responsible for only a small percentage of all pleural effusions, the incidence varying from less than 1 to 13% of all exudative effusions.[38,39] In a study of 1738 cases of pulmonary tuberculosis, 70 patients (4.9%) with tuberculous effusions were identified.[40] In 1991, of all cases that were predominately extrapulmonary, 23.5% were pleural (CDC, Atlanta, unpublished data).

Table 7-2 **Pleural tuberculosis**

Characteristic	Percentage and references
Clinical	
Weight loss (>5 kg)	28–35[42,54]
Night sweats	46[54]
Dyspnea	38–52[42,54]
Cough	55–80[41,42,54]
Chest pain	50–75[41,54]
Leukocytosis (>10,000/mm³)	5–15[41,50]
Insidious onset	33.3[41,50]
Acute onset and pain	66.6[41,50]
Symptoms <1 week	31–62[41,50]
Symptoms <1 month	62[50]
Fever	65–85[41,42,54]
Radiography	
Unilateral effusion	90[41,42,54]
Hemorrhagic effusion	1.5–9[41]
Radiographic pulmonary lesion	
CXR	22–35[41,54]
CT	80[51]
More than 505 lymphocytes in effusion	62–90[41,42]
Stain	
Sputum	7–8[41,55]
Pleural fluid	0–9[42,55]
Pleural biopsy	21–39[41,55]
Pathology	
Pleural biopsy	57–97 [41,42,55]
Culture	
Sputum (without infiltrate)	4–11 [40,42]
Sputum (with infiltrate)	18–89 [40,45,54]
Thoracentesis	23–60 [40-42,54,55]
Pleural biopsy (only culture)	39–65 [41,42,55]
Pleural biopsy (culture and pathology)	90[57]

Pleural TB may affect any age group, although there are peaks at 20–40 years and in the elderly population.[41,42]

B. CLINICAL

The clinical and laboratory characteristics of pleural tuberculosis are included in Table 7-2. Tuberculous pleurisy frequently is associated with primary disease and, in those instances, results from the rupture of a subpleural caseous focus, which may not be evident radiographically.[43,44] It also may result secondarily from intrapulmonary cavitary disease, lymphohematogenous dissemination or spread from an adjacent source, e.g., lymph node or spine.[43] Tuberculous pleuritis has been regarded traditionally as a manifestation of primary tuberculosis. In a study by Antoniskis et al.,[45] tuberculous pleurisy was a manifestation of reactivation in 27 of 59 patients (46%), altering this classic view of the pathogenesis of tuberculous effusions. This study also suggests that perhaps these patients are less capable of mounting an effective immunologic response to the tubercle bacillus.

Delayed hypersensitivity appears to play a pivotal role in the pathogenesis of tuberculous pleuritis. When tuberculin protein is injected into the pleural space of previously immunized laboratory animals a large exudative effusion results within 2 days. It is likely that delayed hypersensitivity also plays a major role in the development of tuberculous pleuritis in humans and explains the small bacterial load seen. Thus the yield of smears and cultures of the pleural fluid is expected to be low. The intense inflammatory reaction obstructs lymphatic pores of parietal pleura and explains the high biopsy yield.[44]

Typically tuberculous pleural effusions occur 3 to 6 months after the primary infection,[46] but they may occur with postprimary or reactivated disease. In HIV-positive patients, it may appear as early as 4 to 12 weeks after the initial infection.[47]

The natural history of an untreated isolated tuberculous effusion is spontaneous resolution, only to recur as active parenchymal disease at a later date.[44] In a Finnish Armed Forces study of 2816 men with undiagnosed pleural effusions, 43% developed tuberculosis during a 7-year follow-up period.[48] In another study by Roper and Waring[49] of 141 military personnel with a positive PPD and a pleural effusion, most patients completely reabsorbed their effusions and became asymptomatic within 2 to 4 months. This response required prolonged bed rest and most recuperated with minimal chest radiographic changes and minimal pleural thickening. Ninety-two of these 141 individuals (65%) developed active tuberculosis within 5 years, 88% of these within 3 years. This proclivity for the development of subsequent active tuberculosis makes it imperative to treat those with documented or presumed tuberculous pleuritis.

The onset of pleurisy is typically abrupt and may resemble bacterial pneumonia with fever and a dry cough. The onset of effusion is acute in about two-thirds and chronic in one-third of patients.[41,50] Effusions usually are small or moderate in size, but may involve the entire hemithorax. Over 90% of effusions are unilateral, and bilateral effusions usually are associated with miliary spread.[41,42] Effusions were present more commonly on the left side in 57% of patients in a study by Berger and Mejia[41] but more commonly on the right side in 65% of patients in a study by Epstein et al.[42] The primary pulmonary focus often is undetectable on chest radiograph, but in a study of 70 patients with pleural tuberculosis 50% had an accompanying infiltrate.[40] The chest CT scan useful especially in those patients with no obvious parenchymal disease on conventional chest radiograph. In one study of 14 such patients, 11 patients (78.5%) had additional cavities or parenchymal infiltrates seen on CT scan. Sites of communication between the parenchyma and pleural space were also demonstrated.[51]

Tuberculous pleuritis has been reported in 9–20% of patients with HIV infection and tuberculosis.[28,52,53] In one study, tuberculous effusions in patients with AIDS often were a manifestation of a disseminated process.[54] In a study of 199 HIV-positive patients with extrapulmonary TB, 32 patients (16%) had pleural effusions; 75% of these had respiratory symptoms including cough, pleuritic chest pain, and dyspnea. Most effusions were present on admission but in 9 patients (28%) the effusions developed during the hospital stay. The effusions were invariably exudative, were bilateral in 6 patients (15.6%), and were more likely to be culture positive (91%).[28]

C. DIAGNOSIS

An unexplained exudative pleural effusion in the presence of a positive PPD skin test may suggest that more aggressive measures are needed to diagnose tuberculous pleurisy, but a negative skin test does not eliminate its possibility. Tuberculin skin test positivity in tuberculous pleurisy, as reflected in several studies, ranges from 47 to 93%.[40-42,45,54,55] In a study of tuberculous pleurisy by Berger and Mejia, 11 of 36 patients (30.5%) had a negative intermediate tuberculin skin test. On retesting, all patients converted their skin test to positive.[41] This skin test negativity has been attributed to sequestration of specific T-lymphocytes in the pleural space.[56] In some patients the negative skin test may represent true anergy. We recommend retesting patients with a suspected tuberculous effusion and a negative tuberculin skin test in 4 to 8 weeks.

The diagnosis is made definitively by a positive culture from pleural tissue or pleural fluid, and presumptively by a positive culture from sputum and appropriate radiographic findings. The effusion almost always is exudative, may be serosanguinous on occasion, and grossly bloody rarely. The protein content invariably is greater than 3 g/dl and greater than 5 g/dl in 77% of patients. The lactate dehydrogenase levels are elevated.[41] Although in the past pleural fluid glucose levels were thought to be low, more recent studies[41,42] demonstrate that most effusions have glucose levels greater than 60 mg/dl and levels less than 30 mg/dl occur rarely. The pleural pH may range from 7.00 to 7.50, parallels pleural glucose levels, but often is nonspecific.[44]

During an early tuberculous effusion, neutrophils (PMNs) predominate. Monocytes increase between day 2 and 5. After 6 days, the classic finding of small lymphocytes, which constitute less than 50% of cells, are present in 90% of effusions.[40,42,44,57] Subsequent thoracenteses show a greater proportion of smaller lymphocytes, as the disease becomes more chronic.[41] The CD4+ lymphocytes are elevated,[56] and eosinophils are seen rarely. Mesothelial cells are typically absent in tuberculous pleurisy. They usually are decreased with extensive pleural inflammation and increased in neoplasia, and therefore their presence or absence is nondiagnostic.[44]

Measurement of adenosine deaminase (ADA) levels in pleural effusions is useful in ascertaining the diagnosis of tuberculous pleuritis, although not readily used in this country. This enzyme is a product of the activated T-lymphocytes and, therefore, is elevated where cellular immunity is stimulated. ADA levels in tuberculous effusions have a sensitivity and specificity of 80%. Levels above 70 U/liter are 90% specific, and levels below 40 U/liter have not been observed in TB.[58,59] Similar results have been reported by Fontan-Bueso et al.[37] in 138 patients with tuberculous and malignant effusions. In the same study a ratio of pleural fluid to serum lysozyme above 1.2 was found to be 80% sensitive and specific and especially helpful when used in conjunction with ADA. Measurement of pleural fluid lysozyme may be useful in differentiating tuberculous from malignant effusions. Gamma interferon levels and SC5b-9, which is generated by the activation of complement and can be measured by a simple and rapid enzyme immunoassay, one day may be useful diagnostic tools.[60,61] Amplification of mycobacterial DNA by the use of the polymerase chain reaction (PCR) is a rapid and sensitive diagnostic test for TB. In a study evaluating 84 patients with pleural effusions, including 53 patients with TB, pleural fluid analysis confirmed a sensitivity of 81% for PCR. The sensitivity for pleural fluid culture, pleural biopsy culture, and histology of the biopsy was 52.8, 69.8, and 77.3%, respectively.[62]

Since a definitive diagnosis of tuberculous pleurisy requires demonstration of the tubercle bacilli in the sputum, pleural fluid, or pleural biopsy, these specimens should be cultured for mycobacteria whenever this condition is suspected. Chan et al.[55] reported 83 patients with tuberculous effusions, of which 7 (8%) were sputum smear positive and 18 (22%) were culture positive. The percentage of positive sputum cultures is dependent largely on the presence or absence of concomitant parenchymal infiltration. Cultures are more likely to be positive if there is underlying parenchymal disease (see Table 7-2).

The recovery of the tubercle bacilli from smear and culture of pleural fluid varies substantially depending on the study (see Table 7-2). They are demonstrable on smear in less than 10% of cases.[42] In most series, pleural fluid cultures show *Mycobacterium tuberculosis* in approximately 25% of cases, but some studies reveal yields of up to 66%.[40-42,54,55]

Parietal pleural biopsy is diagnostic, i.e., positive smear, culture or granuloma formation, in 70–95% of cases depending on the technique employed.[40,55] The smear of the biopsy specimen is positive in 21–39%[41,55] of cases, the culture in 39–65% of cases,[41,42,55] and granulomas can be seen in 57–97% of cases.[41,42,55] When the microscopic examination of the biopsy specimen is combined with biopsy culture, the diagnosis can be achieved in 90% of patients,[57] especially with the use of multiple biopsies.[44,63,64] We recommend that a thoracentesis and a minimum of three pleural biopsy specimens for culture and histology be obtained when tuberculous pleuritis is suspected.

Pleuroscopy or thoracoscopy is a safe, rapid, and useful adjunct to the diagnosis of tuberculous pleurisy by allowing direct visualization of affected tissue. It may obviate the need for open pleural biopsy and as a result may decrease complications.[65,66] In a study by Sarkar et al. of 40 patients with undiagnosed pleural effusions, a diagnosis of tuberculosis was made by pleuroscopic biopsy in 17 patients (42.5%). The yield for tuberculosis was 100% and the overall specific diagnostic yield in this study was 92.5%.[65] The pleuroscopic findings included hyperemia, shiny opalescent pleural thickening, and small white-gray tubercular nodules.[65,67] In another study thoracoscopic pleural biopsy had a yield of 90%.[67] Open thoracotomy for pleural biopsy rarely is necessary today.

D. TREATMENT

The goals of therapy of tuberculous effusions are to prevent the subsequent development of active pulmonary disease, to relieve patient's symptoms, and to prevent associated complications.[44]

Nine-month therapy with isoniazid (INH), 300 mg, and rifampin (RIF), 600 mg daily, is a highly efficacious regimen with no relapses.[68] Standard 6-month therapy probably is equally efficacious,[36] with extension to 9 months in patients with AIDS.[69]

Short-course therapy may be effective in the management of tuberculous effusions. In a study by Dutt et al. 198 patients with tuberculous effusions were treated with INH 300 mg and RIF 600 mg daily for 1 month followed by INH 900 mg plus RIF 600 mg twice weekly for an additional 5 months. There were no relapses in the 161 patients who completed therapy and side effects occurred in only 6.6% of patients. The therapy was efficacious even in the presence of a parenchymal infiltrate.[70]

With appropriate treatment, symptoms and signs of the disease subside slowly. Most patients are afebrile by the second week of therapy, but fever persists for up to 2 months in some patients. Radiologic resolution occurs at about 6 weeks but may take as long as 12 weeks in some patients.[71] Tuberculous effusions have been treated with a combination of antimicrobials and corticosteroids for many years with more rapid improvement in signs and symptoms. Lee et al.[72] in a double-blind, prospective, randomized study showed that resolution of clinical symptoms and pleural fluid was greater in the group receiving the corticosteroids. The development of residual pleural thickening was not influenced by their use. Once a definitive diagnosis is established and therapy is prescribed, corticosteroid therapy may be beneficial if symptoms are severe or if the pleural effusion is particularly large.

E. COMPLICATIONS

The most common sequela of tuberculous pleuritis is residual pleural thickening, which is usually present on diagnosis and may be seen in up to 50% of patients after treatment. Repeated thoracenteses are indicated for relief of symptomatic effusions only, since they do not diminish the amount of residual pleural thickening.[73] Chest tube drainage is useful primarily for the treatment of empyemas and bronchopleural fistulas. Pleurectomy or decortication rarely may be required for a "trapped lung" resulting from a thick fibrin peel.[55,74]

Tuberculous empyema is characterized by a purulent exudate and numerous organisms on smear. Although historically it is a consequence of previous pleurisy, collapse pneumothorax therapy, or thoracoplasty, tuberculous empyema may result from rupture of an underlying cavity.[44] Tuberculous empyema may occur alone or as a "mixed" empyema with superinfection by anaerobic bacteria such as *Bacteroides* species. Repeat thoracentesis or ill-advised chest tube insertion may lead to mixed infection.[75] Closed chest tube drainage or repeated thoracenteses are useful, but surgical intervention with decortication, thoracoplasty, extrapleural pneumonectomy, or Eloesser flap may be required.[44,76] In patients with AIDS, tuberculous empyema may be the result of lymphohematogenous dissemination and a subpleural caseous focus or bronchopleural fistula may not be present.[77] More serious complications include an empyema necessitatis, which may burrow through the parietal pleura, esophagus, retroperitoneum, flank, groin, pericardium, or vertebral column.[78] A chylothorax, due to the obstruction of the thoracic duct, also may be seen with *Mycobacterium tuberculosis*.[79]

Tuberculous bronchopleural fistulas also are uncommon today and usually can be managed with antituberculous therapy. Like tuberculous empyemas, they occur primarily in those who were treated prior to effective chemotherapy.[44,76] Shafer et al. reported 32 HIV-infected patients with pleural tuberculosis and three (9.4%) developed a bronchopleural fistula.[28] A bronchopleural fistula with pneumothorax usually requires closed chest tube drainage but definitive surgical management may be necessary.[76]

III. LYMPH NODES

A. EXTRATHORACIC
1. Epidemiology

Tuberculous lymphadenitis was the most common type of extrapulmonary tuberculosis in the United States in 1991. It accounted for 30.2% (1,475 patients) of all cases of predominantly extrapulmonary disease and 5.6% of all cases of tuberculosis (CDC, Atlanta, unpublished data). Historically, tuberculous lymphadenitis comprises 2–5% of all cases of TB and 31% of extrapulmonary disease, of which approximately 70% is cervical in location.[80-82]

Mycobacterial tuberculous lymphadenitis historically has been a disease of children and especially noted within the first 6 months of infection.[83] Recent studies suggest that the peak incidence now occurs in young adults between the ages of 20 and 40 years.[84-87] This probably reflects the decreasing rate of childhood tuberculosis in developed countries, and, in this age group, atypical mycobacteria now predominate.[86,88]

Both sex and ethnicity play a major role in the development of tuberculous lymphadenitis. Most studies show a female to male predominance of greater than 2:1[81,88,89] and in the developed world, Indian, Asian, and blacks, especially women, appear to be predisposed.[82,84,88,90]

An additional risk factor for development of tuberculous lymphadenitis is HIV infection. In fact, lymphadenopathy is a prominent feature in patients with AIDS and tuberculosis. Peripheral tuberculous lymphadenopathy occurs in 22–31% of patients with AIDS.[27,28,52,53]

2. Clinical

The cervical form of this disease or scrofula was well recognized by the seventeenth century in Europe, where it was called the "King's evil," because of the belief that it could be cured by the hands of a sovereign. Charles II of England is reputed to have applied the "Royal Touch" to the scrofulous over ninety thousand times.[91]

Tuberculous lymphadenitis may represent a localized process or an expression of disseminated disease. Seventy percent of patients with tuberculous lymphadenitis have cervical lymph node involvement. This may include both the anterior and posterior cervical chains.[81,92] Enlarged lymph nodes also may affect the submandibular region, the supraclavicular space, the superior portion of the neck, and the submental and preauricular areas.[84,85] Cervical lymph nodes may be isolated, may extend from an adjacent focus, such as intrathoracic or paratracheal lymph nodes, may develop from subclinical pulmonary disease, or hematogenously from an unrecognized site.[80,90] Infected tonsils or adenoids may be a focus.[80]

Typically, there is slow, painless enlargement in the neck.[85] The nodes are usually discrete and "rubbery-soft" to palpation. As the disease progresses there may significant induration, fluctuance, necrosis, and a sinus tract may form.[82,84,88,93] Progression to draining sinus tracts occur in less than 10% of patients.[81,88,94] In a study by Malik and others the average size of lymph nodes on biopsy was 5×5 cm (range 2–8 cm), and the average number of nodes found was four.[93]

Tuberculous lymphadenitis may be bilateral, but diffuse lymphadenopathy is distinctly uncommon,[88] unless associated with childhood miliary tuberculosis.[95] Systemic symptoms such as fever, weight loss, anorexia, and fatigue occur in less than 20% of patients,[84] but in a recent study of 47 patients (including 10 patients with HIV disease), 43% had systemic symptoms.[94] When isolated peripheral lymphadenopathy is seen, such as in the epitrochlear, axillary, or inguinal regions, a more distal focus must be identified.[96]

Other less common presentations of tuberculous lymphadenopathy may occur. These include chronic abdominal pain from retroperitoneal lymph node involvement, jaundice from biliary tract obstruction, and generalized lymphadenopathy mimicking neoplasia.[97]

In a study by Shafer of 199 HIV-positive patients with extrapulmonary tuberculosis 44 patients (22%) had peripheral lymphadenopathy. Of this group 37 patients (84%) had cervical disease, 8 patients (18%) had axillary disease, and one patient (2.3%) had inguinal disease. In the majority of these patients the clinical presentation was dominated by systemic symptoms. Only 20 of these patients (45%) had symptoms referable to enlarged lymph nodes. This suggests that the lymphadenopathy is only one facet of a more generalized process. An additional 24 patients (12%) had intraabdominal lymphadenopathy, which was present invariably with disseminated tuberculosis.[28]

3. Diagnosis

Since the differential diagnosis of tuberculous lymphadenopathy is vast, many other conditions including infections and neoplasia must be considered before rendering empiric therapy. Careful history taking, a chest radiograph and tuberculin skin testing are important in the evaluation of the patient with suspected tuberculous lymphadenitis. Less than 20% of adults have a history of exposure to tuberculosis[84] and 24–46% of patients have chest radiographic abnormalities consistent with tuberculosis.[81,84,94] Tuberculin skin testing may be positive in 90% of patients unless the patient is HIV positive.[80,81,84,85,90,94] If the diagnosis of tuberculous lymphadenitis remains in doubt, a lymph node biopsy with AFB smear, culture, and histological evaluation is required.

Total excisional biopsy has been long recommended since incomplete excision may result in chronic fistulous tract formation.[82,90] With the chemotherapeutic armamentarium presently available, needle biopsy or aspiration may be safe[98-100] in most cases of cervical tuberculous lymphadenitis. Cervical abscess formation may require total excisional surgery. In a study of 40 patients with tuberculous cervical abscesses, 17 of 22 patients (77%) having a simple drainage procedure required a second operation because of sinus tract formation. Of those having a complete excisional procedure, 17 of 18 patients (94%) required no further surgical intervention.[101]

In a study by Dandapat et al. of 80 cases of peripheral tuberculous lymphadenitis, fine needle aspiration (FNA) provided a positive diagnosis in 66 patients (83%) including a positive culture in 52 patients (65%). Biopsy of the largest affected lymph node gave histological confirmation in 100%.[92] In another study fine needle aspiration or biopsy of cervical lymph nodes showed caseous material and/or granulomas in 80% of patients, and culture positivity in 60% of patients.[102] The yield of AFB smear positivity of tuberculous lymph nodes varies from 35 to 56%.[81,92,94]

Fine needle aspiration of lymph nodes usually is diagnostic in the HIV-positive population. In a study by Shriner et al., all FNA performed were diagnostic for tuberculosis.[80] In HIV-positive patients the smear is positive from 70–90% of patients[28,53,80,103] and culture positivity reaches 90–100%.[28,53,80] This undoubtedly reflects a higher burden of organisms in patients with low CD4+ cell counts.[53] Lymph node biopsy is diagnostic in approximately 90% of patients[28] and offers little advantage over FNA in this group. Lymph node aspiration is a simple, rapid, and inexpensive diagnostic procedure in HIV-positive patients with peripheral nodes equal or larger than 1.5 cm.[103]

Thoracic and abdominal sonography, computed tomography (CT) of the chest and abdomen, and whole-body gallium scanning are useful adjuncts in detecting mediastinal, hilar, and intraabdominal lymph nodes and helpful in directing biopsies or aspiration.[104-107]

4. Treatment

Treatment of tuberculous lymphadenopathy includes antimicrobial therapy and the judicious use of surgical excision in selected patients. Nine months of INH and RIF supplemented initially by 2 months of ethambutol has been shown to be effective therapy with excellent response rates in most studies.[92,98,108,109] Another study showed that 6 months of INH, RIF, pyrazinamide (PZA), and streptomycin was similar to a 9-month 3-drug regimen.[110] However, the incidence of residual enlarged lymph nodes varied from 5 to 14.5%.[92,98,110] In some patients extension of therapy up to 18 months was required before most lymph nodes regressed.[93]

5. Complications

Complete surgical excision can relieve discomfort caused by enlarging lymph nodes and may be helpful with scars or fistulas that do not improve with 6 months of therapy.[94,109] Incision and drainage may be required with cervical abscesses.[101] A second procedure may be necessary when there is persistent discharge, recurrent abscesses, or increasing lymphadenopathy.[99] Excision alone without antituberculous therapy has a relapse rate of 83%.[109,111] During therapy, lymph nodes may enlarge, or new nodes may develop. This often is transient and does not necessarily indicate relapse or treatment failure.[88]

B. INTRATHORACIC

Intrathoracic lymphadenopathy is an uncommon manifestation of adult tuberculosis, although it is quite common in children.[88] In a study by Silver and Steel, intrathoracic tuberculous lymphadenopathy has been found to be more common in Asians and blacks.[112] Although mediastinal nodes are the most common primary regional draining sites, they account for only 5% of lymph node tuberculosis.[91]

In adults, enlarging lymph nodes rarely lead to luminal obstruction with respiratory symptoms such as cough, sputum production, localized wheezing, and dyspnea. Usually fever, weight loss, anorexia, night sweats, and fatigue prevail. The patient may be asymptomatic with an abnormal chest radiograph.[113,114] Two-thirds of mediastinal nodes involve the right paratracheal region.[115]

HIV-positive patients with suspected intrathoracic tuberculous lymphadenopathy frequently have palpable extrathoracic lymph nodes.[103] Hilar lymphadenopathy occurred in 33–40% of patients in several studies.[52,53,116,117] In a study of 199 patients with AIDS and extrapulmonary tuberculosis by Shafer, 28 patients (14%) had mediastinal tuberculosis diagnosed at mediastinoscopy or at autopsy. CT scanning was very useful in assessing the various groups of lymph node involved and the finding of low central density areas consistent with necrosis.[28] Endobronchial obstruction from mediastinal lymphadenopathy, mimicking lung cancer, can occur in patients with AIDS.[118]

In intrathoracic lymphadenopathy due to tuberculosis, mediastinoscopy and especially fiberoptic bronchoscopy may be useful. The latter, when coupled with brush and bronchial biopsy, has a diagnostic yield of 75%.[119] This high yield was explained by the presence of endobronchial disease. Mediastinoscopy or exploratory thoracotomy is rarely required for diagnosis.

Treatment is standard antituberculous chemotherapy including isoniazid, rifampin, and ethambutol (EMB) or pyrazinamide.[109,120]

Severe complications such as rupture of a lymph node into adjacent tissue including esophagus, bronchus, superior vena cava, aorta, and pericardium may occur. Local nerve compression may cause Horner syndrome[110] or unilateral laryngeal palsy with hoarseness.[88]

IV. SKELETAL

A. VERTEBRAL
1. Epidemiology

Skeletal tuberculous was the third most common type of extrapulmonary tuberculosis in the United States in 1991. It accounted for 10.6% (518 patients) of all cases of predominantly extrapulmonary disease and 1.97% of all cases of tuberculosis (CDC, Atlanta, unpublished data). Previously, bone and joint tuberculosis occurred primarily in children afflicted with pulmonary tuberculosis.[83] Today it is a disease of the elderly in America and Europe but is still a disease of children in developing countries.[121] The incidence of skeletal tuberculosis in patients with HIV infection largely is unknown. In several series of HIV-related tuberculosis 0–9% of patients had bone or joint involvement.[21,27,28,52] Skeletal TB remains an important crippling disease worldwide.

Skeletal tuberculosis typically involves the vertebrae and the weight-bearing bones and joints as well. Farer et al. in a retrospective study noted 676 cases of bone and joint tuberculosis. The spine was involved in 40.7% of cases, the hips in 13.3% of cases, the knees in 10.3% of cases, and other areas such as ankles, long bones, wrist, elbow, shoulder, ribs, sacroiliac joint, foot, and hand in 35.7% of cases. This disease process may involve any bone or joint.[91,122]

2. Clinical

Vertebral TB or Pott's disease usually results from lymphohematogenous dissemination from a primary focus such as lung. It also may result from direct invasion of a paravertebral focus, or lymphangitic spread from paravertebral lymph nodes or the pleural space.[122] Mechanical factors seem to play a role in the pathogenesis, and it has been suggested that trauma is responsible for this increased susceptibility of weight-bearing joints.[122]

The basic lesion in skeletal tuberculosis is a combination of osteomyelitis and arthritis. Involvement of the joint space may occur from adjacent epiphyseal bone or through hematogenous dissemination. Early synovitis, granulation tissue, and effusion ensue. Destruction of cartilage, bone demineralization, and caseation necrosis eventually occur. The cartilage is destroyed peripherally first, preserving the integrity of the joint space. The proteolytic enzymes that usually destroy cartilage, as in pyogenic processes, are not produced in tuberculous infections. Focal osteolysis and marginal sclerosis are other features that differentiate it from nontuberculous infections.[123] At this early stage intermittent pain and tenderness over the affected area are seen.[122,124]

Later, as paraosseous abscess and gibbus formation is produced by the collapse of adjacent vertebrae and narrowing of the disk space, an increase in pain is noted.[122,124] Paravertebral abscesses are "cold" without erythema or warmth, may be fluctuant, and either nontender or slightly painful on palpation. They may descend and involve caudal areas, may extend along fascial planes to the retroperitoneal, inguinal, gluteal, or pelvic regions, or rarely as far as the popliteal space. They may form a psoas abscess, and even pleural, cervical, and supraclavicular soft tissue masses have been described.[121] Regardless of location, abscesses may calcify after 1 to 2 years. In the late stage the lesions may disseminate or heal spontaneously with fibrosis and ankylosis.[122,124] Complete destruction with collapse of the vertebral body, kyphosis, and adjacent arthritis eventually ensues.[124]

The midthoracic spine is the area most frequently involved. In the child there is a tendency toward upper or cervical spine involvement, while in the adult infection of the lower thoracic and lumbar spine predominates.[121,124,125] In nonwhites, tuberculous spondylitis has a more atypical presentation involving multiple singular vertebral bodies and affecting the posterior part of the vertebrae.[126]

Pain is the most common complaint noted but sinus drainage, joint swelling, and limitation of motion also may be seen. Systemic symptoms such as fever, chills, weight loss, and fatigue are present in only 20% with skeletal tuberculosis.[121]

Characteristically, the onset is insidious, developing 2–3 years after primary infection.[46] Extensive destruction of the spine may lead to various neurologic syndromes including paralysis.

Skeletal tuberculosis as a manifestation of AIDS has not been well described. Despite frequent bone marrow involvement in patients with AIDS, tuberculous bone and joint infections are uncommon.[28] One case report described a patient with multifocal osteitis,[127] and another study described two patients with psoas abscess formation.[26]

3. Diagnostic

Early diagnosis is critical to the preservation of the cartilage and joint space. Prompt diagnosis and treatment will lead to maintenance of good joint function. The chronicity of the complaints attributable to tuberculous spondylitis may lead to a delay in diagnosis from 4 months to 2 years.[128]

Although skin test results are reported variably in the literature, available data suggest positivity occurs in 76–100% of patients.[121,125]

Radiologic techniques are of benefit in the diagnosis and treatment of tuberculous spondylitis. Up to 58% of patients have normal chest radiographs.[129] The typical radiologic changes of tuberculous spondylitis are beyond the scope of this chapter and are best described in Chapter 10 of this volume. A paravertebral mass can be seen on chest or abdominal roentgenogram, although there is greater likelihood of detection with CT scanning.[124]

Lesions seen on conventional radiographs can be further evaluated by CT scanning or magnetic resonance imaging (MRI) techniques.[129,130] CT findings in 11 patients with tuberculosis of the spine included vertebral body destruction (10 patients), psoas or paraspinous abscesses (10 patients), and intervertebral disk space narrowing in 6 patients.[129] Atypical cases may be seen.[131] Bone scintigraphy with technetium is more sensitive than radiographs and useful at an early stage[124] but may be negative in 35% of patients with spinal tuberculosis.[125] Scanning with ^{67}Ga occasionally may show unsuspected sites not detected by bone scanning and clinical evaluation,[132] but in one study was negative in 70% of patients with tuberculous spondylitis.[125]

Confirmation of tuberculous spondylitis requires microbiological confirmation with smear and culture of obtained material as early as possible if unnecessary delay in treatment is to be avoided. Although historically it is a disease requiring surgical intervention for diagnosis, tuberculosis of the spine may be detected by fine-needle aspiration.[133]

Tuberculous spondylitis is characterized by an uncommonly low mycobacterial population.[134] Even with extensive surgery the yield of culture positivity is approximately 40% even with a large amount of abscess fluid.[121,134] The yield of culture positivity from infected bone is 80–95%.[121] The smear of the biopsy is positive in 30%, and granulomas are found in 90% of specimens obtained.[32] A percutaneous needle biopsy may supplant surgery for diagnosis in early cases.[32]

4. Treatment

In general, response to medical therapy is usually complete although large lesions may require drainage. The British Medical Research Council has undertaken several clinical trials in the treatment of tuberculous spondylitis. Chemotherapy with isoniazid, PAS, and streptomycin plus a radical procedure (Hong Kong operation) with extensive debridement and autologous bone grafting achieved a favorable response at 18 months (89%) and was essentially the same during the 5-year follow-up period. Eighteen months of chemotherapy alone led to a favorable response at 18 months (67%), at 3 years (85%), and at 5 years (88%). On the basis of these results, it has been recommended that tuberculous spondylitis is treated best by a combination of chemotherapy and the Hong Kong procedure.[134] In our opinion this procedure is best left in the hands of a surgeon familiar with the technique.

The chemotherapy used today is clearly superior to the regimens used in the British Medical Research Council trials. Although tuberculosis authorities have recommended treatment of all forms of extrapulmonary tuberculosis with a shorter course regimen employing INH, RIF, and PZA for a period of 6 to 9 months, its efficacy in skeletal tuberculosis is still to be proven.[135] Dutt et al. found that when short-course therapy with INH and RIF was employed in 21 patients with Pott's disease, 4 patients (19%) failed therapy. Six additional patients required radical surgery in the early course of therapy.[34] In another study by Omari et al. of 19 patients with Pott's disease treated with INH, RIF, and EMB, 8 patients (42%) still required surgery for progressive neurologic deficits, spinal deformities, progressive enlargement of psoas abscesses, and poor response to medical therapy.[129]

Most patients with Pott's disease will respond to conventional antituberculous chemotherapy. Standard treatment with INH, RIF, and PZA in the first 2 months and INH and RIF over 6–9 months is sufficient for those without neurologic deficit.[124] Whether therapy should be continued for 2 years for some patients remains to be determined.[124] If medical therapy alone is employed, careful medical and radiologic assessment must be undertaken if treatment failure and progressive neurologic deterioration are to be identified.[121] With acute or progressive neurologic deficits, immediate surgery for decompression is required.[124] Restoration,

especially of the vertebral spine, can be astonishing; however, destruction of the joints is often permanent.[124] A trial of empiric therapy is reasonable if a biopsy or surgery otherwise is contraindicated.

5. Complications

Complications include kyphosis with typical gibbus formation, fistulas, superinfection, myelopathy, cold abscess, and spinal cord compression with radiculopathy or even paraplegia.[121,124]

The paralysis of Pott's disease remains the most serious complication of tuberculous spondylitis and may be of early or late onset. Paralysis of early onset arises in active disease and may respond to medical therapy alone. Paralysis associated with healed disease is problematic and is almost always associated with kyphosis. Surgical success is neither uniform nor complete.[134]

B. OTHER BONES

The rich vascular supply of the epiphysis and metaphysis of long bones explains the predilection for tuberculous infection, particularly the proximal end of the femur, pelvis, ribs, shoulder, elbow, and wrist. Disease of the fingers or the skull is rare.[136] "Spina ventosa" describes the periosteal thickening of finger bones in children.[137] Tuberculosis develops slowly, often without pain, and may be confused with a metastatic carcinoma especially if osteolytic lesions are present. Adjacent monarticular arthritis may be present, presumably due to lymphatic communication.[124] The roentgenographic findings include cartilage destruction, widened joint space, erosions, and cysts. Most lesions are osteolytic, and osteoblastic lesions are seen rarely. Aspiration of the bone usually reveals the diagnosis.[32] Antituberculous chemotherapy is appropriate before resorting to surgical debridement.[32] Abscesses and sinuses are observed frequently.[124]

C. JOINTS

Tuberculous arthritis is a local manifestation of a more systemic disorder, which if left untreated may eventuate in complete destruction of the joint.[138]

Weight-bearing joints are involved most frequently. In a study of 25 patients with tuberculous arthritis, the knees were involved in 6 patients (24%), the hip in 5 patients (20%), the wrist in 5 patients (20%), the ankle in 3 patients (12%), the elbow in 2 patients (8%) and the tarsal–metatarsal, shoulder, carpal–metacarpal, and proximal interphalangeal joint in one each.[138] Although polyarticular involvement has been reported, monarticular infection is the rule.[138]

The most common early symptom of disease is the insidious onset of joint pain and swelling. Twenty percent of patients denied constitutional symptoms and 13 of 25 patients (52%) had local or systemic predisposing factors. These included trauma, narcotic addiction, intraarticular corticosteroid injections, SLE, and diabetes mellitus. Tuberculin skin testing was positive in all patients tested.[138]

Five of 25 patients (20%) had active pulmonary or pleural tuberculosis and an additional 9 patients (36%) had chest radiographic changes of previous pulmonary TB. Nonarticular extrapulmonary foci were seen in 13 patients (52%) and only 4 patients (16%) had joint disease alone.[138] Roentgenograms of the joints reveal metaphyseal and subchondral erosions, however films may be normal in 12% of patients.[138] Narrow joint spaces signal an advanced stage.[124]

Tuberculous arthritis requires aspiration and possible synovial biopsy. Aspiration of the joint space often reveals an exudative effusion fluid with high protein, low glucose, and a leukocyte count of 10,000 to 20,000 cell/mm^3 (predominantly neutrophils). A positive smear is seen in 25% of patients and a positive fluid culture is seen in 94% of patients. Synovial biopsy with histology produces a yield of 95%.[138]

The treatment of tuberculous arthritis is similar to other skeletal tuberculosis but relapse may occur.[68] Surgery should be reserved for failure of medical therapy or the need for decompression, as in the hip joint. Destroyed joints cannot be restored. Ankylosis is an option, but insertion of a prosthetic device should be attempted only after significant chemotherapy is given.[124]

D. PONCET'S DISEASE

Poncet's disease is known otherwise as "tuberculous rheumatism." It originally was described as a rare polyarthritis associated with abdominal TB without evident bacterial joint involvement.[139-141] This differs from monarthritic tuberculous arthritis where the synovial fluid cultures and histology are positive. Since TB may regress and arthritis progress, there is some controversy as to whether this disease represents a coincidental arthritis. Treatment of TB is required for resolution of the syndrome. If no improvement occurs, other diagnoses such as rheumatoid arthritis, osteoarthrosis, acute rheumatic fever, or ankylosing spondylitis should be considered.[142]

V. GENITOURINARY

A. UROLOGICAL TB

1. Epidemiology

Genitourinary tuberculosis was the fourth most common type of extrapulmonary tuberculosis in the United States in 1991. It accounted for 8.7% (425 patients) of all cases of predominantly extrapulmonary disease and 1.6% of all cases of tuberculosis (CDC, Atlanta, unpublished data). Tuberculosis of the genitourinary tract may effect the kidney, ureter, bladder, prostate, and genitalia.

The clinical manifestations of renal tuberculosis are rare in childhood and there is a peak incidence at 20 to 45 years.[143] There is a long latent period between initial pulmonary infection and subsequent clinical urinary disease. The mean interval varies from 8 to 22 years after the primary infection.[144,145] As a result there is a reservoir of disease in the elderly population as well.[145]

The exact incidence of renal tuberculosis is not known in HIV-positive patients with tuberculosis. Several series of patients with HIV infection and tuberculosis, with or without bacteremia, have reported positive urine cultures in 0–44% of patients.[23,27,30,52,53,117,146,147] In one study of 79 patients with HIV infection and disseminated tuberculosis, 18 patients (22.7%) had at least one urine culture positive for MTB.[116]

2. Clinical

Renal tuberculosis originates from a primary lung focus with subsequent lymphohematogenous dissemination leading to bilateral cortical seeding. The subsequent tubercles in the renal cortex may remain silent for years before spreading toward the papillae. Granulomas eventually may rupture into the collecting and calyceal system. Infection descends via the ureter and may involve the contralateral organ or the genitalia. Without therapy the course may be protracted, and eventually fatal. Cavitation, abscess formation, fibrosis, and calcification are typical features. Untreated infection may ultimately lead to ureteral strictures, hydronephrosis, and endstage renal disease. Progressive destruction may be limited to one kidney.[143]

There is no characteristic clinical presentation and symptoms are generally related to local organ involvement. In a study by Simon et al. of 78 patients with genitourinary tuberculosis, 41 patients were identified with active urinary tract disease.[148] The presenting urinary tract signs and symptoms in these 41 patients were dysuria in 34%, hematuria in 27%, flank pain in 10%, and pyuria in 5% of cases. Other presenting signs and symptoms such as a flank mass, recurrent UTIs, and gross hematuria have also been noted.[145] Constitutional symptoms such as fever and weight loss occurred in 14% of patients. No symptoms attributable to tuberculosis were noted in 20% of patients.

Although some patients had physical signs attributable to active or old tuberculous disease, 78% had no findings related to active urinary tract tuberculosis. Of these 41 patients, 66% had an abnormal chest radiograph, representing inactive disease in 58% and active tuberculosis in 7% of patients. Tuberculin skin testing was positive in 20 of 21 patients (95%) in whom it was performed.[148]

In a study by Shafer et al. of 199 HIV-infected patients with extrapulmonary tuberculosis, the genitourinary (GU) tract was a site of disease in 73 patients (37%).[28] Sixty-one patients (83.5%) had positive urine cultures for MTB, 11 patients (15%) had kidney or bladder involvement at autopsy, and the remaining patients had genital disease. Only 3 patients had genitourinary TB without involvement of other sites, indicating that the GU tract was seldom the sole site of infection. Overall, 77% of those patients who had urine specimens cultured grew MTB, suggesting that most had subclinical genitourinary tuberculosis. Presenting localized signs or symptoms rarely indicated genitourinary involvement. Two patients had symptoms referable to involvement of the epididymis and prostate and no patient had gross hematuria or flank pain. Pyuria occurred in 40% of the patients with genitourinary disease.[28]

3. Diagnosis

The diagnosis of renal tuberculosis requires the isolation of the organism from the urinary tract. This can be done by collection of three to six consecutive morning clean catch urine specimens for culture. The direct AFB smear may be misleading since nonpathogenic mycobacteria in the smegma may be confused with MTB. Consecutive morning urine cultures are as reliable as culture of a 24-h urine collection specimen.[143] When the urine specimen is collected and processed properly the yield is very high. In 38 patients with urinary tract tuberculosis who had urine cultures sent, 90% were positive. The few negative results were attributed to inadequate cultures. The urine sediment by microscopic analysis was abnormal in 93% of patients including pyuria and hematuria or both.[148] Percutaneous kidney biopsy may yield the diagnosis.[149]

A plain abdominal film may show punctate calcifications in the renal parenchyma or calyceal system.[150] The intravenous pyelogram (IVP), performed in 30 of 41 patients with urinary tuberculosis, showed an abnormality in 93% of cases.[148] Intravenous pyelography may reveal calcification, cavitation, parenchymal scarring, calyceal dilatation or deformity, calculi, or stricture formation.[148,150] Retrograde pyelography may be safely performed in those with renal dysfunction. Ultrasonography also may reveal the spectrum of morphologic abnormalities of genitourinary tuberculosis.[151] Gallium scanning may show persistent renal uptake after 48 to 120 h.[132]

4. Treatment

Nine-month chemotherapy has been shown to be effective for the treatment of renal tuberculosis.[34] Other studies have shown 4- to 6-month shorter course therapy to be effective in conjunction with adjunctive surgery.[152,153] If concerns remain about persistent bacilli at the end of treatment, cavities may be sampled and cultured by needle aspiration.[154] In persistent infection, isotope renography may show persistent enhancement.[154] At least 1 year of follow-up is required posttreatment, and even longer in the presence of strictures or renal calcifications. The latter may involve the intramural ureters and eventually obliterate the urinary system.[150] Urinalysis should be performed monthly or bimonthly, and excretory urograms or renal scans after 6 and 12 months if structural aberrations are present,[154] although ultrasonography is less invasive. With modern treatment regimens, the majority of patients do not require follow-up for more than 2 years after the completion of therapy.

5. Complications

Complications may include secondary amyloidosis, fistulas, parenchymal destruction, and uremia. Nephrectomy is indicated for relief of intractable pain, unresponsive hypertension due to parenchymal destruction,[155] uncontrollable fever from obstruction, life-threatening hematuria, or resistant disease not amenable to conventional medical treatment.[153] Some advocate nephrectomy as an adjunct to a 4-month course of chemotherapy.[153] Ureteral strictures can be relieved by retrograde dilation or by the use of Double-J ureteral catheters. If strictures progress after 1 month of chemotherapy, prednisolone may be of benefit.[152] Infundibular stenosis, nondraining calyces, and pelvic obstructions all can be manipulated endoscopically.[154] Surgical augmentation can be performed for a shrunken and contracted bladder.[154]

B. GENITAL TB
1. Males

The male genital organs may be affected by urinary, contiguous, or hematogenous spread. The most common sites of involvement are the prostate followed by the seminal vesicles, epididymis, and testes.[156,157] The most common presentation of male genital tuberculosis is that of epididymitis.[158] Abscess formation may lead to a palpable mass and a chronic draining sinus. Orchitis and prostatitis may occur. Other manifestations include painful inflammation of the vas deferens and seminal vesicles; infections of the urethra and penis are rare. Involvement of the epididymis and prostate has been described in patients with HIV infection.[23,28] Constitutional symptoms are seen rarely.[143]

A sonogram is helpful for the evaluation of this condition.[159] The diagnosis of genital tuberculosis may be made by biopsy and culture of the genital mass.[148] Culture of semen may lead to a diagnosis in 11% of patients.[156] Some recommend 9-month short-course therapy but others recommend 18 months of INH and RIF because potential prostatic involvement may require longer therapy.[156] Chemotherapy can be supplemented with surgery if there is abscess formation, stricture formation, or failure to respond to medical therapy. Sterility develops in 50% of patients and all patients with clinical lesions have abnormal semen.[143]

2. Females

Tuberculous infection of the genital tract in women usually is due to lymphohematogenous spread from a pulmonary or abdominal focus or rarely directly by coitus.[143,160] Disease can occur at any age from puberty to menopause. The distal end of the salpinges is affected in approximately 85%, the endometrium in 70–75%, and the ovary in 30–35% of patients. Involvement of the vagina and vulva is rare.[143,160]

Symptoms usually are few or absent. Presenting symptoms are pelvic–abdominal pain, leucorrhea, metrorrhagia, dysmenorrhoea, amenorrhea, and dyspareunia. Abdominal and pelvic examinations are normal in 60% of women.[161] Useful diagnostic tests include first voided early morning urine, premenstrual endometrial culture and biopsy, hysterosalpingography, and laparoscopy.[143,161] The culture of menstrual blood is extremely sensitive and can be used as a screening test.[162,163]

Treatment with isoniazid and rifampin for 15 months supplemented with an initial 3 months of streptomycin led to a 93% response rate in 38 patients.[164] Surgery for large tuboovarian abscesses may be necessary. Fibrotic fallopian tubes may cause sterility. Tuberculosis causes 10% of sterility in women worldwide, and 1% in industrialized countries.[161] Other complications include pelvic inflammatory disease with salpingoooophoritis, endometritis, peritubal abscess, peritonitis, and ascites. Pyometria may develop with an occluded cervical canal.[143]

VI. DISSEMINATED TB

A. EPIDEMIOLOGY

Miliary or disseminated tuberculosis was the fifth most common type of extrapulmonary tuberculosis in the United States in 1991. It accounted for 7.6% (371 patients) of all cases of predominately extrapulmonary disease and 1.4% of all cases of tuberculosis (CDC, Atlanta, unpublished data). Historically, miliary tuberculosis has been a disease

of children, with more than a third of the cases occurring in those under 3 years of age. Today, most cases occur in adults especially over the age of 65 years.[165] Prior to effective antituberculous chemotherapy, dissemination invariably was due to a pulmonary focus. Since the advent of effective antituberculous therapy, an extrapulmonary focus can account for dissemination in approximately 75% of cases.[166] Men and blacks are more likely to be affected than women and caucasians.[166]

Medical risk factors for acute dissemination include immunosuppression, especially cancer and chemotherapy,[167] alcoholism, starvation, chronic hemodialysis,[168] and viral infections (measles, influenza).[162,165] Surgical procedures such as incision and drainage of an abscess, partial resection of a lymph node, tubal surgery,[169] transurethral prostatectomy, urinary instrumentation,[170] lithotripsy treatment,[171] and prosthetic valve replacement[172] on occasion may activate a focus and precipitate dissemination. In the prechemotherapy era, miliary disease was observed after surgery for skeletal tuberculosis.[124] Predictors of mortality from dissemination are age greater than 60 years, lymphopenia, thrombocytopenia, hypoalbuminemia, elevated transaminases, and delay in appropriate therapy.[173] Mortality also has been shown to increase with overwhelming disease, an altered mental status,[174] and HIV infection.[27] One of the most common forms of extrapulmonary tuberculosis in patients with HIV infection is disseminated disease.

B. CLINICAL

Historically, miliary tuberculosis has been defined as disseminated TB, with multiple nodular lesions on chest radiograph that are 1 to 2 mm in diameter. It was first described by Manget who compared the tiny disseminated lesions to millet seeds, hence the term "miliae". The term miliary often has been used mistakenly to characterize dissemination.[174-176] Disseminated lesions can range from miliae to larger nodules to tuberculomas. They originate from a specific focus and spread via the hematogenous route. The lesion may spread from a newly acquired infection or a long standing focus. Indolent forms of disease, e.g., bone, kidney, and lymph node, result only rarely in dissemination.[165]

Disseminated TB is defined by the involvement of two or more noncontiguous tuberculous sites or the presence of bacteremia. It may mimic a variety of diseases and requires a high index of suspicion to diagnose. Of all cases of disseminated TB found at autopsy, 33–80%[177,178] were missed antemortem. In the prechemotherapy era, disseminated TB was rare and invariably fatal.[174]

Miliary tuberculosis may occur in three separate distinct forms:[179] (1) acute (acute primary and late generalized),[166,180] (2) chronic (chronic hematogenous or cryptic),[179,181,182] and (3) nonreactive (typhobacillosis of Landouzy).[183]

The acute form is a rapidly progressive process that is uniformly fatal if not treated. It may occur at the time of primary infection or later as a manifestation of a distant reactivated focus.[166] Several autopsy studies revealed that the lungs, liver, and spleen are involved 75–95% of the time. Next most commonly involved are the kidneys, bone marrow, CNS, adrenal glands, and peritoneum. Less commonly involved are the thyroid, heart, skeleton, genitalia, and gastrointestinal tract.[166,184,185]

Sign and symptoms are nonspecific and frequently include fever, weight loss, malaise, anorexia, and fatigue. Average duration of symptoms before diagnosis varied significantly depending on the series.[166,173,174,180,184,186] Less common symptoms are headache, dyspnea, and abdominal pain. Headache is an ominous sign and signifies meningeal involvement,[180,184] abdominal pain indicates intraabdominal disease,[186] and dyspnea suggests significant pulmonary disease or impairment of lung diffusing capacity.[187] Physical signs include hepatomegaly and less commonly splenomegaly and lymphadenopathy.[173,174,186] Choroidal tubercles have been reported in disseminated disease from "rare" to "almost all cases,"[188] but also may be seen in pulmonary tuberculosis without dissemination.[186,188]

Chronic or cryptic miliary tuberculosis, as defined by Proudfoot et al.,[181] is miliary tuberculosis where the classical and radiological features of miliary TB are not present. The disease is insidious before it becomes acute, typically affects the elderly, presents as a fever of unknown origin, and the diagnosis often is delayed. As a result the diagnosis is frequently made only at postmortem examination. The overall mortality is approximately 80%.[181,182,189] This syndrome rarely is associated with the typical miliary pattern on chest radiograph, and frequently is associated with an underlying malignancy or blood dyscrasias.[181,182]

Nonreactive miliary tuberculosis is a fatal form of the disease where many organs show areas of caseous necrosis surrounded by normal or near normal parenchyma. The clinical spectrum ranges from an acute and overwhelming illness to chronic persistent condition. It is associated with an abnormal blood picture.[183]

Bacteremia is not an uncommon occurrence among patients who are HIV infected with tuberculosis, but is not necessarily synonymous with miliary tuberculosis.[30,116,117,146,147,190] In a study by Shafer et al. of 199 HIV-infected patients and extrapulmonary tuberculosis, 76 patients (38%) had disseminated disease including the bone marrow in 32 patients, the blood in 28 patients, the liver in 25 patients, and greater than 2 noncontiguous extrapulmonary sites in 56 patients.[28] Fever and respiratory symptoms predominated in 67% of patients. Twenty-four patients (32%) had miliary infiltrates on chest radiograph and 9 of these developed the infiltrates during hospitalization. In HIV-positive patients disseminated TB is seen more commonly, and can be rapidly progressive and overwhelming requiring an aggressive diagnostic approach and early therapy.[191] The majority (90%) of patients are anergic.[28,116]

C. DIAGNOSIS

The chest radiograph is the single most important way of detecting miliary tuberculosis. It may be normal in 25–50% of patients[173,192] and may remain that way for several weeks. It also may exhibit a vast array of abnormalities including pleural effusions, hilar adenopathy, interstitial infiltrates, and extensive parenchymal consolidation (ARDS). The retrocardiac space on the lateral view is a very sensitive area for assessment of miliae.[165] This miliary pattern may be confused with congestive heart failure, sarcoidosis, fungal infections, bacterial pneumonia, and even *Pneumocystis carinii* pneumonia in patients with AIDS.[176,193] In one series of patients with HIV infection and tuberculosis, a miliary pattern was seen in 30% of patients.[69] The high resolution CT is a more sensitive indicator of disease.[192] The gallium scan frequently is positive.[194]

The sputum smear is positive in approximately 30% of patients with miliary TB, and increases with additional lesions, e.g., cavitation, in up to 70% of patients. Sputum cultures are positive in almost two-thirds of patients.[173,174,180]

Histologic confirmation of disseminated tuberculosis is achieved best by biopsy of the lung, bone marrow, liver, lymph node, skin, or any other tissue that is clinically involved. Fiberoptic bronchoscopy with bronchoalveolar lavage (BAL) and transbronchial biopsy (TBB) remains an invaluable tool in the immediate diagnosis of miliary TB. Three studies show an immediate (histology and/or +AFB smear) diagnostic rate of 64–79% with cultures providing an additional 4–10% yield. The definitive diagnostic yield from transbronchial biopsy and bronchial washings or lavage is 73–86%.[173,195,196] This procedure is quite useful, provides a high diagnostic yield, and has supplanted the liver biopsy as the initial diagnostic site. In a study including 76 patients with disseminated tuberculosis and HIV infection, only 26% of these patients had histologic evidence of TB on fiberoptic bronchoscopy with transbronchial biopsy.[28] Therefore this procedure cannot be relied upon to exclude disseminated disease in HIV-infected patients.

Percutaneous liver biopsies have been used frequently and reveal granulomata in 50–100% of patients.[173,184,185] Organisms were more likely to be seen when caseation was present, and caseation was seen in 20–45% of cases. In one study of 199 patients with extrapulmonary tuberculosis and HIV infection, 76 patients (38%) had disseminated disease. In those with dissemination, liver biopsy revealed histologic evidence of TB in 14 of 18 (78%) patients where it was performed.[28]

Bone marrow involvement occurs owing to its rich blood supply, and may lead to aplastic anemia, granulocytopenia, leukemoid reaction, a "left shift," and pancytopenia.[197] Bone marrow examination has been reported to be positive in up to 83% of HIV-negative patients with miliary tuberculosis.[173,180,185,198] The marrow is more likely to be positive if a biopsy rather than an aspirate is performed and is improved by culture of the marrow. The yield of a bone marrow biopsy is higher with hematologic abnormalities such as anemia, leukopenia, or thrombocytopenia.[173,197]

Bone marrow aspiration and biopsy also are helpful but less so in HIV-positive patients.[199] AFB stains of the bone marrow are positive in 22% of patients and culture is positive in 29% of patients with disseminated TB.[200] Histologic evidence of tuberculosis is seen in 25–52% of patients having a bone marrow biopsy.[28,200]

Blood cultures are useful in tuberculous bacteremia, especially in patients who are HIV infected, where blood cultures may be positive in up to 38% of cases.[117,146,190] Specimens of gastric washings,[173,174,184] urine,[173,174,184,201] and cerebrospinal fluid[173] should always be cultured and may prove to be useful.

Bronchoscopy with BAL and TBB, bone marrow biopsy, and liver biopsy have a relatively high yield, and, if the diagnosis is suspected, should be performed early to prevent therapeutic delay.[202]

D. TREATMENT

With acute and overwhelming disease, it is reasonable to start early empiric therapy with a 4-drug regimen. This regimen should include isoniazid, rifampin, pyrazinamide, and streptomycin or ethambutol. A delay of even 1 to 8 days contributes to the high mortality rate.[176,203] The decision to embark on empirical therapy without having obtained appropriate tissue can be a difficult one. The effects of early therapy on culture results and the potentially serious adverse effects of antituberculous agents must be weighed against the risk of treatment delay.

Even with appropriate therapy, the mortality rate may reach 16–24%.[173,174,180,184] In one study,

most deaths occurred during the first 2 weeks of admission.[173] This reinforces the fact that patients frequently present late in the natural course of this illness and emphasizes the importance of early diagnosis and treatment. Most cases respond to conventional short-course chemotherapy.[34,173] The practice of the addition of corticosteroids to patients who are severely ill in an attempt to accelerate the clinical response remains controversial.[165]

In a study by Shafer et al. of 76 patients with disseminated tuberculosis, most of the patients treated with antituberculous therapy survived. Thirty-four patients (45%) died during hospitalization and 21 of these died without a definitive diagnosis or specific therapy.[28]

E. COMPLICATIONS

The complications of miliary tuberculosis are numerous and may potentially involve any organ. "Sepsis tuberculosis gravissima" is acute overwhelming septic shock with multiple complications such as respiratory failure,[176] ARDS,[175,204,205] cholestatic jaundice, acute pancreatitis,[206] hepatic and renal failure, and disseminated intravascular coagulation.[173] Multisystem organ failure has a mortality of up to 90%.[207] Autopsy studies in these patients may show extensive necrosis with no granuloma formation and few inflammatory cells,[208] granulomatous inflammation of the interstitial space, exudative alveolitis, or obliterative arteritis.[176]

VII. NEUROLOGIC

A. MENINGES

1. Epidemiology

Although the most frequent type of tuberculosis is pulmonary, among the most dangerous forms is neurotuberculosis. Neurotuberculosis is a life threatening complication that can affect all regions of the CNS, although there is a predilection for the basilar meninges. Tuberculosis of the nervous system can affect the meninges, brain, spinal cord, cranial and peripheral nerves, ears, and eyes.

Tuberculous meningitis was the sixth most common form of extrapulmonary tuberculosis in the United States in 1991. It accounted for 5.4% (264 patients) of all cases of predominately extrapulmonary disease and 1.0% of all cases of tuberculosis reported (CDC, Atlanta, unpublished data).

This disease may occur at any age, but historically is a disease of children in the first 5 years of life. It is uncommon in children less than 6 months of age and rare under age 3 months.[209] Auerbach found that in a series of 97 cases of fatal tuberculosis in children under 13 years of age, 42.2% had tuberculous meningitis.[210] In the same study only

2.7% of 2236 adult deaths due to tuberculosis resulted from meningitis. Riggs et al. found meningeal involvement at postmortem in 19.3% of patients with tuberculosis less than 20 years of age and in 5.9% of patients greater than 20 years of age.[211] The incidence of tuberculous meningitis in adults has been increasing in recent years probably due to later age of acquisition of tuberculous infection.[212] Therefore, it may occur in the elderly patient population.

The most frequent predisposing medical conditions for tuberculous meningitis are alcoholism, substance abuse, corticosteroid use, head trauma, and HIV infection.[213,214]

2. Clinical

Meningitis may develop either from a local activated dormant focus, from a distant site, e.g., lung or paravertebral abscess, through hematogenous spread, or as the result of miliary tuberculosis. Regardless of initial site of origin, there must be rupture of a caseous focus into the arachnoid space. This focus usually lies adjacent to the meninges.[210]

Pathologically only a small number of living bacilli may be seen in the parenchyma, and serous meningitis may result without evident organisms. Hyperemia, capillary damage, scars, and edema are observed. A thick gelatinous exudate may collect at the base of the brain interfering with cranial nerve function, and hydrocephalus may occur. Basal meningeal inflammation may spread focally to adjacent tissue. Granulomas are seen within the choroid plexus in 75% of cases and the ependyma in 90% of cases. Small discrete gray-white tubercles may be visible over the entire surface of the brain.[215]

The onset of tuberculous meningitis is insidious with a 2-week prodromal period before meningeal symptoms occur.[216] The clinical features include fever, anorexia, malaise, nausea, vomiting, headache, apathy, and mental alterations. Physical findings include nuchal rigidity, basilar cranial nerve involvement, focal neurologic deficit, pupillary changes, fundoscopic changes, papilledema, and peripheral adenopathy.[213,215] A waxing and waning course with sudden acceleration may occur especially in children.[215] Nonneurologic tuberculosis is seen in about 37% of patients.[217]

Most cases of tuberculous meningitis progress through three stages. The first stage occurs with low grade fever, personality changes, and irritability, and lasts 1 to 2 weeks. Confusion may be an early sign in the elderly. The cerebrospinal fluid (CSF) shows few neutrophils and a borderline normal glucose and protein. During the second stage there is an increase in the intracranial pressure and nausea, vomiting, nuchal rigidity, photophobia, seizures, and cranial nerve palsies (3rd, 6th, 7th)

are seen. The CSF reveals lymphocytes and an increased protein and decreased glucose content. The last stage is associated with high fever, confusion, stupor, and coma. Decortication and herniation may eventually ensue. Prechemotherapy mortality was 45% in stage 1, 70% in stage 2, and 90% in stage 3.[216,218]

HIV infection may be complicated by tuberculous infection of the nervous system. Bishburg et al. reported tuberculous meningitis in 10 of 52 patients (19.2%) with HIV infection and tuberculosis.[214] In a study of 199 patients with extrapulmonary tuberculosis and HIV infection, 27 patients (14%) had disease of the central nervous system.[28] Of these 21 had meningitis and 6 had tuberculomas. Ninety-six percent of patients had neurologic signs or symptoms and were not dissimilar from the HIV-negative controls, a finding confirmed by two other studies of HIV-related tuberculous meningitis.[19,217] The presence of peripheral, intrathoracic, and intraabdominal lymphadenopathy was more common in patients with HIV infection. Patients with a lower CD4+ count had a poorer prognosis.[217]

3. Diagnosis

The tuberculin skin test can be negative in up to 50% of cases,[213,216,219] but usually becomes positive during chemotherapy.[220] Tuberculin skin testing was positive (greater than 10 mm in induration) in 22.5 and 29% of patients with HIV infection in two studies.[19,217] Hyponatremia is common and is usually secondary to inappropriate secretion of antidiuretic hormone.[216]

Chest radiographs are abnormal and suggestive of tuberculosis in 31–74% of patients.[19,213,221] In a study by Dube et al. of 31 patients with tuberculous meningitis, chest radiographs were abnormal in 81% of HIV-negative patients and 67% of HIV-positive patients.[19] A miliary pattern was predominant in both (44 vs 33%). Abnormal chest radiographs were seen in 54% of patients in another study.[217]

The widespread use of CT and MRI scanning has been useful in the management of tuberculous meningitis. Hydrocephalus, meningeal enhancement (with contrast CT, with gadolinium MRI),[222] thickened basilar meninges, and nonenhancing, enhancing, hyperdense, or isodense lesions, sometimes with surrounding edema, may be seen.[223-226] Abnormalities on CT scan of the head were seen in 60–69% of patients in several studies and they included hydrocephalus, mass lesions, and meningeal enhancement. This yield appears to be increased by the use of MRI scanning.[19,28,217] CT scanning and MRI may be useful in the follow-up process.

Examination of the CSF is the most valuable procedure in the diagnosis of meningeal tuberculosis. Lumbar puncture usually reveals an elevated opening pressure. The CSF protein is elevated and ranges from 100 to 500 mg/dl and may rise considerably if there is a spinal block with xanthochromia.[19,216] An increasing protein concentration is common during therapy and does not necessarily portend treatment failure.[217] The CSF glucose concentration usually is below 40 mg/dl or the CSF/blood glucose ratio is below 0.5 in 50–85% of patients,[216,217] although often normal in diabetics.[123] The glucose concentration declines in untreated cases. Intravenously administered glucose should be avoided 2 h before the lumbar puncture.[209] In two studies of HIV-related tuberculous meningitis, the HIV-positive patients had CSF abnormalities that were comparable to those found in patients without HIV infection. A normal CSF protein concentration was found with higher frequency in patients with HIV infection than in those without.[19,217]

The cellular changes in the CSF reflect a tuberculin reaction provoked by the presence of tuberculoproteins.[216] There may be a moderate degree of pleocytosis usually with less than 500 cells/mm³ and rarely greater than 1200 cells/mm³. Greater than 80–95% are lymphocytes, but a predominance of polymorphonuclear cells may be seen early.[216]

The AFB smear of CSF has been reported to be positive in 10–40% of specimens,[212,219] but the yield may increase up to 85–87% with repeated or centrifuged specimens.[227-229] Serial lumbar punctures even after the onset of therapy may reveal the organism.[230] The AFB smear was reported to be positive in 0–27% of patients with HIV infection.[19,28,217] Tubercle bacilli may be isolated by culture in 50–80% of cases.[124,216,219,221,227]

Achieving the diagnosis at an early stage is critical but often onerous because CSF may be normal in up to 20% of HIV-positive patients.[217] If the CSF remains normal within 2 weeks of presentation, the diagnosis of tuberculous meningitis is unlikely. It may be reasonable to withdraw treatment, and follow the patient over the next few months with repeat lumbar punctures.[123]

More elaborate tests have been utilized in an attempt to establish diagnosis of tuberculous meningitis. Adenosine deaminase (ADA) is elevated in the CSF and 60% of patients have levels of greater than 10 IU/ml. Unfortunately ADA may also be increased in bacterial meningitis and therefore is nondiagnostic.[231] In one study in HIV-infected patients, the sensitivity of ADA was 63% and more sensitive than the AFB smear.[217] Enzyme-linked immunoabsorbent assay (ELISA) to detect soluble mycobacterial antigen (e.g., antigen 5) may be useful with a sensitivity of 80% and a specificity of up to 100%.[232-234] An immunoblot technique using mycobacterial antigen 60 (A60) has been developed. The early appearance of antimycobacterial immunoglobulins to this complex may be seen in the CSF of patients with tuberculous meningitis.[235] Detection of tuberculostearic acid, a fatty acid present only in mycobacteria, in CSF provides a diagnostic test with a high degree of accuracy. This may represent the best approach to the rapid diagnosis of tuberculous meningitis.[236]

The bromide (^{82}Br) partition test,[123] lactate levels[237] are less useful, but polymerase chain reactions (PCR) have sensitivities above 75%, but specificities are lower.[238] A second PCR from stored CSF increases specificity by decreasing possible laboratory contamination.[238] Multicenter trials would be most helpful in establishing the clinical usefulness of these various tests.[239] A meningeal biopsy or brain biopsy may be necessary, on occasion, but carry significant risks, including postoperative epidural hematoma and hydrocephalus.[240]

4. Treatment

Early and immediate treatment are critical in improving outcome. With appropriate chemotherapy, complete recovery is increased to 95, 80, and 20% in stages 1, 2, and 3, respectively.[218] The best agents in tuberculous meningitis are INH, RIF, PZA, and streptomycin, all of which enter the CSF well in the presence of meningeal inflammation,[215] although a recent study raises doubt about the penetrating ability of rifampin.[240a] Ethambutol is less effective in meningeal disease unless used at higher doses.[241] Ethionamide (15 mg/kg/day),[218] cycloserine, and ofloxacin also may be effective.[242] Intrathecal drugs usually are not necessary.

Dutt et al. showed that a 9-month short-course chemotherapy regimen was effective in 18 patients with tuberculous meningitis.[34] Another study showed similar results but emphasized the need for corticosteroids or surgery to treat complications such as hydrocephalus or arachnoiditis.[243] Duration of conventional therapy is 6 to 9 months, although some authors still recommend up to 24 months of therapy.[218,244] Patients who have had meningitis should be kept under medical supervision for a minimum of 2 years.[123] The use of corticosteroids is controversial, and may be indicated in the presence of an elevated intracranial pressure, altered consciousness, focal neurologic findings, or spinal block.[216] The overall mortality is 20%,[217] and probably higher in the elderly. The overall mortality rate for patients with HIV infection and tuberculous meningitis receiving conventional antituberculous therapy was 20–33% in studies.[19,217] Even with appropriate medical therapy and rapid clinical response, patients should be monitored for any complication requiring adjunctive therapy, e.g., anticonvulsants, or surgical intervention.

Surgical intervention for hydrocephalus, tuberculoma, optochiasmatic arachnoiditis, or abscess formation rarely is required. Hydrocephalus, which develops in 20% of patients, or opening pressures greater than 50 cm H_2O, may be improved with diuretics,[123] but most physicians would resort to a ventriculoatrial or ventriculoperitoneal shunt.[162,209] Early shunt placement may improve outcome. External ventricular drainage may be indicated in more severe cases.[245] Hyaluronidase has been tried with spinal arachnoiditis with "excellent" results in more than 15 patients.[246]

Optochiasmatic arachnoiditis is due to an inflammatory reaction in the area of the optic chiasm leading to loss of visual acuity. It may be associated with hydrocephalus and responds well to surgery and corticosteroids.[247]

5. Complications

Complications include hydrocephalus, cranial nerve palsies, and nerve compression (e.g., bilateral 6th nerve palsy), cerebral infarction, and blockage of CSF flow. A steep rise in CSF protein appears before a spinal block develops.[123] Obstruction of capillaries from multiple small tuberculous emboli leads to microinfarcts (tuberculids). They may persist, enlarge, or caseate, and large tuberculomas may lead to focal neurological deficits. An abscess or spinal leptomeningitis may develop and endarteritis may account for focal areas of cerebral infarctions.[216] "Paradoxical" tuberculomas may develop during the course of treatment of sensitive TB.[226,248] Continuation of the same therapy and the addition of corticosteroids have led to good success.[225,248]

Some degree of neurologic deficit remains in 50% of cases, and a decreased IQ is the rule in infantile meningitis.[216] Severe late sequelae such as paralysis or aphasia may persist. Thirty-five percent of survivors have serious disabilities such as memory loss, mental retardation, involuntary movements, paralysis, panhypopituitarism, or epilepsy. Late events are arachnoiditis ossificans and arachnoid cysts.[215] Meningomyeloradiculitis can be life-threatening with advancing paraplegia and rising CSF protein levels.[249]

B. BRAIN/NERVE LESIONS

Hematogenous dissemination leads to perivascular microscopic foci that form tubercles with central caseation, epithelioid and giant cells. Gradually they enlarge to form numerous small macroscopic tuberculomas that then may coalesce. Tuberculomas, which are rare, may be asymptomatic, or present with symptoms and signs of a focal lesion, or el-

evated intracranial pressure.[225] They may mimic almost any disease of the brain including glioma, glioblastoma, metastasis, hemorrhage, or abscesses.[224] Calcification may be present within the contrast-enhanced ring, giving a "target sign," and probably is a sign of reactivation.[224] The CSF may be normal in the presence of parenchymal disease.[215] Tuberculomas may be visualized by CT and MRI scanning techniques in as much as 45% of patients with meningitis[222] and may be more common in patients with HIV infection.[19,28,217]

Surgical intervention is controversial, and generally not required with the use of corticosteroids and antituberculous drugs, but debulking may be necessary if vital structures such as the optic pathway are compromised. Tuberculomas react only slowly to medical therapy and require several months to 1 year for resolution. However, this does not indicate ineffective therapy and partial improvement may be seen within 6 to 8 weeks.[248] Complications include clinical meningitis, spinal cord compression, radiculomyelitis, and seizures.[216]

Brain abscesses are tuberculomas that develop into pus-filled cavities and indicate poor defense mechanisms.[98] They are rare and may require surgical excision.[223] A paravertebral cold abscess may cause local deficits. Rarely the abscess may flow through the intervertebral foramen into the epidural space and cause paraplegia.[225]

Epidural tuberculosis compresses the spine, does not involve bones, and can be confused with carcinomas ("spinal tumor syndrome").[123,209] Spinal cord TB can be focal (with root pain, paraplegia, or loss of bladder control), ascending, or multifocal.[123] Corticosteroids are useful therapy if worsening neurologic deficit occurs secondary to edema (e.g., dexamethasone 0.2 mg/kg/day for the first 2 weeks).

Peripheral polyneuropathy has not been attributed to TB. When described it has been seen with pyridoxine (vitamin B_6) deficiency in malnourished patients on INH therapy or with supranormal supplementation of pyridoxine (greater than 200 mg/day).[250]

C. OCULAR

Ocular manifestations occur in approximately 1% of patients with tuberculosis.[251] Although usually the result of hematogenous dissemination, ocular tuberculosis may extend from surrounding tissues or from direct inoculation with the patient's own sputum.[251] In some developing countries, it accounts for 30% of all uveitis diagnosed.[252]

The cornea and choroidae are most frequently affected, but every segment of the eye and its adnexae (except the lens) including the uvea, retina, sclera, iris, and optic nerve may be involved. External structures, such as lid, orbit, and lacrimal gland, rarely are implicated.[251] The clinical presentation is quite variable. A primary "tuberculous chancre" may occur on the lid and the conjunctiva and may appear as an ulcerated lesion with regional lymphadenopathy.[253] Chronic keratoconjunctivitis, anterior and posterior uveitis, iris nodules, retinal vasculitis, and panophthalmitis have been described.[253]

Phlyctenular (Greek for blister) keratoconjunctivitis was a major cause of visual loss in the United States in the beginning of the century among Eskimos and native Americans. It probably is a hypersensitivity reaction to the presence of tuberculoproteins but may be due to local implantation.[254,255] Careful examination may reveal elevated limbal lesions migrating toward the central cornea carrying a "leash" of vessels and leaving a triangular scar. Phlyctenular lesions may cause intense pain, lacrimation, and photophobia.[256]

Superficial scleritis also is a hypersensitivity reaction, while deep scleritis usually results from direct inoculation. Tuberculous scleritis is characteristically painless.[253]

A classic finding in miliary tuberculosis is multiple bilateral choroidal tubercles (Bouchut's tubercles) or many small discrete yellowish nodules in the posterior pole of the eye.[188] These are normally visible on fundoscopic examination.

Intraocular involvement may include retinal neovascularization and ischemic retinal vasculitis.[252,257] Vitreous hemorrhage may occur from neovascularization and is referred to as Eales' disease. As a result, sudden loss of vision in one eye, or visual impairment with scotoma or floating spots may occur.[251,258] Optic neuropathy may lead to blindness.[251]

A complete evaluation includes funduscopy and a slit-lamp examination. Fluorescein angiography is useful in the follow-up assessment of choroidal lesions.[259] In the absence of a positive ocular culture, the diagnosis of ocular TB may be established by the characteristic findings of ocular TB plus a positive culture from another source and/or the response of lesions to chemotherapy. The bacillus may be recovered directly from cornea or sclera. Chorioretinal endobiopsy or vitreous aspiration with culture is helpful, but rarely necessary.[252]

Antituberculous therapy is effective, but local instillation or systemic use of corticosteroids may be required as adjuvant therapy (e.g., in phlyctenular keratoconjunctivitis). The use of topical corticosteroids may prevent focal corneal scarring.[252] For anterior uveitis, topical mydriatic agents are used.[251] Direct or panretinal[260] photocoagulation is indicated for neovascularization and retinal capillary closure.[251]

Complications of ocular TB usually are reversible, although retinal detachment, glaucoma, and cataract formation have been described. Rarely, exophthalmus may develop secondary to an optochiasmatic tuberculoma. A tuberculoma of the orbit can produce proptosis and therefore mimic other diseases.[256]

D. OTOLOGIC

Historically, tuberculous involvement of the ear has been observed in approximately 2% of all patients with active pulmonary TB.[261] In 1991 there were a total of only 9 patients with tuberculous otitis media in the United States (CDC, Atlanta, unpublished data). However, at the beginning of the century, TB was responsible for up to 20% of all otitis media.[261]

The mucosa of the middle ear thickens and produces a discharge and effusion, which may appear in the nasopharynx. The tympanic membrane may thicken and reveal yellow spots, representing caseating granulomata.[262] The breakdown of a previous tympanoplasty or developing granulation tissue should suggest TB. Large or multiple perforations of the tympanic membrane may develop and produce the characteristic otorrhea. Painless perforation with chronic discharge is characteristic and may linger for many years. Hearing impairment occurs early and may antedate other symptoms. The hearing loss may be conductive and due to ossicle destruction, sensorineural, or both. Mastoiditis also may develop.[261]

The diagnosis is evident by obtaining positive mycobacterial cultures, but the diagnosis may be masked by the presence of bacterial superinfection. The yield of smear and culture from secretions is low although the yield is higher from granulation tissue. Histology frequently is unrevealing and granuloma formation may be lacking. The most sensitive tests are the AFB smear and culture of a biopsy specimen.[261] The possibility of permanent hearing loss makes early diagnosis critical.

Treatment of otologic tuberculosis requires at least INH and RIF for as long as 18 to 24 months.[263] Surgical intervention after failed medical therapy may be necessary for facial nerve palsy, subperiosteal abscess, or persistent fistulas.

Typical complications are postauricular fistula development, preauricular lymphadenopathy, and facial nerve palsy. The most serious complication is arterial invasion and bleeding from spread of a contiguous focus. These complications are rare, occur late, and usually differentiate TB from bacterial otitis.[263] Other rare complications include periosteal abscess formation, labyrinthitis, fistulas, and extension of infection into the CSF.[261]

VIII. ABDOMINAL

A. PERITONEAL TB

1. Epidemiology

Tuberculosis of the abdomen includes disease of the peritoneum, gastrointestinal tract, liver and biliary tract, pancreas, tonsils, tongue, and mouth. At the turn of the century, intraabdominal involvement was present in 25% of patients with far advanced pulmonary disease; it now accounts for about 4% of all cases of extrapulmonary TB.[264] The peritoneum is the major site of intraabdominal involvement, and in a study by Farer from 1969 to 1973, was five times as common as all other forms of abdominal tuberculosis combined.[91] Peritoneal tuberculosis was the seventh most common form of extrapulmonary tuberculosis in the United States in 1991. It accounted for 4.0% (195 patients) of all cases of predominately extrapulmonary disease and 0.74% of all cases of tuberculosis reported (CDC, Atlanta, unpublished data).

Historically, tuberculous peritonitis occurred most commonly in young adults but may be seen at any age. Although it may occur both in men and women, recent studies suggest a male predominance.[265,266] It has been described among blacks, North American Indians, and Asian and West Indian immigrants. Alcoholism, and its associated malnutrition, appears to be a major causative risk factor.[264,266] Tuberculous peritonitis has been described as complicating long-term peritoneal dialysis.[267] Half of all ascites in developing countries is due to tuberculosis.[266]

2. Clinical

Peritoneal tuberculosis occurs from rupture of a latent caseous peritoneal focus that results from hematogenous dissemination from a primary infection. It may result from rupture of a caseous abdominal lymph node or extend from an intestinal source or genitalia.[268,269,270]

The symptoms of peritonitis are insidious over several months, although occasionally may be abrupt if bowel perforation occurs. Symptoms include abdominal pain and swelling, and generalized symptoms of fever, chills, anorexia, and malaise.[271] The physical examination reveals diffuse or local abdominal tenderness, ascites, omental masses, and, on rare occasion, a "doughy abdomen."[266]

There are two forms of tuberculous peritonitis frequently encountered: wet (ascitic) and dry (associated with scant or localized effusion).[264] Ascites almost always is present, although the effusion is large only when complicating hepatic cirrhosis. A pleural effusion, either unilateral or bilateral, is seen in 22–32% of patients.[265,266,268] Cases of tuberculous peritonitis are associated with active

pulmonary tuberculosis up to 50% of the time.[265,268,269,272]

Tuberculin skin testing generally is not helpful and the range of positivity varies significantly depending on age. Nonreactors tend to be older and have coexistent liver disease; younger patients tend to be reactors.[266,268,271]

In a study by Shafer et al., 27 of 199 HIV-positive patients (13.5%) with extrapulmonary tuberculosis had intraabdominal involvement.[28] Of these, 24 patients had lymphadenopathy and 6 had peritoneal involvement. Intraabdominal lymphadenopathy was a universal finding in patients with disseminated tuberculosis. Six patients had pancreatic abscesses originating from peripancreatic lymph nodes and two patients had liver abscesses from portahepatic nodes. Five patients had intestinal perforation from contiguous lymphadenitis. Twenty-one patients (78%) had symptoms of abdominal pain, tenderness, or ascites. Gastrointestinal fistulous tracts from other organs, such as stomach, esophagus, ileum, and rectum, were also seen.

3. Diagnosis

There is leukocytosis in less than 30% of patients and anemia in less than 20% of patients. Liver function tests usually are normal unless there is underlying liver disease.[266,273]

Gallium scanning, ultrasonography, and CT scanning are of considerable diagnostic value. Gallium scanning with prolonged uptake is nonspecific and may merely reflect peritoneal inflammation.[274] Computed tomography reveals no specific findings except lymphadenopathy with low density centers suggesting tuberculosis, especially in patients with HIV infection.[28,275] Ultrasonography facilitates aspiration of localized effusions.[264]

The diagnosis of tuberculous peritonitis may be made by culture of the peritoneal fluid and possibly by biopsy of the peritoneum. The ascitic fluid is exudative and the protein concentration usually is above 2.5–3.0 g/liter, although it may be lower with supervening liver cirrhosis.[273] The ascitic fluid/blood glucose ratio is below 1 in 80% of cases.[276] The ascitic fluid shows lymphocytic predominance, although PMNs may also be present.[272]

In tuberculous peritonitis, the AFB smear is positive in less than 5% of cases,[268,273] while the culture is positive in up to 68% of cases.[266,272] Examining a large amount (1 liter) of centrifuged fluid has a sensitivity of 83%.[268]

Adenosine deaminase (ADA) is increased 5-fold when compared to control groups, but decreased with low protein ascites (false-negative). The ADA ratio of ascitic fluid to serum also is increased.[266,277]

Blind peritoneal needle biopsy has a diagnostic yield of approximately 65%, but rarely is recommended, since bleeding or perforation may occur especially if fibroadhesions are present.[264] Sonogram or CT scan guided fine needle aspiration of an intraabdominal mass or lymph node may be helpful.[278] Peritoneoscopy or laparoscopy is useful, and in one study, peritoneoscopy with biopsy led to a diagnosis of tuberculosis in 77% of cases.[279] Biopsy may reveal a thickened or inflamed peritoneum, miliary yellow-white tubercles of the peritoneum, serosa, and omentum, or fibroadhesions between liver and parietal peritoneum. Procedural complications include a postparacentesis ascitic fluid leakage in 3% of cases, fecal fistulas in 2% of cases, and gastrointestinal hemorrhage.[266]

4. Treatment

Medical therapy usually is adequate and early diagnosis usually averts surgical intervention. In a study by Dutt et al., 17 patients with tuberculous peritonitis were successfully treated with a 9-month short-course therapy.[34]

5. Complications

Late complications of TB peritonitis include retroperitoneal fibrosis with ureteral obstruction,[266] and adhesions between visceral and parietal peritoneum. These adhesions may, on occasion, obstruct the bowel and require surgical resection. Partial obstruction may respond to antituberculous medication. Intestinal obstruction may transpire during or following therapy.[266] Overall mortality of tuberculous peritonitis has decreased from 50 to 10% with appropriate therapy. Mortality is higher with delayed or missed diagnosis, concomitant liver disease, and age above 60 years.[266]

B. ENTERIC TB
1. Epidemiology

Tuberculosis can affect any portion of the gastrointestinal tract. The ileocecal region is most commonly affected but the colon, esophagus, stomach, duodenum, jejunum, appendix, and anorectal area also may be involved.[265,280,281] In a study of 341 cases of abdominal tuberculosis, 21% of patients had ileocecal disease, 20% had anorectal disease, and 1% had involvement of the sigmoid colon.[265] This disease remains more common among immigrants from India, the Middle East, Africa, and Asia, and especially may be seen in women.[265,266]

2. Clinical

Tuberculous enteritis may occur as a result of direct invasion by ingested organisms, lymphohematogenous dissemination, or extension from a contiguous site or biliary secretions.[266] Gastrointestinal involvement due to ingestion of organisms may occur in up to 46% of patients with smear-positive pulmonary TB.[270] With reduced gastric acid production, e.g., postgastrectomy state or achlorhydria, and cavitary lung disease, there is an increased risk of tuberculous enteritis with swallowed organisms reaching the ileum and cecum.[270]

The clinical features of tuberculous enteritis are relatively nonspecific. Symptoms may be acute, associated with obstruction or perforation, chronic for many years, or asymptomatic and found on autopsy.[266,281] There may be crampy abdominal pain, weight loss, fever, anorexia, and diarrhea. On occasion there may be severe gastrointestinal hemorrhage.[281]

Esophageal involvement resulting in dysphagia may occur due to compression by paratracheal and subcarinal nodes. Subcarinal lymph nodes may erode into the esophagus and cause hematemesis, hemorrhage, or fistulous tracts.[282] A fistula to the trachea or the bronchial system or esophageal perforation has been reported in a patient with HIV infection.[283] An intraluminal mass can mimic tumor and an ulceration may cause hemorrhage.[282]

TB of stomach and duodenum may exhibit symptoms of chronic peptic ulceration or may resemble a carcinoma. Gastric outlet or duodenal obstruction may occur.[284]

Jejunal involvement produces malabsorption and may cause severe diarrhea and weight loss. Small bowel disease, especially in the ileocecal region, may lead to chronic weight loss, abdominal cramps, colicky pain, diarrhea, and hematochezia, and mimic Crohn's disease.[266] Intestinal involvement may cause a mass effect, obstruction, perforation, strictures, ileus, bleeding, or diarrhea. Perforation proximal to stricture formation may occur. Up to 2% of appendicitis in India is due to tuberculosis[285] but is a rare finding in this country. Anorectal disease usually presents as an ulceration but may present as a verrucous or lupoid lesion, mass, perirectal abscess especially in males, or fistulous formation.[286]

Tuberculous enteritis may present as an acute abdomen, mimic carcinoma, or complicate hepatic cirrhosis.[287] Thirty percent present as surgical emergencies, another 10% are diagnosed at surgery, and up to 40% are diagnosed postmortem.[266,288]

Stool smears and cultures for *M. tuberculosis* have been described in 16 and 29%, respectively, of patients with HIV infection.[53,117] This may represent swallowed organisms rather than true tuberculous enteritis in these patients.[69] Further workup including barium studies, CT scan, and endoscopy with biopsy may be required.

3. Diagnosis

The diagnosis of tuberculous enteritis requires positive cultures from secretions or biopsy material. Tuberculin skin testing may be negative and represent malnutrition or may be positive in up to 80% of patients.[265]

The barium enema remains relatively nonspecific and may show an irregular coarse mucosal lining said to be suggestive of TB.[289] Computed tomography of the abdomen also is nonspecific but may be suggestive of ileocecal tuberculosis.[266,290]

Upper endoscopy and colonoscopy may reveal nodular areas, ulcerations, fistulas, scarring, mucosal hypertrophy, ileocecal and ascending colon involvement, or pancolitis.[291] Granulomas are submucosal in location, may be missed by the biopsy forceps, and cultures grow mycobacteria in less than 50%. The yield is increased with colonoscopic fine needle aspiration.[292] Arteriograms usually are not required, although they may reveal hypervascularity (with ulcerations), occlusion of arteries (with strictures), stretching, crowding, or encasement.[293] With smear-positive pulmonary TB there is gastrointestinal disease by colonoscopy in up to 45%, mostly in the ileocecal region.[270] Laparoscopy and laparotomy occasionally are useful in the diagnosis.

4. Treatment

Antituberculous therapy is highly effective and adjunctive surgery is indicated only for perforation, abscess formation, or complete obstruction.[266] Nine-month short-course chemotherapy has been successful in a small number of patients.[34] Despite conventional antituberculous chemotherapy up to 50% of patients in one study required surgery for diagnosis or treatment.[294] Narrowing and adhesions generally respond to antituberculous medication, although they may develop even on therapy.[268]

5. Complications

Adhesions and subacute obstruction in acute tuberculous disease may require medical therapy only. Obstruction due to cicatricial healing may occur. Bypass procedures are useful primarily for the treatment of stricture formation and intestinal obstruction. Resection or stricture-plasty is usually preferable.[295]

C. HEPATIC TB

The liver may be involved in all forms of tuberculosis including pulmonary, extrapulmonary, and miliary or disseminated disease. Noncaseating hepatic granulomas have been described in up to 25% of patients with pulmonary tuberculosis without evidence of clinical hepatitis.[296] Percutaneous liver biopsies may reveal granulomata in 50–100% of patients with miliary tuberculosis.[97,173,185] Liver involvement usually occurs with dissemination, but can be an isolated process in 5% of patients.[97] Hepatic tuberculosis may be seen with granulomatous disease, isolated or multiple abscesses, fibrosis, cirrhosis, or chronic hepatitis.[97]

Histologically there is miliary-micronodular, pseudotumoral-macronodular, or pericanalicular involvement with cholestasis. Nonspecific reactive hepatitis can be present with fatty infiltration, inflammatory cell infiltrates, portal inflammation and fibrosis, Kupffer cell hyperplasia, and fatty metamorphosis. The spectrum of hepatic disease extends from granulomas, tuberculids, tuberculomas (coalescing granulomas), abscesses,[297] peliosis hepatis (blood filled lakes), cirrhosis, and hepatic failure.[97]

Hepatic tuberculosis can be asymptomatic, or manifest with fever, right upper quadrant pain, or jaundice, and may mimic a variety of conditions from infections to neoplasms.[97] Often there are no localizing symptoms. Up to 10% of patients with clinically unexplained hepatomegaly have tuberculosis.[270] The alkaline phosphatase is elevated with space occupying granulomas in 30% of patients, transaminases are often normal, and hyperbilirubinemia is absent or minimal.[97] Hepatomegaly is present in 50% of patients and splenomegaly in 30% of patients with hepatic granulomas.[298]

The diagnosis can be established by sonogram-guided percutaneous biopsy in 70% of patients or laparoscopy in 90% of patients, although stains are negative in 50–90% of cases.[298] The sonogram may show periportal lymph nodes that potentially could obstruct the biliary system.[299] Computed tomography of the abdomen may show hepatomegaly or a mass lesion.[290]

Surgery is indicated for diagnosis and possibly for abscess drainage.[300] Mortality due to hepatic tuberculosis is related to respiratory insufficiency, peritonitis, portal vein thrombosis, and portal hypertension with variceal hemorrhage.[97]

D. OTHER DISEASE

TB can involve all sites from the mouth to the anus and atypical presentations such as mouth ulcers, tongue lesions, and tonsillitis have been described.[281,301]

Tuberculosis of the spleen is a rare clinical entity in non-AIDS patients.[302] It may result from lymphohematogenous dissemination or may be an isolated process. Sonography and CT scan of the abdomen may show densities, which are often multiple and 4 to 20 mm in size. These abscesses may be isolated findings without pulmonary tuberculosis in patients with AIDS.[303] Splenic tuberculosis has been diagnosed by needle aspiration, although we would not recommend this in view of bleeding complications.[302] It may take 2 to 4 months for these lesions to resolve on therapy. Splenectomy is indicated only if no improvement with medical therapy occurs.[302] Calcifications represent healed disease and occur in about half the patients.[162]

The biliary tract rarely is involved in tuberculosis. Jaundice is most commonly associated with fulminant intrahepatic disease and only rarely from biliary obstruction.[299] However, on occasion enlarged periportal lymph nodes may obstruct the biliary tract and lead to jaundice.[299] Intrahepatic tubercles may rupture into the ductules.[97] Biliary involvement occurs in up to 7% of patients with abdominal TB and usually is accompanied by multiple small cavities. It is associated with other organs drained by the portal circulation including mesenteric lymph nodes in 89% of patients, gastrointestinal ulcerations in 73% of patients, and peritonitis in 27% of patients.[97] It may be seen only at autopsy, especially in patients with miliary TB. Abdominal symptoms are present in 15% of patients, and hepatomegaly in 30% of patients.[97] Primary tuberculosis of the gallbladder is seen rarely. It usually occurs in women over the age of 30 years and presents as cholecystitis. Treatment includes chemotherapy in conjunction with cholecystectomy or ERCP if there is common bile duct obstruction.[97]

Pancreatic involvement is uncommon and low grade fever, weight loss, and jaundice may be presenting symptoms. A tuberculous mass in the pancreatic head may mimic carcinoma.[304] Peripancreatic tuberculous lymphadenitis may occur and may be found by sonography or CT scan.[305]

In HIV-positive patients, atypical abscess formation has been observed in the pancreatic, retroperitoneal, and subhepatic areas, and even within the abdominal wall.[300] Twenty percent of AIDS patients with TB have abdominal disease. Enlarged lymph nodes (10%), hepatic (10%), and ileal and peritoneal involvement (5%) may be seen.[306] Splenic TB may occur even more often.[302,303]

IX. CARDIOVASCULAR

A. PERICARDIAL
1. Epidemiology
Cardiovascular tuberculosis in industrialized countries is rare and accounts for 1% of all cases of extrapulmonary TB.[307] It is usually a manifestation of disseminated disease in more than 50% of patients.[308] Cardiovascular tuberculosis includes disease of the pericardium, myocardium, and major arteries such as the aorta. The pericardium is the area most frequently involved. In a study of 136 patients with extrapulmonary tuberculosis at Boston City Hospital, 4 patients (3%) had pericardial disease.[309] Tuberculosis accounts for up to 4% of all acute pericarditis and 7% of all cardiac tamponade.[310] In some third-world countries and in a study of patients with AIDS, it was the leading cause of pericarditis.[162,311] It generally occurs in the middle aged[312] and there appears to be a predilection

for black males.[313] Pericardial effusions have been reported in patients with HIV infection[28,314-316] and, in one study, the incidence was approximately 8%.[317]

2. Clinical
Pericardial tuberculosis frequently arises from hematogenous dissemination from a distant focus. It also may arise from other sources such as a contiguous mediastinal or peribronchial lymph node, contiguous pleuritis, or a primary pericardial focus.[162]

It is likely that hypersensitivity to a tuberculoprotein plays a role in the pathogenesis, as in pleuritis and meningitis. The natural course of untreated tuberculous pericarditis includes death during the acute phase, seen in up to 31% of patients, spontaneous reabsorption of the effusion, or progression to constriction.[313] The disease usually is insidious but may present in an acute manner and with cardiac tamponade.[318]

The most common symptoms are weight loss, cough, dyspnea, orthopnea, chest pain, peripheral edema, and night sweats. Tachycardia, increased venous pressure, hepatomegaly, pulsus paradoxicus, and friction rub also may be seen.[313,319,320] A pulmonary infiltrate or a pleural effusion may appear on chest radiograph in 32 and 36% of patients, respectively.[313,321] Cardiomegaly is found with a subacute or chronic effusion, and a small heart size is seen with fibrosis or rapidly evolving effusion. An acute effusion with only 200 ml can cause tamponade and be life threatening, while late and chronic effusions may lead to restrictive disease.[162,313,319,320] Constrictive pericarditis occurs in about 20% of patients and calcification in 50%.[162,313] Cardiomegaly is common, and in one study, 190 of 193 patients had cardiomegaly on chest radiograph.[322]

The tuberculin skin test is positive in most patients with tuberculous pericarditis,[313,322] but yields as low as 54% positivity have been reported.[323]

Tuberculous pericarditis has been described as the first manifestation of AIDS.[324] Kinney et al. reported five patients who presented with tuberculous pericarditis as the initial infectious manifestation of AIDS.[317] All patients had cardiac tamponade and all required a pericardiectomy. The smears and cultures were positive for TB in all cases. In another series, three patients had tuberculous pericarditis with tamponade and all required pericardial windows.[28]

3. Diagnosis
The diagnosis of tuberculous pericarditis is based on finding the tubercle bacilli in the pericardial fluid, on pericardial histology, or proof of TB elsewhere with unexplained pericarditis.

The presence of a thickened pericardium with effusion is characteristic of this disease and the echocardiography is 100% sensitive.[310,312] In the absence of pericardial fluid or if there is only pericardial thickening, the search for disease elsewhere is crucial if a definitive diagnosis is to be made. Calcification of the pericardium may be detected by echocardiography, chest radiograph, fluoroscopy, or CT scan,[325] and usually is associated with chronic or inactive disease. Gallium scanning may be useful in diagnosing tuberculous pericarditis.[326]

The pericardial fluid usually is serosanguinous but may be grossly hemorrhagic or even purulent.[310,327] The fluid is exudative with an increased protein concentration. There is an increased leukocyte count, with lymphocytes and monocytes predominating, but neutrophils may be prevalent in the first 2 weeks.[310]

AFB smears of the pericardial fluid in HIV-negative patients are almost invariably negative.[323,328] However, in patients with HIV infection, one study reported 14.3% smear positivity,[311] and another study reported a yield of 100%.[317] The pericardial fluid may show culture positivity in up to 86% of patients.[310,313,323,328] Pericardial biopsy is a sensitive procedure yielding positive histology in 83 and 100% of patients in two studies.[313,328] Adenosine deaminase levels in tuberculous pericardial fluid are above 60 U/liter and have a sensitivity and specificity of approximately 80%.[329]

4. Treatment

The treatment of tuberculous pericarditis includes both the eradication of the tubercle bacilli and the control of pericardial inflammation. Standard therapy, identical to that for pulmonary tuberculosis, has been recommended.[330] A 9-month short course of chemotherapy appeared to be adequate in a study of 12 patients with pericardial tuberculosis.[34] However, in two studies by Strang et al., 6 months of chemotherapy alone was associated with significant morbidity and mortality.[322,331]

The more difficult task is minimizing the risk of significant pericardial inflammation. Corticosteroid therapy may be useful when the effusion persists or recurs despite adequate chemotherapy, but its use is still controversial. Several studies failed to show its long term benefit.[313,323,328,332] Two controlled prospective studies, using 11 weeks of corticosteroids in addition to a modern 6-month short-course chemotherapy regimen, were undertaken in effusive and constrictive pericarditis.[322,331] Both studies demonstrated a decline in mortality rate and a decrease in the need for pericardiectomy. A significant number still required pericardiectomy.

Pericardiocentesis provides prompt symptomatic relief from accumulation of pericardial fluid and cardiac tamponade but a pericardial window is recommended for a large effusion. If pericardial thickening is found during the window procedure, early pericardiectomy is recommended.[323] Surgical resection of the pericardium is indicated in life-threatening tamponade, persistent elevation of central venous pressure unrelieved by pericardiocentesis, and a nonresolving effusion.[307] As many as 30% of patients will require pericardiectomy despite adequate drug therapy.[331] Since surgical mortality is higher during the late calcific or chronic phase of constrictive pericarditis, early pericardiectomy is recommended.[310] Although some authors recommend pericardiectomy for all patients,[333] most do not.

Both specific antituberculous therapy and adjunctive surgical procedures are required for good therapeutic results.[317,324] The incidence of chronic constrictive pericarditis in patients with HIV infection is largely unknown.

5. Complications

The mortality from tuberculous pericarditis has declined from 80 to 85% prior to the introduction of chemotherapy to below 50% with antituberculous therapy, and as low as 3% in some studies.[309,310,322] The mortality in treated patients is due to cardiac tamponade, congestive heart failure, or advanced TB.[162]

B. CARDITIS

Tuberculosis can also involve the endocardium or the myocardium and in most patients is found in association with disseminated TB.[334] Nodular tuberculomas, miliary nodules, diffuse infiltrations, and focal lymphocytic lesions have been described pathologically.[308,335] In an autopsy study of 243 patients with disseminated tuberculosis, Rose et al. reported myocardial involvement in 8% of patients.[308] It has been described as a tumor mass of the tricuspid valve, and even as congestive heart failure.[334] Carditis may cause arrhythmias, impaired contractility, and even ventricular aneurysm and rupture.[308,336] Endocardial tuberculomas associated with ventricular tachycardia have been described.[337] Involvement of coronary vessels is very rare, and may be due to arteritis, intima lesions, or adjacent mediastinal or pericardial lymph node enlargement.[334]

Although most cases are diagnosed at postmortem, diagnostic tests such as CT scan, MRI, and echocardiogram could be useful.[335] Treatment must be individualized and surgery occasionally may be necessary.[335]

C. AORTITIS

Tuberculous aortitis is a very rare condition and may lead to infectious ("mycotic") aneurysms, rupture, and fatal hemorrhage.[307,338,339] Although usually thought to arise through extension from a lymph node or another contiguous focus, spread from hematogenous dissemination is possible.[340] Aneurysmal dilatation of the thoracic or abdominal aorta occurs in 50% of patients[307,339] and esophagoaortic fistulas[341] also have been described. Transesophageal echocardiogram and abdominal sonogram or CT scan are potentially helpful in suspected aortitis. Treatment includes antituberculous chemotherapy and mindful attention to potential complications. Complications such as aortic valve insufficiency and aneurysm formation and rupture may occur. Surgery usually is indicated. Even the thoracic aorta can be repaired and replaced by prosthetic grafts.[339]

X. UPPER AIRWAYS

Upper airway structures such as the nose, epiglottis, larynx, trachea, and nasopharynx can be infected with *M. tuberculosis*. These structures are continuously bathed by organisms in the expectorated sputum of active cavitary lung disease.[301] Upper airway involvement is associated primarily with severe cavitary pulmonary disease and rarely with miliary tuberculosis.[342] In one North American study of a large number of patients with active tuberculosis, laryngeal lesions were found in 1.5% of patients.[343]

Laryngitis is highly infectious, having a great load of live bacilli, and is accompanied by severe cavitary pulmonary disease or endobronchial disease.[342] The chest radiograph is abnormal in 95% of cases.[342] Hoarseness, cough, and throat pain are common symptoms. The anterior two-thirds of the vocal cords are involved in 70% of patients.[342] There is hypertrophy with a pale or pink appearance, odynophagia, ulceration, edema, and stridor.[342] Pathology may show a superficial lesion, an ulceration, or granuloma. It may mimic a laryngeal cancer or papilloma, although concomitant carcinoma is possible.[342] Unusual presentations mimicking a salivary gland tumor, sebaceous cyst, and carotid body tumor have been reported.[344] Occasionally the epiglottis, the false cords, the aryepiglottic folds, and the hypopharynx are involved.[301] Paralysis of the vocal cords, especially the left, is secondary to lymphatic or pleural disease.[301] There is a dramatic therapeutic response with chemotherapy and pain usually will subside within 1 to 2 weeks.[342] Stenosis secondary to fibrosis or cricoarytenoid fixation is rare.

XI. DERMAL

Tuberculosis of the dermal system includes the skin, subcutaneous tissue, and the breast. A high index of suspicion is necessary to diagnose cutaneous TB. Histology may show only acute and chronic

inflammation, and staining and culture of the biopsy are required.[345] The course is usually benign, but at times may be serious.

There are three distinct categories of disease[346] based on the source including exogenous, endogenous, and hematogenous.

Exogenous infection of the intact skin occurs by inoculation in less than 2% of patients with cutaneous TB.[347] It may appear as a verrucous lesion (prosector's wart, "anatomical tubercle") or a hyperkeratotic papule with hyperplasia and dense inflammation.[346,347] There usually is no lymph node involvement, and it has been previously referred to as "tuberculosis verrucosa cutis" and "tuberculosis cutis verruca et necrogenica."[347] It is acquired primarily in the autopsy room or by touching contaminated specimens.[348] Lesions can be treated with chemotherapy and in some cases by excision alone. Spontaneous resolution in immunocompetent patients may conceivably occur. Primary inoculation may also resemble an ulcer (tuberculous chancre) and is referred to as cutaneous primary complex or cutaneous Ghon complex. Lymph nodes may enlarge 3 to 6 weeks after inoculation. The primary cutaneous infection occurs mostly in children and is associated with regional adenopathy.[347]

Tuberculosis of the skin may occur through contiguous spread, e.g., from cervical lymph nodes, osteomyelitis, or epididymitis. This is called scrofuloderma or tuberculosis colliquativa cutis, and is "the fistulous opening of sinuses originated in glands or bones previously infected with tuberculosis."[349] Disease also may occur secondary to excretion of organisms and autoinoculation and is called orificial tuberculosis. Painful ulcers of the anal, oral, and labial openings and the surrounding skin can be seen. This is referred to as "tuberculosis ulcerosa cutis et mucosae" or "tuberculosis cutis orificialis".[345]

There is a form of cutaneous TB from hematogenous spread that is divided into three subsets: lupus vulgaris, acute dissemination, and nodules or abscesses. Lupus vulgaris is seen primarily in women. It presents with "apple-jelly" plaques or nodules on diascopy, scarring ulcers, and severe deformities of the nose, neck, ear lobe, or face.[346] Its hallmark is chronicity and may be very indolent and missed clinically for years.[345] With long standing chronic ulcers, carcinoma may develop in up to 8% of patients.[350] Antituberculous chemotherapy usually is necessary.

Acute disseminated TB may cause multiple skin lesions (tuberculosis cutis miliaris disseminata),[351] which appear as blue-red to brown papules the size of a pinhead and may be mistaken for folliculitis.[352] It is rare and is primarily a disease of infants and children.[347] Cutaneous vasculitis is rare.

Subcutaneous cold abscesses may be isolated to the breast, chest wall, axilla, buttocks, and extremities.[347] Mastitis or breast abscess may appear in younger women and usually is accompanied by axillary lymphadenopathy.[353] It occurs as the result of retrograde lymphatic extension from adjacent lymph nodes. It may be difficult to diagnose and often is confused with carcinoma.[347] The yield on stain and culture is only 15% and histologic diagnosis is crucial.[353] Pathologically it may be confused with duct ectasia, foreign body, and idiopathic reactions. Surgical excision is the treatment of choice but chemotherapy also may be required.[353] Complications are discharge, ulcer with inflammation, recurring abscess, fistula, and sclerosis with nipple retraction. Open abscesses treated with irrigation may aerosolize organisms and cause infection.[354]

TB may manifest in HIV-positive patients as acneiform papules that mimic folliculitis, indurated crusted plaques, multiple tender skin nodules, abscesses, or swollen lymph nodes with overlying erythema. Sometimes ill-defined macules or ecthymatous lesions are noted.[355] Chronic recurrent perirectal abscesses have been observed. Tuberculosis cutis miliaris disseminata with numerous 2 to 3 mm follicular papules has been described.[352] Lesions with purulent discharge may be infectious.[356] Localized cutaneous disease may respond well to excision and drainage.[355]

Tuberculids are a heterogeneous group of cutaneous lesions with caseation necrosis and perivascular infiltrates (hypersensitivity reaction secondary to dissemination) that includes erythema induratum, papulonecrotic tuberculid, lichen scrofulosorum, and papular lesions of tuberculid hypersensitivity.[347]

XII. ENDOCRINE

A. ADRENAL

In Addison's original description of adrenal insufficiency, 7 of 11 patients had tuberculosis. At least 80–90% of the glands must be destroyed for significant insufficiency to occur.[357] Up to 30% of cases of chronic adrenal insufficiency were considered to be due to TB.[309] The adrenals are involved in approximately 53% of patients with disseminated TB, but adrenal insufficiency is seen in less than 1% of patients, even with severe or chronic disease.[166,358] Nine patients with tuberculosis of the adrenal gland diagnosed at autopsy were reported in one study of extrapulmonary tuberculosis.[28]

Histopathology may show massive caseation and enlargement of both glands in acute disease.[359] Calcification is a sign of chronicity, develops within 6 to 24 months, and is 95% specific for TB.[360] With TB less than 2 years duration, enlarged glands are typical; with more than 2 years, they are normal or small. Therefore, adrenal size can be a clinical clue to the duration of disease. Sonography or CT scan guided fine needle aspiration/biopsy may be helpful in achieving the diagnosis.[361]

HIV-positive patients with miliary TB may develop acute adrenal insufficiency. Rifampin may increase catabolism of corticosteroids and unmask subclinical adrenal insufficiency.[362] With suspected adrenal insufficiency it is prudent first to perform an ACTH stimulation test; start with dexamethasone therapy (to avoid interference with testing), and then change to hydrocortisone 100 mg every 6 h.[363]

B. THYROID

For unknown reasons TB of the thyroid is very unusual despite the relatively high organ perfusion. There were only 2 patients with TB among 75,000 thyroid biopsies.[364] Tuberculosis of the thyroid may present as an abscess, a cold or warm nodule. The patient may have pain, tenderness, hoarseness, dysphagia, or accompanying dyspnea.[359] Only one case of hypothyroidism with myxedema due to TB has been reported; most patients are euthyroid.[364]

In a study by Shafer et al. of 199 cases of extrapulmonary tuberculosis, 3 patients had thyroid involvement at autopsy.[28]

C. PITUITARY

Pituitary gland involvement may cause fever, headache, and visual disturbances, and is usually associated with preexisting pituitary adenomas or meningitis.[209,365] A hypophyseal tuberculoma may impair or destroy function. Diabetes insipidus, hypogonadism, growth failure, and panhypopituitarism are subjects of case reports only.[366] However, hypopituitarism was documented in 10 of 49 patients, years after recovery from tuberculous meningitis in childhood.[367]

REFERENCES

1. Morse, D., Brothwell, D. R., Ucko, P. J., Tuberculosis in ancient Egypt, *Am. Rev. Resp. Dis.*, 90, 524, 1964.
2. Centers for Disease Control/American Thoracic Society, Core curriculum on tuberculosis, American Lung Association, New York, 1990.
3. Rieder, H. L., Snider, D. E., Cauthen, G. M., Extrapulmonary tuberculosis in the United States, *Am. Rev. Resp. Dis.*, 141, 347, 1990.
4. Anonymous, Extrapulmonary tuberculosis in the United States. U.S. Department of Health, Education, and Welfare, Center for Disease Control, Atlanta, GA, 1978.
5. Anon., Cases of specified notifiable diseases, United States, *MMWR*, 38, 241, 1989.

6. Centers for Disease Control, Tuberculosis in developing countries, *MMWR*, 39, 561, 1990.

7. Richter, C., Ndosi, B., Mwammy, A. S., Mbwambo, R. K., Extrapulmonary tuberculosis — a simple diagnosis, *Tropic Geograph. Med.*, 43, 375, 1991.

8. Rieder, H. L., Kelly, G. D., Bloch, A. B., Cauthen, G. M., Snider, D. E., Jr., Tuberculosis diagnosed at death in the United States, *Chest*, 100, 678, 1991.

9. Chastonay, P., Gardiol, D., Extensive active tuberculosis at autopsy: retrospective study of a collection of adult autopsies (1961–1985), *J. Suisse Med.*, 117, 925, 1987.

10. U.S. Department of Health and Human Services, 1990 tuberculosis statistics in the United States, Centers for Disease Control, Atlanta, GA, 1992.

11. Lester, T. W., Extrapulmonary tuberculosis, *Clin. Chest Med.*, 2, 219, 1980.

12. Cuss, F. M. C., Carmichael, D. J. S., Linington, A., Hulme, B., Tuberculosis in renal failure: A high incidence in patients born in the third world, *Clin. Nephrol.*, 25, 129, 1986.

13. Andrew, O. T., Schoenfeld, P., Hopewell, C., Humphries, M. H., Tuberculosis in patients with endstage renal disease, *Am. J. Med.*, 68, 59, 1980.

14. Navari, R. M., Sullivan, K. M., Springmeyer, S. C., Siegel, M. S., Meyers, J. D., Buckner, C. D., Sanders, J. E., Stewart, P. S., Clift, R. A., Fefer, A., Storb, R., Thomas, E. D., Mycobacterial infections in marrow transplant patients, *Transplantation*, 36, 509, 1983.

15. Bruce, R. M., Wise, L., Tuberculosis after jejunoileal bypass for obesity, *Ann. Intern. Med.*, 87, 574, 1977.

16. Snider, D. E., Jejunoileal bypass for obesity: a risk factor for tuberculosis, *Chest*, 81, 531, 1982.

17. Warner, T. T., Khoo, S. H., Wilkins, E. G., Reactivation of tuberculous lymphadenitis during pregnancy, *J. Inf.*, 24, 181, 1992.

18. De Cock, K. M., Soro, B., Coulibaly, I. M., Lucas, S. B., Tuberculosis and HIV infection in Sub-Saharan Africa, *J. Am. Med. Assoc.*, 268, 1581, 1992.

19. Dubé, M. P., Holtom, P. D., Larsen, R. A., Tuberculous meningitis in patients with and without human immunodeficiency virus infection, *Am. J. Med.*, 93, 520, 1992.

20. Raviglione, M. C., Narain, J. P., Kochi, A., HIV-associated tuberculosis in developing countries: clinical features, diagnosis, and treatment, *Bull. WHO.*, 70, 515, 1992.

21. Pitchenik, A. E., Fertel, D., Tuberculosis and nontuberculous mycobacterial disease, *Med. Clin. N. Am.*, 76, 121, 1992.

22. Braun, M. M., Byers, R. H., Heyward, W. L., Ciesielski, C. A., Bloch, A. B., Berkelman, R. L., Snider, D. E., Acquired immunodeficiency syndrome and extrapulmonary tuberculosis in the United States, *Arch. Intern. Med.*, 150, 1913, 1990.

23. Flora, G. S., Modilevsky, T., Antoniskis, D., Barnes, P. F., Undiagnosed tuberculosis in patients with human immunodeficiency virus infection, *Chest*, 98, 1056, 1990.

24. Gilks, C. F., Brindle, R. J., Otieno, L. S., Bhatt, S. M., Newnham, R. S., Simani, P. M., Lule, G. N., Okelo, G. B. A., Watkins, W. M., Waiyaki, P. G., Were, J. O. B., Warrell, D. A., Extrapulmonary and disseminated tuberculosis in HIV-1-seropositive patients presenting to the acute medical services in Nairobi, *AIDS*, 4, 981, 1990.

25. Chaisson, R. E., Slutkin, G., Tuberculosis and human immunodeficiency virus infection, *J. Infect. Dis.*, 159, 96, 1989.

26. Handwerger, S., Mildvan, D., Senie, R., McKinley, F. W., Tuberculosis and the acquired immunodeficiency syndrome at a New York City hospital: 1978–1985, *Chest*, 91, 176, 1987.

27. Chaisson, R. E., Schecter, G. F., Theuer, C. P., et al., Tuberculosis in patients with the acquired immunodeficiency syndrome, *Am. Rev. Resp. Dis.*, 136, 570, 1987.

28. Shafer, R. W., Kim, D. S., Weiss, J. P., Quale, J. M., Extrapulmonary tuberculosis in patients with human immunodeficiency virus infection, *Medicine*, 70, 384, 1991.

29. Hopewell, P. C., Impact of human immunodeficiency virus infection on the epidemiology, clinical features, management, and control of tuberculosis, *Clin. Infect. Dis.*, 15, 540, 1992.

30. Barnes, P. F., Arevalo, C., Six cases of Mycobacterium tuberculosis bacteremia, *J. Infect. Dis.*, 156, 377, 1987.

31. Hartstein, M., Leaf, H. L., Tuberculosis of the breast as a presenting manifestation of AIDS, *Clin. Infect. Dis.*, 15, 692, 1992.

32. Marini, M., Ed., *Tuberculosis of the Bone and Joints,* Springer-Verlag, Berlin, 1988.

33. Edlin, G. P., Active tuberculosis unrecognised until necropsy, *Lancet*, 1, 8076, 650, 1978.

34. Dutt, A. K., Moers, D., Stead, W. W., Short-course chemotherapy for extrapulmonary tuberculosis: nine years' experience, *Ann. Intern. Med.*, 104, 7, 1986.

35. Dutt, A. K., Stead, W. W., Treatment of extrapulmonary tuberculosis, *Sem. Resp. Infect.*, 4, 225, 1989.

36. Cohn, D. L., Catlin, B. J., Peterson, K. L., Judson, F. N., Sbarbaro, J. A., A 62-dose, 6-month therapy for pulmonary and extrapulmonary tuberculosis, a twice-weekly, directly observed, and cost-effective regimen, *Ann. Intern. Med.*, 112, 407, 1990.

37. Bueso, J. F., Hernando, V., Garcia-Buela, J. P., Juncal, L. D., Egaña, M. T. M., Martinez, M. C. M., Diagnostic value of simultaneous determination of pleural adenosine deaminase and pleural lysozyme/serum lysozyme ratio in pleural effusions, *Chest*, 93, 303, 1988.

38. Storey, D. D., Dines, D. E., Coles, D. T., Pleural effusion — a diagnostic dilemma, *J. Am. Med. Assoc.*, 236, 2183, 1976.

39. Light, R. W., Macgregor, I. M., Luchsinger, P. C., Ball, W. C., Pleural effusions, the diagnostic separation of transudates and exudates, *Ann. Intern. Med.*, 77, 507, 1972.

40. Seibert, A. F., Haynes, J., Jr., Middleton, R., Bass, J. B., Jr., Tuberculous pleural effusion. Twenty-year experience, *Chest*, 99, 883, 1991.

41. Berger, H. W., Mejia, E., Tuberculous pleurisy, *Chest*, 63, 88, 1973.

42. Epstein, D. M., Kline, L. R., Albelda, S. M., Miller, W. T., Tuberculous pleural effusions, *Chest*, 91, 106, 1987.

43. Rossman, M. D., Mayock, R. L., Pulmonary tuberculosis, in *Tuberculosis*, Schlossberg, D., Ed., Springer-Verlag, New York, 1988, 61.

44. Light, R. W., Tuberculous pleural effusions, in *Pleural Diseases*, 2nd ed., Light, R. W., Ed., Lea and Febiger, Philadelphia, 1990, 11.

45. Antoniskis, D., Amin, K., Barnes, P. F., Pleuritis as a manifestation of reactivation tuberculosis, *Am. J. Med.*, 22, 447, 1990.

46. Wallgren, A., The timetable of tuberculosis, *Tubercle*, 29, 245, 1948.

47. Fischl, M. A., Uttamchandani, R. B., Daikos, G. L., An outbreak of tuberculosis caused by multiple-drug-resistant tubercle bacilli among patients with HIV infection, *Ann. Intern. Med.*, 117, 177, 1992.

48. Patiala, J., Initial tuberculous pleuritis in the Finnish Armed Forces in 1939–194 with special reference to eventual post pleuritic tuberculosis, *Acta Tuberc. Scand.*, Suppl. 36, 1, 1948.

49. Roper, W. H., Waring, J. J., Primary serofibrinous pleural effusion in military personnel, *Am. Rev. Resp. Dis.*, 71, 616, 1955.

50. Levine, H., Szanto, P. B., Cugell, D. W., Tuberculous pleurisy: an acute illness, *Arch. Intern. Med.*, 122, 329, 1968.

51. Hulnick, D. H., Naidich, D. P., McCauley, D. I., Pleural tuberculosis evaluated by computed tomography, *Radiology*, 149, 759, 1983.

52. Pitchenik, A. E., Burr, J., Suarez, M., Fertel, D., Gonzalez, G., Moas, C., Human T-cell lymphotropic virus-III (HTLV-III) seropositivity and related disease among 71 consecutive patients in whom tuberculosis was diagnosed, *Am. Rev. Resp. Dis.*, 135, 875, 1987.

53. Modilevsky, T., Sattler, F. R., Barnes, P. F., Mycobacterial disease in patients with human immunodeficiency virus infection, *Arch. Intern. Med.*, 149, 2201, 1989.

54. Ankobiah, W. A., Finch, P., Powell, S., Heurich, A., Shivaram, I., Kamholz, S. L., Pleural tuberculosis in patients with and without AIDS, *J. Assoc. Acad. Min. Phys.*, 1, 20, 1990.

55. Chan, C. H., Arnold, M., Chan, C. Y., Mak, T. W., Hoheisel, G. B., Clinical and pathological features of tuberculous pleural effusion and its long term consequences, *Respiration*, 58, 171, 1991.

56. Rossi, G. A., Balbi, B., Manca, F., Tuberculous pleural effusions, *Am. Rev. Resp. Dis.*, 136, 575, 1987.

57. Levine, H., Metzger, W., Lacera, D., Kay, L., Diagnosis of tuberculous pleurisy by culture of pleural biopsy specimen, *Arch. Intern. Med.*, 126, 269, 1970.

58. Bañales, J. L., Pineda, P. R., Fitzgerald, J. M., Rubio, H., Selman, M., Salazar-Lezama, M., Adenosine deaminase in the diagnosis of tuberculous pleural effusions, *Chest*, 99, 355, 1991.

59. Ocaña, I., Martinez-Vazquez, J. M., Segura, R. M., Fernandez-De-Sevilla, T., Capdevila, J. A., Adenosine deaminase in pleural fluids, *Chest*, 84, 51, 1983.

60. Ribera, E., Ocaña, I., Martinez-Vazquez, J. M., Rossell, M., Espanel, T., Ruibal, A., High level of interferon gamma in tuberculous pleural effusion, *Chest*, 93, 308, 1988.

61. Hara, N., Abe, M., Inuzuka, S., Kawarada, Y., Shigematsu, N., Pleural SCb-9 in differential diagnosis of tuberculous, malignant, and other effusions, *Chest*, 102, 1060, 1992.

62. de Wit, D., Maartens, G., Steyn, L., A comparative study of the polymerase chain reaction and conventional procedures for the diagnosis of tuberculous pleural effusion, *Tubercle Lung Dis.*, 73, 262, 1992.

63. Sahn, S. A., The pleura, *Am. Rev. Resp. Dis.*, 138, 184, 1988.

64. Nance, K. V., Shermer, R. W., Askin, F. B., Diagnostic efficacy of pleural biopsy as compared with that of pleural fluid examination, *Mod. Pathol.*, 4, 320, 1991.

65. Sarkar, S. K., Purohit, S. D., Sharma, T. N., Sharma, V. K., Ram, M., Singh, A. P., Pleuroscopy in the diagnosis of pleural effusion using a fiberoptic bronchoscope, *Tubercle*, 66, 141, 1985.

66. Menzies, R., Charbonneau, M., Thoracoscopy for the diagnosis of pleural disease, *Ann. Intern. Med.*, 114, 271, 1991.

67. Boutin, C., Astoul, P., Seitz, B., The role of thoracoscopy in the evaluation and management of pleural effusions, *Lung*, 168, 1113, 1990.

68. Dutt, A. K., Moers, D., Stead, W. W., Short-course chemotherapy for pleural tuberculosis, *Chest*, 90, 112, 1986.

69. Barnes, P. F., Bloch, A. B., Davidson, P. T., Snider, D. E., Tuberculosis in patients with human immunodeficiency virus infection, *N. Engl. J. Med.*, 324, 1644, 1991.

70. Dutt, A. K., Moers, D., Stead, W. W., Tuberculous pleural effusion: 6-month therapy with isoniazid and rifampin, *Am. Rev. Resp. Dis.*, 145, 1429, 1991.

71. Tani, P., Poppius, H., Makiyaja, J., Cortisone therapy for exudative tuberculous pleurisy in the light of the follow-up study, *Acta Tuberc. Scand.*, 44, 303, 1964.

72. Lee, C. H., Wang, W. J., Lan, R. S., Tsai, Y. H., Chiang, Y. C., Corticosteroids in the treatment of tuberculous pleurisy. A double-blind, placebo-controlled, randomized study, *Chest*, 94, 1256, 1988.

73. Large, S. E., Levick, R. K., Aspiration in the treatment of primary tuberculous pleural effusion, *Br. Med. J.*, 1, 112, 1989.

74. Barbas, C. S., Cukier, A., de Varvalho, C. R., Barbas, F. J. V., Light, R. W., The relationship between pleural findings and the development of pleural thickening in patients with pleural tuberculosis, *Chest*, 100, 1264, 1991.

75. Singh, P. P., Sridharan, K. B., Bhagi, R. P., Singla, R., Anaerobic infection of the lung and pleural space in tuberculosis, *Ind. J. Chest Dis. All. Sci.*, 31, 85, 1989.

76. Johnson, T. M., McCann, W., Davey, W. N., Tuberculous bronchopleural fistula, *Am. Rev. Resp. Dis.*, 107, 30, 1973.

77. Cendan, I., Talavera, W., Busillo, C., Garner, G., Mullen, M., Empyema thoracis: a complication of disseminated *Mycobacterium tuberculosis* (MTB) in AIDS, *Am. Rev. Resp. Dis.*, 143(Suppl.), A281, 1991.

78. Glicklich, M., Mendelson, D. S., Gendal, E. S., Teirstein, A. S., Tuberculous empyema necessitatis — computed tomography findings, *Clin. Imag.*, 14, 23, 1990.

79. Vennera, M. C., Moreno, R., Cot, J., Marin, A., Sanchez-Lloret, J., Picado, C., Agusti-Vidal, A., Chylothorax and tuberculosis, *Thorax*, 38, 694, 1983.

80. Shriner, K. A, Mathisen, G. E., Goetz, M. B., Comparison of mycobacterial lymphadenitis among persons infected with human immunodeficiency virus and seronegative controls, *Clin. Infect. Dis.*, 15, 601, 1992.

81. Shikhani, A. H., Hadi, U. M., Mufarrij, A. A., Zaytoun, G. M., Mycobacterial cervical lymphadenitis, *ENT J.*, 68, 660, 1989.

82. Hooper, A. A., Tuberculous peripheral lymphadenitis, *Br. J. Surg.*, 59, 353, 1972.

83. Lincoln, E. M., Sewell, E. M., *Tuberculosis in Children*, McGraw-Hill, New York, 1963.

84. Kent, D. C., Tuberculous lymphadenitis: Not a localized disease process, *Am. J. Med. Sci.*, 118, 866, 1967.

85. Ord, R. J., Matz, G. J., Tuberculous cervical lymphadenitis, *Arch. Otolaryngol.*, 99, 327, 1974.

86. Lai, K. K., Stottmeier, K. D., Sherman, I. H., McCabe, W. R., Mycobacterial cervical lymphadenopathy, *J. Am. Med. Assoc.*, 251, 1286, 1984.

87. Summers, G. D., McNicol, M. W., Tuberculosis of superficial lymph nodes, *Br. J. Dis. Child.*, 74, 369, 1980.

88. Powell, D. A., Tuberculous lymphadenitis, in *Tuberculosis*, Schlossberg, D., Ed., Springer-Verlag, New York, 1988, 99.

89. Huhti, E., Brander, E., Paloheimo, S., Sutinen, S., Tuberculosis of the cervical lymph nodes: a clinical, pathological and bacteriological study, *Tubercle*, 56, 27, 1975.

90. Cantrell, R. W., Jensen, J. H., Reid, D., Diagnosis and management of tuberculous cervical adenitis, *Arch. Otolaryngol.*, 101, 53, 1975.

91. Farer, L. S, Lowell, A. M., Meador, M. P., Extrapulmonary tuberculosis in the United States, *Am. J. Epidemiol.*, 109, 205, 1979.

92. Dandapat, M. C., Mishra, B. M., Dash, S. P., Kar, P. K., Peripheral lymph node tuberculosis: a review of 80 cases, *Br. J. Surg.*, 77, 911, 1990.

93. Malik, S. K., Behera, D., Gilhotra, R., Tuberculous pleural effusion and lymphadenitis treated with rifampin-containing regimen, *Chest*, 92, 904, 1987.

94. Lee, K. C., Tami, T. A., Lalwani, A. K., Schecter, G., Contemporary management of cervical tuberculosis, *Laryngoscope*, 102, 60, 1992.

95. Schuit, K. E., Miliary tuberculosis in children: clinical and laboratory manifestation in 19 patients, *Am. J. Dis. Child.*, 133, 583, 1979.

96. Kecharvarz-Oliai, L., Warren, W. S., Peripheral tuberculous lymphadenitis, *Am. J. Dis. Child.*, 122, 74, 1971.

97. Lewis, J. H., Zimmerman, H. J., Tuberculosis of the liver and biliary tract, in *Tuberculosis*, Schlossberg, D., Ed., Springer-Verlag, New York, 1988, 149.

98. British Thoracic Society Research Committee, Short course chemotherapy for tuberculosis of lymph nodes: a controlled trial, *Br. Med. J.*, 290, 1106, 1985.

99. Campbell, I. A., Dyson, A. J., Lymph node tuberculosis: a comparison of various methods of treatment, *Tubercle*, 58, 171, 1977.

100. Campbell, I. A., Dyson, A. J., Lymph node tuberculosis: a comparison of treatments 18 months after completion of chemotherapy, *Tubercle*, 60, 95, 1979.

101. Cheung, W. L., Siu, K. F., Ng, A., Tuberculous cervical abscess: comparing the results of total excision against simple incision and drainage, *Br. J. Surg.*, 75, 563, 1988.

102. Lau, S. K., Kwan, S., Lee, J., Wei, W. I., Source of tubercle bacilli in cervical lymph nodes: a prospective study, *J. Laryng. Otol.*, 105, 558, 1991.

103. Pithie, A. D., Chicksen, B., Fine-needle extrathoracic lymph node aspiration in HIV-associated sputum-negative tuberculosis, *Lancet*, 340, 1504, 1992.

104. Ganz, W. I., Serafini, A. N., The diagnostic role of nuclear medicine in the acquired immunodeficiency syndrome, *J. Nucl. Med.*, 30, 193, 1989.

105. Radin, D. R., Intraabdominal *Mycobacterium tuberculosis* versus Mycobacterium avium-intracellulare infections in patients with AIDS: distinction based on CT findings, *Am. J. Roentgen.*, 156, 487, 1991.

106. Skarzynski, J. J., Sherman, W., Lee, H. K., Berger, H., Patchy uptake of gallium in the lungs of AIDS patients with atypical mycobacterial infection, *Clin. Nucl. Med.*, 12, 7, 1987.

107. Shiota, Y., Kitade, M., Ueda, N., Furuya, K., Tuberculous mediastinal lymphadenitis in an adult patient, *Jpn. J. Med.*, 28, 382, 1989.

108. Anonymous, Six-months versus nine-months chemotherapy for tuberculosis of lymph nodes: preliminary results, *Resp. Med.*, 86, 15, 1992.

109. Campbell, I. A., The treatment of superficial tuberculous lymphadenitis, [leading article], *Tubercle*, 71, 1, 1990.

110. Cheung, W. L., Siu, K. F., Ng, A., Six-month combination chemotherapy for cervical tuberculous lymphadenitis, *J. R. Coll. Edinb.*, 35, 293, 1990.

111. Illes, P. B., Emerson, P. A., Tuberculous lymphadenitis, *Br. Med. J.*, 1, 143, 1974.

112. Silver, C. P., Steel, S. J., Mediastinal lymphatic gland tuberculosis in Asian and coloured immigrants, *Lancet*, 1, 124, 1961.

113. Dhand, S., Fisher, M., Fewell, J. W., Intrathoracic tuberculous lymphadenopathy in adults, *J. Am. Med. Assoc.*, 241, 505, 1979.

114. Liu, C., Fields, W. R., Shaw, C., Tuberculous mediastinal lymphadenopathy in adults, *Radiology*, 126, 369, 1978.

115. Im, J. G., Song, K. S., Kang, H. S., Park, J. H., Yeon, K. M., Han, M. C., Kim, C. W., Mediastinal tuberculous lymphadenitis: CT manifestations, *Radiology*, 164, 11, 1987.

116. Hill, A. R., Premkur, S., Brustein, S., Vaidya, K., Powell, S., Li, P., Suster, B., Disseminated tuberculosis in the acquired immunodeficiency syndrome era, *Am. Rev. Resp. Dis.*, 144, 1164, 1991.

117. Kramer, F., Modilevsky, T., Waliany, A. R., Leedom, J. M., Barnes, P. F., Delayed diagnosis of tuberculosis in patients with human immunodeficiency virus infection, *Am. J. Med.*, 89, 451, 1990.

118. Wasser, L. S., Shaw, G. W., Talavera, W., Endobronchial tuberculosis in the acquired immunodeficiency syndrome, *Chest*, 94, 1240, 1988.

119. Chang, S. C., Lee, P. Y., Perng, R. P., Clinical role of bronchoscopy in adults with intrathoracic tuberculous lymphadenopathy, *Chest*, 93, 314, 1988.

120. American Thoracic Society, Treatment of tuberculosis and tuberculosis infection in adults and children, *Am. Rev. Resp. Dis.*, 134, 355, 1986.

121. Gorse, G. J., Pais, M. J., Kusske, J. A., Cesario, T. C., Tuberculous spondylitis, *Medicine*, 62, 178, 1983.

122. Davidson, P. T., Horowitz, I., Skeletal tuberculosis: review with patient presentation and discussion, *Am. J. Med.*, 48, 77, 1970.

123. Parsons, M., *Tuberculous Meningitis*, Oxford University Press, Oxford, 1988.

124. Thijn, C. J. P., Steensma, J. T., *Tuberculosis of the Skeleton*, 1st ed., Springer, New York, 1990.

125. Lifeso, R. M., Weaver, P., Harder, E. H., Tuberculous spondylitis in adults, *J. Bone Joint Surg.*, 67A, 1405, 1985.

126. Frankel, D. G., Daffner, R. H., Wang, S. E., Case report 64, *Skeletal Radiol.*, 20, 130, 1991.

127. Gros, T., Soriano, V., Gabarre, E., Tor, J., Sabria, M., Multifocal tubercular osteitis in a female patient infected with the human immunodeficiency virus [Spanish], *Rev. Clin. Esp.*, 191, 3, 1992.

128. Walker, G. F., Failure of early recognition of skeletal tuberculosis, *Br. Med. J.*, 1, 682, 1968.

129. Omari, B., Robertson, J. M., Nelson, R. J., Chiu, L. C., Pott's disease: a resurgent challenge to the thoracic surgeon, *Chest*, 95, 145, 1989.

130. Sharif, H. S., Clark, D. C., Aabed, M. Y., Haddad, M. C., Al Deeb, S. M., Yaqub, B., Al Moutaery, K. R., Granulomatous spinal infections: MR imaging, *Radiology*, 177, 101, 1990.

131. Babhulkar, S. S., Tayade, W. B., Babhulkar, S. K., Atypical spinal tuberculosis, *J. Bone Joint Surg.*, 66, 239, 1984.

132. Sarkar, S. D., Ravikrishnan, K. P., Woodbury, D. H., Carson, J. J., Daley, K., Gallium-67 citrate scanning — a new adjunct in the direction and follow-up of extrapulmonary tuberculosis: concise communication, *J. Nucl. Med.*, 20, 833, 1979.

133. Silverman, J. F., Larkin, E. W., Carney, M., Weaver, M. D., Norris, H. T., Fine needle aspiration cytology of tuberculosis of the lumbar vertebrae (Pott's disease), *Acta Cytol.*, 30, 538, 1986.

134. Griffiths, D. L., Tuberculosis of the spine: a review, *Adv. Tuberc. Res.*, 20, 93, 1980.

135. Medical Section of the American Lung Association, Treatment of tuberculosis and tuberculosis infection in adults and children (joint statement of the American Thoracic Society and the Centers for Disease Control), *Am. Rev. Resp. Dis.*, 134, 355, 1986.

136. Jensen, C. M., Jensen, C. H., Paerregaard, A., A diagnostic problem in tuberculous dactylitis, *J. Hand Surg.*, 16(2), 202, 1991.

137. Rigauts, H., Van Holsbeeck, M., Lechat, A., Spina ventosa: the forgotten diagnosis. Report of one case, review of the literature, *J. Belg. Rad.*, 72, 13, 1989.

138. Berney, S., Goldstein, M., Bishko, F., Clinical and diagnostic features of tuberculous arthritis, *Am. J. Med.*, 53, 36, 1972.

139. Poncet, M. A., Rhumatisme tuberculeux ou pseudo-rhumatisme d'origine bacillaire, *Bull. Acad. Natl. Med.*, 46, 194, 1901; Poncet, M. A., De la polyarthrite tuberculeuse, deformante ou pseudorheumatisme chronic tuberculeux, *Cong. Franc. Chir.*, 1, 732, 1897.

140. Pandy, D., Dubey, A. P., Choudhury, P., Poncet's disease, *Indian Pediatr.*, 26, 828, 1989.

141. Isaacs, A. J., Sturrock, R. D., Poncet's disease — fact or fiction?, *Tubercle*, 55, 135, 1974.

142. Dall, L., Long, L., Stanford, J., Poncet's disease: tuberculous rheumatism, *Rev. Infect. Dis.*, 11, 105, 1989.

143. Weinstein, A. J., Genitourinary tuberculosis, in *Tuberculosis*, Schlossberg, D., Ed., Springer-Verlag, New York, 1988, 108.

144. Cinman, A. C., Genitourinary tuberculosis, *Urology*, 20, 353, 1982.

145. Christensen, W. I., Genitourinary tuberculosis: review of 102 cases, *Medicine*, 53, 377, 1974.

146. Shafer, R. W., Goldberg, R., Sierra, M., Glatt, A. E., Frequency of mycobacterium tuberculosis bacteremia in patients with tuberculosis in an area endemic for AIDS, *Am. Rev. Resp. Dis.*, 140, 1611, 1989.

147. Barber, T. W., Craven, D. E., McCabe, W. R., Bacteremia due to mycobacterium tuberculosis in patients with human immunodeficiency virus infection: a report of 9 cases and a review of the literature, *Medicine*, 69, 375, 1990.

148. Simon, H. B., Weinstein, A. J., Pasternak, M. S., Swartz, M. N., Kunz, L. J., Genitourinary tuberculosis: clinical features in a general hospital population, *Am. J. Med.*, 63, 410, 1977.

149. Shariff, S., Thomas, J. A., Fine needle aspiration cytodiagnosis of clinically suspected tuberculosis in tissue enlargement, *Acta Cytol.*, 35, 333, 1991.

150. Kollins, S. A., Hartman, G. W., Carr, D. T., Segura, J. W., Hattery, R. R., Roentgenographic findings in urinary tract tuberculosis: a 10 year review, *Am. J. Roentgenol.*, 121, 487, 1974.

151. Das, K. M., Indudhara, R., Vaidyanathan., Sonographic features of genitourinary tuberculosis, *Am. J. Roentgenol.*, 18, 327, 1992.

152. Gow, J. G., Genitourinary tuberculosis: a 7-year review, *Br. J. Med.*, 51, 239, 1979.

153. Gow, J. G., Barbosa, S., Genitourinary tuberculosis: a study of 1117 cases over a period of 34 years, *Br. J. Urol.*, 56, 449, 1984.

154. Weinberg, A. C., Boyd, S. D., Short-course chemotherapy and role of surgery in adult and pediatric genitourinary tuberculosis, *Urology*, 31, 95, 1988.

155. Ehrlich, R. M., Lattimer, J. K., Genitourinary tuberculosis, *Surg. Ann.*, 6, 439, 1974.

156. Gorse, G. J., Belshe, R. B., Male genital tuberculosis: a review of the literature with instructive case reports, *Rev. Infect. Dis.*, 7, 511, 1985.

157. Medlar, E. M., Spain, D. M., Holliday, R. W., Post-mortem compared with clinical diagnosis of genito-urinary tuberculosis in adult males, *J. Urol.*, 61, 1079, 1949.

158. Wechsler, H., Westfall, M., Lattimer, J. K., The earliest signs and symptoms in 127 male patients with genitourinary tuberculosis, *J. Urol.*, 83, 801, 1960.

159. Chung, T., Harris, R. D., Tuberculous epididymo-orchitis: sonographic findings, *J. Clin. Ultrasound*, 19, 367, 1991.

160. Davids, A. M., Genital tuberculosis in females, *J. Mt. Sinai Hosp. New York*, 23, 567, 1956.

161. Marana, R., Muzii, L., Lucisano, A., Ardito, F., Muscatello, P., Bilancioni, E., Maniccia, E., Dell'Acqua, S., Incidence of genital tuberculosis in infertile patients submitted to diagnostic laparoscopy: recent experience in an Italian university hospital, *Int. J. Fertil.*, 36, 104, 1991.

162. Rao, K. N., Viswanathan, R., Deshmukh, M. D., Pamra, S. P., Sen, P. K., Bordia, N. L., Dingley, H. B., Eds., *Textbook of Tuberculosis*, 2nd ed., Vikas Publishing, New Delhi, 1981.

163. Margolis, K., Wranz, P. A. B., Kruger, T. F., Joubert, J. J., Odendaal, H. J., Genital tuberculosis at Tyberberg hospital — prevalence, clinical presentation and diagnosis, *S. Afr. Med. J.*, 81, 12, 1992.

164. Sutherland, A. M., Drug treatment of tuberculosis of the female genital tract, *J. Obstet. Gynecol.*, 6, 51, 1985.

165. Menitove, S., Harris, H. W., Miliary tuberculosis, in *Tuberculosis*, Schlossberg, D., Ed., Springer-Verlag, New York, 1988, 179.

166. Slavin, R. E., Walsh, T. J., Pollack, A. D., Late generalized tuberculosis: a clinical pathologic analysis and comparison of 100 cases in the preantibiotic and antibiotic eras, *Medicine*, 59, 352, 1980.

167. Kaplan, M. H., Armstrong, D., Rosen, P., Tuberculosis complicating neoplastic disease: a review of 201 cases, *Cancer*, 33, 850, 1974.

168. Pradhan, R. P., Katz, L. A., Nidus, B. D., Matalon, R., Eisinger, R. P., Tuberculosis in dialyzed patients, *J. Am. Med. Assoc.*, 229, 798, 1974.

169. Ballon, S. C., Clewell, W. H., Lamb, E. J., Reactivation of silent pelvic tuberculosis by reconstructive tubal surgery, *Am. J. Obstet. Gynecol.*, 122, 991, 1975.

170. Yekanath, H., Gross, P. A., Vitenson, J. H., Miliary tuberculosis following ureteral catheterization, *Urology*, 16, 197, 1980.

171. Federmann, M., Kley, H. K., Miliary tuberculosis after extracorporeal shock-wave lithotripsy, *N. Engl. J. Med.*, 323, 1210, 1990.

172. Yamane, H., Fujiwara, T., Doko, S., Inada, H., Nogami, A., Masaki, H., Kanazawa, S., Hara, T., Kondo, J., Yoshida, H., Two cases of miliary tuberculosis following prosthetic valve replacement [Japanese], *Kokyu Junkan — Resp. Circ.*, 37, 803, 1989.

173. Maartens, G., Willcox, P. A., Benatar, S. R., Miliary tuberculosis: rapid diagnosis, hematologic abnormalities, and outcome in 109 treated adults, *Am. J. Med.*, 89, 291, 1990.

174. Kim, J. H., Langston, A. A., Gallis, H. A., Miliary tuberculosis: epidemiology, clinical manifestations, diagnosis, and outcome, *Rev. Infect. Dis.*, 12, 583, 1990.

175. Dyer, R. A., Chappel, W. A., Potgieter, P. D., Adult respiratory distress syndrome associated with miliary tuberculosis, *Crit. Care Med.*, 13, 12, 1985.

176. Heffner, J. E., Strange, C., Sahn, S. A., The impact of respiratory failure on the diagnosis of tuberculosis, *Arch. Intern. Med.*, 148, 1103, 1988.

177. Gee, W. M., The frequency of unsuspected tuberculosis found post-mortem in a geriatric population, *Z. Gerontol.*, 22, 311, 1989.

178. Rossi, S., Reale, D., Grandi, E., Rilievo di patologia tuberculare in una casistica autoptica. Correlazione tra diagnosi clinica e anatomopatologica, *Pathologica*, 80, 449, 1988.

179. Cameron, S. J., Tuberculosis and the blood — a special relationship?, *Tubercle*, 55, 55, 1974.

180. Munt, P. W., Miliary tuberculosis in the chemotherapy era: with a clinical review in 69 American adults, *Medicine*, 51, 139, 1971.

181. Proudfoot, A. T., Akhtar, A. J., Douglas, A. C., Horne, N. W., Miliary tuberculosis in adults, *Br. Med. J.*, 2, 273, 1969.

182. Yu, Y. L., Chow, W. H., Humphries, M. J., Wong, R. W. S., Gabriel, M., Cryptic miliary tuberculosis, *Q. J. Med.*, 228, 421, 1986.

183. O'Brien, J. R., Non-reactive tuberculosis, *J. Clin. Pathol.*, 7, 216, 1954.

184. Gelb, A. F., Leffler, C., Brewin, A., Mascatello, V., Lyons, H. A., Miliary tuberculosis, *Am. Rev. Resp. Dis.*, 108, 1327, 1973.

185. Prout, S., Benatar, S. R., Disseminated tuberculosis: a study of 62 cases, *S. Afr. Med. J.*, 58, 835, 1980.

186. Sahn, S. A., Neff, T. A., Miliary tuberculosis, *Am. J. Med.*, 56, 495, 1974.

187. Williams, N. H., Jr., Kane, C., Yoo, O. H., Pulmonary function in miliary tuberculosis, *Am. Rev. Resp. Dis.*, 107, 858, 1973.

188. Massaro, D., Katz, S., Sachs, M., Choroidal tubercles, *Ann. Intern. Med.*, 60, 231, 1964.

189. Bobrowitz, I. D., Active tuberculosis undiagnosed until autopsy, *Am. J. Med.*, 72, 650, 1982.

190. Saltzman, B. R., Motyl, M. R., Friedland, G. H., McKitrick, J. C., Klein, R. S., Mycobacterium tuberculosis bacteremia in the acquired immunodeficiency syndrome, *J. Am. Med. Assoc.*, 256, 390, 1986.

191. Gachot, B., Wolff, M., Clair, B., Regnier, B., Severe tuberculosis in patients with human immunodeficiency virus infection, *Int. Care Med.*, 16, 491, 1990.

192. McGuinness, G., Naidich, D. P., Jagirdar, J., Leitman, B., McCauley, D. I., High resolution CT findings in miliary lung disease, *J. Comp. Assoc. Tomo.*, 16, 384, 1992.

193. Wasser, L. S., Brown, E., Talavera, W., Miliary PCP in AIDS, *Chest*, 96, 693, 1989.

194. Grieff, M., Lisbona, R., Detection of miliary tuberculosis by Ga-67 scintigraphy, *Clin. Nucl. Med.*, 16, 910, 1991.

195. Willcox, P. A., Potgieter, P. D., Bateman, E. D., Benatar, S. R., Rapid diagnosis of sputum negative miliary tuberculosis using the flexible fibreoptic bronchoscope, *Thorax*, 41, 681, 1986.

196. Pant, K., Chawla, R., Mann, P. S., Jaggi, O. P., Fiberbronchoscopy in smear-negative miliary tuberculosis, *Chest*, 95, 1151, 1989.

197. Cucin, R. L., Coleman, M., Eckhardt, J. J., Silver, R. T., The diagnosis of miliary tuberculosis: utility of peripheral blood abnormalities, bone marrow and liver needle biopsy, *J. Chronic Dis.*, 26, 355, 1973.

198. Heinle, E. W., Jensen, W. N., Westerman, M. P., Diagnostic usefulness of marrow biopsy in disseminated tuberculosis, *Am. Rev. Resp. Dis.*, 91, 701, 1965.

199. Uribe-Botero, G., Prichard, J. G., Kaplowitz, H. J., Bone marrow in HIV infection, *Am. J. Clin. Pathol.*, 91, 313, 1989.

200. Nichols, J., Florentine, B., Lewis, W., Sattler, F., Rarick, M. U., Brynes, R. K., Bone marrow examination for the diagnosis of mycobacterial and fungal infections in the acquired immunodeficiency syndrome, *Arch. Pathol. Lab. Med.*, 115, 1125, 1991.

201. Bentz, R. R., Dimcheff, D. G., Nemiroff, M. J., Tsang, A., Weg, J. G., The incidence of urine cultures positive for MTB in a general tuberculosis patient population, *Am. Rev. Resp. Dis.*, 111, 647, 1975.

202. Kissner, D. G., Missed opportunities, *Arch. Intern. Med.*, 147, 2037, 1987.

203. Counsell, S. R., Tan, J. S., Dittus, R. S., Unsuspected pulmonary tuberculosis in a community teaching hospital, *Arch. Intern. Med.*, 149, 1274, 1989.

204. Huseby, J. S., Hudson, L. D., Miliary tuberculosis and adult respiratory distress sndrome, *Ann. Intern. Med.*, 85, 609, 1976.

205. Murray, H. W., Tuazon, C. U., Kirmani, N., Sheagren, J. N., The adult respiratory distress syndrome associated with miliary tuberculosis, *Chest*, 73, 37, 1978.

206. Knowles, K. F., Saltman, D., Robson, H. G., Lalonde, R., Tuberculous pancreatitis, *Tubercle*, 71, 65, 1990.

207. Piqueras, A. R., Marruecos, L., Artigas, A., Rodriguez, C., Miliary tuberculosis and adult respiratory distress syndrome, *Int. Care Med.*, 13, 175, 1987.

208. Ahuja, S. S., Ahuja, S. K., Phelps, K. R., Thelmo, W., Hill, A. R., Hemodynamic confirmation of septic shock in disseminated tuberculosis, *Crit. Care Med.*, 20, 901, 1992.

209. Tandon, P. N., Tuberculous meningitis (cranial and spinal), in *Handbook of Clinical Neurology: Infections of the Nervous System*, Vinken, P. J., Bruyn, G. W., Klawans, H. L., Eds., North Holland, Amsterdam, 1978, 195.

210. Auerbach, O., Tuberculous meningitis: correlation of therapeutic results with the pathogenesis and pathologic changes, *Am. Rev. Tuberc.*, 64, 408, 1951.

211. Riggs, H. E., Rupp, C., Ray, H., Clinicopathologic study of tuberculous meningitis in adults, *Am. Rev. Tuberc.*, 74, 830, 1956.

212. Hinman, A. R., Tuberculous meningitis at Cleveland Metropolitan General Hospital 1959–1963, *Am. Rev. Resp. Dis.*, 95, 670, 1967.

213. Ogawa, S. K., Smith, M. A., Brennessel, D. J., Lowy, F. D., Tuberculous meningitis in an urban medical center, *Medicine*, 66, 317, 1987.

214. Bishburg, E., Sunderam, G., Reichman, L. B., Kapila, R., Central nervous system tuberculosis with the acquired immunodeficiency syndrome and its related complex, *Ann. Intern. Med.*, 105, 210, 1986.

215. Kasik, J. E., Central nervous system tuberculosis, in *Tuberculosis*, Schlossberg, D., Ed., Springer-Verlag, New York, 1988, 87.

216. Molavi, A., LeFrock, J. L., Tuberculous meningitis, *Med. Clin. N. Am.*, 69, 315, 1985.

217. Berenguer, J., Moreno, S., Laguna, F., Vicente, T., Adrados, M., Ortega, A., González-LaHoz, J., Bouza, E., Tuberculous meningitis in patients infected with the human immunodeficiency virus, *N. Engl. J. Med.*, 326, 668, 1992.

218. Humphries, M., The management of tuberculous meningitis [editorial], *Thorax*, 47, 577, 1992.

219. Haas, E. J., Madhavan, T., Quinn, E. L., Cox, F., Fisher, E., Burch, K., Tuberculous meningitis in an urban general hospital, *Arch. Intern. Med.*, 137, 1518, 1977.

220. Rooney, J. J., Jr., Crocco, J. A., Kramer, S., Lyons, H. A., Further observations on tuberculin reactions in active tuberculosis, *Am. J. Med.*, 60, 517, 1976.

221. Klein, N. C., Damsker, B., Hirschman, S. Z., Mycobacterial meningitis: retrospective analysis from 1970 to 1983, *Am. J. Med.*, 79, 29, 1985.

222. Offenbacher, H., Fazekas, F., Schmidt, R., Kleinert, R., Payer, F., Kleinert, G., Lechner, H., MRI in tuberculous meningoencephalitis: Report of four cases and review of the neuroimaging literature, *J. Neurol.*, 238, 340, 1991.

223. Whitener, D. R., Tuberculous brain abscess, *Arch. Neurol.*, 35, 148, 1978.

224. Jinkins, J. R., Computed tomography of intracranial tuberculosis, *Neuroradiology,* 33, 126, 1991.

225. Lees, A. J., Marshall, J., MacLeod, A. F., Cerebral tuberculomas developing during treatment of tuberculous meningitis, *Lancet*, 2, 1208, 1970.

226. van Bommel, E. F., Stiegelis, W. F., Schermers, H. P., Paradoxical response of intracranial tuberculomas during chemotherapy: an immunologic phenomenon?, *Neth. J. Med.*, 38, 126, 1991.

227. Kennedy, D. H., Fallon, R. J., Tuberculous meningitis, *J. Am. Med. Assoc.*, 241, 264, 1979.

228. Illingworth, R. S., Miliary and meningeal tuberculosis: difficulties in diagnosis, *Lancet*, 271, 646, 1956.

229. Stewart, S. M., Technical methods: the bacteriological diagnosis of tuberculous meningitis, *J. Clin. Pathol.*, 6, 241, 1953.

230. Leonard, J. M., Des Prez, R. M., Tuberculous meningitis, *Infect. Dis. Clin. N. Am.*, 4, 769, 1990.

231. Chawla, R. K., Seth, R. K., Raj, B., Saini, A. S., Adenosine deaminase levels in cerebrospinal fluid in tuberculosis and bacterial meningitis, *Tubercle*, 72, 190, 1991.

232. Daniel, T. M., New approaches to the rapid diagnosis of tuberculous meningitis, *J. Infect. Dis.*, 155, 599, 1987.

233. Kadival, G. V., Mazarelo, T. B. M. S., Chaparas, S. D., Sensitivity and specificity of enzyme-linked immunosorbent assay in the detection of antigen in tuberculous meningitis cerebrospinal fluids, *J. Clin. Microbiol.*, 23, 901, 1986.

234. Kadival, G. V., Samuel, A. M., Mazarelo, T. B. M. S., Chaparas, S. D., Radioimmunoassay for detection of *Mycobacterium tuberculosis* antigen in cerebrospinal fluids of patients with tuberculous meningitis, *J. Infect. Dis.*, 155, 608, 1987.

235. Cocito, C. G., Properties of the mycobacterial antigen complex A60 and its applications to the diagnosis and prognosis of tuberculosis, *Chest*, 100, 1687, 1991.

236. Daniel, T. M., The rapid diagnosis of tuberculosis: a selective review, *J. Lab. Clin. Med.*, 116, 277, 1990.

237. Tang, L. M., Serial lactate determinations in tuberculous meningitis, *Scand. J. Infect. Dis.*, 20, 81, 1988.

238. Shankar, P., Manjunath, N., Mohan, K. K., Prasad, K., Behari, M., Shriniwas, Ahuja, G. K., Rapid diagnosis of tuberculous meningitis by polymerase chain reaction, *Lancet*, 337, 5, 1991.

239. Cameron, D., Ansari, B. M., Boyce, J. M. H., Rapid diagnosis of tuberculous meningitis, *J. Infect.*, 24, 334, 1992.

240. Bouchama, A., Al-Kawi, M. Z., Kanaan, I., Coates, R., Jallu, A., Rahm, B., Siqueira, E. B., Brain biopsy in tuberculoma: the risks and benefits, *Neurosurgery*, 28, 405, 1991.

240a. Ellard, G. A., Humphries, M. J., Allen, B. W., Cerebrospinal fluid drug concentrations and the treatment of tuberculous meningitis, *Am. Rev. Respir. Dis.,* 148, 650, 1993.

241. Bobrowitz, I. D., Ethambutol in tuberculous meningitis, *Chest*, 61, 629, 1972.

242. Alegre, J., Fernández de Sevilla, T., Falcó, V., Martinez Vazquez, J. M., Ofloxacin in miliary tuberculosis, *Eur. Resp. J.*, 3, 238, 1990.

243. Parenti, F., New experimental drugs for the treatment of tuberculosis, *Rev. Infect. Dis.,* 11(Suppl.), S479, 1989.

244. Goel, A., Pandya, S. K., Satoskar, A. R., Whither short-course chemotherapy for tuberculous meningitis?, *Neurosurgery*, 27, 418, 1990.

245. Palur, R., Rashekhar, V., Chandy, M. J., Joseph, T., Abraham, J., Shunt surgery for hydrocephalus in tuberculous meningitis: a long-term follow-up study, *J. Neurosurg.*, 74, 64, 1991.

246. Gourie-Devi, M., Satish, P., Hyaluronidase as an adjuvant in the treatment of cranial arachnoiditis complicating meningitis, *Acta Neurol. Scand.*, 62, 368, 1980.

247. Navarro, I. M., Peralta, V. H. R., Leon, J. A. M., Varela, E. A. S., Cabrera, J. M. S., Tuberculous optochiasmatic arachnoiditis, *Neurosurgery*, 9, 654, 1981.

248. Chambers, S. T., Hendrickse, W. A., Record, C., Rudge, P., Smith, H., Paradoxical expansion of intracranial tuberculomas during chemotherapy, *Lancet*, 2, 181, 1984.

249. Naidoo, D. P., Desai, D., Kranidiotis, L., Tuberculous meningomyeloradiculitis — a report of two cases, *Tubercle*, 72, 65, 1991.

250. Marcus, R., Coulston, A. M., Water-soluble vitamins, in *The Pharmacological Basis of Therapeutics*, Gilman, A. G., Rall, T. W., Nies, A. S., Taylor, E., Eds., W. B. Saunders, Philadelphia, 1992, 1539.

251. Albert, D. M., Dehm, E. J., Ocular tuberculosis, in *Tuberculosis*, Schlossberg, D., Ed., Springer-Verlag, New York, 1988, 81.

252. Rosen, P. H., Spalton, D. J., Graham, E. M., Intraocular tuberculosis, *Eye*, 4, 486, 1990.

253. Duke-Elder, S., Summary of systemic ophthalmology, in *System of Ophthalmology*, Vol. 15, Duke-Elder, S., Ed., C. V. Mosby, St. Louis, 1976, 160.

254. Philip, R. N., Comstock, G. W., Phlyctenular keratoconjunctivitis among Eskimos in southwestern Alaska. I. Epidemiologic characteristics, *Am. Rev. Resp. Dis.*, 91, 171, 1965.

255. Philip, R. N., Comstock, G. W., Phlyctenular keratoconjunctivitis among Eskimos in southwestern Alaska. II. Isoniazid prophylaxis, *Am. Rev. Resp. Dis.*, 91, 188, 1965.

256. Friedlaender, M. H., *Allergy and Immunology of the Eye,* Raven Press, New York, 1993, 139.

257. Fountain, J. A., Werner, R. B., Tuberculous retinal vasculitis, *Retina*, 4, 48, 1984.

258. Eales, H., Cases of retinal haemorrhage associated with epistaxis and constipation, *Birmingham Med. Rev.,* 9, 262, 1880.

259. Gur, S., Silverstone, B. Z., Sylberman, R., Berson, D., Chorioretinitis and extrapulmonary tuberculosis, *Ann. Opthalmol.*, 19, 112, 1987.

260. Magargal, L. E., Walsh, A. W., Magargal, H. O., Robb-Doyle, E., Treatment of Eales' disease with scatter laser photocoagulation, *Ann. Ophthalmol.*, 21, 300, 1989.

261. Skolnik, P. R., Nadol, J. B., Baker, A. S., Tuberculosis of the middle ear: review of the literature with an instructive case report, *Rev. Infect. Dis.*, 8, 403, 1986.

262. Vomero, E., Ratner, S. J., Diagnosis of miliary tuberculosis by examination of middle ear discharge, *Arch. Otolaryng. Head Neck Surg.*, 114, 1029, 1988.

263. Pankey, G. A., Otologic tuberculosis, in *Tuberculosis*, Schlossberg, D., Ed., Springer-Verlag, New York, 1988, 77.

264. Israel, H. L., Tuberculous peritonitis, in *Tuberculosis*, Schlossberg, D., Ed., Springer-Verlag, New York, 1988, 143.

265. Jakubowski, A., Elwood, R. K., Enarson, D. A., Clinical features of abdominal tuberculosis, *J. Infect. Dis.*, 158, 687, 1988.

266. Fitzgerald, J. M., Menzies, R. I., Elwood, R. K., Abdominal tuberculosis: a critical review, *Dig. Dis.*, 9, 269, 1991.

267. Cheng, I. K., Chan, P. C., Chan, M. K., Tuberculous peritonitis complicating long-term peritoneal dialysis: report of 3 cases and review of the literature, *Am. J. Nephrol.*, 9, 155, 1989.

268. Singh, M. M., Bhargave, A. N., Jain, K. P., Tuberculous peritonitis: an evaluation of pathogenetic mechanisms, diagnostic procedures and therapeutic measures, *N. Engl. J. Med.*, 281, 1091, 1969.

269. Sochocky, S., Tuberculous peritonitis: a review of 100 cases, *Am. Rev. Resp. Dis.*, 95, 398, 1967.

270. Pettengell, K. E., Larsen, C., Garb, M., Mayet, F. G. H., Simjee, A. E., Pirie, D., Gastrointestinal tuberculosis in patients with pulmonary tuberculosis, *Q. J. Med.*, 74, 303, 1990.

271. Bastani, B., Shariatzadeh, M. R., Dehdashti, F., Tuberculous peritonitis — report of 30 cases and review of the literature, *Q. J. Med.*, 56, 549, 1985.

272. Sherman, S., Rohwedder, J. J., Ravikrishman, K. P., Weg, J. G., Tuberculous enteritis and peritonitis: report of 36 general hospital cases, *Arch. Intern. Med.*, 140, 506, 1980.

273. Karney, W. W., O'Donoghue, J. M., Ostrow, J. H., Holmes, K. K., Beaty, H. N., The spectrum of tuberculous peritonitis, *Chest*, 72, 310, 1977.

274. Lerer, S., Romano, T., Denmark, L., Gallium-67-citrate scanning in tuberculous peritonitis, *Am. J. Gastroenterol.*, 71, 264, 1979.

275. Hulnick, D. H., Megibow, A. J., Naidich, D. P., Hilton, S., Cho, K. C., Balthazar, E. J., Abdominal tuberculosis: CT evaluation, *Radiology*, 157, 199, 1985.

276. Wilkens, E. G., Tuberculous peritonitis: Diagnostic value of the ascitic/blood glucose ratio, *Tubercle*, 6, 47, 1984.

277. Voigt, M. D., Trey, C., Lombard, C., Kalvaria, I., Berman, P., Kirsch, R. E., Diagnostic value of ascites adenosine deaminase in tuberculous peritonitis, *Lancet*, 1, 71, 1989.

278. Thapa, B. R., Yachha, S. K., Mehta, S., Abdominal tuberculosis, *Ind. Ped.,* 28, 1093, 1991.

279. Geake, T. M. S., Spitaels, J. M., Moshal, M. G., Simjee, A. E., Peritoneoscopy in the diagnosis of tuberculous peritonitis, *Gastrointest. Endosc.*, 27, 66, 1981.

280. Bhansali, S. K., Abdominal tuberculosis: experience with 300 cases, *Am. J. Gastroenterol.*, 67, 324, 1977.

281. Paustian, F. F., Stahl, M. G., Tuberculosis enteritis, in *Tuberculosis*, Schlossberg, D., Ed., Springer-Verlag, New York, 1988, 139.

282. Eng, J., Sabanathan, S., Tuberculosis of the esophagus (4 cases), *Dig. Dis. Sci.*, 36, 536, 1991.

283. Allen, C. M., Craze, J., Grundy, A., Case report: tuberculous broncho-oesophageal fistula in the acquired immunodeficiency syndrome, *Clin. Rad.*, 43, 60, 1991.

284. Vijayraghavan, M., Arunabh, K., Sarda, A. K., Sharma, A. K., Chatterjee, T. K., Duodenal tuberculosis: a review of the clinicopathologic features and management of twelve cases, *Jpn. J. Surg.*, 20, 526, 1990.

285. Gupta, S. C., Gupta, A. K., Keswani, N. K., Singh, P. A., Tripathi, A. K., Krishna, V., Pathology of tropical appendicitis, *J. Clin. Pathol.*, 42, 1169, 1989.

286. Sen, P., Kapila, R., Salaki, J., Louria, D. B., The diagnostic enigma of extra-pulmonary tuberculosis, *J. Chron. Dis.*, 30, 321, 1977.

287. Gilinsky, N. H., Marks, I. N., Kottler, R. E., Price, S. K., Abdominal tuberculosis: a 10-year review, *S. Afr. Med. J.*, 84, 849, 1983.

288. Aston, N. O., de Costa, A. M., Abdominal tuberculosis, *Br. J. Clin. Pract.*, 44, 58, 1990.

289. Thoeni, R. F., Margulis, A. R., Gastrointestinal tuberculosis, *Sem. Roentgenol.*, 14, 283, 1979.

290. Balthazar, E. J., Gordon, R., Hulnick, D., Ileocoecal tuberculosis: CT and radiologic evaluation, *Am. J. Roentgenol.*, 154, 499, 1990.

291. Shah, S., Thomas, V., Mathan, M., Chacko, A., Chandy, G., Ramakrishna, B. S., Rolston, D. D. K., Colonoscopic study of 50 patients with colonic tuberculosis, *Gut*, 33, 347, 1992.

292. Kochhar, R., Rajwanshi, A., Goenka, M. K., Nijhawan, R., Sood, A., Nagi, B., Kochhar, S., Mehta, S. K., Colonoscopic fine needle aspiration cytology in the diagnosis of ileocecal tuberculosis, *Am. J. Gastroenterol.*, 86, 102, 1991.

293. Shah, P., Ramakantan, R., Role of vasculitis in the natural history of abdominal tuberculosis — evaluation by mesenteric angiography, *Ind. J. Gastroenterol.*, 10, 127, 1991.

294. Palmer, K. R., Patil, D. H., Basran, G. S., Riordan, J. F., Silk, D. B. A., Abdominal tuberculosis in urban Britain — a common disease, *Gut*, 26, 1296, 1985.

295. Goldman, M., The surgical management of abdominal tuberculosis, *Surg. Ann.*, 21, 363, 1989.

296. Bowry, S., Chan, C. H., Weiss, H., Katz, S., Zimmerman, H. J., Hepatic involvement in pulmonary tuberculosis: histologic and functional characteristics, *Am. Rev. Resp. Dis.*, 101, 941, 1970.

297. Weinberg, J. J., Cohen, P., Malhotra, R., Primary tuberculous abscess associated with the human immunodeficiency virus, *Tubercle*, 69, 145, 1988.

298. Harrington, P. T., Gutiérrez, J. J., Ramírez-Ronda, C. H., Quiñones-Soto, R., Bermúdez, R. H., Chaffey, J., Granulomatous hepatitis, *Rev. Inf. Dis.*, 4, 638, 1982.

299. Ratanarapee, S., Pausawasdi, A., Tuberculosis of the common bile duct [case report], *HPB Surg.*, 3, 205, 1991.

300. Lupatkin, H., Braeu, N., Flomenberg, P., Simberkoff, M. S., Tuberculous abscesses in patients with AIDS, *Clin. Infect. Dis.*, 14, 1040, 1992.

301. Rohwedder, J. J., Upper respiratory tract tuberculosis, in *Tuberculosis*, Schlossberg, D., Ed., Springer-Verlag, New York, 1988, 71.

302. Khalil, T., Uzoaru, I., Nadimpalli, V., Wurtz, R., Splenic tuberculous abscess in patients positive for HIV: report of two cases and review, *Clin. Infect. Dis.*, 14, 1265, 1992.

303. Wolff, M. J., Bitran, J., Northland, R. G., Levy, I. L., Splenic abscesses due to *M. tuberculosis* in patients with AIDS, *Rev. Infect. Dis.*, 13, 373, 1991.

304. Desai, D. C., Swaroop, V. S., Mohandas, K. M., Borges, A., Dhir, V., Nagral, A., Jagannath, P., Sharma, O. P., Tuberculosis of the pancreas: report of three cases, *Am. J. Gastroenterol.*, 86, 761, 1991.

305. Allen, J. R., Bauer, L. A., Evans, L., Watson, K., Primary pancreatic tuberculosis, *Miss Med.*, 88, 766, 1991.

306. Soriano, E., Mallolas, J., Gatell, J. M., Latorre, X., Miró, J. M., Pecchiar, M., Mensa, J., Trilla, J., Moreno, A., Characteristics of tuberculosis in HIV-infected patients. a case-control study, *AIDS*, 2, 429, 1988.

307. Crocco, J. A., Cardiovascular tuberculosis, in *Tuberculosis*, Schlossberg, D., Ed., Springer-Verlag, New York, 1988, 133.

308. Rose, A. G., Cardiac tuberculosis, *Arch. Pathol. Lab. Med.*, 111, 422, 1987.

309. Alvarez, S., McCabe, W. R., Extrapulmonary tuberculosis revisited: a review of experience at Boston City and other hospitals, *Medicine*, 63, 25, 1984.

310. Fowler, N. O., Tuberculous pericarditis, *J. Am. Med. Assoc.*, 266, 99, 1991.

311. Reynolds, M. M., Hecht, S. R, Berger, M., Kolokathis, A., Horowitz, S. F., Large pericardial effusions in the acquired immunodeficiency syndrome, *Chest*, 102, 1746, 1992.

312. Larrieu, A. J., Tyers, F. O., Williams, E. H., Derrick, J. R., Recent experience with tuberculous pericarditis, *Ann. Thorac. Surg.*, 29, 464, 1980.

313. Rooney, J. J., Crocco, J. A., Lyons, H. A., Tuberculous pericarditis, *Ann. Intern. Med.*, 72, 73, 1970.

314. Cegielski, J. P., Ramaiya, K., Lallinger, G. J., Mtulia, I. A., Mbaga, I. M., Pericardial disease and human immunodeficiency virus in Dar es Salaam, Tanzania, *Lancet*, 335, 209, 1990.

315. D'Cruz, I. A., Sengupta, E. E., Abrahams, C., Reddy, H. K., Turlapati, R. V., Cardiac involvement, including tuberculous pericardial effusion, complicating acquired immune deficiency syndrome, *Am. Heart J.*, 112, 1100, 1986.

316. de Miguel, J., Pedreira, J. D., Campos, V., Gomez, A. P., Porto, J. A. L., Tuberculous pericarditis and AIDS, *Chest*, 97, 1273, 1990.

317. Kinney, E. L., Monsuez, J. J., Kitzis, M., Vittecoq, D., Treatment of AIDS-associated heart disease, *Angiology*, 40, 970, 1989.

318. Guberman, B. A., Fowler, N. O., Engel, P. J., Gueron, M., Allen, J. M., Cardiac tamponade in medical patients, *Circulation*, 3, 633, 1981.

319. Desai, H. N., Tuberculous pericarditis, *S. Afr. Med. J.*, 55, 877, 1979.

320. Hageman, J. H., D'Esopo, N. D., Glenn, W. W. L., Tuberculosis of the pericardium, *N. Engl. J. Med.*, 270, 327, 1964.

321. Fowler, N. O., Manitsas, G. T., Infectious pericarditis, *Prog. Cardiovasc. Dis.*, 16, 323, 1973.

322. Strang, J. I. G., Gibson, D. J., Mitchison, D. A., Girling, D. J., Kakaza, H. H. S., Allen, B. W., Evans, D. J., Nunn, A. J., Controlled clinical trial of complete open surgical drainage and of prednisolone in treatment of tuberculous pericardial effusion in Transkei, *Lancet*, 2(8614), 759, 1988.

323. Quale, J. M., Lipschik, G. Y., Heurich, A. E., Management of tuberculous pericarditis, *Ann. Thorac. Surg.*, 43, 653, 1987.

324. Dalli, E., Quesada, A., Juan, G., Navarro, R., Payá, R., Tormo, V., Tuberculous pericarditis as the first manifestation of acquired immunodeficiency syndrome, *Am. Heart J.,* 114, 905, 1987.

325. Suchet, I. B., Horwitz, T. A., CT in tuberculous constrictive pericarditis, *J. Comp. Assoc. Tomogr.*, 16, 391, 1992.

326. Haase, D., Marrie, T. J., Martin, R., Hayne, O., Gallium scanning in tuberculous pericarditis, *Clin. Nucl. Med.*, 6, 275, 1981.

327. Schepers, G. W. H., Tuberculous pericarditis, *Am. J. Cardiol.*, 9, 248, 1962.

328. Sagristá-Sauleda, J., Permanyer-Miralda, G., Soler-Soler, J., Tuberculous pericarditis: ten year experience with a prospective protocol for diagnosis and treatment, *J. Am. Coll. Cardiol.*, 11, 724, 1988.

329. Telenti, M., Fdez, J., de Quiros, B., Susano, R., Moreno, T. A., Tuberculous pericarditis: diagnostic value of adenosine deaminase, *Presse Med. Paris*, 20, 637, 1991.

330. Bass, J. B., Farer, L. S., Hopewell, P. C., Jacobs, R. F., Treatment of tuberculosis and tuberculous infection in adults and children, *Am. Rev. Resp. Dis.*, 134, 355, 1986.

331. Strang, J. I. G., Gibson, D. G., Nunn, A. J., Kakaza, H. H. S., Girling, D. J., Fox, W., Controlled trial of prednisolone as adjuvant in treatment of tuberculous constrictive pericarditis in Transkei, *Lancet*, 2, 1418, 1987.

332. Gooi, H. C., Smith, J. M., Tuberculous pericarditis in Birmingham, *Thorax*, 33, 94, 1978.

333. Carson, T. J., Murray, G. F., Wilcox, B. R., Starek, P. J. K., The role of surgery in tuberculous pericarditis, *Ann. Thorac. Surg.*, 17, 163, 1974.

334. Kannangara, D. W., Salem, F. A., Rao, B. S., Thadepalli, H., Cardiac tuberculosis: tb of the endocardium, *Am. J. Med. Sci.*, 287, 45, 1984.

335. Halim, M. A., Mercer, E. N., Guinn, G. A., Myocardial tuberculoma with rupture and pseudoaneurysm formation — successful surgical treatment, *Br. Heart J.*, 54, 603, 1982.

336. Wallis, P. J. W., Branfoot, A. C., Emerson, P. A., Sudden death due to myocardial tuberculosis, *Thorax*, 39, 155, 1984.

337. O'Neill, P. G., Rokey, R., Greenberg, S., Pacifico, A., Resolution of ventricular tachycardia and endocardial tuberculoma following antituberculosis therapy, *Chest*, 100, 1467, 1991.

338. Abaskaron, M., Multiple pseudoaneurysms in a tuberculous patient, *South Med. J.*, 79, 1582, 1986.

339. Sandron, D., Patra, P., Lelann, P., Bouillard, S., Pioche, D., Tuberculous pseudo-aneurysm of the descending thoracic aorta, *Eur. Resp. J.*, 1, 565, 1988.

340. Felson, B., Akers, P. V., Hall, G. S., Schreiber, J. T., Greene, R. E., Pedrosa, C. S., Mycotic tuberculous aneurysm of the thoracic aorta, *J. Am. Med. Assoc.*, 237, 1104, 1977.

341. Catinella, F. P., Kittle, C. F., Tuberculous oesophagus with aortic aneurysm fistula, *Ann. Thorac. Surg.*, 45, 87, 1988.

342. Rupa, V., Bhanu, T. S., Laryngeal tuberculosis in the eighties — an Indian experience, *J. Laryngol. Otol.*, 103, 864, 1989.

343. Brodovsky, D. M., Laryngeal tuberculosis in an age of chemotherapy, *Can. J. Otol.*, 4, 168, 1977.

344. el-Hakim, I. E., Langdon, J. D., Unusual presentation of tuberculosis of the head and neck region, *Int. J. Oral Maxillofac. Surg.*, 18, 194, 1989.

345. Sehgal, V. N., Wagh, S. A., Cutaneous tuberculosis, *Int. J. Dermatol.*, 29, 237, 1990.

346. Beyt, B. E., Jr., Ortbals, D. W., Santa Cruz, D. J., Cutaneous mycobacteriosis: analysis of 34 cases, *Medicine*, 60, 95, 1981.

347. Beyt, B. E., Cutaneous tuberculosis, in *Tuberculosis*, Schlossberg, D., Ed., Springer-Verlag, New York, 1988, 171.

348. Minkowitz, S., Brandt, L. J., Rapp, Y., Radlauer, C. B., "Prosector's wart" (cutaneous tuberculosis) in a medical student, *Am. J. Clin. Pathol.*, 51, 260, 1969.

349. Michelson, H. E., Scrofuloderma gummosa (tuberculosis colliguativa), *Arch. Dermatol.*, 10, 565, 1924.

350. Forstrom, L., Carcinomatous changes in lupus vulgaris, *Ann. Clin. Res.*, 1, 213, 1969.

351. Rietbrok, R. C., Dahlmans, R. P. M., Smedts, F., Frantzen, P. J., Koopman, R. J. J., van der Meer, J. W. M., Tuberculosis cutis miliaris disseminata as a manifestation of miliary tuberculosis; literature review and report of a case of recurrent skin lesions, *Rev. Infect. Dis.*, 13, 265, 1991.

352. Rohatgi, P. K., Palazzolo, J. V., Saini, N., Acute miliary tuberculosis of the skin in acquired immunodeficiency syndrome, *J. Am. Acad. Dermatol.*, 26, 356, 1992.

353. Sharma, P. K., Babel, A. L., Yadav, S. S., Tuberculosis of breast (study of 7 cases), *J. Postgrad. Med.*, 37, 24, 1990.

354. Hutton, M. D., Nosocomial transmission of tuberculosis associated with a draining abscess, *J. Infect. Dis.*, 161, 286, 1990.

355. Zalla, M. J., Su, W. P. D., Fransway, A. F., Dermatologic manifestations of human immunodeficiency virus infection, *Mayo Clin. Proc.*, 67, 1096, 1992.

356. Frampton, M. W., An outbreak of tuberculosis among hospital personnel caring for a patient with a skin ulcer, *Ann. Intern. Med.*, 117, 312, 1992.

357. Sarma, G. R., Immanuel, C., Ramachandran, G., Krishnamurthy, P. V., Kumaraswani, V., Prabhakar, R., Adrenocortical function in patients with pulmonary tuberculosis, *Tubercle*, 71, 277, 1990.

358. Barnes, D. J., Naraqui, S., Temu, P., Turtle, J. R., Adrenal function in patients with active tuberculosis, *Thorax*, 44, 422, 1989.

359. Arnstein, A. R., Endocrine and metabolic aspects of tuberculosis, in *Tuberculosis*, Schlossberg, D., Ed., Springer-Verlag, New York, 1988, 191.

360. Vita, J. A., Silverberg, S. J., Goland, R. S., Austin, J. H. M., Knowlton, A. I., Clinical clues to the cause of Addison's disease, *Am. J. Med.*, 78, 461, 1985.

361. Des Prez, R. M., Mycobacterial infections, in *The Year Book of Medicine*, Rogers, D. E., Des Prez, R. M., Cline, M. J., Braunwald, E., Greenberger, N. J., Wilson, J. D., Epstein, F. H., Malawista, S. E., Eds., Year Book Medical, Chicago, 1986, 201.

362. Wilkins, E. G. L., Hnizdo, E., Cope, E., Addisonian crisis induced by treatment with rifampicin, *Tubercle*, 70, 69, 1989.

363. Orth, D. N., Kovacs, W. J., DeBold, C. R., The adrenal cortex, in *Williams Textbook of Endocrinology*, Wilson, J. D., Foster, D. W., Eds., W. B. Saunders, Philadelphia, 1992, 552.

364. Barnes, P., Weatherstone, R., Tuberculosis of the thyroid: two case reports, *Br. J. Dis. Chest.*, 73, 187, 1979.

365. Berger, S. A., Edberg, S. C., David, G., Infectious disease in the sella turcica, *Rev. Infect. Dis.*, 8, 747, 1986.

366. Shenoi, A., Deshpande, S. A., Marwaha, R. K., Diabetes insipidus and growth hormone deficiency following tubercular meningitis, *Ind. Ped.*, 27, 624, 1990.

367. Lam, K. S. L., Sham, M. M. K., Tam, S. C. F., Ng, M. M. T., Ma, H. G. T., Hypopituitarism after tuberculous meningitis in childhood, *Ann. Intern. Med.*, 118, 701, 1993.

Chapter 8

Tuberculosis in Childhood and Pregnancy

Jeffrey R. Starke, M.D.

CONTENTS

0-8493-4825-0/94/$0.00+$.50
© 1994 by CRC Press, Inc.

I. TUBERCULOSIS IN CHILDREN

A. INTRODUCTION

Tuberculosis remains a significant cause of morbidity and mortality for children throughout the world. In many developing countries, tuberculous infection and disease have remained commonplace among children. The incidence appears to be increasing in many countries also experiencing the epidemic of infection due to the human immunodeficiency virus (HIV).[1] In most industrialized countries, the incidence of childhood tuberculosis declined substantially between the 1920s and the 1980s, due in part to improved social conditions, the widespread use of antituberculosis drugs, and, perhaps, to the use of certain bacillus Calmette–Guérin (BCG) vaccines. Unfortunately, several industrialized countries are experiencing a resurgence in pediatric tuberculous infection and disease.[2,3]

Beyond the profound health consequences for the affected child due to tuberculosis, the occurrence of tuberculosis in children represents a sentinel health marker for ongoing transmission of tuberculosis in a community. Infected children also are a large portion of the pool from which future tuberculosis cases will arise. However, childhood tuberculosis has a limited influence on the immediate epidemiology of the disease because children rarely are a source of infection to others. Programs that target children for treatment of tuberculosis will have few short-term effects on disease rates but will have a profound impact on the long-term control of the disease.[4]

B. EPIDEMIOLOGY
1. Worldwide Tuberculous Disease

The worldwide scope of tuberculosis in children is difficult to assess because data are scarce and poorly organized. Reports of disease rates usually grossly underestimate the true incidence. The prevalence of tuberculous infection without disease in children is completely unknown in most areas of the world due to the lack of surveillance testing. In many areas of Africa and Asia, the annual new tuberculous infection rate for all ages is approximately 2%, which would yield an estimated 220 cases of tuberculosis per 100,000 population per year.[5] Approximately 15–20% of these cases occur in children younger than 15 years of age. In addition, between 10 and 20% of deaths caused by tuberculosis in the developing world occur among children. The World Health Organization recently has estimated that the developing world has 1.3 million cases of tuberculosis and 400,000 tuberculosis-related deaths annually among children younger than 15 years of age.[6] There is no indication that tuberculosis rates among

children in developing nations are declining; in several surveys it is clear that infection and disease rates are increasing, especially in areas where HIV infection is prevalent.[1]

2. Tuberculous Disease in the United States

Between 1953 and 1980 the number of cases of childhood tuberculosis in the United States declined by approximately 6% per year.[7] Case rates declined in a similar fashion, from 10 per 100,000 children less than 15 years of age in 1962 to 2.4 per 100,000 children in 1985. Between 1980 and 1987 the case rates remained relatively flat, but they began to increase steadily in 1988. In 1992, 1707 cases of tuberculosis were reported in children less than 15 years of age, a 39% increase over 1987 cases (Figure 8-1).

The source of tuberculous infection for children usually is an adult in the environment who has infectious pulmonary tuberculosis. Therefore, the risk of a child developing tuberculous infection or disease depends on the likelihood that he or she will come in contact with an adult at high risk for tuberculosis (Table 8-1). Determining the risk level for tuberculosis in a child can be difficult since it is dependent on determining the risk level of all the adults with whom a child has significant contact. Children with tuberculosis rarely, if ever, infect other children or adults.[8] In tuberculous children, tubercle bacilli are sparse in endobronchial secretions, and cough often is absent. When young children do cough they rarely produce sputum and they lack the tussive force of adults. Adolescents with reactivation forms of pulmonary tuberculosis may be infectious to others. Occasionally, transmission of *Mycobacterium tuberculosis* from a child may occur by direct contact with infected fluids and discharges such as urine or purulent sinus tract drainage. Fomites such as syringes, gastric lavage tubes, or bronchoscopes are rare sources of infection.[9]

Age and gender are important variables for tuberculosis among children. While there is no evidence that the likelihood of infection with *M. tuberculosis* is influenced by age or gender, both probably influence the risk of developing active disease in an infected child. Approximately 60% of the pediatric tuberculosis cases in the United States occur in children younger than 5 years of age, the group traditionally at highest risk for disease. The interval between ages 5 and 14 years often has been referred to as the "favored age" since usually these children have the lowest rates of tuberculous disease in any population. Age also affects the anatomic site of involvement of tuberculosis.[10,11] Younger children are more likely to develop meningeal, disseminated, or lymphatic tuberculosis, whereas

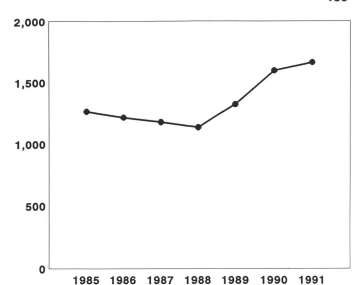

Figure 8-1 The annual number of cases of tuberculosis in children less than 15 years of age in the United States, 1985 to 1991.

Table 8-1 Adults at highest risk for tuberculosis in the United States

Persons with HIV coinfection
Foreign-born persons from high-prevalence
  countries
Current or former residents of correctional
  institutions
Homeless persons
Substance abusers
Socioeconomically disadvantaged persons,
  especially within cities
Healthcare workers in high-risk settings
Persons with immunosuppressive conditions
  or medications

Table 8-2 Major sites of extrapulmonary tuberculosis among children in the United States[a]

Sites	Percentage	Average Age (Years)
Lymphatic	67	5
Meningeal	13	3
Pleural	6	16
Miliary	5	1
Skeletal	4	5
Other	5	—
	100	

[a] Adapted from Smith, M. H. D., *Clin. Chest. Med.*, 10, 381, 1989 and Reider, H. L., Snider, D. E., Jr., Cauthen, G. M., *Am. Rev. Resp. Dis.*, 141, 347, 1990.

adolescents more frequently present with pleural, genitourinary, or peritoneal disease (Table 8-2). Among younger children, the gender ratio for tuberculous disease usually is approximately 1:1, but girls may have a slightly higher incidence of tuberculosis than boys during adolescence.

Historically, pediatric tuberculosis case rates in the United States have been the highest between January and June, possibly due to more extensive indoor contact with infectious adults during the colder months. The disease also is geographically focal with seven states — California, Florida, Georgia, Illinois, New York, New Jersey, and Texas — accounting for 72% of reported cases among children less than 5 years of age. As expected, disease rates are highest in cities with more than 250,000 residents.

Childhood tuberculosis case rates in the United States are strikingly higher among ethnic and racial minority groups and the foreign-born than among whites. Approximately 85% of cases occur among African-American, Hispanic, Asian, and Native American children, which probably reflects the

increased risk of transmission within the living conditions of these children.[7] Although most of these children were born in the United States, from 1986 to 1991, the proportion of foreign-born children with tuberculosis rose from 13 to 16% among children less than 5 years of age, and from 40 to 49% among adolescents aged 15 to 19 years.[2]

Most children with tuberculosis become infected with *M. tuberculosis* in their home, but outbreaks of childhood tuberculosis centered in elementary and high schools, nursery schools, family daycare homes, churches, school buses, and stores still occur.[12-14] In most cases, a high-risk adult working in the area has been the source of the outbreak. In certain environments, these outbreaks can be quite widespread; during a recent outbreak in a St. Louis, Missouri elementary school, almost 50% of the students in the school developed tuberculous infection and 11% had radiographic evidence of tuberculous disease after a teacher was found to have extensive pulmonary tuberculosis.

3. Human Immunodeficiency Virus-Related Tuberculosis

The recent epidemic of HIV infection has had a profound effect on the epidemiology of tuberculosis among children in the United States, by two major mechanisms:[1,15,16] (1) HIV-infected adults with tuberculosis may transmit *M. tuberculosis* to children, a portion of whom will develop tuberculous disease; and (2) children with HIV infection may be at increased risk of progressing from tuberculous infection to disease.

The infectiousness of HIV-infected adults with pulmonary tuberculosis depends mostly on the proportion who have acid-fast sputum smear-positive disease. Pulmonary involvement is common among HIV-infected adults with tuberculosis especially when the tuberculosis precedes other opportunistic infections.[17] Although many HIV-infected adults with pulmonary tuberculosis have a positive sputum smear, one study showed that they were slightly less likely to have a positive sputum smear than non-HIV-infected adults with pulmonary tuberculosis.[18] However, studies from Africa and New York City have suggested that HIV-seronegative and HIV-infected patients with smear-positive pulmonary tuberculosis infect similar proportions of their contacts with *M. tuberculosis*.[1] One retrospective study in Florida showed that an observed increase in pediatric tuberculosis cases was linked to an increase in pulmonary tuberculosis cases among HIV-infected adults in the same population.[19] Across the United States, the largest increases in pediatric tuberculosis cases over the last several years have occurred in cities with high rates of HIV infection among the adult population. It appears as though the increased case load of infectious adult tuberculosis associated with the HIV is at least partly responsible for rising tuberculosis case rates among children.

Information about the risk of tuberculous disease in HIV-infected children is surprisingly meager. Prior to 1991 in the United States, less than 10 children with HIV infection and extrapulmonary tuberculosis had been reported. Only several case reports and small series of pulmonary tuberculosis in HIV-infected children in the United States have been published.[20,21] In countries where tuberculous infection rates in children generally are higher than in the United States, HIV-infected pediatric cohorts have a risk of developing tuberculosis that exceeds background rates.[1,22] In both developing and technically advanced nations tuberculosis probably is underdiagnosed in HIV-infected children because of the similarity of its clinical presentation to other opportunist infections, the frequency of anergy, and the difficulty in confirming the diagnosis with positive mycobacterial cultures. In the United States, all children with suspected tuberculous disease should have HIV serological testing, because the two infections are linked epidemiologically and recommended treatment for tuberculosis may be prolonged for HIV-infected patients.

4. Tuberculous Infection

While data on tuberculous disease among children are available, data on tuberculous infection without disease are lacking. Although there are estimates that approximately 20% of the world's population is infected with *M. tuberculosis*, it is impossible to determine how many children actually have asymptomatic tuberculous infection.[6] All countries but two (United States and The Netherlands) have used BCG vaccine extensively, and population surveys for tuberculous infection using the tuberculin skin test rarely are performed and may be difficult to interpret. In the United States, tuberculous infection without disease is a reportable condition in only three states — Kentucky, Indiana, and Missouri — and national surveys of tuberculous infection rates in children were discontinued in 1971.

The most efficient method of finding children infected with *M. tuberculosis* is through contact investigation of adults with infectious pulmonary tuberculosis. On average, 30–50% of household contacts of an index case will have a reactive skin test.[23] Even among children who have received BCG vaccine, a positive tuberculin skin test in a child who has had close contact with an adult with suspected tuberculosis probably represents infection with *M. tuberculosis*, and preventive therapy to halt progression of infection to disease should be given.

In the United States, most children have a risk of less than 1% of acquiring asymptomatic tuberculous infection. However, in some urban populations the risk appears to be much greater. In a 1990 study of Boston public schools, 5.1% of 7th graders and 8.9% of 10th graders were tuberculin skin test positive; approximately 85% of the infections occurred among foreign-born children.[24] Similar studies in Los Angeles[25] and Houston[26] revealed tuberculous infection rates between 2 and 10% for elementary and high school children. However, surveys in some other large cities have revealed infection rates in public schools of less than 1%.

The performance of optimal contact investigations should have a large impact on the incidence of tuberculous disease among children since these investigations identify recently infected children who are most likely to develop disease within a short time period. In general, community programs of tuberculin testing for school aged children are unlikely to have a significant impact on the incidence of childhood tuberculosis since most childhood cases occur in children less than 5 years of age and many of the "positive" tuberculin skin test reactions found among low-risk children in large screening programs actually represent false-positive cross-reactions. For high incidence populations, targeted testing and preventive chemotherapy programs will be necessary to diminish the pool of infected children and prevent future adolescent and adult cases of tuberculous disease.

C. CLINICAL MANIFESTATIONS
1. Asymptomatic Infections

The vast majority of children with tuberculous infection develop no signs or symptoms, nor radiographic abnormalities at any time. Occasionally, the initiation of the infection is marked by several days of low grade fever and mild cough. Rarely, the child experiences clinically significant disease with high fever, cough, malaise, and flu-like symptoms that resolve within 1 to 2 weeks. Other children, at the onset of tissue hypersensitivity, experience a fever and mild systemic symptoms that resolve over 1 to 3 weeks. The asymptomatic presentation of tuberculous infection is more common among school-aged children than among younger infants. Approximately 80–90% of infected older children have completely asymptomatic infection, whereas only 50–60% of infected infants less than 1 year of age remain free of symptoms or radiographic abnormalities with tuberculous infection.[27]

2. Intrathoracic Disease
a. Pulmonary

The primary pulmonary complex includes the lung parenchymal focus and regional lymphadenopathy. Approximately 70% of primary foci are subpleural, and localized pleurisy is a common part of the primary complex. During the initial infection, all lobar segments are at equal risk of being involved, and 25% of cases have multiple primary lung foci.[28] The initial parenchymal inflammation usually is not visible on chest radiograph but a localized, nonspecific infiltrate may be seen. Within days the infection spreads to regional lymph nodes. As tuberculin hypersensitivity develops, within 3 to 10 weeks after infection, the inflammatory reaction in the lung tissue and lymph nodes often intensifies. The hallmark of primary tuberculosis is the relatively large size and importance of the hilar, mediastinal, or subcarinal adenitis compared with the relatively small size of the initial lung focus.

In most children, the parenchymal infiltrate and adenitis resolve early, often by the time the chest radiograph is obtained. In some children, particularly

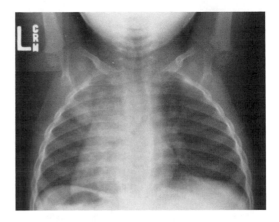

Figure 8-2 Hilar and mediastinal adenopathy in a child with primary tuberculosis.

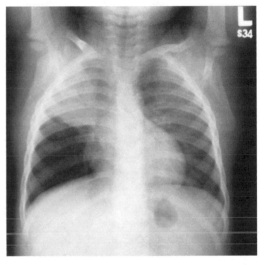

Figure 8-3 A child with right-sided adenopathy and a collapse-consolidation lesion of the right upper lobe due to tuberculosis.

infants, the lymph nodes continue to enlarge (Figure 8-2). Bronchial obstruction caused by external compression may begin as the nodes impinge on the neighboring regional bronchus, compressing it and causing diffuse inflammation of its outer wall.[29] If the inflammation intensifies, the lymph nodes may erode through the bronchial wall leading to perforation and formation of thick caseous material within the lumen. This process may result in partial or complete obstruction of the bronchus.[30,31] The common radiographic sequence is adenopathy followed by localized hyperinflation and, eventually, atelectasis.[32] These radiographic shadows have been called "collapse-consolidation" or "segmental" lesions (Figure 8-3). The radiographic picture is similar to that caused by aspiration of a foreign body but usually is quite different from a bacterial or viral pneumonia. In pulmonary tuberculosis, the lymph nodes act as the foreign body.

Obstructive emphysema of a lobar segment may accompany bronchial obstruction.[33] This rare complication occurs most often in children younger than 2 years of age. The obstruction usually resolves spontaneously, but this may take several months. Rarely, surgical removal of the lymph nodes is necessary to hasten the clinical improvement. The most common complication of bronchial obstruction is the fan-shaped segmental lesion that results from a combination of the primary pulmonary focus, the caseous material from an eroded bronchus, the host inflammatory response, and the subsequent atelectasis. Up to 45% of children younger than 1 year of age who are infected with *M. tuberculosis* develop a segmental lesion compared with 25% of children aged 1 to 10 years and 16% of children aged 11 to 15 years.[27] Usually a single segmental lesion is present, but lesions may occur simultaneously in several different pulmonary lobes.

The symptoms and physical signs of pulmonary tuberculosis in children usually are surprisingly meager considering the degree of radiographic changes often seen. The physical manifestations of disease tend to differ by the age of onset. Young infants and adolescents are more likely to have significant signs and/or symptoms while school aged children usually have clinically silent disease. More than 50% of infants and children with radiographically moderate to severe pulmonary tuberculosis have no symptoms or physical findings, and they are discovered only via contact tracing of an adult with pulmonary tuberculosis. Infants are more likely to experience signs and symptoms probably because of their smaller airway diameters relative to the parenchymal and lymph node changes in pulmonary tuberculosis. Nonproductive cough and mild dyspnea are the most common symptoms in infants. Systemic complaints such as fever, night sweats, anorexia, and decreased activity are less common. Some infants present with difficulty gaining weight or failure to thrive and these signs may not improve significantly until several months into therapy. Pulmonary signs are even less common. Some infants and young children with bronchial obstruction show signs of air trapping such as localized wheezing or decreased breath sounds that may be accompanied by tachypnea or, rarely, respiratory distress. A double-headed stethoscope may reveal delayed exhalation of air on the affected side. Occasionally these nonspecific symptoms and signs are alleviated by antibiotics, suggesting that bacterial superinfection distal to the focus of tuberculous bronchial obstruction contributes to the clinical presentation of disease.

Enlargement of other groups of intrathoracic lymph nodes can cause additional clinical manifestations. Enlarged subcarinal nodes, which cause splaying of the large bronchi, may impinge on the esophagus causing difficulty swallowing or leading to the development of a bronchoesophageal fistula. Enlarged nodes may compress the subclavian vein producing edema of the hand or arm. Occasionally nodes rupture into the mediastinum causing left or right sided supraclavicular adenitis.

The majority of cases of pulmonary tuberculosis in children resolve radiographically with or without antituberculosis chemotherapy. In the pretreatment era, up to 60% of children had residual anatomic sequelae not apparent on radiographs. With delayed or no treatment, calcification of the caseous lesions is common but usually takes at least 6 months to occur. Healing of the pulmonary segment can be complicated by scarring or contraction associated with cylindrical bronchiectasis or bronchostenosis. When these complications occur in the upper lobes they often are clinically silent. They appear to be rare in children who have successfully completed current regimens of chemotherapy.

A rare but serious complication of primary pulmonary tuberculosis occurs when the parenchymal focus enlarges and develops a large caseous center. The radiographic and clinical picture of progressive primary tuberculosis is closest to that of bronchial pneumonia, the child having high fever, moderate to severe cough, night sweats, dullness to percussion, rales, and decreased breath sounds. Liquefaction in the center of the lesion may result in formation of a thin-walled cavity, which may become a tension cavity as a result of a valve-like mechanism allowing air to enter but not escape (Figure 8-4). The enlarging focus may slough debris into adjacent bronchi leading to intrapulmonary dissemination of infection. Rupture of this cavity into the pleural space causes a bronchopleural fistula or pyopneumothorax. Rupture into the pericardium can cause acute pericarditis with constriction. Prior to the advent of antituberculosis chemotherapy, the mortality of progressive primary pulmonary tuberculosis in children was 30–50%; with current treatment the prognosis is excellent for full recovery.

Older children and adolescents may develop chronic reactivation pulmonary tuberculosis that resembles disease in adults. Even before the discovery of antituberculosis drugs, chronic pulmonary tuberculosis complicated infection in only 6–7% of pediatric patients.[34] Children with a healed primary tuberculous infection acquired before 2 years of age rarely develop chronic pulmonary disease. Chronic pulmonary tuberculosis is more common among children who acquire the initial

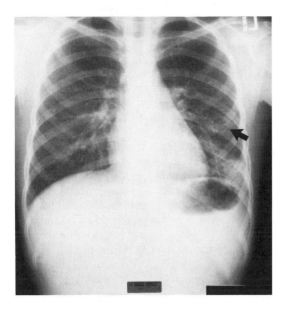

Figure 8-4 A 12-year-old girl with a thin-walled cavity (arrow) and pleural reaction due to tuberculosis.

infection after 7 years of age, particularly if they become infected close to the onset of puberty. The most common sites of chronic pulmonary tuberculosis are the original parenchymal focus, the regional lymph nodes, or the apical seedings (Simon foci). Typical symptoms are fever, anorexia, malaise, weight loss, night sweats, productive cough, chest pain, and hemoptysis. However, the findings on physical examination usually are minor or absent even when cavities or large infiltrates are present. Most signs and symptoms improve within several weeks of starting effective treatment, although cough may last for several months. This form of tuberculous disease usually remains localized to the lungs because the presensitization of tissue to tuberculin evokes an immune response that prevents further lympho-hematogenous spread.

b. Pleural

Tuberculous pleural effusions are caused by the hypersensitivity response to the discharge of bacilli into the pleural space from a subpleural pulmonary focus or from subpleural caseous lymph nodes.[35] The discharge usually is small and the subsequent pleuritis is localized and asymptomatic. Occasionally a larger discharge causes a generalized pleural effusion, usually within 6 months after initial infection. The effusion usually is unilateral in children.[36] A clinically significant pleural effusion occurs in 10–30% of tuberculosis cases in young adults but is infrequent in children younger than 6 years of age and extremely rare in children below

2 years of age.[11] It is most common among adolescents. It virtually is never associated with a segmental pulmonary lesion and occurs only rarely with miliary tuberculosis.

The onset of symptoms and signs usually is abrupt with fever, chest pain, shortness of breath, dullness to percussion, and diminished breath sounds on the affected side. Fever can be high and may last for several weeks even after antituberculosis chemotherapy has been started. The diagnosis may be difficult to make as the acid-fast stain of the pleural fluid virtually is always negative and the culture is positive in only 30–50% of cases. The best material for diagnosis is a biopsy of the pleura, which will reveal caseating granulomas in up to 90% of cases and a positive culture in up to 70% of cases.

c. Cardiac

Involvement of the myocardium may occur during miliary tuberculosis. Direct extension of tuberculosis into the myocardium from adjacent lymph nodes or lung parenchyma is rare. Tuberculous endocarditis has been described in several children.

The most common form of cardiac tuberculosis is pericarditis, which occurs in 0.4–4% of tuberculosis cases in children.[37] Pericarditis usually arises by direct invasion or lymphatic drainage from subcarinal lymph nodes. Early in the course, the pericardial fluid is serofibrinous or, occasionally, hemorrhagic. Echocardiography often reveals thin strands of fibrinous material in the pericardial space. In approximately 10–20% of cases, fibrosis leads to obliteration of the pericardial sac with development of constrictive pericarditis over a period of months to years. The presenting symptoms of serofibrinous pericarditis are nonspecific and include low grade fever, malaise, and weight loss; in children, chest pain is unusual. A pericardial friction rub with distant heart sounds and with pulsus paradoxicus may be present, especially if constrictive changes have occurred. The acid-fast smear of the pericardial fluid rarely reveals the organism but cultures of the fluid are positive in 30–70% of cases. Pericardial biopsy may be necessary to confirm the diagnosis; typical findings of caseating granulomas are present in 50–75% of cases. Partial or complete pericardiectomy may be required when constrictive pericarditis is present.

3. Lymphohematogenous

Tubercle bacilli are disseminated to distant anatomic sites virtually in all cases of asymptomatic tuberculous infection. Autopsy cultures from people who died of other causes within days to weeks after initial infection with *M. tuberculosis* have demonstrated the organisms in many tissues, most commonly liver, spleen, skin, and lung apices. The clinical picture produced by lymphohematogenous dissemination depends on the quantity of organisms released from the primary focus and the host immune response. Individuals who have a diminished immune response, such as infants and those with HIV infection, are more likely to develop severe forms of disseminated disease.[38]

The occult dissemination of tubercle bacilli during the initial infection usually produces no symptoms, but it is the event that results in extrapulmonary foci that can become the site of disease months to years after the initial infection. Rare patients experience protracted hematogenous tuberculosis caused by the intermittent release of tubercle bacilli as a caseous focus erodes through the wall of a blood vessel in the lung. The clinical picture may be acute but often is indolent and prolonged, with spiking fevers accompanying the release of organisms into the blood stream. Multiple organ involvement is common, often leading to hepatomegaly, splenomegaly, lymphadenitis in superficial or deep nodes, or papulonecrotic tuberculids appearing in crops on the skin. Bones and joints or the kidneys may become involved. Meningitis occurs only late in the course and often was the cause of death in the prechemotherapy era. Pulmonary involvement is surprisingly mild early in the course, but diffuse lung involvement usually becomes apparent if treatment is not given early. Culture confirmation of this complication can be difficult; bone marrow or liver biopsy with appropriate stains and cultures may be necessary and should be performed if the diagnosis is considered and other tests are unrevealing. The tuberculin skin test usually is reactive.

The most common clinically significant form of disseminated tuberculosis is miliary disease, which occurs when massive numbers of tubercle bacilli are released into the blood stream causing disease in two or more organs. Miliary tuberculosis usually is an early complication of the primary infection occurring within 3 to 6 months of the primary inoculation. While this form of disease is most common among infants and young children, it also is common in older adults as a result of the breakdown of a previously healed or calcified primary pulmonary lesion that formed years earlier.

The clinical manifestations of miliary tuberculosis are protean and depend on the load and the final location of disseminated organisms.[39] Tissues have varying susceptibility to infection. Lesions usually are larger and more numerous in the lungs, spleen, liver, and bone marrow than other organs. The distribution may be caused both by blood sup-

ply and by the numbers of reticuloendothelial cells and tissue phagocytes.

The onset of clinical disease may be explosive with the patient becoming gravely ill over several days. More often, the onset is insidious and the patient may not be able to accurately pinpoint the time of initial symptoms. Early systemic signs include malaise, anorexia, weight loss, and low grade fever. At this time abnormal physical signs usually are absent. Within several weeks, hepatosplenomegaly and generalized lymphadenopathy develop in approximately 50% of patients. The fever may become higher and more sustained although the chest radiograph usually is normal and respiratory symptoms are few. Within several weeks the lungs often become filled with tubercles, accompanied by the onset of dyspnea, cough, rales, or wheezing.[38] As the pulmonary disease progresses, an alveolar air block syndrome may result in frank respiratory distress, hypoxia, and pneumothorax or pneumomediastinum. Signs or symptoms of meningitis or peritonitis are found in only 20–40% of patients with advanced disease. Chronic or recurrent headache in a child with miliary tuberculosis usually indicates the presence of meningitis while the onset of abdominal pain or tenderness often heralds tuberculous peritonitis. Cutaneous lesions such as papulonecrotic tuberculids or nodules often occur in crops. Choroid tubercles occur in 13–87% of patients.

The early diagnosis of miliary tuberculosis can be difficult, requiring a high index of suspicion by the clinician. Up to 30% of children have a negative tuberculin skin test. A biopsy of liver or bone marrow may facilitate a rapid diagnosis. In one recent review, the diagnosis could be confirmed by culture in only 33% of cases in children.[38] With proper treatment, the prognosis of miliary tuberculosis in children is excellent. However, resolution of signs and symptoms may be slow with fever declining in 2 to 3 weeks and chest radiograph abnormalities persisting for several months.

4. Lymphatic

Tuberculosis of the superficial lymph nodes — historically referred to as scrofula — is the most common form of extrapulmonary tuberculosis among children, accounting for approximately 67% of cases.[11,40] Historically, scrofula was often caused by drinking unpasteurized cow's milk laden with *Mycobacterium bovis*. However, through effective veterinary control, *M. bovis* has been nearly eliminated from North America.

Most current cases of tuberculous lymphadenitis occur within 6 to 9 months of the initial tuberculous infection, although some cases arise years later. The tonsillar, anterior cervical, and submandibular nodes become involved secondary to extension of a primary lesion of the upper lung fields or abdomen. Infected lymph nodes in the inguinal, epitrochlear, or axillary regions are rare in children and result from regional adenitis associated with tuberculosis of the skin or skeletal system.

In the early stages of infection the lymph nodes usually enlarge gradually. The nodes are firm but not hard and they are discrete and nontender. The nodes usually feel fixed to underlying or overlying tissues. The disease most often is unilateral, but bilateral involvement may occur because of crossover drainage patterns of lymphatic vessels in the chest and lower neck. As infection progresses, multiple nodes usually become involved, often resulting in a mass of matted nodes. Other than low grade fever, systemic signs and symptoms usually are absent. The tuberculin skin test usually is reactive. Although a primary pulmonary focus virtually always is present, it is visible radiographically in only 30–70% of cases. Pulmonary signs and symptoms usually are lacking. Occasionally the illness is more acute with rapid enlargement of lymph nodes associated with high fever, tenderness, and fluctuance. Rarely, the initial presentation will be a fluctuant mass with overlying cellulitis and skin discoloration.

If left untreated, the lymph node infection may resolve but more often progresses to caseation and necrosis of the node.[41] The capsule of the node breaks down leading to spread of infection to adjacent nodes. The skin overlying the mass of nodes becomes thin, shiny, and erythematous. Rupture through the skin results in a draining sinus tract that may require surgical removal.

The most difficult issue in the differential diagnosis of tuberculous adenitis is distinguishing this condition from adenitis due to nontuberculous mycobacteria, which are especially prevalent in the southern United States. Both conditions tend to cause chronic, nontender adenopathy with overlying skin changes and the eventual creation of tissue breakdown and sinus tracts. The chest radiograph often is negative in both conditions and skin test reactions may be positive in either condition. The most important diagnostic clue for tuberculous lymphadenitis is the identification of an adult source case in the child's environment. Often, excisional biopsy and culture of the lymph nodes are required to definitively establish the etiology; however, the cultures are negative in approximately 50% of reported cases of both tuberculous and nontuberculous mycobacterial lymphadenitis.

5. Central Nervous System
a. Meningitis

Central nervous system tuberculosis is the most serious complication in children and is uniformly fatal without effective treatment. It usually arises from the formation of a metastatic caseous lesion in the cerebral cortex or meninges that is established during the occult lymphohematogenous dissemination of the primary infection.[42] This lesion, often called a Rich focus, increases in size and discharges small numbers of tubercle bacilli into the subarachnoid space. The resulting gelatinous exudate may infiltrate the cortical or meningeal blood vessels producing inflammation, obstruction, and subsequent infarction of the cerebral cortex. The brain stem is the area most commonly affected, accounting for the frequent involvement of cranial nerves III, VI, and VII. This exudate interferes with the normal flow of cerebrospinal fluid (CSF) in and out of the ventricular system at the level of the basilar cisterns, leading to a communicating hydrocephalus. This combination of vasculitis, infarction, cerebral edema, and hydrocephalus results in the severe damage that can occur gradually or rapidly with this disease. Profound abnormalities in electrolyte metabolism, especially hyponatremia secondary to the inappropriate secretion of antidiuretic hormone, are common and may contribute to the pathophysiology.[43] Salt wasting may make correction of the electrolyte disturbances difficult.

Tuberculous meningitis complicates approximately 0.5% of untreated primary infections.[44] It is extremely rare in infants less than 4 months of age because it usually takes that long for the pathologic events to take place. It is most common among children between 6 months and 4 years of age. Since it is an early manifestation of the primary infection, the adult source case usually can be identified fairly quickly.

The clinical progression of tuberculous meningitis may be rapid or gradual.[45] Rapid progression tends to occur more often among infants and young children who may experience symptoms for only days before the onset of acute hydrocephalus, seizures, or cerebral edema.[46] More often, the signs and symptoms progress slowly over several weeks and can be divided into three stages. The first stage typically lasts 1 to 2 weeks and is characterized by nonspecific symptoms such as fever, headache, irritability, drowsiness, and malaise. Focal neurologic signs are absent but infants may experience a stagnation or loss of developmental milestones. The second stage usually begins more abruptly with lethargy, nuchal rigidity, Kernig or Brudzinsky signs, seizures, hypertonia, vomiting, cranial nerve palsies, and other focal neurologic signs. The clinical picture usually correlates with the early development of hydrocephalus with subsequent increased intracranial pressure and vasculitis. Some children do not have signs of meningeal irritation but have signs of encephalitis such as disorientation, abnormal movements, and speech impairment.[47] The third stage is marked by coma, hemiplegia or paraplegia, hypertension, decerebrate posturing, deterioration in vital signs and, eventually, death. The prognosis of tuberculous meningitis correlates most closely with the clinical stage of illness at the time antituberculosis chemotherapy is started;[48] the vast majority of patients in the first stage have an excellent outcome, while most patients in the third stage who survive have permanent disabilities that include blindness, deafness, paraplegia, diabetes insipidus, and mental retardation. It is imperative that antituberculosis treatment be considered strongly for any child who develops basilar meningitis and hydrocephalus with no other apparent etiology. The key to the diagnosis in children often is identifying the adult source case.

The initial diagnosis of tuberculous meningitis may be extremely difficult. The tuberculin skin test is negative in up to 40% of cases and the chest radiograph is normal in up to 50% of cases.[49] The CSF leukocyte cell count ranges from 10 to 500 cells/mm³. Polymorphonuclear cells may be the major cell type early, but a lymphocyte preponderance is more typical. The CSF glucose level usually is between 20 and 40 mg/dl whereas the CSF protein concentration is elevated and occasionally markedly high (>400 mg/dl). The success of microscopic examination of stained CSF and mycobacterial cultures is related directly to the size of the CSF sample. When 10 ml of CSF is available, the acid-fast stain is positive in up to 30% of cases and the culture is positive in up to 70% of cases. Computed tomography or magnetic resonance scans may help establish the diagnosis of tuberculous meningitis and can aid in evaluating the success of therapy.

b. Tuberculoma

Another manifestation of central nervous system tuberculosis is the tuberculoma, which usually presents clinically as a brain tumor. They occur most often in children less than 10 years of age and are usually singular. While the lesions in adults are most often supratentorial, in children they are often infratentorial, located at the base of the brain near the cerebellum. Tuberculomas account for up to 40% of brain "tumors" in some areas of the world but they are rare in North America. The most common symptoms are headache, fever, and convulsions. The tuberculin skin test usually is reactive, but the chest radiograph often is unremarkable. Surgical excision may be necessary to distinguish tuberculoma from other causes of brain tumors.

A phenomenon that has been recognized since the advent of computerized tomography is the paradoxical development of tuberculomas in patients with tuberculous meningitis while on ultimately effective chemotherapy.[50,51] The cause and nature of these tuberculomas are poorly understood. Their development is not thought to be a failure of drug treatment and does not necessitate a change in the therapeutic regimen. This phenomenon should be considered whenever a child with tuberculous meningitis deteriorates or develops focal neurologic findings while on treatment. Corticosteroids may help alleviate the occasionally severe clinical signs and symptoms these lesions cause. They may be very slow to resolve, persisting for months or even years. It is unclear how long antituberculosis treatment or corticosteroids should be given when these lesions appear.

6. Skeletal

Skeletal tuberculosis usually results from lymphohematogenous seeding of tubercle bacilli during the primary infection. Bone infection also may originate from direct extension of a caseous regional lymph node or by extension from a neighboring infected bone. The time interval between infection and disease can be as short as 1 month in cases of tuberculous dactylitis or 30 months or longer for tuberculosis of the hip. The infection usually begins in the metaphysis (Figure 8-5). Granulation tissue and caseation develop, which destroy bone both by direct infection and pressure necrosis. Soft tissue abscess and extension of the infection through the epiphysis into the nearby joint often complicate the bone lesion. Frequently, the infection becomes clinically apparent when the joint involvement progresses. Weight-bearing bones and joints are affected most commonly. Most cases of bone tuberculosis occur in the vertebrae causing tuberculosis of the spine, known as Pott's disease.[52] Although any vertebral body can be involved, there is a predilection for the lower thoracic and upper lumbar vertebrae. Involvement of two or more vertebrae is common; they usually are contiguous but there may be skip areas between lesions. The infection is in the body of the vertebra leading to bony destruction and collapse. The usual progression of tuberculous spondylitis is from initial narrowing of one or several disc spaces to collapse and wedging of the vertebral body with subsequent angulation of

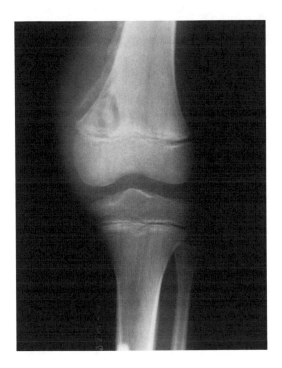

Figure 8-5 Tuberculosis in a long bone of a child.

the spine (gibbus) or kyphosis. The infection may extend out from the bone causing a paraspinal (Pott's), psoas, or retropharyngeal abscess.

The most frequent clinical signs and symptoms of tuberculous spondylitis in children are low grade fever, irritability and restlessness (especially at night), back pain usually without significant tenderness, and abnormal positioning and gait or refusal to walk. Rigidity of the spine may be caused by profound muscle spasm resulting from the patient's involuntary effort to immobilize the spine.

Other sites of skeletal tuberculosis, in approximate order of frequency, are the knee, hip, elbow, and ankle.[53] The degree of involvement ranges from joint effusion without bone destruction to frank destruction of bone and restriction of the joint caused by chronic fibrosis of the synovial membrane. The process usually evolves over months to years, most commonly causing mild pain, stiffness, limping, and restricted movement. The tuberculin skin test is reactive in 80–90% of cases. Culture of joint fluid or bone biopsy usually yields the organism. Tuberculosis should be considered in any child with a persistent bone or joint lesion.

One form of bony tuberculosis peculiar to infants is tuberculous dactylitis. Affected children develop distal endarteritis followed by painless swelling and cystic bone lesions. Abscesses are rare but the tuberculin skin test usually is reactive.

D. DIAGNOSTIC TESTS
1. General Approach

Many children with tuberculosis are discovered via contact investigations of adults with infectious pulmonary tuberculosis. Many of these children have asymptomatic disease that would have progressed or escaped detection if the contact tracing had not occurred. Some children are discovered after a symptomatic illness begins. A strong index of suspicion for tuberculosis is required to correctly identify the cause of illness in children since the signs and symptoms of most forms of tuberculosis are similar to those of many other infections and conditions. The importance of the epidemiologic setting of the child in establishing the diagnosis of tuberculosis cannot be overemphasized.

Routine laboratory tests such as a complete blood count and cell differential, erythrocyte sedimentation rate, urinalysis, and blood chemistries are usually normal in children with tuberculous disease. Abnormalities in liver enzymes or function tests may indicate hepatic involvement in miliary tuberculosis.

2. Tuberculin Skin Tests

The principles for tuberculin skin testing for children are the same as those for adults.[54] A positive tuberculin skin test is the hallmark of the primary infection with *M. tuberculosis*. In children, the tuberculin reaction persists for many years, even after successful completion of chemotherapy.[55] However, young infants generally produce less induration and response to tuberculin than do older children and adults. A variety of factors common in children such as malnutrition, viral infections (especially varicella, influenza, and measles), and, perhaps, administration of live virus vaccines, can lower tuberculin reactivity. Approximately 10% of immunocompetent children with culture-documented tuberculosis initially do not react to tuberculin, although most become reactive after several months of therapy.[28,56] Parents should not be allowed to interpret their children's skin test results because of unreliable interpretation and reporting.

Two techniques are used for tuberculin skin testing in children — multiple puncture tests and the Mantoux test. The multiple puncture tests utilize either purified protein derivative (PPD) or Old Tuberculin as the antigen, which is delivered intradermally via metal or plastic prongs. These devices became popular in 1960s and 1970s because of the speed and ease with which they can be administered. Unfortunately, several technical and practice-related problems severely limit their usefulness. First, the exact dose of tuberculin introduced into the skin cannot be precisely controlled so interpretation of the reaction size is difficult to standardize. As a result, a reactive test cannot be considered diagnostic of infection unless a vesicular reaction occurs.[54] The need to verify a positive multiple puncture test with a Mantoux test leads to the second problem, called boosting.[57] Boosting is an increase in the reaction size to a skin test in a person already sensitized to mycobacterial antigens caused by repetitive tests. This phenomenon is caused in older adults by stimulation of a waned immunologic response to *M. tuberculosis* and in children and young adults by cross-reactions due to nontuberculous mycobacteria or prior vaccination with BCG.[58] The booster reaction may occur for tuberculin tests performed several days to 12 or more months apart, resulting in a subsequent positive Mantoux skin test that may not represent infection with *M. tuberculosis*.

The third problem with multiple puncture skin tests is that the sensitivity and specificity compared with the Mantoux test are quite variable and in some studies quite low. False-positive rates may be as high as 30% or greater and false-negative results may be greater than 10%.[59] The final problem is that many clinicians allow parents and families to interpret their own tuberculin skin tests, a practice that should be condemned.[60]

In general, multiple puncture skin tests should not be used in children. They are absolutely contraindicated for children who have had BCG vaccine, known contacts of persons with infectious tuberculosis, ill children, or testing of children in high-risk groups for tuberculosis.

The effect of BCG vaccination on the subsequent Mantoux skin test in children is highly variable, and is partly dependent on the strain of BCG used.[61] Several studies have shown that at least 50% of infants who received BCG vaccine do not convert their tuberculin skin test to reactive, and 80–90% of those who react initially become tuberculin skin test negative within 2 to 3 years after BCG vaccination.[62,63] Prior BCG vaccination in a child is never a contraindication to subsequent tuberculin skin testing, and, in general, the results of the skin test should be interpreted as if the child had never received BCG vaccination.

3. Acid-Fast Stain and Culture

Generally, the most important laboratory tests for the diagnosis and management of tuberculosis are the acid-fast stain and mycobacterial culture. The best culture specimen for children with suspected pulmonary tuberculosis is the early morning gastric aspirate obtained before the child has arisen and peristalsis has emptied the stomach of the pooled, swallowed overnight respiratory secretions. Unfortunately, even under optimal conditions three consecutive morning gastric aspirates yield the organism in less than 50% of cases; negative cultures never exclude the diagnosis of tuberculosis in a child. The yield from culture obtained via flexible bronchoscopy is significantly less than that from properly obtained gastric aspirates.[64]

Fortunately, there is usually little need for culture confirmation for most children with suspected pulmonary tuberculosis. If the child has a positive tuberculin skin test, clinical and/or radiographic findings suggestive of tuberculosis and previous contact with an adult source case with infectious tuberculosis, the child should be treated for tuberculous disease. The drug susceptibility test results from the source case isolate can be used to determine the best therapeutic regimen for the child. However, cultures should be obtained and susceptibility tests performed on specimens from the child with suspected tuberculosis under three conditions: (1) the source case is unknown, (2) the source case has a drug-resistant organism, and (3) the child has extrapulmonary tuberculosis (since the differential diagnosis for the condition is somewhat broader than it usually is for pulmonary tuberculosis). The yield from gastric aspirate acid-fast stains is much lower than for culture, but a markedly positive stain of gastric fluid usually is indicative of pulmonary tuberculosis. Unfortunately, while acid-fast stains of gastric contents may have a specificity for tuberculosis greater than 90%, the sensitivity usually is below 25%.[65] Acid-fast stain and mycobacterial culture of urine may be helpful for children with suspected miliary tuberculosis or in some cases of primary pulmonary tuberculosis.

4. New Techniques

The serodiagnosis of tuberculosis has been envisioned since 1898, when the first agglutination test was developed. In the past 15 years, there have been numerous studies using both whole-cell and specific antigens in various antibody detection systems. For adults, most serologic tests have a sensitivity and specificity approaching those of a sputum acid-fast smear. Several studies have used samples from children. One study of a small number of children with pulmonary tuberculosis in Argentina, which used a specific mycobacterial antigen in an enzyme-linked immunosorbent assay (ELISA) system, found a sensitivity of 86% and specificity of 100%.[66] Another study of children with tuberculosis, using whole-cell *M. tuberculosis* as the antigen in an ELISA test, found a sensitivity of 62% and specificity of 98%.[67] However, a different study that used various whole mycobacterial sonicates had a sensitivity of only 26% and specificity of 40%.[68] It is unlikely that serodiagnosis will make a substantial contribution to the diagnosis of tuberculosis in children in the near future.

Several new techniques have been designed to detect the presence of mycobacterial antigens or DNA in patient specimens. The polymerase chain reaction (PCR) has been used to detect the DNA of *M. tuberculosis*, while high-pressure liquid chromatography has been used to detect the cell wall constituent mycolic acids. The sensitivity of PCR for children with pulmonary tuberculosis in two published studies has been approximately 50%.[69,70] Both studies showed that some children with recent infection with *M. tuberculosis* but no radiographic evidence of disease had positive PCR tests from gastric aspirate samples. This is not surprising since these children had recent infection and probably had active multiplication of *M. tuberculosis* within the lungs, even though no radiographic disease was apparent. It is unlikely that PCR of gastric acid samples will distinguish between asymptomatic tuberculous infection and tuberculous disease. However, this test may be useful for the child who has radiographic pneumonia to determine whether the cause of that pneumonia is tuberculosis.

E. TREATMENT
1. Principles

The general principles that have determined the development of antituberculosis chemotherapy regimens in adults generally apply to infants and children. However, there are several special considerations for children with tuberculosis based on microbiology, natural history of the disease, and product availability. First, children usually develop tuberculous disease as an immediate complication of the primary infection. They typically have closed caseous lesions with relatively few mycobacteria. The large bacterial populations found within cavities or infiltrates that are characteristic of adult reactivation pulmonary tuberculosis usually are absent in children. Since the likelihood of developing resistance to any antimycobacterial drug is proportional to the size of the bacillary population, children generally are less likely than adults to develop secondary drug resistance while receiving therapy, even if adherence is poor.[71]

A related problem concerns the natural history of primary tuberculosis in children. All children with tuberculous infection have involvement of the hilar or mediastinal lymph nodes; however, the involvement is visible radiographically in less than 20% of children. While asymptomatic infection and pulmonary disease usually are easily distinguishable events in adults, the range of microbiologic and host response events lays more on a continuum in children. Pediatric radiographs can be difficult to interpret and there are no standards for what constitutes significant intrathoracic adenopathy in a child. In general, the clinician considers the child to have tuberculous disease if adenopathy is readily visible on the chest radiograph, even if the child has no signs or symptoms of tuberculosis. When determining the best treatment regimen for a child, it usually is safer to overestimate rather than underestimate the extent of disease, particularly in a child known to be at high risk for recent acquisition of tuberculous infection.

Third, children have a higher propensity than adults to develop extrapulmonary forms of tuberculosis, especially disseminated disease and meningitis. It is important that antituberculosis drugs for children penetrate into a variety of tissues and fluids, especially across the meninges. Isoniazid, rifampin, pyrazinamide, and ethionamide cross both inflamed and uninflammed meninges adequately to kill virtually all strains of drug-susceptible *M. tuberculosis*.

Fourth, the pharmacokinetics of antituberculosis drugs differ between children and adults.[72] In general, children tolerate larger doses per kilogram of body weight and have fewer adverse reactions than adults.[73,74] It is unclear whether the higher serum concentration of drugs achieved in children has any therapeutic advantage.[75] The lower rates of toxicity in children usually mean that fewer interruptions in treatment will occur. In general, children with more severe forms of tuberculosis, especially disseminated disease and meningitis, experience more significant hepatotoxic effects than less severely ill children treated with the same doses per kilogram of isoniazid and rifampin, especially if the isoniazid dose exceeds 10 mg/kg per day.[76] However, many hepatoxic "reactions" in children taking antituberculosis medications really are caused by intercurrent infections with hepatitis A and B viruses or other viruses.[77]

Finally, an important difference between children and adults concerns the administration of medications. Most available dosage forms were designed for use in adults. Giving these preparations to children may involve crushing pills or making suspensions that are neither standardized nor well studied. Some dosage forms may lead to inadequate absorption of oral medications.[78] Many children experience difficulty taking the several antituberculosis medications required at the beginning of therapy. If these problems are not anticipated and addressed, they may cause significant delays and interruptions of treatment. Currently, fixed dose combination preparations are not readily usable in children. Technical problems may be difficult to solve; one recent study demonstrated a marked decline in rifampin concentration over time in suspensions also containing isoniazid or pyrazinamide.[79]

Table 8-3 Antituberculosis drugs in children

Drugs	Dosage Forms	Daily Dose (mg/kg)	Twice-Weekly Dose (mg/kg/per dose)	Maximum Dose
Isoniazid[a]	Scored tablets 100 mg 300 mg Syrup: 10 mg/ml[b]	10–15	20–40	Daily: 300 mg; twice-weekly: 900 mg
Rifampin[a]	Capsules 150 mg 300 mg Syrup formulated in syrup from capsules[c]	10–20	10–20	600 mg
Pyrazinamide	Scored tablets 500 mg	20–40	50–70	2 g
Streptomycin	Vials 1 g, 4 g	20–40 (im)	20–40 (im)	1 g
Ethambutol	Scored tablets 100 mg 400 mg	15–25	50	2.5 g
Ethionamide	Tablets 250 mg	10–20		1 g
Kanamycin	Vials 1 gm	15 (im)	15–25 (im)	1 g
Cycloserine	Capsules 250 mg	10–20		1 g

[a] Rifamate is a capsule containing 150 mg of isoniazid and 300 mg of rifampin. Two capsules provide the usual adult(more than 50 kg) daily dose of each drug.

[b] Many experts recommend not using isoniazid syrup, as it is unstable and is associated with frequent gastrointestinal complaints, especially diarrhea.

[c] Merrill Dow issues directions for preparation of this "extemporaneous" syrup.

2. Antituberculosis Drugs for Children (Table 8-3)

Isoniazid is familiar to pediatricians as it is effective and well tolerated by children. Although it is metabolized by acetylation in the liver, there is no correlation in children between acetylation rate and either efficacy or adverse reactions.[80] The major toxic effects of isoniazid in adults are very rare in children. Pyridoxine levels are decreased in children taking isoniazid, but peripheral neuritis is exceedingly rare.[81] However, certain children — especially teenagers with inadequate diets, children from ethnic groups with low meat and milk intake, and breast-feeding babies — should receive pyridoxine supplementation. Hepatoxicity among children taking isoniazid also is rare with only 3–10% experiencing transiently elevated liver enzyme levels; clinically significant hepatitis occurs in far less than 1% of children.[74] Adolescents are more likely than younger children to experience hepatoxicity.[82] For most children and adolescents, toxicity can be monitored using only clinical signs and symptoms; routine biochemical monitoring is not necessary.

Rifampin is well tolerated by children. Hepatoxicity is infrequent and other adverse reactions that occur in adults, such as leukopenia, thrombocytopenia, and the immunologically mediated flu-like syndrome, are rare. Pyrazinamide has been used extensively in children over the past decade. Formal pharmacokinetic studies in children have not been reported but a daily dose of 30 mg/kg results in adequate CSF levels, is well tolerated, produces little toxicity, and appears to be effective.[83] Hepatitis and complications of hyperuricemia are exceedingly rare among children. Streptomycin is used less frequently than in the past but is well tolerated by children. Although safe in infants, it cannot be given to pregnant women because it causes damage to the eighth cranial nerve of the fetus.

Ethambutol has not been used widely among children because of its potential toxicity to the eye and the relative difficulty monitoring ophthalmological signs and symptoms in young children. However, there is no published evidence of optic toxicity in children and there is no damage to the fetus when the pregnant woman takes ethambutol.[84] Ethambutol is not recommended for general use in children, but should be considered strongly for children with suspected drug-resistant tuberculosis. Ethionamide is well tolerated by children and is probably underutilized in this population. Children experience much less gastrointestinal distress than adults. Ethionamide can be used as a fourth antituberculosis medication for initial treatment in children with possible or suspected resistance to either isoniazid or rifampin.

3. Specific Treatment
a. Thoracic Disease
During the past decade, several treatment trials for tuberculosis in children have been reported. One study from Arkansas reported successful treatment of 50 children with tuberculosis using isoniazid and rifampin daily for 1 month, then twice weekly for 8 months, a total treatment duration of 9 months.[85] Some patients with only hilar adenopathy were successfully treated with a 6-month regimen of isoniazid and rifampin.[86] One study from Brazil reported successful treatment of 117 children with pulmonary tuberculosis using isoniazid and rifampin daily for 6 months.[87] Although these results are impressive, this 6-month regimen in children has not been adopted widely because of limited data and the growing problem of isoniazid and rifampin resistance in many areas of the world. The Brazilian study also demonstrated the difficult problem of nonadherence among children since, even with this fairly simple regimen, 17% of the patients did not complete treatment.

There have been several studies of 6-month duration of antituberculosis therapy in children using at least three drugs initially for drug-susceptible tuberculosis.[88-92] Although the exact regimens used in these trials differed slightly, the most common was a 6-month regimen of isoniazid and rifampin supplemented during the first 2 months with pyrazinamide. The success of these regimens was the same whether or not streptomycin also was given. Most trials used daily therapy for the first 1 to 2 months followed by daily or twice weekly, directly observed therapy for the last 4 months. Regimens using twice weekly therapy under the direct observation of a healthcare worker were as safe and effective as those using daily self-administered therapy. In all trials, the overall success rate was greater than 95% for complete clinical and radiographic cure and 99% for significant radiographic improvement during a 2-year period of follow-up. The incidence of clinically significant

adverse reactions, most commonly gastrointestinal upset or mild skin rash, was less than 2%.

The current recommendations of the American Academy of Pediatrics,[93] Centers for Disease Control and Prevention, and the International Union Against Tuberculosis and Lung Disease,[4] suggest that standard therapy for drug-susceptible thoracic tuberculosis in children should be 6 months of isoniazid and rifampin supplemented during the first 2 months with pyrazinamide. Although daily administration of medications during the first 2 months is preferable, two studies have shown that 6 months of twice or thrice weekly medications yielded results equivalent to regimens that used an initial phase of daily self-administered treatment.[89,91] If the risk of initial isoniazid- or rifampin-resistant tuberculosis is significant for a child, a fourth drug, usually ethambutol, streptomycin, or ethionamide, should be given initially until drug susceptibility patterns can be established.

b. Extrathoracic Disease
Controlled trials comparing treatment regimens for various forms of extrapulmonary tuberculosis in children are virtually nonexistent. Several of the 6-month, 3-drug regimen trials in children included cases of lymph node and disseminated tuberculosis, both of which responded favorably to these regimens.[90,91] Most data come from series of extrathoracic tuberculosis in adults. In general, the 6-month regimen using isoniazid, rifampin, and pyrazinamide initially is recommended for most forms of extrathoracic tuberculosis. One exception may be bone and joint tuberculosis, which may require a treatment duration of 9 to 12 months, especially if surgical intervention has not been undertaken.[94]

Tuberculous lymphadenitis responds well to antituberculosis chemotherapy, although involved nodes may remain enlarged for months to years.[95] Surgical removal alone is not adequate treatment since the lymph node disease is only part of a systemic infection. However, surgical biopsy and culture may be necessary to distinguish tuberculous adenitis from other entities, especially cat-scratch disease or infection due to nontuberculous mycobacteria. Excisional biopsy is preferred over incisional biopsy because of an increased risk of subsequent sinus tract formation or severe scarring with the latter procedure.

Tuberculous meningitis has not been included in trials of extrapulmonary tuberculosis because of its serious nature and low incidence. As with other forms of extrapulmonary tuberculosis, the number of mycobacteria causing disease usually is small. Treatment with isoniazid and rifampin daily for 12 months generally is effective for drug-susceptible disease.[96] Several recent reports have suggested that 6 to 9 months of therapy is effective if isoniazid, rifampin, and pyrazinamide are administered during the initial phase of treatment.[97] At present, there probably are not sufficient data to recommend the 6-month treatment duration for most children with tuberculous meningitis. The recommendation of the American Academy of Pediatrics for tuberculous meningitis is 12 months of treatment that includes at least isoniazid and rifampin and usually one or two other drugs in the initial phase of treatment.[93] However, some experts believe that a treatment duration of 6 to 9 months is adequate, if pyrazinamide is included in the initial treatment. Many experts add a fourth drug during initial treatment — usually streptomycin or another aminoglycocide, ethambutol or ethionamide — to protect against unsuspected initial drug resistance.

c. Human Immunodeficiency Virus-Related

The optimal treatment of tuberculosis in HIV-infected children has not been established. Adults with tuberculosis who are HIV infected usually can be treated successfully with standard regimens that include isoniazid, rifampin, and pyrazinamide, if the total duration of therapy is extended to 9 months, or to 6 months after cultures of sputum become sterile, whichever is longer.[98] Although this therapy has been shortened to 6 months, in cases where the response to therapy is good (see Chapter 6, this volume), this may not be wise in children.

It may be difficult to determine whether a pulmonary infiltrate is due to *M. tuberculosis* in an HIV-infected child who has a positive tuberculin reaction or history of exposure to an adult with infectious tuberculosis. It is likely, as in immunocompetent children, that gastric aspirate or bronchoscopy cultures may be sterile even when tuberculous disease is present. The radiographic appearance of other pulmonary complications of HIV infection in children, such as lymphoid interstitial pneumonitis, may be similar to that of tuberculosis. Treatment usually is empiric, based on epidemiologic and radiographic information, and it should be considered when tuberculosis cannot be excluded.

Most experts believe that HIV-infected children with drug-susceptible tuberculous disease should receive isoniazid, rifampin, and pyrazinamide for 2 months followed by isoniazid and rifampin to complete a total treatment duration of 9 to 12 months. All children with tuberculous disease should be evaluated for HIV infection since its presence may necessitate a longer duration of treatment.

d. Drug-Resistant Tuberculosis

The incidence of drug-resistant tuberculosis appears to be increasing in North America, particularly in large cities such as New York and Miami, and along the Mexican border. For the entire United States, approximately 10% of isolates of *M. tuberculosis* are resistant to at least one drug, while many countries in Latin America and Asia routinely report drug resistance rates of 20–30%. Patterns of drug resistance among children tend to mirror those found among adults in the same population.[99,100] Certain epidemiologic factors such as being an Asian or Latin American immigrant, homelessness, coinfection with HIV, or history of prior antituberculosis treatment correlate with drug resistance in adults and their childhood counterparts.

Treatment for drug-resistant tuberculosis is successful only when at least two bactericidal drugs to which the infecting strain of *M. tuberculosis* is susceptible are given. When a child has possible drug-resistant tuberculosis at least three and usually four or five drugs should be given initially until the exact susceptibility pattern is determined and a more specific regimen can be designed. The specific regimen must be individualized for each patient according to the results of susceptibility testing on the isolates from the child or the adult source case. Although primary resistance to pyrazinamide is rare, pyrazinamide may not be effective in preventing the emergence of rifampin resistance during treatment when isoniazid resistance initially is present. Therefore, the combination of isoniazid, rifampin, and pyrazinamide may not be adequate for children if initial isoniazid or rifampin resistance is present. A fourth drug — usually streptomycin, ethambutol, or ethionamide — also should be given initially. When isoniazid or rifampin resistance is present, the total duration of therapy usually is extended to 12 to 18 months.

Recently, several outbreaks of tuberculosis caused by strains that have become resistant to both isoniazid and rifampin with or without resistance to other drugs have been reported in hospitals and several North American cities. The strains are now referred to as multiple drug-resistant strains. The reported outbreaks have affected primarily HIV-infected adults but tuberculous infection and disease also have occurred among their childhood counterparts. Optimal treatment regimens for these children can be determined only after complete drug susceptibility information from their, or the adult source case, isolate is available.

e. Corticosteroids

Corticosteroids are useful in the treatment of some children with tuberculosis but only when used with effective antituberculosis drugs. They are beneficial

Table 8-4 **Manifestations of tuberculosis that may benefit from corticosteroid therapy**

Tuberculous meningitis
Tuberculoma with edema
Endobronchial disease
Miliary disease with alveolar-capillary block
Constrictive pericarditis
Massive pleural effusion
Pott's disease with nerve compression

---

for tuberculosis in children when the host inflammatory reaction is contributing significantly to tissue damage or impairment of organ function (Table 8-4). There is convincing evidence that corticosteroids decrease mortality rates and long-term neurologic sequelae in children with tuberculous meningitis by reducing vasculitis, inflammation, and, ultimately, intracranial pressure.[101] Lowering the intracranial pressure not only limits tissue damage but also favors the circulation of antituberculosis drugs through the brain and meninges. Short courses of corticosteroids may be effective for children with enlarged hilar lymph nodes that compress the tracheobronchial tree causing respiratory distress, localized emphysema, or segmental pulmonary lesions.[102,103] There also is evidence that corticosteroids can help ameliorate the chronic sequelae associated with acute tuberculous pericardial effusion.[103a] In patients with tuberculous pleural effusion in whom there is shift of the mediastinum and acute respiratory compromise, corticosteroids may cause dramatic improvement in symptoms, although the long-term course probably is unaffected.[35] Some children with severe miliary tuberculosis have dramatic improvement with corticosteroids if the inflammatory reaction is so severe that alveolocapillary block is present. There is no convincing evidence that one corticosteroid is better than another. The most commonly prescribed regimen is prednisone at 1 to 2 mg/kg/day for 4 to 6 weeks, with gradual tapering.

f. Asymptomatic Tuberculous Infection

The treatment of children with asymptomatic tuberculous infection to prevent the development of tuberculous disease is an established practice. The effectiveness of isoniazid preventive therapy in children has approached 100% and the effect has lasted for at least 30 years.[104] Tuberculin-positive children with contact to an infectious adult are at the highest risk of developing disease and always should be given preventive therapy. Almost all tuberculin-positive children without known contact also should receive therapy, especially adolescents and children younger than 6 years of age.

Children who are tuberculin negative, including newborn infants, who have had contact with an infectious adult should receive isoniazid therapy until 10 to 12 weeks after contact has been broken by either physical separation from the source case or chemotherapy. If the repeat tuberculin skin test is negative, isoniazid can be discontinued; if the test is positive, a full course of isoniazid therapy should be given. The American Academy of Pediatrics recommends treatment with isoniazid for 9 months,[93] although 12 months may be more effective (see Chapter 13, this volume). Rifampin is recommended for preventive therapy for children with asymptomatic infection due to an isoniazid-resistant strain of *M. tuberculosis*. Although controlled trials are lacking, either isoniazid or rifampin probably will be effective if given twice weekly under direct observation when adherence with daily therapy cannot be ensured. There are no available data concerning the effectiveness of any therapy regimen in children infected with isoniazid and rifampin resistant strains of *M. tuberculosis*.

g. Supportive and Follow-Up Care

In the prechemotherapy era, supportive care was all the clinician was able to offer children with tuberculosis. With proper chemotherapy, supportive care plays a small role in the management of the child with tuberculosis. Activity need not be restricted unless the child develops respiratory embarrassment or immobilization is necessary for treatment, as in some cases of vertebral tuberculosis. Adequate nutrition is important, although many small children who present with failure to thrive and tuberculosis will not begin to gain weight until several months after effective chemotherapy has been started.

Nonadherence with treatment is a major problem in tuberculosis control due to the long-term nature of treatment and sometimes difficult social circumstances of the patients.[105] Several factors may influence adherence among children with tuberculosis. Many children with significant disease have relatively few symptoms and therefore do not receive the feedback of improvement in symptoms as treatment progresses. Since the initial diagnosis often cannot be confirmed by a positive culture, there is no opportunity to inform the patient and family that the cultures have gone from positive to negative during treatment. Many children in socially disrupted families have multiple caregivers and assurance of administration of medications is lacking. Finally, the lack of dosage preparations suitable for use in children makes the administration of several medications difficult, especially for small infants and toddlers.

An assessment of potential nonadherence should be made at the initiation of therapy. During treatment, if the physician suspects any chance of non-adherence with daily self-administered medications, directly observed therapy should be instituted with the help of the local health department. Responsible adults in the child's environment such as grandparents, teachers, school nurses, or church workers often can be used to help ensure that medication is properly given. Twice weekly directly observed therapy is extremely effective in children and most experts would consider it part of standard antituberculosis treatment.

It is important that the physician and other healthcare workers take an active role in the care of children with tuberculosis. Children should be followed carefully to ensure adherence with treatment, to monitor for toxic reactions to medications, and to ensure that the tuberculosis is coming under adequate control. It is extremely important for the family that a single healthcare provider be identified as the person primarily responsible for care. Nonadherence rates are significantly higher in clinical situations where several physicians care for the child on a rotating basis, as frequently occurs in teaching hospitals with housestaff clinics. In general, children on treatment should be seen at monthly intervals and should be given enough medication at each visit to last until the next scheduled visit.

Anticipatory guidance in taking the several antituberculosis medications is crucial when treating children. Children may receive little medication in the first several weeks due to vomiting and difficult administration until the family develops a dosing scheme that works for them. Commercially available preparations of antituberculosis medications may be difficulty to administer to small children. A liquid suspension of isoniazid is available but its stability is variable and many children have diarrhea and gastrointestinal upset while taking this preparation. Rifampin can be made into a stable suspension by a pharmacist, which is helpful for treating small children who cannot swallow capsules. Isoniazid, pyrazinamide, and other pills can be crushed and given with small amounts of food but rifampin should be taken on an empty stomach, if possible.

The rates of adverse reactions to antituberculosis medications are low enough in children that routine biochemical monitoring is not necessary. If there is any history of previous hepatitis or other chronic illness, it is advisable to obtain a baseline set of serum liver enzyme and uric acid levels. If the patient or family reports any symptoms that could be toxic reactions to antituberculosis medications, the child should have a complete physical examination and a set of serum hepatic enzymes and bilirubin determinations. Serum liver enzyme elevations of two to three times normal are fairly common and do not necessitate discontinuation of medications if all other findings are normal. Mild arthralgias or arthritis could be due to pyrazinamide, but usually are transient even when pyrazinamide is continued. All children taking ethambutol should have regular monitoring of visual acuity and color discrimination.

Radiographic changes with intrathoracic tuberculosis in children occur very slowly and frequent chest radiography is not necessary. A common practice is to obtain a chest radiograph at diagnosis and 1 to 2 months after the beginning of treatment to be sure that no unusual changes in radiographic appearance have occurred. If these radiographs are satisfactory it is not necessary to repeat a chest radiograph until the completion of 6 months of treatment. A normal chest radiograph at this time is not necessary to discontinue treatment. The majority of children with significant intrathoracic adenopathy have abnormal radiographic findings for 1 to 3 years, long after effective antituberculosis treatment has been stopped. If improvement has occurred after 6 months of treatment, medications can be discontinued and the child can be followed at intervals of 3 to 6 months with appropriate chest radiographs to determine continued improvement in radiographic appearance.

II. TUBERCULOSIS IN PREGNANT WOMEN AND THE NEWBORN

A. INTRODUCTION

Before 1985, tuberculosis in the pregnant woman and her newborn infant had become an infrequent event in the United States. Although specific statistics concerning tuberculosis in pregnancy are not reported, the recent increase in total cases and the shift to young adults and children imply that tuberculosis in pregnancy may become an increasing problem. This problem should affect minority urban populations disproportionately because this group has very high tuberculosis rates, a greater relative shift in cases to childbearing-aged adults, and, in general, poor access to prenatal care and testing for tuberculous disease and infection.

The influence of pregnancy on the incidence and prognosis of tuberculosis has been debated since antiquity.[106] At various times, pregnancy has been thought to improve, worsen, or have no effect on the prognosis of tuberculosis. This controversy has lost some of its importance since the advent of effective antituberculosis chemotherapy. Although it generally is accepted that with adequate treatment a pregnant woman with tuberculosis has a prognosis equivalent to that of a comparable nonpregnant woman, debate remains about the use of

Table 8-5 **Potential modes of inoculation of the newborn with *Mycobacterium tuberculosis***

Maternal Focus	Mode of Spread
Pneumonitis	Airborne
Placentitis	Hematogenous (umbilical vessel)
Amniotic	Aspiration of infected fluid
Cervicitis	Direct contact, aspiration

preventive therapy for tuberculous infection during pregnancy and the postpartum period.

B. PATHOGENESIS

The pathogenesis of pulmonary tuberculosis during pregnancy is similar to that for nonpregnant individuals. Shortly after the initiation of infection, some organisms enter the lymphatic and blood vessels and disseminate throughout the body. During this phase of infection, the genitalia, endometrium, or placenta may become involved. Tuberculous endometritis and salpingeal tuberculosis have become rare in the United States. Genital tuberculosis is most likely to start around the time of menarche and can have a very long and relatively asymptomatic course. The fallopian tubes most often are involved (90–100%), followed by the uterus (50–60%), ovaries (20–30%), and cervix (5–15%).[107] Sterility often is the presenting complaint of tuberculous endometritis, which diminishes the likelihood of congenital tuberculosis occurring.[108] When infection of the placenta occurs it results more frequently from disseminated tuberculosis in the mother than from a local endometritis. However, tuberculous endometritis can lead to congenital infection in the newborn.[109,110]

The potential modes of inoculation of the newborn infant with tuberculosis from the mother are shown in Table 8-5. Infection of the neonate through the umbilical cord has been rare with fewer than 200 cases reported in the English language literature. These infants' mothers frequently suffer from tuberculous pleural effusion, meningitis, or disseminated disease during pregnancy or soon after.[111-113] However, in some series of congenital tuberculosis, fewer than 50% of the mothers were known to be suffering from tuberculosis at the time of delivery.[113,114] In most of these cases, diagnosis of the child led to the discovery of the mother's tuberculosis. The intensity of lymphohematogenous spread during pregnancy is one of the factors that determines if congenital tuberculosis will occur. Hematogenous dissemination in the mother leads to infection of the placenta with subsequent transmission to the fetus. Tubercle bacilli have been demonstrated in the decidua, amnion, and chorionic villi of the placenta.[108] However, even massive involvement of the placenta with tuberculosis does not always give rise to congenital infection. It is not clear whether the fetus can be directly infected from the mother's bloodstream without a caseous lesion forming first in the placenta, although this phenomenon has been reported in experimental animal models.[115]

In hematogenous congenital tuberculosis, *M. tuberculosis* reaches the fetus via the umbilical vein. If some bacilli infect the liver, a primary focus develops with involvement of the periportal lymph nodes. However, the bacilli can pass through the liver into the main circulation leading to a primary focus in the fetus' lung. The tubercle bacilli in the lung often remain dormant until after birth when oxygenation and circulation increase significantly, leading to pulmonary tuberculosis in the young infant.

Congenital infection of the infant also might occur via aspiration or ingestion of amniotic fluid.[116] If the caseous lesion in the placenta ruptures directly into the amniotic cavity, the fetus can inhale or ingest the tubercle bacilli. Inhalation or ingestion of infected amniotic fluid is the most likely cause of tuberculosis if the infant has multiple primary foci in the lung, gut, or middle ear.[117]

The pathology of tuberculosis in the fetus and newborn usually demonstrates the predisposition to dissemination and fatal disease.[118] The liver and lungs are the primary involved organs with bone marrow, bone, the gastrointestinal tract, adrenal glands, spleen, kidney, abdominal lymph nodes, and skin also involved frequently.[119] The histologic patterns of involvement are similar to those in adults; tubercles and granulomas are common. Central nervous system involvement occurs in fewer than 50% of cases. In most recent series, the mortality of congenital tuberculosis has been close to 50% due primarily to the failure to suspect the correct diagnosis. Most fatal cases are diagnosed at autopsy.[113,114]

Postnatal acquisition of tuberculosis via airborne inoculation is the most common route of infection for the neonate. It may be impossible to differentiate postnatal infection from prenatal acquisition on clinical grounds alone. It is important to remember that any adult in the neonate's environment can be a source of airborne tuberculosis. Since newborns infected with tuberculosis are at extremely high risk of developing severe forms of disease, investigation of an adult with tuberculosis whose household contains a pregnant woman or newborn infant should be considered a public health emergency. In addition, all adults in contact with an infant suspected of having tuberculous infection or disease should undergo a thorough investigation for tuberculosis.

C. EPIDEMIOLOGY: INTERACTION OF TUBERCULOSIS AND PREGNANCY

The current epidemiology of tuberculosis in pregnant women and the newborn largely is unknown. From 1966 to 1972, the incidence of tuberculosis during pregnancy at New York Lying-in Hospital ranged from 0.6 to 1%.[107] During this time, 2.3% of the patients with culture-proven pulmonary tuberculosis were diagnosed first during pregnancy, a rate equal to that of nonpregnant women of comparable age. There has been no reported large series of pregnant women with tuberculosis in the last two decades.

From ancient times, medical opinions regarding the interaction of pregnancy and tuberculosis have varied considerably. Hippocrates believed that pregnancy had a beneficial effect on tuberculosis, a view that persisted virtually unchallenged into the nineteenth century, when an opposite view emerged. In 1850, Grisolle[120] reported 24 cases of tuberculosis that developed during pregnancy. In all patients the progression of tuberculosis during pregnancy was more severe than usually seen in nonpregnant individuals of the same age. Shortly thereafter, several papers were published that implied that pregnancy had a deleterious effect on tuberculosis. This view gained so much support that by the early twentieth century, the concept of induced abortion to deal with the consequences of tuberculosis during pregnancy became widely accepted.

The opinion that pregnancy had a deleterious effect on tuberculosis predominated until the late 1940s. In 1943, Cohen[121] detected no increased rate of progression of tuberculosis among 100 pregnant women with abnormal chest radiographs. In 1953, Hedvall[122] presented a comprehensive review of published studies concerning tuberculosis in pregnancy in the prechemotherapy era. He cited studies totaling over 1000 cases that reported negative effects of pregnancy on tuberculosis. However, he discovered a nearly equal number of reported cases in which a neutral or favorable relationship between pregnancy and tuberculosis was observed. In his own study of 250 pregnant women with abnormal chest radiographs consistent with tuberculosis, he noted that 9% improved, 7% worsened, and 84% remained unchanged during pregnancy. During the first postpartum year, 9% improved, 15% worsened, and 76% were stable. Crombie[123] noted that 31 of 101 pregnant women with quiescent tuberculosis experienced a relapse after delivery; 20 of the 31 relapses occurred in the first postpartum year. Several other investigators observed a higher risk of relapse during the puerperium. However, other studies failed to support an increased risk of progression of tuberculosis in the postpartum period.[124] Cohen's study failed to show a major increase in activity of tuberculosis during pregnancy or any postpartum interval.[121] Other studies had similar results and, although they did not have control populations, it was estimated that the rates of progression would be comparable to nonpregnant age-matched control subjects.[125,126] From these and other studies it became clear that the anatomic extent of disease, the radiographic pattern, and the susceptibility of the individual patient to tuberculosis are more important than pregnancy itself in determining the course and prognosis of the pregnant woman with tuberculosis.

The controversy concerning the effect of pregnancy or the postpartum period on tuberculosis has lost most of its importance since the advent of effective chemotherapy. With adequate treatment, pregnant women with tuberculosis have the same excellent prognosis as nonpregnant women. Several studies could document no adverse affects of pregnancy, birth, the postpartum period, or lactation on the course of tuberculosis in women receiving chemotherapy.[107,127]

Most of the studies cited previously dealt with the risk of reactivation of tuberculosis among women with abnormal chest radiographs but no evidence of active tuberculous lesions. It is not as clear if women with asymptomatic tuberculous infection but no radiographic disease are at increased risk of developing tuberculous disease during pregnancy or the postpartum period. In 1959, Pridie and Stradling[128] found that the incidence of pulmonary tuberculosis among pregnant women was the same as in the nonpregnant female population of the area. From 1966 to 1972, Schaefer et al.[107] found that the annual pulmonary tuberculosis case rate among pregnant women at New York Lying-in Hospital was 18 to 29 per 100,000 population, comparable to the incidence during the same period in women of child-bearing age in New York City of 19 to 39 per 100,000. Although no definitive study has been reported, it appears unlikely that progression from asymptomatic tuberculous infection to active tuberculosis is accelerated during pregnancy or the postpartum period.

In the prechemotherapy era, active tuberculosis at an advanced stage carried a poor prognosis for both mother and child. Schaefer et al.[107] reported that the infant and maternal mortality from untreated tuberculosis was between 30 and 40%. In the chemotherapy era, the outcome of pregnancy rarely is altered by the presence of tuberculosis in the mother, except in the rare cases of congenital tuberculosis. One study from Norway revealed a higher incidence of toxemia, postpartum hemorrhage, and difficult labor in mothers with tuberculosis compared with control subjects.[129] The incidence of miscarriage was almost 10 times higher in tuberculous mothers, but there was no significant difference in the rate of congenital malformations between children born to mothers with and without tuberculosis. One study reported an incidence of prematurity among infants born to untreated mothers in a tuberculosis sanatarium ranging from 23 to 64%, depending on the severity of tuberculosis in the mother.[130] However, most experts now believe that with adequate treatment of the pregnant tuberculous woman, the prognosis of pregnancy should not be affected adversely by the presence of tuberculosis. Because of the excellent prognosis for both mother and child, the recommendation for therapeutic abortion has been abandoned.

D. CLINICAL MANIFESTATIONS
1. Pregnant Woman

In general, the clinical manifestations of tuberculosis in the pregnant woman are the same as those in nonpregnant individuals of the same age and with the same disease severity. In one series of 27 pregnant and postpartum women with pulmonary tuberculosis, the most common clinical findings were cough, weight loss, fever, malaise, fatigue, and hemoptysis.[131] Almost 20% of the patients had no significant symptoms. The tuberculin skin test was positive in 26 of 27 patients. Diagnosis was established in all cases by culture of sputum for *M. tuberculosis*. A total of 16 of these patients had drug-resistant tuberculosis and their clinical course was marked by more extensive pulmonary involvement, higher incidence of pulmonary complications, longer sputum conversions times, and a higher incidence of death. In other series, approximately 5–10% of pregnant women with tuberculosis have had extrapulmonary disease, a rate comparable to the nonpregnant population. [132]

The indications for treatment and the basic principles for management of tuberculous disease in the pregnant woman are really no different from those in the nonpregnant patient. However, the recommended regimens and drugs used are slightly different, mostly due to possible effects of several drugs on the developing fetus. There is no doubt that untreated tuberculous disease represents a far greater risk to the pregnant woman and her fetus than does appropriate treatment of the disease.[133] The recommended treatment for drug-susceptible tuberculosis in pregnancy is 9 months of isoniazid and rifampin daily, with ethambutol added to the initial regimen until the drug susceptibility pattern is known. Pyridoxine also should be given because of increased requirements for this vitamin in pregnancy.[134] Extensive experience with isoniazid, rifampin, and ethambutol has shown that they are

Table 8-6 **Most frequent signs and symptoms of congenital tuberculosis**

Sign or Symptom	Frequency (in percentage)
Respiratory distress	77
Fever	62
Hepatic and/or splenic enlargement	62
Poor feeding	46
Lethargy or irritability	42
Lymphadenopathy	35
Abdominal distention	27
Failure to thrive	19
Ear discharge	15
Skin lesions	12

[a] Adapted from Hageman, J., Shulman, S., Schreiber, M., Luck, S., Rogeu, R., *Pediatrics*, 66, 980, 1980.

safe to both the mother and fetus.[135] Streptomycin should be avoided during pregnancy, if possible, since almost 20% of infants will have eighth nerve damage if the drug is given to their mothers during pregnancy.[136] The safety of pyrazinamide during pregnancy is unknown. Treatment of drug-resistant tuberculosis in pregnancy is difficult because some of the "contraindicated" or "unknown safety" drugs may be required for adequate treatment; under these conditions, an expert in tuberculosis should be consulted.

2. Newborn

The clinical manifestations of tuberculosis in the fetus or newborn are shown in Table 8-6. Most patients have an abnormal chest radiograph and approximately 50% have a miliary pattern. Some infants with a normal chest radiograph early in the course develop profound radiographic abnormalities as the disease progresses. The most common findings are adenopathy and parenchymal infiltrates. Occasionally, the pulmonary involvement progresses very rapidly, leading to development of a thin-walled cavity.

The clinical presentation of tuberculosis in the newborn is similar to that caused by bacterial sepsis and other congenital infections such as syphilis and cytomegalovirus. The diagnosis of congenital tuberculosis should be suspected in any infant with appropriate signs and symptoms who does not respond to vigorous antibiotic therapy and whose evaluation for other congenital infections is unrevealing. Of course, suspicion also should be high if the mother has or has had tuberculosis or if she is in a high-risk group for tuberculosis.

The timely diagnosis of congenital or neonatal tuberculosis often is difficult. The tuberculin skin test reaction usually is negative initially, although it may become positive after 1 to 3 months. The diagnosis must be established by finding acid-fast bacilli in body fluids or tissue and by culturing *M. tuberculosis*. A positive acid-fast smear of an early morning gastric aspirate in a newborn should be considered indicative of tuberculosis, although false-positive smears occur. Direct acid-fast smears from middle ear fluid, bone marrow, tracheal aspirate, or biopsy tissue can be useful and should be attempted more frequently. One study found positive cultures for *M. tuberculosis* in 10 of 12 gastric aspirates, 3 of 3 liver biopsies, 3 of 3 lymph nodes biopsies, and 2 of 4 bone marrow aspirations from children with congenital tuberculosis.[113] Open lung biopsy also has been used to establish the diagnosis.[137] The CSF should be examined and cultured, although the yield for isolating *M. tuberculosis* is low.[113,114]

The most important clue to rapidly establish the diagnosis of congenital or neonatal tuberculosis is the maternal and family history. Suspicion should increase if the mother or other family members suffer from unexplained pneumonia, bronchitis, pleural effusion, meningeal disease, or endometritis during, shortly before, or after pregnancy. Testing of both parents and other family members can yield important clues about the presence of tuberculosis within the family. The importance of this epidemiologic information cannot be overemphasized. The need for thorough investigation of the mother was emphasized by Hageman et al.,[113] who found that only 10 of 26 mothers who gave birth to neonates with congenital tuberculosis were diagnosed prior to their infants; the other 16 were discovered as part of the investigation of the infant.

The optimal treatment of congenital tuberculosis has not been established since the rarity of the condition precludes formal treatment trials. It would appear that the basic principles for treatment of other children and adults also apply to the treatment of congenital tuberculosis. Although the optimal duration of therapy has not been established, many experts would treat infants with congenital tuberculosis for a total duration of 9 to 12 months due to the decreased immunologic capability of the young infant. Isoniazid given alone is known to be safe in the neonate.[113,114] There are no comparable data for isoniazid given in combination with other drugs or for other drugs alone. Rifampin, pyrazinamide, streptomycin, and kanamycin appear to be safe in neonates. Young infants taking these drugs should have biochemical monitoring of serum liver enzymes and uric acid performed on a regular basis. Although the pharmacokinetics of antituberculosis drugs in the neonate are basically unknown, the doses listed in Table 8-3 appear to be effective and relatively safe.

E. TESTING FOR TUBERCULOSIS DURING PREGNANCY

For all pregnant women, the history obtained in an early visit should include questions about a previously positive tuberculin skin test, previous treatment for tuberculosis, current symptoms compatible with tuberculosis, and known exposure to other adults with the disease. Membership in a high risk group is a sufficient reason for a tuberculin skin test. For many high-risk women, prenatal or peripartum care represents their only contact with the healthcare system and the opportunity to test them for tuberculous infection or disease should not be lost. Some experts believe that all pregnant women should receive a tuberculin skin test. However, it must be emphasized that women coinfected with HIV and *M. tuberculosis* may show no reaction to a tuberculin skin test. Pregnant women at high risk for or with known HIV infection should have a thorough investigation for tuberculosis.

The effect of pregnancy on tuberculin hypersensitivity as measured by the tuberculin skin test is controversial.[138] Some studies have shown a decrease in *in vitro* lymphocyte reactivity to PPD during pregnancy.[139] However, *in vivo* studies using patients as their own controls have demonstrated no effect of pregnancy on cutaneous delayed hypersensitivity to tuberculin.[140,141] Most experts believe the tuberculin test by the Mantoux technique is valid throughout pregnancy. There is no evidence that the tuberculin skin test has adverse affects on the pregnant mother or fetus or that skin testing reactivates quiescent foci of tuberculous infection.

Routine chest radiography is not currently advisable as a screening test for pregnant women because the prevalence of tuberculosis remains fairly low.[142] However, with appropriate shielding, pregnant women with a positive tuberculin skin test result should have a chest radiograph to rule out active tuberculosis. In addition, a thorough review of systems and physical examination should be carried out to exclude extrapulmonary tuberculosis.

The principles of treatment of asymptomatic tuberculous infection are similar for pregnant women and other adults of comparable age. Although treatment of tuberculous disease during pregnancy is unquestioned, the treatment of the pregnant woman who has an asymptomatic tuberculous infection is more controversial. Some clinicians prefer to delay preventive therapy until after delivery because pregnancy does not seem to increase the risk of developing active tuberculosis. Others believe that because recent infection can be accompanied by hematogenous spread to the placenta, it is preferable to treat without delay or to wait until the second trimester to start chemotherapy.[143] Certainly, the benefits of immediate treatment are greater in high risk patients such as HIV-positive women or close contacts who are recent convertors.

Recent reports suggest that the risk of isoniazid-associated hepatitis and death is higher in women than men, and that women in the postpartum period are especially vulnerable to isoniazid hepatotoxicity.[144,145] The authors of these studies suggest that it might be prudent to avoid isoniazid during the postpartum period or at least to monitor postpartum women taking isoniazid with frequent examinations and laboratory studies. The possible increased risk of isoniazid hepatoxicity must be weighed against the risk of developing active tuberculosis as well as the consequences to both mother and baby should tuberculous disease develop in the mother.

Because treatment of tuberculosis in pregnant women often continues after delivery, the question arises whether it is safe for the mother to breast-feed her infant. Snider and Powell[146] concluded that a breast-feeding infant would receive no more than 20% of the usual therapeutic dosage of isoniazid for infants and less than 11% for other antituberculosis drugs. Potential toxic affects of drugs delivered via breast milk have not been reported. However, because pyridoxine deficiency in the neonate can cause seizures,[147] and breast milk has relatively low levels of pyridoxine, an infant whose breast-feeding mother is taking isoniazid probably should receive supplemental pyridoxine.

F. MANAGEMENT WHEN THE MOTHER HAS A POSITIVE TUBERCULIN SKIN TEST

1. Negative Chest Radiograph

If the mother is well, no separation of infant and mother is needed. The child needs no special evaluation or therapy if he remains asymptomatic. Because the mother's skin test result may be a marker that there is infectious tuberculosis within the household, all other household members should receive a Mantoux skin test and further evaluation as indicated. The mother usually is a candidate for therapy for tuberculous infection.

2. Abnormal Chest Radiograph

In general, the newborn should be separated from the mother until the chest radiograph is taken, hopefully a matter of only hours. If the mother's radiograph is abnormal, separation should be maintained until the mother has been evaluated thoroughly. Examination of the mother's sputum always is necessary even if obtaining a sample requires vigorous measures.

If the mother's chest radiograph is abnormal but the history, physical examination, sputum examination, and evaluation of the radiograph reveal no evidence of active tuberculosis, it is reasonable to assume that the infant is at low risk. The radiographic abnormality is due to another cause or a quiescent focus of past tuberculosis. However, if the mother remains untreated, she may develop active tuberculosis and expose her infant.[148,149] The untreated mother should receive appropriate treatment, and she and her infant receive careful follow-up care. In addition, all household members should be evaluated for tuberculosis.

If the mother's chest radiograph or acid-fast sputum smear reveals evidence of active tuberculosis, additional steps will be necessary to protect the infant. Isoniazid preventive therapy for newborn infants has been so efficacious that separation of the mother and infant no longer is considered mandatory.[150,151] Separation should occur only if the mother is ill enough to require hospitalization, she has been or is expected to become nonadherent with her treatment, or she has or is suspected of having a resistant strain. Because isoniazid resistance is increasing, it is not always clear that isoniazid therapy for the neonate will be effective. If, due to epidemiologic factors, isoniazid resistance is suspected or the mother's adherence with medication is in question, rigorous separation of the infant from the mother must be considered. The duration of separation will vary but must be at least as long as it takes to render the mother noninfectious. Although modern chemotherapy often eliminates infectivity within several weeks, it takes several more weeks to document sterility of the mother's sputum culture. A conservative suggestion for duration of separation would be 6 to 12 weeks of culture negativity for the mother.[115] In cases where the organism is drug susceptible, isoniazid should be continued in the infant at least until the mother has been shown to be sputum culture negative for 3 months. At that time, a Mantoux tuberculin skin test is placed on the child; if positive, isoniazid is continued for a total duration of 9 to 12 months, but if negative, isoniazid can be discontinued.

If a family member has tuberculosis and cannot be relied on to receive proper treatment, then BCG vaccination of the infant should be considered.[152] Vaccination with BCG appears to decrease the risk of tuberculosis in the infant but the effect is variable. Kendig[149] reported 117 infants born to mothers with active tuberculosis around the time of delivery; none of the 30 BCG-vaccinated infants developed tuberculosis, while 38 cases of tuberculosis and 3 deaths occurred among the 75 infants who received neither BCG vaccine nor isoniazid. Similar studies in England and Canada also described the apparent efficacy of BCG given to neonates.[152,153] BCG has some protective effect against the development of tuberculosis in newborns and appears to decrease the incidence of life-threatening forms of disease. Many experts recommend that the child be kept out of the household until the skin test becomes reactive, although there is poor correlation between skin test status and the presence or absence of infection. While routine BCG vaccination of newborns is not appropriate in the United States, it should be considered for the neonate whose household is chaotic and cannot be made free from tuberculosis, or who is likely to be lost to follow-up. For further information on this matter, please refer to Chapter 15 (this volume).

REFERENCES

1. Braun, M. M., Cauthen, G., Relationship of the human immunodeficiency virus epidemic to pediatric tuberculosis and bacille Calmette-Guerin immunization, *Pediatr. Infect. Dis. J.*, 11, 220, 1992.
2. Centers for Disease Control, CDC surveillance summaries. Tuberculosis morbidity in the United States: final data, 1990, *MMWR*, 40 (SS-3), 23, 1991.
3. Starke, J. R., Jacobs, R. F., Jereb, J., Resurgence of tuberculosis in children, *J. Pediatr.*, 120, 839, 1992.
4. International Union Against Tuberculosis and Lung Disease, Tuberculosis in children: guidelines for diagnosis, prevention and treatment, *Bull. Int. Union Tuberc. Lung Dis.*, 66, 61, 1991.
5. Murray, C. J. L., Styblo, K., Rouillon, A., Tuberculosis in developing countries: burden, intervention, and cost, *Bull. Int. Union Tuberc. Lung Dis.*, 65, 6, 1990.
6. Kochi, A., The global tuberculosis situation and the new control strategy of the World Health Organization, *Tubercle*, 72, 1, 1991.
7. Snider, D. E., Rieder, H. L., Combs, D., Bloch, A. B., Hayden, C. H., Smith, M. H. D., Tuberculosis in children, *Pediatr. Infect. Dis. J.*, 7, 271, 1988.
8. Wallgren, A., On contagiousness of childhood tuberculosis, *Acta Paediatr. Scand.*, 22, 229, 1937.
9. Smith, M. H. D., Marquis, J. R., Tuberculosis and other mycobacterial diseases, in *Textbook of Pediatric Infectious Diseases*, 2nd ed., Feigin, R. D., Cherry, J. D., Eds., W.B. Saunders, Philadelphia, 1987.
10. Smith, M. H. D., Tuberculosis in children and adolescents, *Clin. Chest Med.*, 10, 381, 1989.
11. Reider, H. L., Snider, D. E., Jr., Cauthen, G. M., Extrapulmonary tuberculosis in the United States, *Am. Rev. Resp. Dis.*, 141, 347, 1990.
12. Lincoln, E. M., Epidemics of tuberculosis, *Adv. Tuberc. Res.*, 14, 157, 1965.
13. Nolan, C. M., Barr, H., Elarth, A. M., Boase, J., Tuberculosis in a daycare home, *Pediatrics*, 79, 630, 1987.
14. Leggiadro, R. J., Gallory, B., Dowdy, S., Larkin, J., An outbreak of tuberculosis in a family daycare home, *Pediatr. Infect. Dis. J.*, 8, 52, 1989.
15. Bloch, A. B., Reider, H. L., Kelly, G. D., Cauthen, G. M., Hayden, C. H., Snider, D. E., Jr., The epidemiology of tuberculosis in the United States, *Clin. Chest Med.*, 10, 297, 1989.
16. Braun, M., Badi, N., Ryder, R., Baende, E., Mukadi, Y., Nsuami, M., Matela, B., Williams, J. C., Kaboto, M., Heyward, W., A retrospective cohort study of the risk of tuberculosis among women of childbearing age with HIV infection in Zaire, *Am. Rev. Resp. Dis.*, 143, 501, 1991.
17. Chaisson, R. E., Slutkin, G., Tuberculosis and human immunodeficiency virus infection, *J. Infect. Dis.*, 159, 96, 1989.
18. Klein, N. C., Duncanson, F. P., Lenox, T. H., Pitta, A., Cohen, S. C., Wormser, G. P., Use of mycobacterial smears in the diagnosis of pulmonary tuberculosis in AIDS/ARC patients, *Chest*, 95, 1190, 1989.
19. Jones, D. S., Malecki, J. M., Bigler, W. J., Witte, J. J., Oxtoby, M. J., Pediatric tuberculosis and human immunodeficiency virus infection in Palm Beach County, Florida, *Am. J. Dis. Child.*, 146, 1166, 1992.
20. Moss, W. J., Dodyo, T., Suarez, M., Nicholas, S. W., Abrams, E., Tuberculosis in children infected with human immunodeficiency virus: a report of five cases, *Pediatr. Infect. Dis. J.*, 10, 114, 1992.
21. Varteresian-Karanfil, L., Josephson, A., Fikrig, S., Kauffman, S., Steiner, P., Pulmonary infection and cavity formation caused by *Mycobacterium tuberculosis* in a child with AIDS, *N. Engl. J. Med.*, 319, 1018, 1988.
22. Chintu, C., Bhat, G., Luo, C., Raviglione, M., Diwan, V., Dupont, H. L., Zumla, A., Seroprevalence of human immunodeficiency virus type 1 infection in Zambian children with tuberculosis, *Pediatr. Infect. Dis. J.*, 12, 499, 1993.
23. Hsu, K. H. K., Contact investigation: a practical approach to tuberculosis eradication, *Am. J. Public Health*, 53, 1761, 1963.

24. Barry, M. A., Shirley, L., Grady, M. T., Etkind, S. W., Almeida, C., Bernardo, J., Lamb, G. A., Tuberculous infection in urban adolescents: results of a school-based testing program, *Am. J. Public Health*, 80, 439, 1990.

25. Davidson, P. T., Ashkar, B., Salem, N., Tuberculosis testing of children entering school in Los Angeles County, California, *Am. Rev. Resp. Dis.*, 141 (Suppl.), 336, 1990.

26. Starke, J. R., Taylor, K. T., Martindill, C. A., Pyle, N. D., Herrin, C. M., Extremely high rates of tuberculin reactivity among young school children in Houston, *Am. Rev. Resp. Dis.*, 137 (Suppl.), 22, 1988.

27. Miller, F. J. W., Seale, R. M. E., Taylor, M. D., *Tuberculosis in Children*, Little Brown, Boston, 1963.

28. Starke, J. R., Taylor-Watts, K. T., Tuberculosis in the pediatric population of Houston, Texas, *Pediatrics*, 84, 28, 1989.

29. Daly, J. F., Brown, D. S., Lincoln, E. M., Wilkins, V. N., Endobronchial tuberculosis in children, *Dis. Chest*, 22, 380, 1952.

30. Lorriman, G., Bentley, F. J., The incidence of segmental lesions in primary tuberculosis of childhood, *Am. Rev. Tuberc.*, 79, 756, 1959.

31. Morrison, J. B., Natural history of segmental lesions in primary pulmonary tuberculosis, *Arch. Dis. Child.*, 48, 90, 1973.

32. Stansberry, S. D., Tuberculosis in infants and children, *J. Thorac. Imaging*, 5, 17, 1990.

33. Giammona, S. T., Poole, C. A., Zelowitz, P., Skrovan, C., Massive lymphadenopathy in primary pulmonary tuberculosis in children, *Am. Rev. Resp. Dis.*, 100, 480, 1969.

34. Lincoln, E. M., Gilbert, L., Morales, S. M., Chronic pulmonary tuberculosis in individuals with known previous primary tuberculosis, *Dis. Chest*, 38, 473, 1960.

35. Smith, M. H. D., Matsaniotis, N., Treatment of tuberculous pleural effusions with particular reference to adrenal corticosteroids, *Pediatrics*, 22, 1074, 1958.

36. Lincoln, E. M., Davies, P. A., Bovornkitti, S., Tuberculous pleurisy with effusion in children. A study of 202 children with particular reference to prognosis, *Am. Rev. Tuberc.*, 77, 271, 1958.

37. Boyd, G. L., Tuberculous pericarditis in children, *Am. J. Dis. Child.*, 86, 293, 1953.

38. Hussey, G., Chisholm, T., Kibel, M., Miliary tuberculosis in children: a review of 94 cases, *Pediatr. Infect. Dis. J.*, 10, 832, 1991.

39. Schuitt, K. E., Miliary tuberculosis in children. Clinical and laboratory manifestations in 19 patients, *Am. J. Dis. Child.*, 133, 583, 1979.

40. Margileth, A. M., Chandra, R., Altman, R. P., Chronic lymphadenopathy due to mycobacterial infection. Clinical features, diagnosis, histopathology and management, *Am. J. Dis. Child.*, 138, 917, 1984.

41. Appling D., Miller, R. H. Mycobacterial cervical lymphadenopathy: 1981 update, *Laryngoscope*, 91, 1259, 1981.

42. Rich, A. R., McCordock, H. A., The pathogenesis of tuberculous meningitis, *Bull. Johns Hopkins Hosp.*, 52, 5, 1933.

43. Cotton, M. F., Donald, P. R., Schoeman, J. F., Aalbers, C., VanZyl, L. E., Lombard, C., Plasma arginine vasopressin and the syndrome of inappropriate antidiuretic hormone secretion in tuberculous meningitis, *Pediatr. Infect. Dis. J.*, 10, 837, 1991.

44. Jaffe, I. P., Tuberculous meningitis in childhood, *Lancet*, 1, 738, 1982.

45. Waecker, N. J., Jr., Conners, J. D., Central nervous system tuberculosis in children: a review of 30 cases, *Pediatr. Infect. Dis. J.*, 9, 539, 1990.

46. Idriss, Z. H., Sinno, A., Kronfol, N. M., Tuberculous meningitis in childhood: 43 cases, *Am. J. Dis. Child.*, 130, 364, 1976.

47. Udani, P. M., Parekh, U. C., Dastur, D. K., Neurologic and related syndromes in CNS tuberculosis: clinical features and pathogenesis, *J. Neurol. Sci.*, 14, 341, 1971.

48. Ramachandran, P., Duraipandian, M., Nagarajan, M., Probhakar, R., Ramakrishnan, C. V., Tripathy, S. P., Three chemotherapy studies of tuberculous meningitis in children, *Tubercle*, 67, 17, 1986.

49. Zarabi, M., Sane, S., Girdany, B. R., Chest roentgenogram in the early diagnosis of tuberculous meningitis in children, *Am. J. Dis. Child.*, 121, 389, 1971.

50. Chambers, S. T., Hendrickse, W. A., Record, C., Rudge, P., Smith, H., Paradoxical expansion of intracranial tuberculomas during chemotherapy, *Lancet*, 2, 181, 1984.

51. Teoh, R., Humphries, M. J., O'Mahony, S. G., Symptomatic intracranial tuberculoma developing during treatment of tuberculosis: a report of 10 patients and review of the literature, *Q. J. Med.*, 63, 449, 1987.

52. Janssens, J. P., deHaller, R., Spinal tuberculosis in a developed country, *Clin. Ortho. Rel. Res.*, 257, 67, 1990.

53. Bavadekar, A., Osteoarticular tuberculosis in children, *Prog. Pediatr. Surg.*, 15, 131, 1982.

54. American Thoracic Society, Diagnostic standards and classification of tuberculosis, *Am. Rev. Resp. Dis.*, 142, 725, 1990.

55. Hsu, K. H. K., Tuberculin reaction in children treated with isoniazid, *Am. J. Dis. Child.*, 137, 1090, 1983.

56. Steiner, P., Rao, M., Victoria, M. S., Jabbar, H., Steiner, M., Persistently negative tuberculin reactions: their presence among children culture positive for *Mycobacterium tuberculosis*, *Am. J. Dis. Child.*, 134, 747, 1980.

57. Seibart, A. F., Bass, J. B., Jr., Tuberculin skin testing: guidelines for the 1990's, *J. Resp. Dis.*, 11, 225, 1990.

58. Sepulveda, R. L., Burr, C., Ferrer, X., Sorensen, R. U., Booster effect of tuberculin testing in healthy 6-year old school children vaccinated with bacille Calmette-Guerin at birth in Santiago, Chile, *Pediatr. Infect. Dis. J.*, 7, 578, 1988.

59. Catanzaro, A., Multiple-puncture skin test and Mantoux test in Southeast Asian refugees, *Chest*, 87, 346, 1985.

60. Howard, T. P., Soloman, D. A., Reading the tuberculin skin test: who, when and how?, *Arch. Intern. Med.*, 148, 2457, 1988.

61. Ashley, M. J., Siebenmann, C. O., Tuberculin skin sensitivity following BCG vaccination with vaccines of high and low viable counts, *Can. Med. Assoc. J.*, 97, 1335, 1967.

62. Lifschitz, M., The value of the tuberculin skin test as a screening test for tuberculosis among BCG-vaccinated children, *Pediatrics*, 36, 264, 1965.

63. Karalliede, S., Katugha, L. P., Uragoda, C. G., The tuberculin response of Sri Lankan children after BCG vaccination at birth, *Tubercle*, 68, 33, 1987.

64. Abadco, D. L., Steiner, P., Gastric lavage is better than bronchoalveolar lavage for isolation of *Mycobacterium tuberculosis* in childhood pulmonary tuberculosis, *Pediatr. Infect. Dis. J.*, 11, 735, 1992.

65. Klotz, S. A., Penn, R. L., Acid-fast staining of urine and gastric contents is an excellent indicator of mycobacterial disease, *Am. Rev. Resp. Dis.*, 136, 1197, 1987.

66. Alde, S. L. M., Pinasco, H. M., Pelosi, F. R., Budani, H. F., Palma-Beltran, O. H., Gonzalez-Montaner, L. J., Evaluation of an enzyme-linked immunosorbent assay using an IgG antibody to *Mycobacterium tuberculosis* antigens in the diagnosis of active tuberculosis in children, *Am. Rev. Resp. Dis.*, 139, 748, 1989.

67. Hussey, G., Kibel, M., Dempster, W., The serodiagnosis of tuberculosis in children: an evaluation of an ELISA test using IgG antibodies to *Mycobacterium tuberculosis*, strain H37RV, *Ann. Tropic. Med.*, 11, 113, 1991.

68. Rosen, E. U., The diagnostic value of an enzyme-linked immune sorbent assay using absorbed mycobacterial sonicates in children, *Tubercle*, 71, 127, 1990.

69. Starke, J. R., Ong, L. T., Eisenach, K. D., Connelly, K. K., Detection of *Mycobacterium tuberculosis* in gastric aspirate samples from children using a polymerase chain reaction, *Am. Rev. Resp. Dis.*, 147 (Suppl.), 801, 1993.

70. Pierre, C., Oliver, C., Lecossier, D., Boussougont, Y., Yeni, P., Hance, A. J., Diagnosis of primary tuberculosis in children by amplification and detection of mycobacterial DNA, *Am. Rev. Resp. Dis.*, 147, 420, 1993.

71. Starke, J. R., Multidrug therapy for tuberculosis in children, *Pediatr. Infect. Dis. J.*, 9, 785, 1990.

72. Reed, M. D., Blumer, J. L., Clinical pharmacology of antitubercular drugs, *Pediatr. Clin. North Am.*, 30, 177, 1983.

73. Stein, M. T., Liang, D., Clinical hepatotoxicity of isoniazid in children, *Pediatrics*, 64, 499, 1979.

74. O'Brien, R. J., Long, M. W., Cross, F. S., Lyle, M. A., Snider, D. E., Jr., Hepatotoxicity from isoniazid and rifampin among children treated for tuberculosis, *Pediatrics*, 72, 491, 1983.

75. Olson, W. A., Pruitt, A. W., Dayton, P. G., Plasma concentrations of isoniazid in children with tuberculous infections, *Pediatrics*, 67, 876, 1981.

76. Tsagarpoulou-Stinga, H., Mataki Emmanouilidou, T., Karida-Kavalioti, S., Manios, S., Hepatotoxic reactions in children with severe tuberculosis treated with isoniazid-rifampin, *Pediatr. Infect. Dis. J.*, 4, 270, 1985.

77. Kumar, A., Misra, P. K., Mehotra, R., Govil, Y. C., Rana, G. S., Hepatotoxicity of rifampin and isoniazid: is it all drug-induced hepatitis?, *Am. Rev. Resp. Dis.*, 143, 1350, 1991.

78. Notterman, D. A., Nardi, M., Saslow, J. G., Effect of dose formulation on isoniazid adsorption in two young children, *Pediatrics*, 77, 850, 1986.

79. Seifart, H. I., Parkin, D. P., Donald, P. R., Stability of isoniazid, rifampin, and pyrazinamide in suspensions used for the treatment of tuberculosis in children, *Pediatr. Infect. Dis. J.*, 10, 827, 1991.

80. Martinez-Roig, A., Roig, A., Cami, J., Llorens-Terol, J., de la Torre, R., Perich, F., Acetylation phenotype and hepatotoxicity in the treatment of tuberculosis in children, *Pediatrics*, 77, 912, 1986.

81. Pellock, J. M., Howell, J., Kendig, E. L., Jr., Baker, H., Pyridoxine deficiency in children treated with isoniazid, *Chest*, 87, 658, 1985.

82. Litt, I. F., Cohen, M. I., McNamara, H., Isoniazid hepatitis in adolescents, *J. Pediatr.*, 89, 133, 1976.

83. Donald, P. R., Seifart, H., Cerebrospinal fluid pyrazinamide concentrations in children with tuberculous meningitis, *Pediatr. Infect. Dis. J.*, 7, 469, 1988.

84. Snider, D. E., Jr., Layde, P. M., Johnson, M. W., Treatment of tuberculosis during pregnancy, *Am. Rev. Resp. Dis.*, 122, 65, 1980.

85. Abernathy, R. S., Dutt, A. K., Stead, W. W., Doers, D. L., Short-course chemotherapy for tuberculosis in children, *Pediatrics*, 72, 801, 1983.

86. Jacobs, R. F., Abernathy, R. S., The treatment of tuberculosis in children, *Pediatr. Infect. Dis. J.*, 4, 513, 1985.

87. Reis, F. J. C., Bedran, M. R. M., Moura, J. A. R., Assis, I., Rodrigues, M. E., Six-month isoniazid-rifampin treatment for pulmonary tuberculosis in children, *Am. Rev. Resp. Dis.*, 142, 996, 1990.

88. Ibanez, S., Ross, G., Quimioterapia abreviado de 6 meses en tuberculosis pulmonar infantil, *Rev. Chil. Pediatr.*, 51, 249, 1980.

89. Varudkar, B. L., Short-course chemotherapy for tuberculosis in children, *Indian J. Pediatr.*, 52, 593, 1985.

90. Biddulph, J., Short-course chemotherapy for childhood tuberculosis, *Pediatr. Infect. Dis. J.*, 9, 794, 1990.

91. Kumar, L., Dhand, R., Singhi, P. D., Rao, K. L. N., Katariya, S., A randomized trial of fully intermittent and daily followed by intermittent short — course chemotherapy for childhood tuberculosis, *Pediatr. Infect. Dis. J.*, 9, 802, 1990.

92. Tsakalidis, D., Pratsidou, P., Hitoglou-Makedou, A., Tzouvelekis, G., Sofroniadis, I., Intensive short course chemotherapy for treatment of Greek children with tuberculosis, *Pediatr. Infect. Dis. J.*, 11, 1036, 1992.

93. American Academy of Pediatrics Committee on Infectious Diseases, Chemotherapy for tuberculosis in infants and children, *Pediatrics*, 89, 161, 1992.

94. Dutt, A. K., Doers, D., Stead, W. W., Short-course chemotherapy for extrapulmonary tuberculosis, *Ann. Intern. Med.*, 107, 7, 1986.

95. Jawahar, M. S., Sivasubramanian, S., Vijayan, V. K., Ramakrishnan, C. V., Paramasivan, C. N., Selvakumar, V., Paul, S., Tripathy, S. P., Prabhakar, R., Short-course chemotherapy for tuberculous lymphadenitis in children, *Br. Med. J.*, 301, 359, 1990.

96. Visudhiphan, P., Chiemchanya, S., Tuberculous meningitis in children: treatment with isoniazid and rifampin for twelve months, *J. Pediatr.*, 114, 875, 1989.

97. Jacobs, R. F., Sunakorn, P., Chotpitayasunonah, T., Pope, S., Kelleher, K., Intensive short-course chemotherapy for tuberculous meningitis, *Pediatr. Infect. Dis. J.*, 11, 194, 1992.

98. Barnes, P. F., Bloch, A. B., Davidson, P. T., Snider, D. E., Jr., Tuberculosis in patients with human immunodeficiency virus infection, *N. Engl. J. Med.*, 324, 1644, 1991.

99. Steiner, P., Rao, M., Victoria, M. S., Hunt, J., Steiner, M., A continuing study of primary drug-resistant tuberculosis among children observed at Kings County Hospital Medical Center between the years 1961–1980, *Am. Rev. Resp. Dis.*, 128, 425, 1983.

100. Steiner, P., Rao, M., Mitchell, M., Steiner, M., Primary drug-resistant tuberculosis in children. Correlation of drug-susceptibility patterns of matched patient and source case strains of *Mycobacterium tuberculosis*, *Am. J. Dis. Child.*, 139, 780, 1985.

101. Girgis, N. I., Farid, Z., Kilpatrick, M. E., Sultan, Y., Mikhail, I. A., Dexamethasone adjunctive treatment for tuberculous meningitis, *Pediatr. Infect. Dis. J.*, 10, 179, 1991.

102. Nemir, R. L., Cordova, J., Vaziri, F., Toledo, F., Prednisone as an adjunct in the chemotherapy of lymph node-bronchial tuberculosis in childhood: a double-blinded study. II. Further term observation, *Am. Rev. Resp. Dis.*, 95, 402, 1967.

103. Toppet, M., Malfroot, A., Derde, M. P., Toppet, V., Spehl, M., Dab, I., Corticosteroids in primary tuberculosis with bronchial obstruction, *Arch. Dis. Child.*, 65, 1222, 1990.

103a. Strang, J. I. G., Kakaza, H. H. S., Gibson, D. G., Allen, B. W., Mitchison, D. A., Evans, D. J., Girling, D. J., Nunn, A. J., Fox, W., Controlled clinical trial of complete open surgical drainage and prednisolone in treatment of tuberculous pericardial effusion in Transkei, *Lancet*, 2, 759, 1988.

104. Hsu, K. H. K., Thirty years after isoniazid. Its impact on tuberculosis in children and adolescents, *J. Am. Med. Assoc.*, 251, 1283, 1984.

105. Sbarbaro, J. A., Compliance: Inducements and enforcements, *Chest*, 76 (Suppl.), 750, 1979.

106. Snider, D. E., Jr., Pregnancy and tuberculosis, *Chest*, 86, 11, 1984.

107. Schaefer, G., Zervoudakis, I. A., Fuchs, F. F., Pregnancy and pulmonary tuberculosis, *Obstet. Gynecol.*, 46, 706, 1975.

108. Bazaz-Malik, G., Maheshwari, B., Lal, N., Tuberculous endometritis: a clinicopathologic study of 1000 cases, *Br. J. Obstet. Gynaecol.*, 90, 84, 1983.

109. Hallum, J. L., Thomas, H. E., Full term pregnancy after proved endometrial tuberculosis, *J. Obstet. Gyneaecol. Br. Emp.*, 62, 548, 1955.

110. Kaplan, C., Benirschke, K., Tarzy, B., Placental tuberculosis in early and late pregnancy, *Am. J. Obstet. Gynecol.*, 137, 858, 1980.

111. Centeno, R. S. , Winter, J., Bentson, J. R., Central nervous system tuberculosis related to pregnancy, *J. Comput. Tomogr.*, 6, 141, 1982.

112. Grenville-Mathers, R., Harris, W. C., Trenchard, H. J., Tuberculous primary infection in pregnancy and its relation to congenital tuberculosis, *Tubercle*, 41, 181, 1960.

113. Hageman, J., Shulman, S., Schreiber, M., Congenital tuberculosis: critical reappraisal of clinical findings and diagnostic procedures, *Pediatrics*, 66, 980, 1980.

114. Nemir, R. L., O'Hare, D., Congenital tuberculosis, *Am. J. Dis. Child.*, 139, 284, 1985.

115. Smith, M. H. D., Teele, D. W., Tuberculosis, in *Infectious Diseases of the Fetus and Newborn*, 3rd ed., Remington, J. S., Klein, J. O., Eds., W.B. Saunders, Philadelphia, 1990.

116. Hertzog, A. J., Chapman, S., Herring, J., Congenital pulmonary aspiration-tuberculosis, *Am. J. Clin. Pathol.*, 19, 1139, 1940.

117. Hughesdon, M. R., Congenital tuberculosis, *Arch. Dis. Child.*, 21, 131, 1946.

118. Jacobs, R. F., Abernathy, R. S., Management of tuberculosis in pregnancy and the newborn, *Clin. Perinatol.*, 15, 305, 1988.

119. Siegel, M., Pathologic findings and pathogenesis of congenital tuberculosis, *Am. Rev. Tuberc.*, 29, 297, 1934.

120. Grisolle, A., De l'influence que la grossesse et la phthisie pulmonaire excercent reciproquement l'une sur l'autre, *Arch. Gener. Med.*, 22, 41, 1850.

121. Cohen, R. C., Effect of pregnancy and parturition on pulmonary tuberculosis, *Br. Med. J.*, 2, 775, 1943.

122. Hedvall, E., Pregnancy and tuberculosis, *Acta Med. Scand.*, 147 (Suppl. 286), 1, 1953.

123. Crombie, J. B., Pregnancy and pulmonary tuberculosis, *Br. J. Tuberc.*, 48, 97, 1954.

124. Rosenbach, L. M., Gangemi, C. R., Tuberculosis and pregnancy, *J. Am. Med. Assoc.*, 161, 1035, 1956.

125. Cohen, J. D., Patton, E. A., Badger, T. L., The tuberculous mother, *Am. Rev. Resp. Dis.*, 65, 1, 1952.

126. Edge, J. R., Pulmonary tuberculosis and pregnancy, *Br. Med. J.*, 2, 845, 1952.

127. De March, P., Tuberculosis and pregnancy, *Chest*, 68, 800, 1975.

128. Pridie, R. B., Stradling, P., Management of pulmonary tuberculosis during pregnancy, *Br. Med. J.*, 3, 78, 1961.

129. Bjerkedal, T., Bahna, S. L., Lehmann, E. H., Course and outcome of pregnancy in women with pulmonary tuberculosis, *Scand. J. Resp. Dis.*, 56, 245, 1975.

130. Ratner, B., Rostler, A. E., Salgado, P. S., Care, feeding and fate of premature and full term infants born of tuberculous mothers, *Am. J. Dis. Child.*, 81, 471, 1951.

131. Good, J. T., Jr., Iseman, M. D., Davidson, P. T., Tuberculosis in association with pregnancy, *Am. J. Obstet. Gynecol.*, 140, 492, 1981.

132. Wilson, E. A., Thelin, T. J., Dilts, P. V., Tuberculosis complicated by pregnancy, *Am. J. Obstet. Gynecol.*, 115, 526, 1972.

133. Lowe, C. R., Congenital defects among children born to women under supervision or treatment for pulmonary tuberculosis, *Br. J. Prev. Soc. Med.*, 18, 14, 1964.

134. Atkins, J. N., Maternal plasma concentration of pyridoxal phosphate during pregnancy: adequacy of vitamin B_6 supplementation during isoniazid therapy, *Am. Rev. Resp. Dis.*, 126, 714, 1982.

135. Lewit, T., Nebel, L., Terracina, S., Ethambutol in pregnancy: observations on embryogenesis, *Chest*, 68, 25, 1974.

136. Robinson, G. C., Cambon, K. G., Hearing loss in infants of tuberculous mothers treated with streptomycin during pregnancy, *N. Engl. J. Med.*, 271, 949, 1964.

137. Stallworth, J. R., Brasfield, D. M., Tiller, R. E., Congenital miliary tuberculosis proven by open lung biopsy specimen and successfully treated, *Am. J. Dis. Child.*, 134, 320, 1980.

138. Gillum, M. D., Maki, D. G., Brief report: tuberculin testing, BCG in pregnancy, *Infect. Control Hosp. Epidemiol.*, 9, 119, 1988.

139. Smith, J. K., Caspary, E. A., Field, E. J., Lymphocyte reactivity to antigen in pregnancy, *Am. J. Obstet. Gynecol.*, 113, 602, 1972.

140. Montgomery, W. P., Young, R. C., Jr., Allen, M. P., The tuberculin test in pregnancy, *Am. J. Obstet. Gynecol.*, 100, 829, 1968.

141. Present, P. A., Comstock, G. W., Tuberculin sensitivity in pregnancy, *Am. Rev. Resp. Dis.*, 112, 413, 1975.

142. Bonebrake, C. R., Noller, K. L., Loehnen, P. C., Routine chest radiography in pregnancy, *J. Am. Med. Assoc.*, 240, 2747, 1978.

143. Vallejo, J. G., Starke, J. R., Tuberculosis and pregnancy, *Clin. Chest Med.*, 13, 693, 1992.

144. Franks, A. L., Binkin, N. J., Snider, D. E., Jr., Isoniazid hepatitis among pregnant and post-partum hispanic patients, *Public Health Rep.*, 104, 151, 1989.

145. Snider, D. E., Jr., Caras, G. J., Isoniazid-associated hepatitis deaths: a review of available information, *Am. Rev. Resp. Dis.*, 145, 494, 1992.

146. Snider, D. E., Jr., Powell, K. E., Should mothers taking antituberculosis drugs breast-feed?, *Arch. Intern. Med.*, 144, 589, 1984.

147. McKenzie, S. A., Macnab, A. J., Katz, G., Neonatal pyridoxine responsive convulsions due to isoniazid therapy, *Arch. Dis. Child.*, 51, 567, 1976.

148. Kendig, E. L., Rogers, W. L., Tuberculosis in the neonatal period, *Am. Rev. Tuberc.*, 77, 418, 1958.

149. Kendig, E. L., The place of BCG vaccine in the management of infants born to tuberculous mothers, *N. Engl. J. Med.*, 281, 520, 1969.

150. Dormer, B. A., Swarit, J. A., Harrison, I., Prophylactic isoniazid protection of infants in a tuberculosis hospital, *Lancet*, 2, 902, 1959.

151. Light, I. J., Saidleman, M., Sutherland, J. M., Management of newborns after nursery exposure to tuberculosis, *Am. Rev. Resp. Dis.*, 109, 415, 1974.

152. Young, T. K., Hershfield, E. S., A case-control study to evaluate the effectiveness of mass neonatal BCG vaccination among Canadian Indians, *Am. J. Public Health*, 76, 783, 1986.

153. Curtis, H. M., Bamford, F. N., Leck, I., Incidence of childhood tuberculosis after neonatal BCG vaccination, *Lancet*, 1, 145, 1984.

Chapter 9

Nontuberculous Mycobacteria With and Without HIV Infection

Paul W. Wright, M.D. and Richard J. Wallace, Jr., M.D.

CONTENTS

I. INTRODUCTION

The family of bacteria called Mycobacteriaceae, of the order Actinomycetales, contains the single genus *Mycobacterium*. This group of aerobic, nonmotile, nonspore-forming rods is resistant to decolorization by alcohol-acid decolorizing agents (acid-fast), is a slow grower (generation time of 2 to over 20 h compared to 20 min for *Escherichia coli*), and has high lipid concentrations in its cell walls.

The first description of the mycobacteria occurred in 1873 when the Norwegian physician G. H. Armauer Hansen described some rod-shaped bodies (*Mycobacterium leprae*) frequently observed in skin preparations of leprosy patients. In 1882, the German physician Robert Koch isolated the tubercle bacillus, *Mycobacterium tuberculosis*. Three years later Alvarez and Tavel described the smegma bacillus[1]. Following these discoveries, many other mycobacteria were discovered, most of which were not pathogenic in animal models, e.g., the guinea pig. Only *M. tuberculosis, M. bovis,* and *M. leprae* consistently were considered pathogenic to humans until the 1940s and 1950s. Currently 54 species of mycobacteria are described in the ninth edition of *Bergey's Manual of Systematic Bacteriology*.[2] Approximately half of these species are associated with human disease. The remainder are saprophytic or are associated with animal disease only. Some of these mycobacteria, such as *M. genavense* and *M. haemophilum,* are newly isolated and their pathogenicities are yet to be well defined. Rapid advancements in the taxonomic separation of mycobacterial species has occurred with the development of nucleic acid probes, high-performance liquid chromatography (HPLC) of mycolic acid esters, and other laboratory techniques that facilitate more rapid and accurate identification.

Nontuberculous mycobacteria (NTM) are differentiated from *M. tuberculosis* in colony morphology and pigment, nucleic acid composition, growth rate, biochemical behavior, and pathogenicity. They are stained readily with acid-fast dye techniques (Kinyoun or Ziehl-Neelsen) and also the fluorochrome procedure. However, only *M. kansasii* and *M. marinum* can be distinguished occasionally from other mycobacteria on stain identification alone by their larger and more beaded appearance. Clinical sputum samples for NTM are digested and decontaminated in a technique similar to that used for *M. tuberculosis,* but the NTM require greater care in the decontamination process since they are killed more easily by the alkaline agents used in decontamination.

The NTM may be cultured on the same media as *M. tuberculosis,* i.e., an egg-potato-based medium such as Lowenstein–Jensen or an agar-based medium such as Middlebrook 7H10 or 7H11. Culture onto a broth medium, such as Middlebrook 7H9 or radiolabeled 7H12 broth (BACTEC system, Becton-Dickinson, Sparks, MD), also is standard in most laboratories. The slow-growing NTM grow in 2 to 4 weeks on solid media and in 5 to 7 days with the BACTEC system. Most of the NTM are cultured best at 35°C, while *M. marinum, M. chelonae,* and *M. haemophilum* usually grow at lower temperatures of 28 to 30°C. *M. haemophilum* requires the addition of hemin (X factor) to the culture media for growth and identification. Currently commercially available DNA probes (Accu-Probe) (Gen-Probe Inc., San Diego, CA) are useful in rapid identification (1 day) of pure cultures of *M. tuberculosis, M. avium, M. intracellulare, M. gordonae,* and *M. kansasii.*

In 1954 Timpe and Runyon[3] classified the nontuberculous mycobacteria into four groups according to their colony growth rate, morphology, and pigmentation. The first three groups contain slowly growing organisms whose colonies show (I, photochromogens) yellow pigmentation when grown in light, (II, scotochromogens) yellow to orange pigmentation when grown in darkness, and (III, nonphotochromogens) little or no pigmentation when grown in light or dark. Group IV, the rapid growers, are similar to the nonphotochromogens except that individual colonies grow in less than 5–7 days instead of 10–21 days. Runyon's classification was quite helpful in developing a global understanding of the mycobacteria by relating the morphologic qualities of the mycobacteria to their clinical presentation. However, with increased understanding and complexity of the taxonomy and pathogenicity of the mycobacteria, it is evident that a number of mycobacteria species do not fit well into the Runyon classification. Consequently, it has been replaced and the mycobacteria now are classified according to their species designation and by the clinical disease syndromes they produce, i.e., pulmonary, cutaneous, disseminated disease, or lymphadenitis (see Table 9-1). This newer organ-system classification provides a more clinical and pathologic basis for understanding the etiology, diagnosis, clinical course, and management of mycobacteria disease.

In 1935, Pinner[4] referred to the nontuberculosis isolates of mycobacteria causing human disease as "atypical acid-fast microorganisms." Timpe and Runyon[3] continued this same designation when they developed their system of classification mentioned above. However, many have objected to the concept of "atypical" because it tends to demand a comparison with *M. tuberculosis* that limits the description of many of the mycobacteria. The term "nontuberculous mycobacteria" (NTM) will be the designated term in this article. "Mycobacteria other than tuberculosis" (MOTT) and "environmental mycobacteria" are other terms that have been used collectively to describe these organisms. The major differences between *M. tuberculosis* and the other mycobacteria involve not only the issue of human pathogenicity and tubercles, but also the mode of transmission, i.e., human to human versus environmental, and the relative responsiveness to drug therapy.

II. NONTUBERCULOUS MYCOBACTERIA: NON-HIV

A. EPIDEMIOLOGY

The prevalence and incidence of the NTM are difficult to characterize because infections due to the NTM rarely cause death and are not routinely reported to public health departments. Although state laboratories provide data concerning the isolation of the NTM, many private laboratories isolate these organisms without referring the specimens to the state laboratories for further identification. This results in the lack of documentation of these infections. Furthermore, it often is difficult from single cultures to determine whether the isolation of NTM indicates a state of disease, infection without apparent disease (i.e., colonization), or environmental contamination. Nevertheless, much work is being accomplished on our understanding of the epidemiology of NTM infections, not only with studies of the organism as it exists in the environment (primarily for *M. avium* complex), but also with our ability to separate different strains of the same species. These techniques utilize primarily DNA fingerprinting methods such as large restriction fragment (LRF) pattern analysis using pulse field gel electrophoresis.[5] Studies using this identification system have shown that isolates of a specific NTM such as *M. fortuitum, M. abscessus,* or *M. avium* complex (MAC) recovered from a single individual have the same LRF pattern, even when

Table 9-1 Clinical sites of infection with the nontuberculous mycobacteria

	Common Organism	Less Common Organism	
Lung	M. avium complex M. kansasii M. abscessus	M. gordonae M. malmoense M. simiae M. szulgai M. smegmatis	M. xenopi M. fortuitum
Skin/ soft tissue	M. marinum M. fortuitum M. abscessus M. chelonae	M. avium complex M. kansasii M. smegmatis M. nonchromogenicum	M. ulcerans M. haemophilum
Lymph node	M. avium complex M. scrofulaceum	M. kansasii M. fortuitum M. abscessus M. chelonae M. marinum	
Postoperative catheter- related	M. fortuitum M. abscessus	M. chelonae M. chelonae-like organism	
Disseminated	M. avium complex M. kansasii M. chelonae M. abscessus M. haemophilum	M. xenopi M. genavense	
Bone/joint	M. avium complex M. marinum M. abscessus M. fortuitum	M. kansasii M. chelonae M. haemophilum	

it comes from different body fluids of the same person and are cultured several years apart.[6]

Although the method of initial infection with the NTM is poorly understood, these opportunistic pathogens probably enter the human host from environmental sources. There is little evidence to support human-to-human transmission. Support for environmental sources of infection derives from matching serotypes of MAC with isolates from the soil as well as patients living in areas where the soil was sampled.[7,8] Support for animal-to-human infection comes from West Germany,[7] but similar studies from South Africa fail to support the concept of this mode of transmission.[9]

Skin tests with complex mixtures of mycobacterial-soluble antigens demonstrate that the prevalence of infection due to NTM is very high.[10] Unfortunately, these skin test antigens give relatively blurred pictures of the rate of infection for any given species because of cross-reactivity to various specific antigens.[11] One interesting aspect of the skin test reactivity to MAC as measured by PPD-B (intradermal skin test for MAC) is that it tends to be lower in older age groups. This contrasts to reactivity to PPD-S (standard tuberculin skin test), which tends be higher in higher age groups.[12] The reason for the lower reactivity to PPD-B with age is unclear.

The prevalence of NTM disease has been studied locally, nationally, and also internationally. The average yearly incidence of NTM disease varies from 0.7 per 100,000 in South Carolina[13] to an estimated annual incidence of 2 per 100,000 per year in Australia.[14] MAC was the most commonly isolated NTM species in studies from South Carolina (86%),[13] the United States (60%),[15,16] and British Columbia (73%).[17]

The pathogenesis of NTM infection is unclear but is thought to be similar to tuberculosis. Pulmonary patients are thought to inhale the aerosolized organisms from infected soil, dust, and natural water supplies such as estuaries. Sometimes the source is thought to be nosocomial, as MAC of the serotype causing human disease has been found in the hot water systems of hospitals.[18] Mycobacterial organisms in desiccated water droplets (so called droplet nuclei) are thought to localize in the heavily ventilated portions of the lung, namely the middle or lower lung zones or the anterior segments of the upper lobes.[19] Following this primary infection, there is lymphohematogenous dissemination of NTM to the lungs and (perhaps) to the rest of the body, causing a mild self-limited disease in most nonimmunocompromised patients.[20]

Ingestion of the NTM provides a possible second possible mode for disease entry, especially in patients with extrapulmonary infection. These sources are felt to be water and foodstuffs contaminated with the NTM. Direct entry across the protective skin barrier is a third method of infection seen in penetrating skin and soft tissue injuries, as well as postoperative wounds.

The evidence above would support the concept that this organism is inhaled by the susceptible human host. Very little is known about the pathogenesis of *M. kansasii*, but some evidence would suggest that the organism is inhaled by the susceptible human host with potable (tap) water as a likely source.

Mycobacterium avium complex (MAC) includes several phenotypically similar species: *M. avium, M. intracellulare, M. paratuberculosis,* and *M. lepraemurium*. These organisms are serologically different, but have been considered collectively as one entity because of the difficulty in separating them in the laboratory.[21] Separate commercial DNA probes now are available for *M. avium* and *M. intracellulare* that allow for rapid and accurate separation of these two species. *M. avium* strains appear to be more virulent than *M. intracellulare*,[22] but both organisms can cause significant human illness. *M. lepraemurium* is associated with animal illness only. Some include *M. scrofulaceum* in this group, calling the group "MAIS",[23] but we will consider *M. scrofulaceum* separately. MAC contains at least 28 separate serovars that can be differentiated by seroagglutination testing.[24] Such serotyping is not available readily and has no utility in the evaluation of individual patients. With the currently available commercial DNA probes, *M. avium* and *M. intracellulare* are readily separable.

In the early 1980s, NTM accounted for approximately one-third of all mycobacteria isolated by state laboratories, with MAC comprising 61% of the NTM isolates.[15,16,25] Other commonly isolated species of NTM include *M. fortuitum* complex (19%), *M. kansasii* (10%), and *M. scrofulaceum, M. marinum,* and *M. xenopi*. Unpublished data currently (i.e., 1990s) suggest that NTM (primarily MAC) now are more common than *M. tuberculosis* in most large private or state laboratories, especially in areas of high endemicity for MAC. The majority of these isolates are respiratory, and are considered to be non-HIV related based on the usual patient populations evaluated by nonhospital laboratories. In laboratories that see HIV-related opportunistic infections, MAC also is the most common mycobacterial isolate.

MAC commonly is found in water sources as demonstrated by Wolinsky and Rynearson[26] who isolated at least one species of NTM from 86% of soil samples collected from the eastern United States. MAC has been recovered from soil,[26] fresh and brackish water,[27] house dust,[28] chickens,[29] birds,[30] food,[31] and animals.[32] MAC tends to grow better in water with warmer temperatures, low salinity, low pH, and low dissolved oxygen.[33] Water is considered to be a major reservoir for these organisms. MAC together with *M. scrofulaceum* have been recovered from one-third of sampled aquatic environments in the southeastern United States.[34] Waters, aerosols, and soils associated with the acidic swamp waters of the southeastern United States are optimal sources for MAC recovery.[33] Correspondingly, the greatest number of human isolates of MAC and the highest prevalence of skin test reactivity to an MAC-purified protein derivative come from this same geographic area.[33]

Diagnostic criteria for pulmonary disease due to MAC and other NTM have been somewhat controversial. Recent American Thoracic Society criteria[34a] suggest that anyone with two of more positive respiratory cultures containing moderate numbers of organisms as determined by positive AFB smears and/or culture and an abnormal chest X-ray not explained by other diseases should be considered as having NTM lung disease. Tsukamura suggests that patients with a new pulmonary cavitary with two or more (and perhaps only one) sputum culture positive for MAC should be considered as having MAC pulmonary disease.[35] This latter criterion is more specific, but excludes the almost one-third of current patients with noncavitary disease.

The typical non-HIV-infected patient with MAC disease is an older (late 50s to 60s) white male living in a rural area of the southeastern United States with a long history of cigarette abuse and resultant pulmonary disease.[36] The male-to-female ratio varies from 3:2 in Texas[37] to 7:1 in Australia.[38] Occupation does not seem to be a risk factor for MAC infection except for the fact that its rural association puts farmers and ranchers at higher risk. Patients with MAC infection, especially males, have a history of chronic pulmonary disease related to long-term smoking. Other potential pulmonary risk factors include previously treated mycobacterial disease including tuberculosis, cystic fibrosis, and some forms of pneumoconiosis. In Wales, for example, MAC disease occurs more often in coal miners[39] and, along with tuberculosis, is found more often in patients with silicosis ("sand-blaster's" disease). Some chronic systemic diseases such as alcoholism, cancer, rheumatoid arthritis, and diabetes also may carry some risk.[40] However, at the time of diagnosis, as many as one-third of patients with MAC disease (especially women) have no definable predisposing condition.[41]

M. kansasii is a slow growing mycobacterium that forms yellow-colored colonies when exposed to light (photochromogen). Unlike MAC, this species is recovered only rarely from the natural environment (no isolations from soil and only one from fresh water).[42] It has been isolated from samples of municipal water supplies,[27] biofilm from water treatment plants, domestic water supply systems, aquaria,[43] and tap waters sources.[42,44] (These sites of isolation fit well with the general urban character of clinical disease.) Rarely, *M. kansasii* has been recovered from dust[38] and animals (cattle and swine).[45] Infection from *M. kansasii* occurs most commonly in the central and southern United States; the more common states include Texas, Louisiana, Illinois, and Florida. Infection from this organism is reported in England and Wales.[46] Its incidence in Japan has increased to 0.34 per 100,000 per year.[47]

The average age for the patient with *M. kansasii* infection is 50 years for males and 42 years for females.[37] The male-to-female ratio is 3:1[37] to 2:1.[25] In the United States, the ethnic distribution of this disease corresponds to that of the population being studied, with more disease usually found in white rather than in black or Hispanic populations. The typical patient is a 50-year-old white male living in an urban area of one of the above states.[25]

Patients who develop *M. kansasii* disease seem to have less predisposing disease than those infected with MAC. Occupation has not been established as a risk factor, but some studies suggest that *M. kansasii* disease occurs more commonly in the setting of both nonindustrial and industrial dust exposure,[39,47-49] including patients with clinical silicosis. In a bacteriological survey of gold miners, NTM were recovered from 8–12% of collected sputums, with *M. kansasii* being the commonest NTM isolated (67–79%).[48] NTM were isolated from 16.9% of sputums from gold miners with silicosis, but only 5.7% of those without silicosis.[48]

The mode of transmission of *M. kansasii* is unclear, but infection probably originates from inhaled environmental sources. In spite of the limited recovery of this organism in the environment, and the major concentration of disease within the urban setting, there has been little evidence for human-to-human transmission of this organism.

Clinical disease due to rapidly growing mycobacteria (RGM) is almost always due to a member of the *M. fortuitum* complex. The clinically important members of this group are *M. fortuitum*, *M. chelonae* (formerly *M. chelonae* subspecies *chelonae*), and *M. abscessus* (formerly *M. chelonae* subspecies *abscessus*). *M. fortuitum* complex is responsible for the majority of mycobacterial skin and soft tissue infections as well as an increasing number of pulmonary infections. There are 23 other RGM species including pigmented species such as *M. gadium*, *M. thermoresistible*, *M. vaccae*, *M favescens*, and *M. neoaurum*, and nonpigmented species such as *M. peregrinum*, *M. fortuitum* third biovariant complex, *M. chelonae*-like organisms (MCLO),[49a] and *M. smegmatis*, which rarely are associated with human disease.[50] *M. fortuitum* complex species are recovered commonly from water and soil samples.[25] They also have been isolated from such nosocomial sources as procedural instruments,[51,52] tap water, surgical marking solutions, ice, distilled water, and surgical cleansing solutions,[34a] with water the almost universal common denominator. In a series of 125 cases of RGM infection reported in 1983, 74 cases (59%) were cutaneous infections and over half of these followed surgical procedures.[54]

The mode of transmission of *M. fortuitum* complex lung disease is unclear but probably parallels that of MAC, both commonly recovered from the environment. Direct inoculation is the usual mode of transmission for localized cutaneous and/or bone disease, while nosocomial infections usually relate to contamination from colonized distilled water or tap water.

M. marinum forms a yellow colony when exposed to light, grows more rapidly (within 5 days) than most other slow growers, and requires incubation at room temperature or, slightly higher, for primary isolation (25–30°C). Skin infections due to this organism have been reported from the United States,[55] Europe,[56] Japan,[57] Israel,[58] Hong Kong,[59] New Zealand,[60] Australia,[61] and Canada.[62] This infection occurs typically in patients exposed to water, particularly with saltwater activities and the cleaning of freshwater fish tanks.[56] It also has been associated with saltwater and freshwater fish,[27] soil,[27] natural bathing pools, dolphins, shrimp, snails, water fleas, and rarely freshwater sources such as tributaries, lakes, and a well.[58] *M. marinum* exhibits powerful fucosidase activity[27] that may enable it to derive its carbon requirement from aquatic algae containing fucose. This may explain its recovery in certain types of waters such as aquaria, swimming pools, and biofilms.[27]

Patients infected with *M. marinum* usually are young (mean age, approximately 36 years), men (male-to-female ratio of 1.5:1) who typically present with a history of skin trauma prior to exposure and infection.[58] They typically present with an indolent papule, nodule, or ulcerated skin lesion on the extremity with no systemic symptoms. Ascending nodules (lymphocutaneous syndrome), as with sporotrichosis and Nocardia, occasionally can be seen. Most patients are considered to be in excellent health before acquiring this infection, with only a few having a history of immunosuppression from HIV infection or renal transplantation therapy. Johnston and Izumi reviewed 42 case reports involving 590 patients and found that 493 (84%) patients came from four large series of cases.[63] The largest series involved 290 patients who were infected due to a poorly chlorinated swimming pool in Glenwood Springs, Colorado. The other four large series were from New Orleans (31 patients), Japan (75 cases), the Centers for Disease Control (79 patients), and Maryland (18 cases).

Transmission of *M. marinum* occurs when susceptible hosts are exposed to penetrating skin trauma in an aquatic environment containing the organism, or place their hands in the water before healing of a cutaneous injury (such as cleaning a household fish tank). Eighty-five percent of Glenwood Springs patients had reactive skin tests to PPD-S, with 91% of these patients having negative PPD skin tests within 2 years prior to their illness.[63] In a study of 12 patients with culture-proven *M. marinum* infection of deep tissues, 11 patients showed antigen-specific T-cell anergy to *M. marinum* while having normal responses to other antigens.[64] This study suggests that patients may have a narrow immune defect causing susceptibility to *M. marinum* infection.

Environmental recovery of *M. xenopi* has been from hot water systems almost exclusively, most often in hospitals where the species has been associated with nosocomial outbreaks. It has not been isolated from intake water pipes, but only with hot water pipe systems. It grows optimally in temperatures from 43 to 45°C and recently was shown to be the most heat stable of five mycobacterial species tested.[65] It was the most commonly isolated NTM that caused mycobacterial disease in southeast England from 1977 to 1984.[66] In a 1992 study from Brooklyn, New York, *M. xenopi* was the second (MAC was first) most common pathogenic NTM isolated from 86 hospitalized patients of whom only 41% were seropositive for HIV.[67] Simor et al.[68] noted most isolates of this organism come from the respiratory tract. In their study, only 9 of 28 isolates of *M. xenopi* recovered were considered to be causing disease.

M. haemophilum infection of the skin and subcutaneous tissues recently has been recognized, almost exclusively in immunocompromised patients such as organ transplant patients or patients with AIDS.[69] The incidence of infection, the natural habitat, and route of infection are unknown. The organism has been isolated in patients from widely diverse geographic areas, (e.g., Australia, Israel, the United States), but has yet to be isolated from the environment. The majority of United States isolates have occurred in New York City. *M. haemophilum* requires growth media enriched with iron (ferric) salts (hence its name), a feature that may explain its previous lack of growth and attention.

B. CLINICAL MANIFESTATIONS

In the HIV-negative populations, pulmonary disease accounts for almost 90% of disease due to NTM, followed by lymph node, skin, bone and joint, and disseminated illness.[25] MAC and *M. kansasii* are the most frequently isolated species in patients with NTM pulmonary disease in the United States.[16,25]

1. Pulmonary

Patients with MAC pulmonary infection typically present with nonspecific and variable signs and symptoms, which may include productive cough, malaise, weakness, dyspnea, and hemoptysis. These patients typically are older males with underlying pulmonary disease and a history of cigarette smoking. They usually present with less fever and weight loss than patients with pulmonary tuberculosis. Ahn and colleagues reported that 76.5% of 226 patients with MAC pulmonary disease had cavitary disease.[70] In one study of 244 patients with lung disease caused by MAC, four clinical patterns of chest radiographic presentations are described in decreasing order of frequency as follows: solitary nodules, bronchitis–bronchiectasis pattern, tuberculosis-like infiltrates, and diffuse infiltrates as seen in patients with AIDS.[71] However, in our experience and the experience of others, solitary nodules are a relatively rare form of radiographic presentation[45] (Figure 9-1). The presence of multiple small (<5 mm) nodules in patients with bronchiectasis on computed tomography (CT) scans of the lung has recently been shown to be highly specific for MAC,[71a] and appears to be the typical radiographic pattern among nonsmokers, especially women.

Reich and Johnson[72] recently described six elderly female patients with MAC pulmonary infection involving the middle lobe or lingula portions of the lung. Hilar adenopathy, volume loss, cavitary disease, and predisposing pulmonary disease were absent in all these elderly female patients. The authors postulated that these patients may have

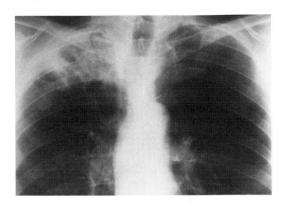

Figure 9-1 Chest X-ray of patient with MAC infection, right upper lobe fibronodular infiltrate.

suppressed their cough reflexes and developed nonspecific inflammatory processes in areas of the lung with poor drainage. They labeled this the "Lady Windermere's syndrome."

Pulmonary disease is the most common presentation of *M. kansasii* infection, followed by disseminated disease, lymph node disease, bone and joint disease, and skin and soft tissue disease. Patients with pulmonary infection with *M. kansasii* typically present with a clinical picture indistinguishable from that of pulmonary tuberculosis. Underlying lung disease is present in 62% of patients with *M. kansasii* infection, 95% of which is chronic obstructive pulmonary disease.[73] Cavitary disease is found in 85–95%[70,73] of patients with pulmonary infection with *M. kansasii*, and 20% have bilateral cavitary disease.[73] Clinical symptoms are similar to that of pulmonary tuberculosis, except that they are generally less intense. Pulmonary disease due to *M. kansasii* or other NTM rarely is seen in children.[74]

Pulmonary disease due to RGM is not uncommon and involves primarily *M. abscessus* (approximately 80% of cases) and *M. fortuitum* (approximately 15% of cases).[54,75] Unlike other mycobacterial lung diseases, typical patients with RGM pulmonary disease are female nonsmokers without underlying lung disease. As with other mycobacterial lung disease, the patients typically are white and over age 50. In a 1993 study of 154 patients with RGM pulmonary disease, most patients were white (83%), female (65%), and nonsmokers (66%), with a mean age of 54 years.[75] In this study, cough was the most common presenting symptom and constitutional symptoms appeared only after disease progression. Other symptoms included recurrent episodes of acute bronchitis, fatigue, mild fever, weight loss, and occasional hemoptysis. The radiographic appearance differed from tuberculosis or pulmonary disease due to MAC or *M. kansasii* in that cavitary

disease was rare (16% of cases).[75] The commonly seen interstitial (37%), reticulonodular (36%), or interstitial/alveolar (40%) infiltrates typically involved three or four lobes (greater than 50%) and was bilateral in 77% of cases.[75] Upper lobe disease was seen most frequently with right upper lobe (77%) being more common than left upper lobe disease (61%).[75] The disease may be easily confused clinically and/or radiographically with fibrotic lung disease or bronchiectasis. The diagnosis is confirmed in patients who have compatible radiographic abnormalities and multiple sputum cultures that are positive for the same organism.

Pulmonary disease due to *M. xenopi* has been reported predominantly in England and Canada.[66,68,76,77] It typically occurs in the elderly male patient who has a history of COPD, past tuberculosis, or a similar underlying condition. In a study of 19 patients with this pulmonary illness, 12 presented with mild symptoms of cough, fever, and increased sputum production.[77] Three patients had hemoptysis and 7 were asymptomatic, having only a change on chest film. Roentgenographic features included, either singly or in combination, a nodular or mass shadow (14/19), single or multiple cavities (9/19), and a tuberculosis type presentation with multifocal, nodular densities.

2. Extrapulmonary
a. Lymph Node

Lymph node disease due to NTM infection in the non-HIV-infected patient is typically seen in young children, from 1 to 10 years of age. The unilateral enlarged (often painless) lymph node or group of nodes is usually the only presenting complaint, with occasional low-grade fever and malaise. The lymph nodes most frequently encountered are the submandibular, submaxillary, cervical, and preauricular nodes. The majority of infections currently are due to MAC (80%) and *M. scrofulaceum; M. kansasii, M. fortuitum,* and *M. abscessus* are only occasionally cultured from infected lymph nodes. Only 10% of mycobacterial lymphadenitis in children is due to *M. tuberculosis,* whereas it is responsible for 90% of adult mycobacterial lymphadenitis.[77,78]

A definitive diagnosis of mycobacterial lymphadenitis is made by culturing the organism from the lymph node, a procedure that yields a positive culture in cervical lymph nodes in only 50–85% of cases.[79] The reason for the negative cultures is unknown, but could reflect the presence of more fastidious mycobacterial species such as *M. haemophilum* or *M. genavense.* The use of the polymerase chain reaction (PCR) followed by DNA sequencing or restriction endonuclease analysis of these noncultureable cases may allow for a better diagnosis in these cases in the future. A presumptive diagnosis is made with a typical histopathologic finding of caseating granulomata with or without positive acid-fast bacteria (AFB) smears but with negative cultures. Differential diagnosis includes cat-scratch disease, tuberculosis, drug reactions, malignancies, nocardiosis, brucellosis, mononucleosis, sarcoidosis, toxoplasmosis, and others. Without treatment, spontaneous drainage usually occurs, but spontaneous resolution may be more common than reported, especially in children. Lymph nodes infected with NTM should be excised to facilitate both diagnosis and therapy. Incomplete or incisional biopsies of lymphadenitis due to mycobacteria should be avoided to prevent problems with fistulae and chronic drainage.

b. Cutaneous Disease

Cutaneous disease due to NTM is caused most commonly by *M. fortuitum, M. abscessus, M chelonae, M. marinum, M. haemophilum,* and (in selected areas of the world) *M. ulcerans.* Patients with cutaneous manifestations of NTM infection usually present with local symptoms; systemic symptoms and disease are uncommon. In the immunocompetent patient, these skin lesions usually are the site of primary disease (as opposed to disseminated disease) and typically occur after trauma to the skin. These skin lesions have been classified into the following seven clinical–histological categories:[80] (1) abscess, (2) tuberculoid granulomas, (3) diffuse histiocytic infiltration, (4) panniculitis, (5) nonspecific chronic inflammation, (6) sarcoid-like granulomas, and (7) rheumatoid-like nodules.

Skin disease due to *M. marinum* commonly presents as a nodular or ulcerative sporotrichosis-like lesions on the elbows, fingers, hands, and knees. Systemic disease, lymphadenitis, and disseminated disease are uncommon in the immunocompetent host. The time interval between exposure and the appearance of lesions varied from 10 days to 2 years with an average of 3 to 8 weeks.[63] Without treatment the lesions usually persist for 14 or 15 months. Most lesions (80%) spontaneously resolve by 36 months.[81]

The most common site of presentation for infection due to RGM is the skin or soft tissue. Most infections produce lesions of the lower extremity in healthy hosts, usually following trauma such as nail or other puncture wounds. In community acquired skin infection due to RGM, one-third involves *M. chelonae* or *M. abscessus,* with the remainder due to *M. fortuitum.*[82] Typically there is a long incubation period averaging 1 month and extending up to 6 months. Symptoms include pain, local swelling, and

serous-bloody drainage. Disseminated skin disease, usually due to *M. chelonae* in the setting of low dose corticosteroid therapy, may occur but is uncommon. Diagnosis is made by culturing the organism from the wound, which usually can be accomplished without a tissue biopsy by the use of a vigorously applied swab. Nosocomial infections due to RGM can occur in association with the use of indwelling catheters, especially long-term intravenous catheters, and certain surgical procedures such as augmentation mammaplasty and cardiac bypass surgery.[83] *M. fortuitum* has been associated with 80% of the breast and sternum wound infections due to RGM. Sporadic disease is more common than epidemic disease. Geographic location is important since 80% of these infections occur in the southern coastal states.[82]

Skin infection due to *M. haemophilum* is a newly described cause of rash, papules, nodules, and draining sinuses in immunocompromised patients. Most infections have occurred in patients who are post-renal transplantation or who are infected with HIV. One case presented as a chronic erythematous papular eruption, mimicking tinea corporis, in a patient who underwent coronary artery bypass surgery who was otherwise healthy.[83]

While skin and soft tissue infections due to *M. ulcerans* have not been reported in the United States, they are endemic and relatively common in parts of Asia, Africa, Mexico, and Australia. The natural reservoir and mode of transmission are unknown. The typical patient is a child 5 to 8 years of age who develops a painless nodule on his leg without other signs or symptoms. This nodule will develop into a shallow ulcer with a necrotic base. Spontaneous resolution may occur in 6 to 9 months, but others will persist, spread, and eventually cause serious deformity. Other satellite nodules may develop, but lymphadenitis is absent.[84]

Posttraumatic, localized bone and joint infections due to mycobacteria occasionally are due to MAC and *M. kansasii.* In a review of 25 non-HIV-infected patients with granulomatous synovitis and bursitis, mycobacteria were identified in 20 patients. The isolates were *M. tuberculosis* (4 cases), *M. kansasii* (6 cases), MAC (2 cases), and one case each of *M. marinum, M. chelonae, and M. gordonae.*[85] MAC infection also has been reported in patients with reactive arthritis,[86] acute mastoiditis,[87] and prostatitis.[88] Synovitis of the hands, fingers, and wrists due to infection with *M. marinum* is common.[89]

c. Disseminated Disease

Disseminated disease due to NTM was rare before 1970.[91] Today, most cases occur in AIDS patients, less frequently in other immunosuppressed patients, and rarely in normal children or adults.[92-94] Diagnosis of disseminated disease is made when the organism is isolated from closed sterile sites, such as blood, bone marrow, or liver or from multiple skin sites. Organisms causing disseminated disease include MAC, *M. kansasii, M. chelonae,*[90,94] *M. scrofulaceum, M. abscessus,*[54] *M. haemophilum,*[69,92] and, most recently, *M. genavense.*

In 1984, Horsburgh et al. described 37 non-AIDS patients with disseminated MAC infection and found 20 to have immunosuppression, mostly from corticosteroid therapy.[92] The clinical presentation of these patients included fever, bone pain, weight loss, lymphadenopathy, hepatosplenomegaly, and cutaneous lesions.

Disseminated disease due to *M. kansasii, M. chelonae,* and *M. haemophilum* generally presents with cutaneous disease such as nodules or abscesses rather than the systemic disease presentation of MAC.

Mortality due to disseminated NTM disease depends on the organism and the status of the underlying disease. In 1972 Lincoln and Gilbert[93] reported 12 fatal cases of disseminated NTM (most were MAC) disease in children. They also describe nine cases of meningitis due to NTM with at least 4 fatalities.

Disseminated disease due to RGM usually involves immunosuppressed patients with chronic renal failure, renal transplantation, those treated with low-dose corticosteroids, but not from HIV infection.[82] Ninety percent of disseminated cutaneous RGM infection is due to *M. chelonae* or *M. abscessus.* Initial reports that included only about 10 patients suggested that most infections were due to *M. abscessus.*[54] However, recently 52 cases of cutaneous disease due to disseminated *M. chelonae* have been reported,[94] suggesting that this species is responsible for most of the current cases. The majority of these patients have disseminated disease with little or no systemic symptoms. The remainder, especially those with dialysis-dependent renal failure, have systemic disease, positive blood cultures, and are seriously ill.

C. DIAGNOSIS

The cornerstone of diagnosis of disease due to NTM is the isolation of the organism from sputum, tissue, or body fluid in patients presenting with histories, physical examinations, and radiographic findings suggestive of NTM disease. Single positive sputum cultures, usually with low numbers of organisms, may occur as a consequence of transient contamination or colonization of the respiratory tract, or even from specimen contamination. Therefore, the diagnosis of lung disease caused by MAC or other NTM (with the possible exception

of *M. kansasii*) requires more than one positive acid-fast sputum smear and/or culture positivity (moderate or heavy growth) for acid-fast bacteria. However, recovery of *M. kansasii* from sputum and other human tissue and fluids usually indicates the infection because this organism rarely is a contaminant.[26] Nonetheless, a minimum of two positive cultures is preferred. Other causes of lung disease such as tuberculosis, fungal disease, and malignancy should be excluded. Bronchial washings seem to have greater sensitivity and less specificity in diagnosing NTM lung disease than routinely expectorated sputums.[34a] Suggested criteria for the diagnosis for NTM disease are shown in Table 9-2.

D. TREATMENT

Therapy for NTM disease is both difficult and controversial because first line antituberculous drugs are variably active against NTM depending on the species and there are few if any controlled clinical trials of antibiotic therapy. A summary of the authors' recommended therapy for NTM disease is shown in Table 9-3.

Therapy for MAC infection is challenging because of the increasing number of patients who require therapy and the resistance of MAC to first line antituberculous agents. Antituberculous drugs like cycloserine and ethionamide have excellent *in vitro* activity against MAC but seldom are used because of their toxicity. In non-AIDS patients with MAC pulmonary disease, the American Thoracic Society[34a] recommended initial daily therapy with four drugs followed by three drugs for a total of 18 to 24 months of therapy: isoniazid 300 mg, rifampin 600 mg, and ethambutol (25 g/kg, followed by 15 mg/kg on the third month); streptomycin therapy (usual adult dose is 0.5–1.0 g, or 10–15 mg/kg/day) consists of five daily doses per week for 6 to 12 weeks followed by two to three doses per week for 3 to 6 months of therapy as tolerated. Dosing modifications are required in patients over age 50, patients with small body mass, and those with altered renal function.

This ATS recommendation was published in 1990,[34a] and antedated the availability of the newer macrolides and rifabutin. The new macrolides, clarithromycin and azithromycin, are structurally similar to their parent compound erythromycin, but are unique in their striking microbiologic activity against NTM. In increasing situations involving MAC lung disease, one of these agents is being used in place of isoniazid, because of the former's greater antimicrobial activity against MAC and the lower toxicity. Clarithromycin concentrates well in both lung tissue and in macrophages, and probably remains active in the acid environment of the phagolysosomes.[95] Clarithromycin has inhibited

Table 9-2 **Diagnostic criteria for skin and lung nontuberculous mycobacterial disease**

Usual History		Minimum Number of Cultures	Chest X-ray
Non-HIV related			
Cutaneous			
M. marinum	Water/fish tank exposure, typical skin lesions	1	NA
M. fortuitum	Penetrating/open trauma or prior surgery		
M. abscessus	Same as *M. fortuitum*	1	NA
M. chelonae	On low dose steroids	1	NA
Pulmonary			
MAC	Rural male smoker or female over age 40 with chronic cough	2	Abnormal, not explained by other diseases, (bronchiectasis not an acceptable explanation); 2/3 cavitary
M. abscessus	Adult, no prior lung disease, prior granulomatous lung disease, or cystic fibrosis	2	Same as above except 10–20% cavitary
M. kansasii	Urban male smoker over age 50	2	Same as above
Lymph node disease			
MAC	Child, age 1–10 years, cervical node	0–1 Compatible histopathology, negative culture for *M. tuberculosis*	Should be negative
M. scrofulaceum	Cervical node	Same as above	Same as above
M. fortuitum	Regional drainage from trauma/surgical site		
M. chelonae	Same as above		
HIV Related			
Pulmonary			
M. kansasii			
MAC	Not helpful	(?) 2	Cavitary upper lobe disease, miliary disease, some nonspecific
Disseminated			
MAC	Blood, bone marrow, liver, (sputum, and stool are not diagnostic)	1	NA

NA = Not applicable.

90% of strains of MAC at MICs of 1 to 8 μg/ml.[95] However, controlled studies using the newer macrolides for MAC lung disease are not complete yet. Rifabutin (ansamycin), a derivative of rifampin, has better *in vitro* activity against MAC than rifampin[96,97] and recently was shown to be effective as prophylactic monotherapy against disseminated MAC in patients with advanced AIDS.[98] Controlled trials of this agent in lung disease have not been performed, but may occur in the near future as the drug has recently (1993) been released by the FDA. The impact of these drugs on the currently recommended (ATS) therapeutic regimen has not been established. It seems likely that these two agents are more active than isoniazid and rifampin and will replace them in the drug regimen.

The use of surgery in conjunction with chemotherapy has been highly effective in some patients with MAC lung disease but remains controversial.[99] It should be considered in all patients with localized disease (such as an unilateral cavity) and adequate cardiopulmonary reserve. Ideally, patients should be culture negative for several months prior to resection. With expanded future knowledge of rifabutin and clarithromycin, surgery to prevent disease relapse/recurrence may be indicated less often or no longer may be necessary.

While drug susceptibility testing is very helpful in the therapeutic management of tuberculosis, it is not as useful in directing the therapy of most NTM infections.[34a] Isolates of MAC almost are always resistant to the standard low drug concentrations currently used for *M. tuberculosis* testing. Susceptibility testing may be useful clinically at higher concentrations, but this has not been established yet. Hence routine susceptibility testing of MAC is not recommended and most laboratories have stopped doing them.

Most strains of *M. kansasii* are moderately susceptible to standard first line antituberculous agents, except pyrazinamide. Currently, rifampin is the cornerstone of multiple drug therapy. Prior to rifampin therapy, the 6-month sputum conversion rates for pulmonary patients infected with *M. kansasii* were only 52–81% with 10% relapse rates.[100,101] With multidrug therapy using rifampin, 100% of sputums converted within 4 months of therapy with only 1.1% relapse.[101] The current recommendation of the American Thoracic Society for pulmonary infection caused by *M. kansasii* is the regimen of isoniazid (300 mg), rifampin (600 mg), and ethambutol (15 mg/kg) given daily for 18 months.[34a] Susceptibilities of untreated strains of *M. kansasii* are highly predictable and routine susceptibility testing (except for rifampin) is not needed.

In patients who develop rifampin-resistant *M. kansasii*, a daily regimen, lasting 18 to 24 months, of isoniazid (900 mg plus pyridoxine), ethambutol (25 mg/kg for the duration), trimethoprim–sulfamethoxazole (160/800 mg three times/day), and streptomycin (3 to 6 months only) has been used with excellent success.[102] (The hepatotoxicity

with isoniazid is idiosyncratic, and there is no evidence that it is more likely with 900 mg than with 300 mg dose.) The follow-up report from this study indicates that long-term sputum conversion can be accomplished in 90% of treatments (mean onset of negative cultures after 11 weeks) using the above therapy.[103] However recent data indicate that clarithromycin is highly active against both rifampin-susceptible and rifampin-resistant strains of *M. kansasii* with mean MICs of ≤0.25 µg/ml. Given its success with other mycobacterial disease, clarithromycin would seem to be a reasonable agent to include in future retreatment regimens, perhaps in place of the more toxic streptomycin.

Lymphadenitis due to MAC and *M. scrofulaceum* (MAIS) infection should be treated with excisional surgery. This usually establishes the diagnosis as well as resulting in a 95% cure rate.[104] Although clinically unproven, a course of clarithromycin should be considered in children with recurrent lymph node disease after surgical resection.

More than 90% of clinical disease caused by the RGM is caused by *M. fortuitum, M. abscessus,* and *M. chelonae.*[34a] These three mycobacteria are resistant to most antituberculous agents, but variably susceptible (*M. fortuitum* > *M. abscessus* > *M. chelonae*) to a number of traditional antibiotics including amikacin, fluorinated quinolones, sulfonamides, cefoxitin, imipenem, and doxycycline. Isolates of *M. fortuitum* are susceptible to clarithromycin (80%),[105] ciprofloxacin, ofloxacin (100%), amikacin (100%), sulfonamides (90%), imipenem (100%), cefoxitin (80%), and doxycycline (50%). Isolates of M. abscessus are less susceptible than *M. fortuitum,* but only 20% or fewer of *M. chelonae* isolates were susceptible to doxycycline, ciprofloxacin, ofloxacin, and sulfamethoxazole. However, 100% of both *M. chelonae* and *M. abscessus* are susceptible *in vitro* to low concentrations of clarithromycin.[106] A recent clinical trial showed monotherapy with clarithromycin 500 mg bid for 6 months to be highly successful for patients with cutaneous (disseminated) infection due to *M. chelonae.*[106a]

M. marinum disease has been treated according to the following approaches: (1) simple observation for minor cutaneous infection, (2) surgical excision, and (3) single and multiple drug therapy. Isolates of *M. marinum* are susceptible to antituberculous concentrations of rifampin and ethambutol. They have intermediate susceptibility to sulfonamides, doxycycline, amikacin, kanamycin, and streptomycin, and are resistant to isoniazid.[106-108] Recent studies have shown 100% of isolates to be susceptible to 4 µg/ml or less of clarithromycin.[109] Acceptable single drug regimens includes minocycline or doxycycline at 100 mg

Table 9-3 **Therapy**[a]

Organism	First Line (Oral, Except Where Specified)	Injectable or Alternative Drugs (Oral Except Where Specified)	Surgery Potentially Beneficial
Therapy for Non-HIV-Related Disease			
Cutaneous			
M. marinum	Doxycycline (100 mg bid); or minocycline (100 mg bid); or TMP (160 mg)/SMX (800 mg) bid; or rifampin(600 mg) + ethambutol (15 mg/kg)	Clarithromycin (500 mg bid)	+
M. fortuitum	Doxycycline (100 mg bid) or minocycline (100 mg bid): 50% susceptible; or sulfamethoxazole (1.0 g bid); or ciprofloxacin (750 mg bid); or ofloxacin (400 mg bid); or clarithromycin (500 mg bid)	Amikacin (5 mg/kg bid) im/iv,[b] imipenem-cilastin 0.5–1.0 g qid) iv, cefoxitin (2.0 g q 4 h or 3.0 g q 6 h) iv	+
M. chelonae	Clarithromycin (500 mg bid); or doxycycline (100 mg bid): 25% susceptible	Tobramycin (1.0–1.5 mg/kg tid) im/iv,[b] imipenem-cilastin (0.5–1.0 g qid) iv	++
M. abscessus	Clarithromycin (500 mg bid)	Amikacin (5 mg/kg bid) im/iv,[b] imipenem-cilastin (0.5–1.0 g qid) iv, cefoxitin (2.0 g q 4 h or 3.0 g q 6 h) iv	++
Pulmonary Disease			
MAC	Clarithromycin (500 mg bid) + rifampin (600 mg qd) + ethambutol (15 mg/kg) + streptomycin (0.5–1.0 g qd) im	Rifabutin (300 mg qd), cycloserine (250 mg tid), ciprofloxacin (750 mg bid), ethionamide (250 mg bid or qid)	++
M. abscessus	Clarithromycin (500 mg bid)	Amikacin (5 mg/kg bid) im/iv,[b] imipenem-cilastin (0.5–1.0 g qid) iv, cefoxitin (2.0 g q 4–8 h) iv	++
M. kansasii	INH (300 mg qd) + rifampin (600 mg qd) + ethambutol (15 mg/kg)	Streptomycin (0.5–1.0 g qd) im, clarithromycin (500 mg bid), sulfamethoxazole (1.0 g bid), TMP(160mg)/SMX(800mg) bid	–
M. xenopi	INH (300 mg qd)+ rifampin (600 mg qd) + ethambutol(15mg/kg)	Clarithromycin (500 mg bid), streptomycin (0.5–1.0 g qd) im	++
M. fortuitum	Same as cutaneous	Same as cutaneous	–
M. simiae	(?) Clarithromycin (500 mg bid)	Unknown	?++
Lymph Node			
M. scrofulaceum	Surgery	Clarithromycin (500 mg bid)	+++
MAC	Surgery	Clarithromycin (500 mg bid)	+++
M. fortuitum	Same as cutaneous	Same as cutaneous	+
M. chelonae	Same as cutaneous	Same as cutaneous	++
M. abscessus	Same as cutaneous	Same as cutaneous	++
Disseminated			
M. chelonae	Clarithromycin (500 mg bid)	Doxycycline (100mg bid) or minocycline (100 mg bid)): 25% susceptible	

Table 9-3 **Therapy[a] (continued)**

Organism	First Line (Oral, Except Where Specified)	Injectable or Alternative Drugs (Oral Except Where Specified)	Surgery Potentially Beneficial
M. abscessus	Clarithromycin (500 mg bid)	Amikacin (5 mg/kg bid) im/iv[b] + imipenem-cilastin (0.5–1.0 g qid) iv, or amikacin (5 mg/kg bid) im/iv + cefoxitin (2.0 g q 4 or 3.0 g 96 h) iv	
M. haemophilum	Clarithromycin (500 mg bid) + rifampin (600 mg qd)	Sulfamethoxazole (1.0 g bid), TMP (160 mg)/SMX (800 mg) bid, ciprofloxacin (750 mg bid), ofloxacin (400 mg bid)	
M. kansasii	Same as pulmonary	Same as pulmonary	

Therapy for HIV-Related Disease
Disseminated

MAC (prophylaxis)	Rifabutin (300 mg q d)	Clarithromycin (500 mg bid), azithromycin (500 mg first dose, then 250 mg qd)	
MAC (disease)	Clarithromycin (500 mg bid) [or azithromycin (500 mg first dose, then 250 mg qd)] + rifabutin (300 mg qd) + ethambutol (15 mg/kg)	Streptomycin (0.5–1.0 g qd) im, amikacin (5 mg/kg qd) im or iv, clofazamine (50–100 mg qd), rifampin (600 mg qd)	
M. chelonae	Same as non-HIV	Same as non-HIV	
M. kansasii	Same as non-HIV	Same as non-HIV	
M. haemophilum	Same as non-HIV	Same as non-HIV	
M. abscessus	Same as non-HIV	Same as non-HIV	

[a] See text for clarification of dosing schedules; [b]Administration of the total daily dose as a single once a day dose is probably equally efficacious.

twice a day, trimethoprim–sulfamethoxazole at 160/800 mg two to three times a day, and perhaps clarithromycin. Acceptable dual drug therapy is rifampin (600 mg) and ethambutol (15 mg/kg) daily. The optimal duration of therapy is unknown, but a minimum of 3 months, or 4 weeks after clearing of symptoms, seems acceptable.[34a] Surgical debridement sometimes is indicated and most prescribe antibiotics during the perioperative period. Since the clinical response rate varies, additional therapeutic options should not be started any earlier than 3 weeks following initiation of therapy. As many as 80% of skin lesions may spontaneously resolve without therapy within 36 months.[80] Drug therapy for *M. xenopi* disease, usually pulmonary, often includes isoniazid, rifampin, and ethambutol.[68,76,110,111] Results from drug therapy are unpredictable, sometimes poor, and not related to the results of *in vitro* drug sensitivity tests.[111] Most isolates show varying resistance to first line antitubercular agents, but are sensitive to streptomycin, kanamycin, ethionamide, cycloserine,[110] the

macrolides,[112] and the quinolones (ciprofloxacin and ofloxacin).[113] Parrot and Grosset[111] studied the outcome of surgery in 57 patients with *M. xenopi* disease who failed to respond adequately to chemotherapy. Only 21 of these patients were cured of their *M. xenopi* infection without experiencing significant complications. These complications included death (12), relapse of *M. xenopi* infection (12), cancer (9), and postoperative complications requiring additional surgery (19).

Skin infections due to *Mycobacterium haemophilum* are typically the result of disseminated disease, often involving the extremities. The lesions require months to years for healing and it is unclear whether drug therapy is effective.[2] Isolates of *M. haemophilum* have shown *in vitro* resistance to most drugs tested with the exception of rifampin, the newer quinolones, and clarithromycin. Drugs tested include rifampin, isoniazid, streptomycin, ethambutol, *p*-aminosalicylic acid, capreomycin, kanamycin, gentamicin, amikacin, cefoxitin, sulfamethoxazole, ciprofloxacin, and clofazimine.[114]

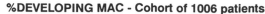

%DEVELOPING MAC - Cohort of 1006 patients

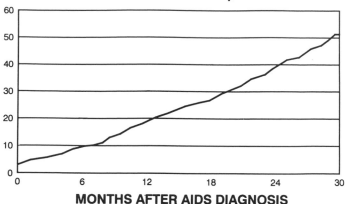

MONTHS AFTER AIDS DIAGNOSIS

Figure 9-2 The percentage of patients developing MAC bacteremia by month after the diagnosis of AIDS. (From Nightingale et al.,[122] reproduced with permission.)

III. NONTUBERCULOUS MYCOBACTERIA: HIV

A. EPIDEMIOLOGY

Since the advent and recognition of the AIDS epidemic in the early 1980s, the prevalence of mycobacterial disease has risen concurrently with the proliferation of patients infected with HIV. In 1985, the incidence of disease due to *M. tuberculosis* in the United States increased for the first time in more than two decades, and has continued to rise.[115] Infection due to MAC has risen in a spectacular fashion. Before the AIDS epidemic, MAC disease essentially was limited to lymph node disease in children and chronic pulmonary disease in elderly patients with underlying lung illnesses such as chronic bronchitis, emphysema, or bronchiectasis. Extrapulmonary MAC disease and, in particular, disseminated MAC disease was rare. Before 1980, only 24 cases of disseminated MAC disease had been reported in the medical literature.[116] By the end of 1990, 7.6% (12,202 of 161,073) of all AIDS patients reported to the Centers for Disease Control had disseminated nontuberculous mycobacterial infection.[116]

Disseminated MAC disease (D-MAC) accounts for over 96% of NTM disseminated illness, followed by *M. kansasii* (2.9%), *M. gordonae, M. fortuitum, M. chelonae,*[117] *M. xenopi, M. haemophilum,*[118] and newer mycobacteria such as *M. genavense.*[119] However, case-surveillance information appears to underestimate markedly the true prevalence of D-MAC infection in AIDS patients as reporting occurs often only at the time of diagnosis. Premortem diagnosis rates for this illness vary from 18 to 28% and postmortem prevalences range above 50%.[120,121] Figure 9-2 shows by month the percentage of patients developing MAC bacteremia after the diagnosis of AIDS has been made.[122] In the United States and other developed countries, MAC is the most commonly

isolated mycobacteria in patients infected with HIV.[118]

B. DISSEMINATED DISEASE DUE TO *M. AVIUM* COMPLEX (MAC)

The distribution of D-MAC among AIDS patients in the United States appears to be fairly uniform in that it relates to the distribution of AIDS cases and not the geographic location of the cases. This is in striking contrast to the localized geographic distribution seen in non-AIDS patients with lung disease. The latter parallels the environmental recovery of the organism (e.g., commonly recovered in coastal states of the southeast). In Europe and Australia a similar pattern of distribution is seen in the AIDS patient populations. Only in Africa has there been a seeming dearth of AIDS patients with disseminated MAC disease. In a 1990 report from Uganda, all of 50 severely ill AIDS patients were blood culture negative for MAC.[123]

A CD4 cell count of less than 60 cells per cubic millimeter is the major risk factor for this illness[116,120] (Figure 9-3).[122] The majority of patients have CD4 counts less than 20 at the time of D-MAC diagnosis. This corresponds to the late development of MAC infection in patients with AIDS, and to a shortened survival time (median, 7.5 months) compared with other AIDS patients (median, 13.3 months).[117] Disseminated NTM disease has been seen less in AIDS cases with Kaposi's sarcoma than in other AIDS cases.[117] The frequency of D-MAC infection is similar for both sexes and for persons with various HIV risk factors. Overall Hispanics have less infection compared to non-Hispanic whites and blacks. This infection is more common in younger age groups and the frequency of infection decreases with age.[116]

Based on the use of the species-specific DNA probe, almost 90% of AIDS patients in the United States have been shown to be infected with strains of *M. avium*. These isolates most commonly are

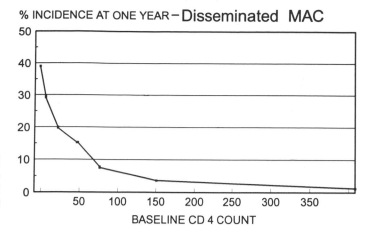

% INCIDENCE AT ONE YEAR – Disseminated MAC

BASELINE CD 4 COUNT

Figure 9-3 The incidence of MAC bacteremia at 1 year in relationship to the baseline CD4 cell count. (From Nightingale et al.,[122] reproduced with permission.)

serotypes 4 and 8 of *M. avium*.[116,124] This is in contrast to pulmonary disease, where equivalent numbers of *M. avium* and *M. intracellulare* are involved with numerous different serotypes.

The *M. avium* strains recovered from AIDS patients tend to be more virulent than other MAC isolates in animal models.[125] Yamori and Tsukamura[22] compared pulmonary disease due to *M. avium* and *M. intracellulare* in 55 patients and found progressive disease and death more common with *M. intracellulare* infection. They concluded that pulmonary disease due to *M. avium* has a better prognosis than pulmonary disease due to *M. intracellulare.*

While the pathogenesis of D-MAC infection in the AIDS patient is incompletely understood, it appears this infection results from primary infection rather than reactivation of infection as is the case for tuberculosis. The portal of entry for MAC infection in the AIDS patients appears to be the gastrointestinal tract rather than the respiratory tract. This may be supported by common gastrointestinal symptoms in AIDS patients such as nausea, diarrhea, abdominal pain, and biliary tract obstruction. Further support comes from studies that more frequently recover MAC from lymph tissue in the gastrointestinal tract than from respiratory tissues.[126,127]

Since AIDS patients are uniquely and highly vulnerable to MAC infection, cell-mediated immunity is considered to be the main defense against infection with this organism. Phagocytosis seems to be intact while macrophage-mediated killing seems to be defective. This may be related to the role of lymphokines such as interleukin-2, tumor necrosis factor, and granulocyte–macrophage colony-stimulating factor.[116]

Diagnosis of MAC or other NTM disease in the AIDS patient typically is made when the organism is cultured from normally sterile body fluid or tissue. Blood, bone marrow, liver, and lymph nodes are the most common sites of positive cultures. Less common sites include the spleen, eyes, brain, meninges, cerebrospinal fluid, tongue, skin, heart, stomach, lungs, thyroid, breasts, parathyroids, adrenals, kidneys, pancreas, prostate, testes, and urine.[126,127] Because of the ease of acquisition and almost uniform positivity in D-MAC, blood cultures for MAC are the usual method for making or excluding the diagnosis. When the organism is cultured from nonsterile sites such as feces or sputum, colonization or localized disease must be differentiated from D-MAC disease. Direct examination of blood films can provide rapid diagnosis of mycobacteremia in some AIDS patients. Eng and colleagues[128] found 13 of 15 patients who were culture positive for mycobacteria (14 with MAC, 1 with *M. tuberculosis)* and had identifiable organisms on Kinyoun- or auramine-stained buffy coat blood smears.

On autopsy the infected organ may be enlarged and colored yellow because of pigmentation from great quantities of the organism (nearly 10^{10} colony-forming units per gram).[116] Microscopic exam reveals many organisms, reduced inflammatory reaction, and few and poorly formed granulomas.

The clinical presentation of D-MAC varies and often mimics other signs and symptoms associated with AIDS. Persistent fever, weight loss, night sweats, abdominal pain, and diarrhea are the most common and significant presenting symptoms. Severe anemia, often requiring transfusions, and neutropenia also are important finding in this illness.[127] A few patients with positive blood cultures for MAC may (at least initially) be asymptomatic.

Therapy for D-MAC has been difficult because the organism is resistant to standard antimycobacterial agents and controlled studies have been difficult to perform. This is especially true where antiretroviral agents such as zidovudine or drugs for other opportunistic infections are used concurrently. Early trials of therapy for D-MAC

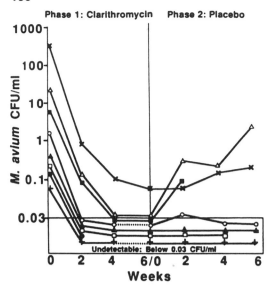

Figure 9-4 Changes in levels of *M. avium* bacteremia (colony-forming units, CFU) in eight patients initially receiving clarithromycin alone for 6 weeks (phase 1) and then receiving placebo plus a four-drug regimen (rifampin, isoniazid, ethambutol, and clofazimine) for 6 more weeks (phase 2). (From Dautzenberg et al.,[132] reproduced with permission.)

were discouraging in part because the expected response times probably were unrealistic. However, newer trials even without the macrolides have demonstrated a decrease in days of bacteremia and improvement in clinical response.[95,129] To date, no controlled studies have demonstrated improved survival in patients with AIDS and disseminated MAC infection receiving drug therapy. One retrospective chart review of this group of patients showed increased median survival (from 80 days to 191 days).[130]

A dramatic improvement in early clinical and microbiologic responses has been seen with monotherapy trials with the newer macrolides, azithromycin[131] and clarithromycin.[132] In a randomized, double blind, placebo-controlled trial, Dautzenberg et al. showed that clarithromycin alone was more effective against D-MAC than placebo plus four other drugs (Figure 9-4).[132] A recent dose–response study comparing daily doses of 1.0, 2.0, and 4.0 g of clarithromycin showed that patients cleared their mycobacteremia more rapidly at the higher dose, but limiting side effects (gastrointestinal and hepatic) were greater[133] (Figure 9-4). At present, clarithromycin, 1.0 g twice a day, is the most commonly used regimen. The development of MAC resistance to clarithromycin with clinical and microbiologic relapse appears to occur in most patients who receive macrolide monotherapy, in contrast to about 20% who receive clarithromycin as part of a multidrug regimen.

Several different multidrug regimens have been used for therapy. Currently there is no consensus for either the number of drugs, the selection of drugs, the length of therapy or therapy for suppression of established illness. Regimens have included ciprofloxacin (750 mg twice daily), ethambutol (1000 mg or 15 mg/kg daily), and rifampin (600 mg daily) with either amikacin (7.5 mg/kg body weight),[134] or clofazimine (100 mg once daily),[129] or all five drugs.[135] In 1993, Centers for Disease Control and Prevention recommended oral therapy with rifabutin (300 mg daily) for the life of the patient as a primary prophylaxis against DMAC for patients with advanced (<100 CD4 + T-lymphocytes/μL) HIV disease.[135a]

Uncontrolled studies[95,130] recently have tested multidrug regimens using the newer macrolides. In one study, 12 patients with AIDS and MAC bacteremia were treated with amikacin (7.5 mg/kg of body weight intravenously, twice daily for only 3 weeks), clarithromycin (1 g orally twice daily), and ciprofloxacin (500 mg orally three times daily) indefinitely. Mycobacteremia cleared without recurrence in all patients within 2 to 8 weeks.[95] Uncontrolled studies have shown decreased mycobacteremia and improvement in systemic symptoms; however, it is unknown whether therapy for NTM will prolong life in these patients.[95,130]

It is the authors' opinion that a regimen of clarithromycin, rifabutin, and ethambutol is the most reasonable long-term treatment for D-MAC, although the addition of several other drugs such as amikacin (or streptomycin) and clofazimine during the early phase of treatment is reasonable.

New drugs showing promise as beneficial therapy include the new rifampin derivative rifabutin (oral) and intravenously administered liposome-encapsulated aminoglycosides. This latter group appears as effective as standard aminoglycosides (amikacin, gentamicin, or streptomycin) and may be much less toxic.

Given the problems with therapy, the ideal or preferred approach to D-MAC would be disease prevention. A recently completed randomized, double-blind placebo-controlled trial of rifabutin 300 mg/day in patients with CD4 counts of less than 200 showed that this drug was highly effective both in delaying and preventing D-MAC.[98] Given the low incidence of D-MAC in patients with CD4 counts above 50, it would seem reasonable to begin this drug as a prophylactic agent at this point. The newer macrolides may also be useful prophylactic agents, but randomized comparative trials are still ongoing (as of early 1994).

C. DISEASE DUE TO *M. KANSASII*

In the United States, *M. kansasii*, is a distant second to MAC as a cause of NTM infection in the

AIDS patient.[117] Two retrospective studies[136,137] describe a total of 28 AIDS patients infected with *M. kansasii*, 22 with pulmonary disease, 4 with pulmonary and extrapulmonary disease, 5 with extrapulmonary disease only, and 10 with positive blood cultures or disseminated disease. The extrapulmonary disease involved one case of osteomyelitis and two cases of gastrointestinal involvement. Only three patients had normal chest roentgenograms. Thin-walled cavitary lesions were present in 9 of 19 patients in one study and in none of 9 patients in the other study. Other chest film patterns were heterogeneous with focal upper lobe infiltrates or diffuse interstitial infiltrates being somewhat common. The infection occurred late in the AIDS illness with a median CD4 lymphocyte count of 49 in the larger study.[137] In this study treatment with conventional therapy for *M. kansasii* (isoniazid, rifampin, and ethambutol) resulted in a clearing of symptoms, radiographic infiltrates, and bacteremia while on therapy.

D. DISEASE DUE TO *M. XENOPI*

In a study[67] from Brooklyn, New York, 23 patients with AIDS and pulmonary *M. xenopi* infection were described briefly. Only one of these patients had bacteremia due to *M. xenopi*. Six of these patients had clearing of pulmonary symptoms without therapy; none was treated for their pulmonary infections due to *M. xenopi*. In this same study, only 5 of 34 (15%) patients with disease due to *M. fortuitum* or *M. chelonae* had concomitant HIV infection.

E. DISEASE DUE TO *M. HAEMOPHILUM*

Infection due to *M. haemophilum* occurs primarily in immunocompromised hosts, but only a few cases (less than 20) have been reported in patients infected with the HIV.[69] Recently (1992) a larger number of patients have been recognized in New York City. In the reported cases, the median age of diagnosis was 34 years.[138] The organism had been isolated in this group of patients from multiple sites and blood, suggesting disseminated disease. CD4 cell counts were markedly depressed with *M. haemophilum* infection being the AIDS-defining illness in only one case. Therapy using a variety of antimycobacterial agents showed favorable response to therapy with decreased symptoms, but all relapsed shortly after discontinuation of antibiotic therapy.

F. DISEASE DUE TO *M. CELATUM*

The use of DNA probes has recently allowed the identity of a new slowly growing *Mycobacterium* species of the proposed name *"Mycobacterium celatum."*[138a] Although its clinical disease mimics MAC, the organism fails to react with the MAC probe and biochemically most closely resembles *M. xenopi*. It has been isolated from patients from throughout the United States. While most isolates come from bronchial washings and sputum, some strains have also been isolated from stool, bone, and blood. In patients from whom *M. celatum* has been isolated, seven were HIV positive while four were HIV negative. As more information develops about this organism, it may prove to be very clinically significant because it is resistant (*in vitro*) to most antituberculosis drugs (including high-level resistance to rifabutin).

G. DISEASE DUE TO *M. GENAVENSE*

Mycobacterium genavense is the name proposed for a recently recovered mycobacterium that has been isolated from blood, bone marrow, liver, spleen, lymph node, and intestinal cultures in 2,[139] 7,[119] and 18[140] patients with AIDS in Australia, Seattle, and Europe, respectively. The first patients were from Geneva, Switzerland, hence the organism's name. These patients had advanced AIDS with low CD4 counts and presented typically with fever, weight loss, and diarrhea. The organism is quite fastidious and grows in liquid media (such as BACTEC 12B and/or 13A), but not on routine solid media (Lowenstein–Jensen medium or egg yolk agar). Recently it has been subcultured on special solid media such as 7H9/CYE[139] and M7H11-MJ.[141] This organism may account for many of the unidentified mycobacteria isolated from blood cultures of patients with AIDS. Mycobacterial blood cultures should include a broth medium incubated for at least 8 weeks to allow identification of this newly discovered *Mycobacterium*.

IV. DISEASE DUE TO *M. BOVIS* AND BACILLUS CALMETTE–GUÉRIN (BCG)

Technically, BCG and *M. bovis* are not NTMs, but are part of the tuberculosis spectrum of diseases.

A. *M. BOVIS*

Although common 100 years ago, disease with *M. bovis* is rare today, due to the pasteurization of milk, the slaughter of infected cattle, and the absence of a common wild animal host. In the recent past, reports from various hospitals have shown only a handful of cases.[142-146] However, England and Wales have had a slightly higher percentage of cases, and from January 1986 to October 1991, 117 isolates, or 1.2% of the total number of mycobacterial isolates, were identified as *M. bovis*.[147] Furthermore, in San Diego, Dankner et al. reported 73 cases (48 adults, 25 children) of *M. bovis* during the 12-year period from 1980 to 1991, accounting for almost 3% of all cases in San Diego during that time period.[148] Hispanics comprised the majority of cases, and Mexican cattle were thought to be a likely source. AIDS was present in 25% of adults and 4% of children with *M. bovis* disease. Pulmonary disease was present in 25 (52%) of the adults, and in 3 (12%) of the children.

Humans can become infected by drinking contaminated milk or by sharing a closed air space with a group of cows with pulmonary disease.[148] In cattle, the respiratory route is thought to be the primary route of infection.[149]

Extrapulmonary tuberculosis is present in a higher percentage of persons diseased with *M. bovis* than in those diseased with *M. tuberculosis*. The disease is not difficult to cure, but the treatment regimen should not rely on pyrazinamide, since classically, the organism is resistant to this drug. There has been some confusion on this issue because of the similarity between *M. bovis* and *M. africanum*, and there has been discussion about whether *M. africanum* is actually a subvar of *M. bovis*. Collins et al., in a series of 137 cases from southeast England, divided *M. bovis* into "classical" strains ($n = 63$), resistant to pyrazinamide, and "Afro-Asian" strains ($n = 74$), sensitive to pyrazinamide, and stated that the organisms in the "Afro-Asian" group that were also nitratase positive might be considered *M. africanum*.[150]

In general, treatment of this disease should be based on a non-pyrazinamide-containing regimen. It would be wise to use 9-month therapy starting with initial isoniazid, rifampin, and ethambutol followed by maintenance isoniazid and rifampin.

B. BACILLUS CALMETTE–GUÉRIN

Immunization and cancer therapy with bacillus Calmette–Guérin (BCG) has produced localized lymphadenitis with and without abscess formation, pulmonary infection, osteomyelitis, cutaneous nodules, and other disseminated disease sometimes referred to as "BCGosis" and "BCGitis." BCG vaccine, a live attenuated vaccine derived from *M. bovis*, is used worldwide (except in the United States) to prevent tuberculosis.

Intravesical instillation of BCG for bladder cancer therapy can produce localized cystitis, as well as disseminated disease involving the lungs and liver, and, less frequently, the bone marrow, brain, kidney, prostate, and spleen.[151] There are 45,000 new cases of bladder cancer each year in the United States.[151] From retrospective studies[151] it is estimated that up to 1% of these cases treated with BCG therapy may experience BCGosis. Only a small number of treated cases have been reported, but some have responded well to standard two-drug antituberculous therapy (isoniazid 300 mg/day and rifampin 600 mg/day) (BCG is resistant to pyrazinamide).

When BCG is administered to young infants, 0.5–5.0% will experience a localized injection abscess or regional (axillary) lymphadenitis.[152] This complication usually is benign, but often persists for 6 to 12 months. Therapy may, in some cases, shorten the duration of disease. Therapeutic options include erythromycin (50 g/kg/day in four divided doses) for 1 month, INH 5–10 mg/kg/day for 1 to 3 months, surgical removal, or local INH instillation (50 mg) into the abscess. Disseminated disease occurs rarely (3.4 per 1,000,000) in newborns immunized with BCG, but when it does occur, it often is resistant to therapy and often is fatal.[153] Apparently, infants born to women infected with HIV are not at appreciably higher risk of adverse effects to BCG vaccine.[154] However, infants with other immunodeficiency syndromes probably are at severe risk of BCGosis and death from BCG vaccination.[153] Further information may be found in Chapter 15 (this volume).

REFERENCES

1. Alvarez, E., Tavel, E., Recherches sur le bacille de Lustgarten, *Arch. Physiol. Norm. Pathol.*, 3rd series, 6, 303, 1885.

2. Wayne, L. G., Kubica, G. P., Mycobacteria, in *Bergey's Manual of Systematic Bacteriology*, Sneath, P. H. A., Mair, N. S., Sharpe, M. E., Holt, J. G., Eds., Vol. 2., Williams & Wilkins, Baltimore, 1986, 1436.

3. Timpe, A., Runyon, E. H., The relationship of "atypical acid-fast" bacteria to human disease: a preliminary report, *J. Lab. Clin. Med.*, 44, 202, 1954.

4. Pinner, M., Atypical acid-fast microorganisms, *Am. Rev. Tuberc.*, 32, 424, 1935.

5. Hector, J. S. R., Pang, Y., Mazurek, G. H., Zhang, Y., Brown, B., Wallace, R. J., Jr., Large restriction fragment patterns of genomic *Mycobacterium fortuitum* DNA strain-specific markers and their use in epidemiologic investigation of four nosocomial outbreaks, *J. Clin. Microbiol.*, 30, 1250, 1992.

6. Mazurek, G. H., Hartman, S. L., Zhang, Y., Brown, B. A., Hector, J. S. R., Murphy, D., Wallace, R. J. Jr., Large DNA fragment polymorphism in the *Mycobacterium avium-M. intracellulare* complex: a potential epidemiologic tool, *J. Clin. Microbiol.*, 31(2), 390, 1993.

7. Meissner, G., Anz, W., Sources of *Mycobacterium avium* complex infection resulting in human diseases, *Am. Rev. Resp. Dis.*, 116, 1057, 1977.

8. Reznikov, M., Dawson, D. J., Mycobacteria of the *intracellulare-scrofulaceum* group in soils from the Adelaide area, *Pathology*, 12, 525, 1980.

9. Nel, E. E., *Mycobacterium avium-intracellulare* complex serovars isolated in South Africa from humans, swine, and the environment, *Rev. Infect. Dis.*, 3, 1013, 1981.

10. Edwards, L. B., Acquaviva, F. A., Livesay, V. T., Palmer, C. E., An atlas of sensitivity to tuberculin, PPD, and histoplasmin in the United States, *Am. Rev. Resp. Dis.*, 99, 1, 1969.

11. Huebner, R. E., Schein, M. F., Cauthen, G. M., Geiter, L. J., Selin, M. J., Good, R. C., O'Brien, R. J., Evaluation of the clinical usefulness of mycobacterial skin test antigens in adults with pulmonary Mycobacterioses, *Am. Rev. Resp. Dis.*, 145, 1160, 1992.

12. Wijsmuller, G., Erickson, P., The reaction to PPD-Battey: a new look, *Am. Rev. Resp. Dis.*, 29, 109, 1974.

13. Krajnack, M. A., Dowda, H., Nontuberculous mycobacteria in South Carolina, 1971–1980, *J. S. C. Med. Assoc.*, 77, 551, 1981.

14. Edwards, F. G. B., Disease caused by "atypical" (opportunistist) mycobacteria: a whole population review, *Tubercle*, 51, 285, 1970.

15. Good, R. C., Isolation of nontuberculous mycobacteria in the United States, 1979, *J. Infect. Dis.*, 142, 779, 1980.

16. Good, R. C., Snider, D. E., Jr., Isolation of nontuberculous mycobacteria from the United States, 1980, *J. Infect. Dis.*, 146, 829, 1982.

17. Issac-Renton, J. L., Allen, E. A., Chao, C. W., Grzybowski, E., Black, W. A., Isolation and geographic distribution of *Mycobacterium* other that *M. tuberculosis* in British Columbia, 1972–1981, *Can. Med. Assoc. J.*, 133, 573, 1985.

18. Du Moulin, G. C., Stottmeier, K. D., Pelletier, P. A., Tsang, A. Y., Hedley-Whyte, J., Concentration of *Mycobacterium avium* by hospital hot water system, *J. Am. Med. Assoc.*, 260, 1599, 1988.

19. Geppert, E. F., Feff, A., The pathogenesis of pulmonary and miliary tuberculosis, *Arch. Intern. Med.*, 139, 1381, 1979.

20. Woodring, J. H., MacVandiviere, H., Pulmonary disease caused by nontuberculous mycobacteria, *J. Thorac. Imaging*, 5, 64, 1990.

21. Wayne, L. G., Sramek, H. A., Agents of newly recognized or infrequently encountered mycobacterial diseases, *Clin. Microbiol. Rev.*, 5, 1, 1992.

22. Yamori, S., Tsukamura, M., Comparison of prognosis of pulmonary diseases caused by *Mycobacterium avium* and by *Mycobacterium intracellulare*, *Chest*, 102, 89, 1992.

23. Tsang, A. Y., Drupa, I., Goldberg, M., McClatchy, J. K., Brennan, P. J., Use of serology and thin-layer chromatography for the assembly of an authenticated collection of serovars within the *Mycobacterium-avium-Mycobacterium intracellulare-Mycobacterium scrofulaceum* complex, *Int. J. Syst. Bacteriol.*, 33, 285, 1983.

24. Shaefer, W. B., Serologic identification and classification of the atypical mycobacteria by their agglutination, *Am. Rev. Tuberc.*, 96, 115, 1967.

25. O'Brien, R. J., Geiter, L. J., Snider, D. E., Jr., The epidemiology of nontuberculous mycobacterial diseases in the United States, *Am. Rev. Resp. Dis.*, 135, 1007, 1987.

26. Wolinsky, E., Rynearson, T. K., Mycobacteria in soil and their relation to disease-associated strains, *Am. Rev. Resp. Dis.*, 97, 1032, 1968.

27. Collins, C. H., Grange, J. M., Yates, M. D., Mycobacteria in water, *J. Appl. Bacteriol.*, 57, 193, 1984.

28. Reznikov, M., Leggo, J. H., Dawson, D. J., Investigation by seroagglutination of strains of the *Mycobacterium intracellulare-M. scrofulaceum* group from house dusts and sputum in southeastern Queensland, *Am. Rev. Resp. Dis.*, 104, 951, 1974.

29. Thoen, C. O., Karson, A. G., Tuberculosis, in *Disease of Poultry*, Hoffstead, M. S., Calnek, B. W., Helmboldt, C. F., Eds., 7th ed., Iowa State University Press, Ames, 1978, 209.

30. Montali, R. J., Bush, M., Thoen, C. O., Smith, E., Tuberculosis in captive exotic birds, *J. Am. Vet. Med. Assoc.*, 169, 920, 1976.

31. Chapman, J. S., Isolation of atypical mycobacteria from pasteurized milk, *Am. Rev. Resp. Dis.*, 98, 1052, 1968.

32. Engbaek, H. C., Vergmann, B., Baiss, I., Bentzon, M. W., *Mycobacterium avium*: a bacteriological and epidemiological study of *M. avium* isolated from animals and man in Denmark. II. Strains isolated from man, *Acta Pathol. Microbiol. Scand.*, 72, 295, 1968.

33. Kirschner, R. A., Parker, B. C., Falkinham, J. O., III., Epidemiology of infection by nontuberculous mycobacteria, *Am. Rev. Resp. Dis.*, 145, 271, 1992.

34. Falkinham, J. O., III., Parker, B. C., Gruft, H., Epidemiology of infection by infection by nontuberculous mycobacteria. I. Geographic distribution in the eastern United States, *Am. Rev. Resp. Dis.*, 121, 931, 1980.

34a. Wallace, R. J., Jr., O'Brien, R., Glassroth, J., Raleigh, J., Dutt, A., Diagnosis and treatment of disease caused by nontuberculous mycobacteria (official statement ATS), *Am. Rev. Resp. Dis.*, 142, 940, 1990.

35. Tsukamura, M., Diagnosis of disease caused by *Mycobacterium avium* complex, *Chest*, 99, 667, 1991.

36. Yeager, H., Raleigh, J. W., Pulmonary disease due to *Mycobacterium intracellulare*, *Am. Rev. Resp. Dis.*, 108, 547, 1979.

37. Mammo, A., Epidemiologic trends of lung disease due to *Mycobacterium kansasii* and *Mycobacterium avium-intracellulare* in Texas, 1977–1983, Doctoral thesis, University of Texas Health Science Center at Houston, 1983, 1.

38. Reznikow, M., Leggo, J. H., Dawson, D. J., Investigation by sero-agglutination of strains of *Mycobacterium intracellulare-Mycobacterium scrofulaceum* group house dusts and sputum in southeastern Queensland, *Am. Rev. Resp. Dis.*, 104, 951, 1971.

39. Kamat, S. R., Rossiter, C. E., Gilson, J. C., A retrospective clinical study of pulmonary disease due to "Anonymous Mycobacteria in Wales," *Thorax*, 16, 297, 1961.

40. Davidson, P. T., Khanijo, V., Goble, M., Moulding, T. S., Treatment of disease due to *Mycobacterium intracellulare*, *Rev. Infect. Dis.*, 3, 1052, 1981.

41. Rosenzweig, D. Y., Pulmonary mycobacterial infections due to *Mycobacterium intracellulare-avium* complex: clinical features and course in 100 consecutive cases, *Chest*, 75, 115, 1979.

42. Engel, H. W. B., Berwald, L. G., Havelaar, A. H., The occurrence of *Mycobacterium kansasii* in tap water, *Tubercle*, 61, 21, 1980.

43. Janning, R. S. B., Fischeder J. R., Occurrence of mycobacteria in biofilm samples, *Tubercle Lung Dis.*, 73, 141, 1992.

44. Bailey, R. K., Wyles, S., Dingley, M., Hesse, F., Kent, G. W., The isolation of high catalase *Mycobacterium kansasii* from tap water, *Am. Rev. Resp. Dis.*, 101, 430, 1970.

45. Wolinsky, E., State of the art — nontuberculous mycobacteria and associated diseases, *Am. Rev. Resp. Dis.*, 199, 107, 1979.

46. Banks, J., Hunter, A. M., Campbell, I. A., Jenkins, P. A., Smith, A. P., Pulmonary infection with *Mycobacterium kansasii* in Wales, 1970–9: review of treatment and response, *Thorax*, 38, 271, 1983.

47. Tsukamura, M., Kita, N., Shimoide, H., Arakawa, H., Kuze, A., Studies on the epidemiology of nontuberculous mycobacteriosis in Japan, *Am. Rev. Resp. Dis.*, 137, 1280, 1988.

48. Cowie, R. L., The mycobacteriology of pulmonary tuberculosis in South African gold miners, *Tubercle*, 71, 39, 1990.

49. Chapman, J. S., *The Atypical Mycobacteria and Human Mycobacteriosis*, Plenum Medical Book Co., New York, 1977, chap. 5.

49a. Wallace, R. J., Jr., Silcox, V. A., Tsukamura, M., Brown, B. A., Kilburn, J. O., Butler, W. R., Onyi, G., Clinical significance, biochemical features, and susceptibility patterns of sporadic isolates of the *Mycobacterium chelonae*-like organism, *J. Clin. Microbiol.*, 31, 3231, 1993.

50. Wayne, L. G., Sramek, H. A., Agents of newly recognized or infrequently encountered mycobacterial disease, *Clin. Microbiol. Rev.*, 5, 1, 1992.

51. Fraser, V. J., Jones, M., Murray, P. R., Medoff, G., Zhang, Y., Wallace, R. J., Jr., Contamination of flexible fiberoptic bronchoscopes with *Mycobacterium chelonae* linked to an automated bronchoscope disinfection machine, *Am. Rev. Resp. Dis.*, 145, 853, 1992.

52. Raad, I. I., Vartivarian, S., Khan, A., Bodey, G. P., Catheter-related infections caused by the *Mycobacterium fortuitum* complex: 15 cases and review, *Rev. Infect. Dis.*, 13, 1120, 1991.

53. Safranek, T. J., Jarvis, W. R., Carson, L. A., Cusick, L. B., Bland, L. A., Swenson, J. M., Silcox, V. A., *Mycobacterium chelonae* wound infections after plastic surgery employing contaminated gentian violet skin-marking solution, *N. Engl. J. Med.*, 317, 197, 1987.

54. Wallace, R. J., Jr., Swenson, J. M., Silcox, V. A., Good, R. C., Tschen, J. A., Stone, M. S., Spectrum of disease due to rapidly growing mycobacteria, *Rev. Infect. Dis.*, 5, 657, 1983.

55. Philpott, J. A., Woodburne, A. R., Philpott, O. S., Schaefer, O. S., Mollohan, C. S., Swimming pool granuloma: a study of 290 cases, *Arch. Dermatol.*, 88, 94, 1963.

56. Keczkes, K., Tropical fish tank granuloma, *Br. J. Dermatol.*, 91, 709, 1974.

57. Arai, H., Nakajima, H., Nagai, R., *Mycobacterium marinum* infections of the skin in Japan, *J. Dermatol.*, 11, 37, 1984.

58. Huminer, D., Pitlik, S. D., Block, C., Kaufman, L., Amit, S., Rosenfeld, J. B., Aquarium-borne *Mycobacterium marinum* skin infection, *Arch. Dermatol.*, 122, 698, 1986.

59. Chow, S. P., Stroebel, A. B., Lau, J. K., Collins, R. J., *Mycobacterium marinum* infection of the hand involving deep structures, *J. Hand Surg.*, 8, 568, 1983.

60. Faoagali, J. L., Muir, A. D., Sears, P. J., Paltridge, G. P., Tropical fish tank granuloma, *N. Z. Med. J.*, 85, 332, 1977.

61. MacLellan, D. G., Moon, M., Fish tank granuloma: A diagnostic dilemma, *Aust. N. Z. J. Surg.*, 8, 568, 1982.

62. Brown, J., Kelm, M., Bryan, L. E., Infection of the skin by *Mycobacterium marinum*: Report of five cases, *Can. Med. Assoc. J.*, 117, 912, 1989.

63. Johnston, J. M., Izumi, A. K., Cutaneous *Mycobacterium marinum* infection ("swimming pool granuloma"), *Clin. Dermatol.*, 5, 68, 1987.

64. Dattwyler, R. J., Thomas, J., Hurst, L. C., Antigen-specific T-cell anergy in progressive *Mycobacterium marinum* infections in Humans, *Ann. Intern. Med.*, 107, 675, 1987.

65. Schulze-Robbecke, R., Buchholtz, K., Heat susceptibility of aquatic mycobacteria, *Am. Soc. Microbiol.*, 58, 1869, 1992.

66. Yates, M. D., Grange, J. M., Collins, C. H., The nature of mycobacterial disease in southeast England, 1977–84, *J. Epidemiol. Commun. Health*, 40, 295, 1986.

67. Shafer, R. W., Sierra, M. F., *Mycobacterium xenopi, Mycobacterium fortuitum, Mycobacterium kansasii,* and other nontuberculous mycobacteria in an area of endemicity for AIDS, *Clin. Infect. Dis.*, 15, 161, 1992.

68. Simor, A. E., Salit, I. E., Vellend, H., The role of *Mycobacterium xenopi* in human disease, *Am. Rev. Resp. Dis.*, 129, 435, 1984.

69. Dever, L. L., Martin, J. W., Seaworth, B., Jorgensen, J. H., Varied presentations and responses to treatment of infections caused by *Mycobacterium haemophilum* in patients with AIDS, *Clin. Infect. Dis.*, 14, 1195, 1992.

70. Ahn, C. H., McLarty, J. W., Ahn, S. S., Ahn, S. I., Hurst, G. A., Diagnostic criteria for pulmonary disease caused by *Mycobacterium kansasii* and *Mycobacterium intracellulare*, *Am. Rev. Resp. Dis.*, 125, 388, 1982.

71. Teirstein, A. S., Damsker, B., Kirschner, P. A., Krellenstein, D. J., Robinson, B., Chuang, M. T., Pulmonary infection with MAI: diagnosis, clinical patterns, treatment, *Mt. Sinai J. Med.*, 57, 209, 1990.

71a. Swensen, S. J., Hartman, T. E., Williams, D. E., Computed tomographic diagnosis of *Mycobacterium avium-intracellulare* complex in patients with bronchiectasis, *Chest,* 105, 49, 1994.

72. Reich, J. M., Johnson, R. E., *Mycobacterium avium* complex pulmonary disease presenting as an isolated lingular or middle lobe pattern, *Chest*, 101, 1605, 1992.

73. Johanson, W., Jr., Nicholson, D., Pulmonary disease due to *Mycobacterium kansasii, Am. Rev. Resp. Dis.*, 99, 73, 1969.

74. Herrod, H. G., Rourk, M. H., Jr., Spock, A., Pulmonary disease in children caused by nontuberculous mycobacteria, *J. Pediatr.*, 94, 915, 1979.

75. Griffith, D. E., Girard, W. M., Wallace, R. J., Jr., Clinical features of pulmonary disease caused by rapidly growing mycobacteria: an analysis of 154 patients, *Am. Rev. Resp. Dis.*, 147, 1271, 1993.

76. Thomas, P., Liu, F., Weiser, W., Characteristics of *Mycobacterium xenopi* disease, *Bull. Int. Union Tuberc. Lung Dis.*, 6, 12, 1988.

77. Costrini, A. M., Mahler, D. A., Gross, W. M., Hawkins, J. E., Yesner, R., D'Esposo, E., Clinical and roentgenographic features of nosocomial pulmonary disease due to *Mycobacterium xenopi, Am. Rev. Resp. Dis.,* 123, 104, 1981.

78. Lai, K. K., Stottmeir, K. D., Sherman, I. H., McCabe, W. R., Mycobacterial cervical lymphadenopathy: relation of etiologic agents to age, *J. Am. Med. Assoc.*, 251, 1286, 1984.

79. Schaad, H. B., Votteler, P., McCracken, G. H., Jr., Nelson, J. D., Management of atypical mycobacterial lymphadenitis in childhood: a review based on 380 cases, *J. Pediatr.*, 95, 356, 1979.

80. Santa Cruz, D. J., Strayer, D. S., The histologic spectrum of the cutaneous mycobacterioses, *Hum. Pathol.*, 13, 485, 1982.

81. Feingold, D., *Mycobacterium marinum* granuloma, *Arch. Dermatol.,* 114, 1564, 1978.

82. Wallace, R. J., Jr., The clinical presentation, diagnosis, and therapy of cutaneous and pulmonary infections due to the rapidly growing mycobacteria, *M. fortuitum* and *M. chelonae*, *Clin. Chest Med.*, 10, 419, 1989.

83. McBride, M. E., Rudolph, A. H., Tschen, J. A., Cernoch, P., Davis, J., Brown, B. A., Wallace, R. J., Jr., Diagnostic and therapeutic considerations for cutaneous *Mycobacterium haemophilum* infections, *Arch. Dermatol.*, 127, 276, 1991.

84. Radford, A. J., *Mycobacterium ulcerans* in Australia, *Aust. N. Z. J. Med.*, 5, 162, 1975.

85. Sutker, W. L., Lankford, L. L., Tompsett, R., Granulomatous synovitis: the role of atypical mycobacteria, *Rev. Infect. Dis.*, 1, 729, 1979.

86. Maricic, M. J., Alepa, E. P., Reactive arthritis after *Mycobacterium avium-intracellulare* infection: Poncet's disease revisited, *Am. J. Med.*, 88, 549, 1990.

87. Wardrop, P. A., Pillsbury, H. C., III., *Mycobacterium avium* acute mastoiditis, *Arch. Otolaryngol.*, 110, 686, 1984.

88. Mikolich, D. J, Mates, S. M., Granulomatous prostatitis due to *Mycobacterium avium* complex, *Clin. Infect. Dis.*, 14, 589, 1992.

89. Beckman, E. N., Pankey, G. A., McFarland, G. B., The histopathology of *Mycobacterium marinum* synovitis, *J. Clin. Pathol.*, 83, 457, 1985.

90. Bennett, C., Vardiman, J., Golomb, H., Disseminated atypical mycobacterial infection in patients with hairy cell leukemia, *Am. J. Med.*, 80, 891, 1986.

91. Horsburgh, C. R., Jr., Mason, U. G., III., Farhi, D. C., Iseman, M. D., Disseminated infection with *Mycobacterium avium-intracellular*: a report of 13 cases and a review of the literature, *Medicine*, 64, 36, 1985.

92. Lichtenstein, I. H., MacGregor, R. R., Mycobacterial infections in renal transplant recipients: report of five cases and review of the literature, *Rev. Infect. Dis.*, 5, 216, 1983.

93. Lincoln, E. M., Gilbert, L. A., Disease in children due to *Mycobacteria* other than *Mycobacterium tuberculosis*, *Am. Rev. Resp. Dis.*, 105, 683, 1972.

94. Wallace, R. J., Jr., Brown, B. A., Onyi, G. O., Skin, soft tissue, and bone infections due to *Mycobacterium chelonae chelonea*: importance of prior corticosteroid therapy, frequency of disseminated infections, and resistance to oral antimicrobials other than clarithromycin, *J. Infect. Dis.*, 166, 405, 1992.

95. de Lalla, F., Maserati, R., Scarpellini, P., Marone, P., Nicolin R., Caccamo F., Rigoli R., Clarithromycin-ciprofloxacin-amikacin for therapy of *Mycobacterium avium-Mycobacterium intracellulare* bacteremia in patients with AIDS, *J. Antimcrob. Chemother.*, 36, 1567, 1992.

96. Woodley, C. L., Kilburn, J. O., *In vitro* susceptibility of *Mycobacterium avium* complex and *Mycobacterium tuberculosis* strains to a spiropiperidyl rifamycin, *Am. Rev. Resp. Dis.*, 126, 586, 1982.

97. Heifets, L. B., Iseman, M. D., Determinations of *in vitro* susceptibility of mycobacteria to ansamycin, *Am. Rev. Resp. Dis.*, 132, 710, 1985.

98. Nightingale, S. D., Cameron, D. W., Gordin, F. M., Sullam, P. M., Cohn, D. L., Chaisson, R. E., Eron, L. J., Sparti, P. D., Bihari, B., Kaufman, D. L., Stern, J. J., Pearce, D. D., Weinberg, W. G., LaMarca, A., Siegal, F. P., Two controlled trials of rifabutin prophylaxis against *Mycobacterium avium* complex infection in AIDS, *N. Engl. J. Med.*, 329, 828, 1993.

99. Corpe, R. F., Surgical management of pulmonary disease due to *Mycobacterium-avium-intracellulare*, *Rev. Infect. Dis.*, 35, 597, 1981.

100. Pezzia, W., Raleigh, J. W., Bailey, M. C., Toth, E. A., Sliverblatt, J., Treatment of pulmonary disease due to *Mycobacterium kansasii*: Recent experience with rifampin, *Rev. Infect. Dis.*, 3, 1035, 1981.

101. Jenkins, D. E., Bahar, D., Chofuas, I., Pulmonary disease due to atypical mycobacterial: current concepts, *Transact. 19th Conf. Chemother. Tuberc.*, 224, 1960.

102. Ahn, C. H., Wallace, R. J., Jr., Steele, L. C., Murphy, D. T., Sulfonamide-containing regimens for disease caused by rifampin-resistant *Mycobacterium kansasii*, *Am. Rev. Resp. Dis.*, 135, 10, 1987.

103. Wallace, R. J., Jr., Dunbar, D., Brown, B. A., Onyi, G., Dunlap, R., Ahn, C. H., Murphy, D. T., Rifampin resistant *M. kansasii*, *Clin. Inf. Dis.*, in press, 1994.

104. Taha, A. M., Davidson, P. T., Bailey, W. C., Surgical treatment of atypical mycobacterial lymphadenitis in children, *Pediatr. Infect. Dis.*, 111, 816, 1985.

105. Brown, B. A., Wallace, R. J., Jr., Onyi, G. O., de Rosas, V., Wallace, R. J., III, Activities of four macrolides, including clarithromycin, against *Mycobacterium fortuitum, Mycobacterium chelonae,* and *M. chelonae*-like organisms, *Antimicrob. Agents Chemother.*, 36, 180, 1992.

106. Donta, S. T., Smith, P. W., Levitz, R. E., Quinitiliani, R., Therapy of *Mycobacterium marinum* infections use of tetracyclines vs. rifampin, *Arch. Intern. Med.*, 146, 902, 1986.

106a. Wallace, R. J., Jr., Tanner, D., Brennan, P. J., Brown, B. A., Clinical trial of clarithromycin for cutaneous (disseminated) infection due to *Mycobacterium chelonae*, *Ann. Intern. Med.*, 119, 482, 1993.

107. Sanders, W. J., Wolinsky, E., *In vitro* susceptibility of *Mycobacterium marinum* to eight antimicrobial agents, *Antimicrob. Agents Chemother.*, 18, 529, 1980.

108. Stone, M. S., Wallace, R. J., Jr., Swenson, J. M., Thornsberry, C., Christensen, L. A., Agar disk elution method for susceptibility testing of *Mycobacterium marinum* and *Mycobacterium fortuitum* complex to sulfonamides and antibiotics, *Antimicrob. Agents Chemother.*, 4, 486, 1983.

109. Brown, B. A., Wallace, R. J., Jr., Onyi, G. O., Activities of clarithromycin against eight slowly growing species of nontuberculous mycobacteria, determined by using a broth microdilution MIC system, *Antimicrob. Agents Chemother.*, 36, 1987, 1992.

110. Thomas, P., Liu, F., Weiser, W., Characteristics of *Mycobacterium xenopi* disease, *Bull. Int. Union Tuberc. Lung Dis.*, 6, 12, 1988.

111. Parrot, R. G., Grosset, J. H., Post-surgical outcome of 57 patients with *Mycobacterium xenopi* pulmonary infection, *Tubercle*, 69, 47, 1988.

112. Maugein, J., Fourche, J., Mormede, M., Pellegrin, J. L., Sensibliite *in vitro* de *Mycobacterium avium* et *Mycobacterium xenopi* a l'erythromycine, roxithromycine et doxycycline, *Pathol. Biol.*, 37, 565, 1989.

113. Leysen, D. C., Haemers, A., Pattyn, S. R., Mycobacteria and the new quinolones, *Antimicrob. Agents Chemother.*, 33, 1, 1989.

114. Kristjanson, M., Bieluch, V. M., Byeff, P. D., *Mycobacterium haemophilum* infection in immunocompromised patients: case report and review of the literature, *Rev. Infect. Dis.*, 13, 906, 1991.

115. Centers for Disease Control: Tuberculosis — United States, 1985 — and the possible impact of human T-lymphtropic virus type III/lymphadenopathy-associated virus infection, *MMWR*, 35, 74, 1986.

116. Horsburgh, C. R., Jr., Current concepts: *Mycobacterium avium* complex infection in the acquired immunodeficiency syndrome, *N. Engl. J. Med.*, 324, 1332, 1991.

117. Horsburgh, C. R., Selik, R. M., The epidemiology of disseminated nontuberculous mycobacterial infection in the acquired immunodeficiency syndrome (AIDS), *Am. Rev. Resp. Dis.*, 139, 4, 1989.

118. Pitchenik, A. E., Fertel, D., Medical management of AIDS patients: tuberculosis and nontuberculous mycobacterial disease, *Med. Clin. North Am.*, 76, 121, 1992.

119. Wald, A., Coyle, M. B., Carlson, L. C., Thompson, R. L., Hooten, T. M., Infection with a fastidious mycobacterium resembling *Mycobacterium simiae* in seven patients with AIDS, *Ann. Intern. Med.*,7, 586, 1992.

120. Hoy, J., Mijch, A., Sandland, M., Grayson, L., Lucas, R., Dwyer, B., Quadruple-drug therapy for *Mycobacterium avium-intracellulare* bacteremia in AIDS patients, *J. Infect. Dis.*, 161, 801, 1990.

121. Meduri, G. U., Stein, D. S., Pulmonary manifestations of acquired immunodeficiency syndrome, *Clin. Infect. Dis.*, 14, 98, 1992.

122. Nightingale, S. D., Byrd, L. T., Southern, P. M., Jockusch, J. D., Cal, S. X., Wynne, B. A., Incidence of *Mycobacterium avium-intracellulare* complex bacteremia in human immunodeficiency virus-positive patients, *J. Infect. Dis.*, 165, 1082, 1992.

123. Okello, D. O., Sewankambo, N., Goodgame, R., Aisu, T. O., Kwezi, M., Morrissey, A., Ellner, J. J., Absence of bacteremia with *Mycobacterium avium-intracellulare* in Ugandan patients with AIDS, *J. Infect. Dis.*, 162, 208, 1990.

124. Yakrus, M. A., Reeves, M. W., Hunter, S. B., Characterization of isolates of *Mycobacterium avium* serotypes 4 and 8 from patients with AIDS by multilocus enzyme electrophoresis, *J. Clin. Micro.*, 30, 1474, 1992.

125. Gangadharam, P. R. J., Perumal, V. K., Crawford, J. T., Bates, J. H., Association of plasmids and virulence of *Mycobacterium avium* complex, *Am. Rev. Resp. Dis.*, 137, 212, 1988.

126. Klatt, E. C., Jensen, D. F., Meyer, P. R., Pathology of *Mycobacterium avium-intracellulare* infection in acquired immune deficiency syndrome (AIDS), *Hum. Pathol.*, 18, 709, 1987.

127. Wallace, J. M., Hannah, J. B., *Mycobacterium avium* complex infection in patients with the acquired immunodeficiency syndrome, *Chest,* 93, 926, 1988.

128. Eng, R. H. K., Bishburg, E., Smith, S. M., Mangia, A., Diagnosis of *Mycobacterium* bacteremia in patients with acquired immunodeficiency syndrome by direct examination of blood films, *J. Clin. Microbiol.*, 27, 768, 1989.

129. Kemper, C. A., Meng, T., Nussbaum, J., Chiu, J., Feigal, D. F., Bartok, A. E., Leedom, J. M., Tilles, J. G., Deresinski, S. C., McCutchan, J. A., The California Collaborative Treatment Group, Treatment of *Mycobacterium avium* complex bacteremia in AIDS with a four-drug oral regimen, *Ann. Intern. Med.*, 116, 466, 1992.

130. Kerlikowske, K. M., Katz, M. H., Chan, A. K., Perez-Stable, E. J., Antimycobacterial therapy for disseminated *Mycobacterium avium* complex infection in patients with acquired immunodeficiency syndrome, *Arch. Intern. Med.*, 152, 813, 1992.

131. Young, L. S., Wiviott, L., Wu, M., Kolonoski, P., Bolan, R., Inderlied, B. B., Azithromycin for treatment of *Mycobacterium avium-intracellulare* complex infection in patients with AIDS, *Lancet*, 338, 1107, 1991.

132. Dautzenberg, B., Truffot, C., Legris, S., Meyohas, M., Berlie, H. C., Mercat, A., Chevret, S., Grosset, J., Activity of clarithromycin against *Mycobacterium avium* infection in patients with the acquired immune deficiency syndrome, *Am. Rev. Resp. Dis.*, 144, 564, 1991.

133. Chaisson, R. E., Benson, C., Dube, M., Korvick, J., Wu, A., Lichter, S., Dellerson, M., Smith, T., Sattler, F., *Program and Abstracts ICCAC 32nd Intersci. Conf. Antimicrob. Agents Chemother.*, 891, 259, 1992.

134. Chiu, J., Nussbaum, J., Bozzette, S., Tilles, J. G., Young, L. S., Leedom, J., Heseltine, N. R., McCutchan, J. A., The California Collaborative Treatment Group, Treatment of disseminated *Mycobacterium avium* complex infection in AIDS with amikacin, ethambutol, rifampin, and ciprofloxacin, *Ann. Intern. Med.*, 113, 358, 1990.

135. Benson, C. A., Kessler, H. A., Pottage, J. C., Trenholme, G. M., Successful treatment of acquired immunodeficiency syndrome-related *Mycobacterium avium* complex disease with a multiple drug regimen including amikacin, *Arch. Intern. Med.*, 151, 582, 1991.

135a. Centers for Disease Control and Prevention, Recommendations on prophylaxis and therapy for disseminated *Mycobacterium avium* complex for adults and adolescents infected with human immunodeficiency virus, *MMWR*, 42 (No. RR-9), 17, 1993.

136. Carpenter, J. L., Parks, J. M., *Mycobacterium kansasii* infections in patients positive for human immunodeficiency virus, *Rev. Infect. Dis.*, 13, 789, 1990.

137. Levine, B., Chaisson, R. E., *Mycobacterium kansasii*: A cause of treatable pulmonary disease associated with advanced human immunodeficiency virus (HIV) infection, *Ann. Intern. Med.*, 114, 861, 1991.

138. Armstrong, D., Kiehn, T., Boone, N., White, M., Pursell, K., Lewin, S., Sordillo, E. M., Schneider, N., Grieco, M. H. et al., *Mycobacterium haemophilum* infections — New York City metropolitan area, 1990–1991, *MMWR*, 40, 636, 1991.

138a. Butler, W. R., O'Connor, P. O., Yakrus, M. A., Smithwick, R. W., Plikaytis, B. B., Moss, C. W., Floyd, M. M., Woodley, C. L., Kilburn, J. O., Vadney, F. S., Gross, W. M., *Mycobacterium celatum sp. nov.*, *Int. J. Syst. Bacteriol.*, 43, 539, 1993.

139. Jackson, K., Sievers, A., Ross, B. C., Dwyer, B., Isolation of a fastidious *Mycobacterium* species from two AIDS patients, *J. Clin. Microbiol.*, 30, 11, 1992.

140. Bottger, E. C., Teske, A., Kirschner, P., Bost, S., Chang, H. R., Beer, V., Hirshcel, B., Disseminated "*Mycobacterium genavense*" infection in patients with AIDS, *Lancet*, 340, 76, 1992.

141. Coyle, M. B., Carlson, L. C., Wallis, C. K., Leonard, R. B., Raisys, V. A., Kilburn, J. O., Samadpour, M., Bottger, E. C., Laboratory aspects of "*Mycobacterium genavense*," a proposed species isolated from AIDS patients, *J. Clin. Microbiol.*, 30, 3206, 1992.

142. Karlson, A. G., Carr, D. T., Tuberculosis caused by *Mycobacterium bovis*: report of six cases: 1954–1968, *Ann. Intern. Med.*, 73, 979, 1970.

143. Wilkins, E. G. L., Griffiths, R. J., Roberts, C., Pulmonary tuberculosis due to *Mycobacterium bovis*, *Thorax*, 41, 685, 1986.

144. Damsker, B., Bottone, E. J., Schneierson, S. S., Human infections with *Mycobacterium bovis*, *Am. Rev. Resp. Dis.*, 110, 446, 1974.

145. Wigle, W. D., Ashley, M. J., Killough, E. M., Cosens, M., Bovine tuberculosis in humans in Ontario: the epidemiologic features of 31 active cases occurring between 1964 and 1970, *Am. Rev. Resp. Dis.*, 106, 528, 1972.

146. Sauret, J., Jolis, R., Ausina, V., Castro, E., Cornudella, R., Human tuberculosis due to *Mycobacterium bovis*: report of 10 cases, *Tubercle*, 73, 388, 1992.

147. Hardie, R. M., Watson, J. M., *Mycobacterium bovis* in England and Wales: past, present and future, *Epidemiol. Infect.*, 109, 23, 1992.

148. Dankner, W. M., Waecker, J. J., Essey, M. A., Moser, K., Thompson, M., Davis, C. E., Mycobacterium bovis infections in San Diego: a clinicoepidemiologic study of 73 patients and a historical review of a forgotten pathogen, *Medicine*, 72, 11, 1993.

149. Collins, C. H., Grange, J. M., A review: the bovine tubercle bacillus, *J. Appl. Bacteriol.*, 55, 13, 1983.

150. Collins, C. H., Yates, M. D., Grange, J. M., A study of bovine strains of Mycobacterium tuberculosis isolated from humans in southeast England, 1977–1979, *Tubercle*, 62, 113, 1981.

151. McParland, C., Cotton, D. J., Gowda, K. S., Hoeppner, V. H., Martin, W. T., Weckworth, P. F., Miliary *Mycobacterium bovis* introduced by intravesical *Bacillus Calmette-Guérin* immunotherapy, *Am. Rev. Resp. Dis.*, 146, 1330, 1992.

152. Lotte, A., Wasz-Hockert, P., Poisson, N., Dumitresau, N., Venon, M., Couvet, E., BCG complications, *Adv. Tuberc. Res.*, 21, 107, 1984.

153. Gonzalez, B., Moreno, S., Burdach, R., Valenzuela, M. T., Henriquez, A., Ramos, M. I., Sorenson, R. U., Clinical presentation of *Bacillus Calmette-Guérin* infections in patients with immunodeficiency syndromes, *Pediatr. Infect. Dis. J.*, 8, 201, 1989.

154. Braun, M. M., Cauthen, G., Relationship of the human immunodeficiency virus epidemic to pediatric tuberculosis and *Bacillus Calmette-Guérin* immunization, *Pediatr. Infect. Dis. J.*, 11, 220, 1992.

Chapter 10

Radiology of Mycobacterial Disease

Anne McB. Curtis, M.D.

CONTENTS

I. PRIMARY TUBERCULOSIS

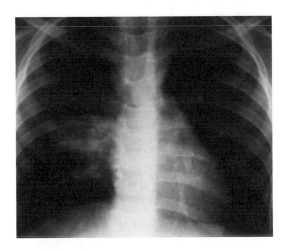
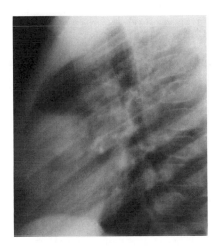

1a   1b

Figure 10-1a,b A 12-year-old female who presented with a fever and cough. Her grandmother had active tuberculosis. The location of the infiltrate and the adenopathy are typical for primary infection.

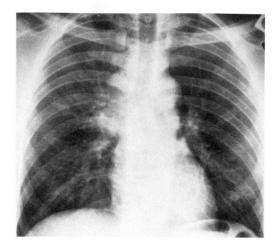

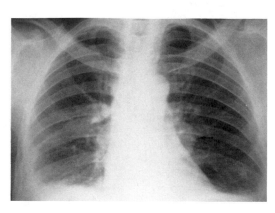

Figure 10-2 A 43-year-old male with carpal tunnel syndrome and right paratracheal and hilar adenopathy. The carpal tunnel syndrome was the result of caseating granulomas found at surgery. In the non-HIV-positive population, adenopathy is more common in children and noncaucasian adults, particularly in African-Americans and persons from India. Although asymmetric adenopathy is uncommon in sarcoidosis, the patterns of tuberculous adenopathy may mimic exactly those of sarcoid and lymphoma.

Figure 10-3 A 25-year-old male with fever and weight loss. The pleural effusion and adenopathy (arrows) are characteristic of primary infection.

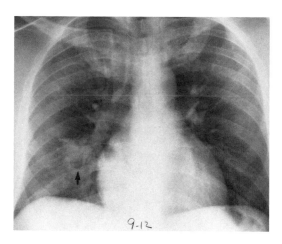

4a

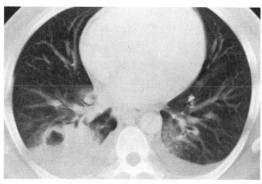

4b

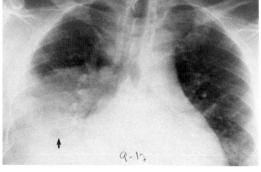

4c

Figure 10-4a–c A 40-year-old male diabetic with a fever, chills, and cough of 3 weeks duration. An ill-defined infiltrate with a cavity is present on the admission film (a) and is seen easily on computed tomography (b). A tuberculous pleural effusion developed as well (c). The patient was anergic at admission and the diagnosis was made initially by a positive smear at bronchoscopy. He then remembered that a friend had been sick with tuberculosis several months earlier (Figure 10-11).

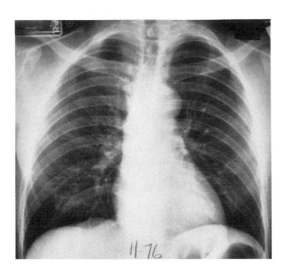

5a

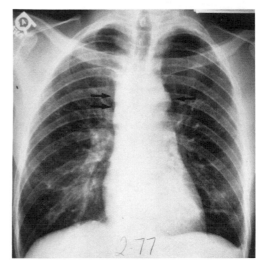

5b

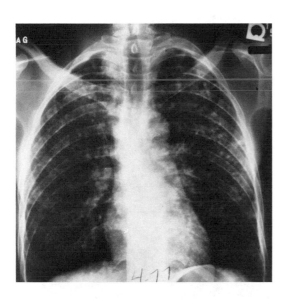

5c

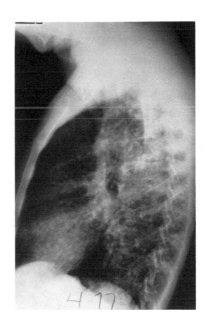

5d

Figure 10-5a–d A 25-year-old male presenting with a cough and fever in February 1977 (b). In comparison with an earlier film in November 1976 (a), there now is right paratracheal, right hilar, and aortopulmonary adenopathy as well as a left pleural effusion (b). All of these findings favor primary infection. The patient was lost to follow-up until he returned in April 1977 with continued fevers and a 30 pound weight loss. The adenopathy and pleural effusion resolved, but nodules disseminated throughout both lungs; the sputum was positive for AFB (c,d). No apparent cavitary focus is present, and nodules, now larger than 3 mm, are too big to be considered miliary. Presumably, this represents progression of the hematogenously disseminated primary disease.

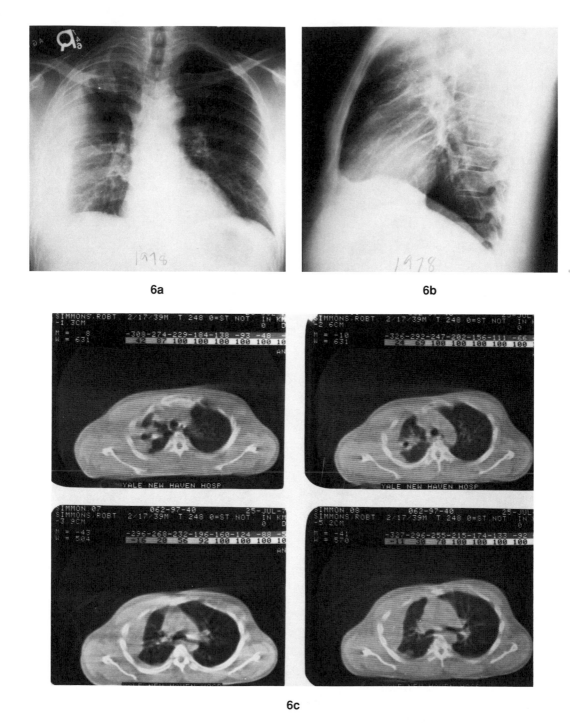

6a

6b

6c

Figure 10-6a–c A 32-year-old asymptomatic male routine chest radiograph. No parenchymal focus is evident on posteroanterior and lateral chest radiographs in the presence of a large effusion (a,b). Computed tomography of the chest shows an apical focus of parenchymal disease (c). *Mycobacterium tuberculosis* was found on pleural biopsy and culture. In cases of pleural effusion, a parenchymal lesion that ruptures into the pleural space to produce the effusion usually is found on computed tomography. Effusions are more frequent with primary infection.

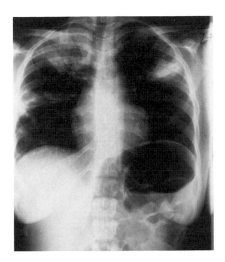

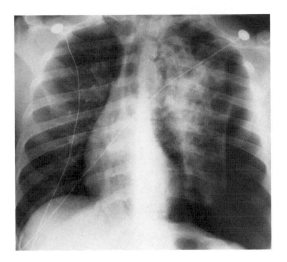

Figure 10-7 A 23-year-old female, 7 weeks post-partum, who presented with fever. The tuberculin skin test was negative and septic emboli were suspected. Angiography was negative and the diagnosis of tuberculosis was made at open lung biopsy. The skin test converted 6 weeks after admission.

Figure 10-8 A 32-year-old male who presented with chest pain, fever, and a 20 pound weight loss the day his sister was discharged from the hospital for treatment of active pulmonary tuberculosis. Multiple areas of cavitation are noted in the left lung, which is partially collapsed in the presence of a pneumothorax. The pneumothorax probably resulted from rupture of a necrotic focus into the pleural space. Smear and culture were positive for *M. tuberculosis*.

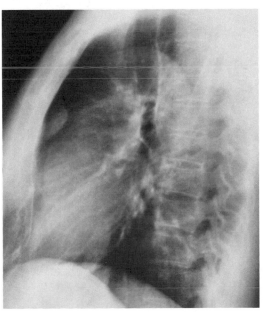

9a

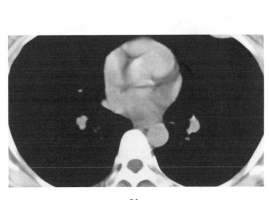

9b

Figure 10-9a,b Residual pleural focus. A 45-year-old female with a history of fever and pleurisy 7 years earlier treated in China for 3 months with streptomycin, isoniazid, and penicillin. A lateral chest film and computed tomography show a pleural based soft tissue mass without evidence of bony destruction. No parenchymal lesions or adenopathy were evident. A needle biopsy was negative; caseating granulomas were found at surgery and *M. tuberculosis* was cultured. The differential diagnosis includes pleural tumors, both benign and malignant.

II. REACTIVATION TUBERCULOSIS

A. PULMONARY

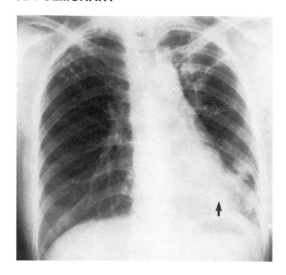

Figure 10-10 A 28-year-old laboratory worker with a chronic cough. Bilateral upper lobe volume loss with nodular opacities of varying sizes are seen. Poorly marginated larger opacities are noted in the left lower lobe with a central lucency (arrow) representing cavitary disease. This lesion probably is of bronchogenic origin with proliferation of inflammatory foci.

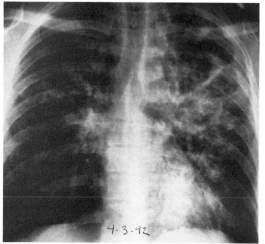

11b

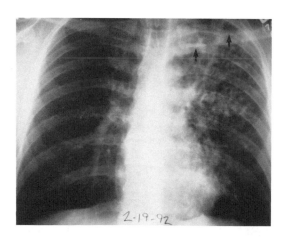

11a

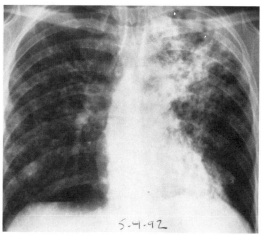

11c

Figure 10-11a–c Bronchogenic spread. A 31-year-old male with a fever and cough. Cavities at the left apex (arrow) were not observed initially and the patient was treated for a presumed community acquired infection (a). Progressive cavitation developed with bronchogenic spread to both lungs (b,c). The sputum smear was markedly positive for *M. tuberculosis*. This patient is the contact for patient in Figure 10-4.

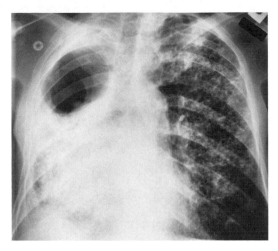
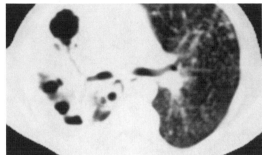

12a   12b

Figure 10-12a,b Multiple cavities with bronchogenic spread. A 52-year-old alcoholic male with a cough and weight loss. The sputum smear was markedly positive for *M. tuberculosis*. There is extensive destruction of the right upper lobe with consolidation of the rest of the right lung and bronchogenic spread to the left lung (a). Computed tomography demonstrates much more destruction with multiple irregular cavities in the right lung, as well as bronchogenic spread to the left lung (b). If untreated, destruction of the lung can be complete, with gangrene resulting.

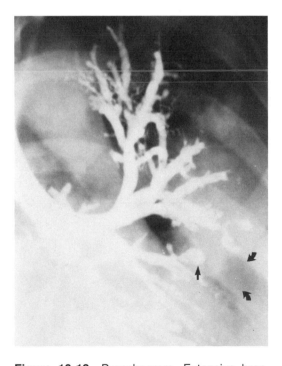

Figure 10-13 Bronchogram. Extensive bronchiectasis with small cavity formation (arrows). Note the lucency peripherally that represents a cavity that did not fill (curved arrows). The smear was markedly positive for *M. tuberculosis*.

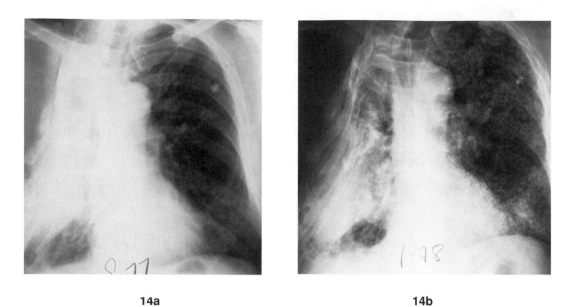

14a   14b

Figure 10-14a,b A 60-year-old male who had had a thoracoplasty for tuberculosis 30 years earlier (a). He presented with a fever in January 1978. Miliary dissemination had occurred (b).

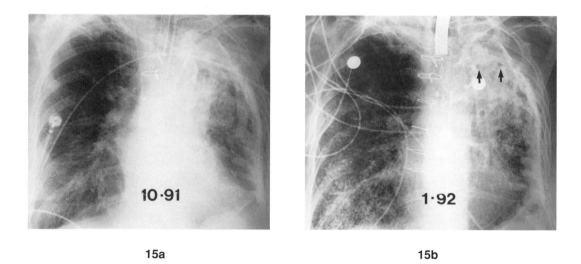

15a   15b

Figure 10-15a,b A 55-year-old female with diabetes who underwent a thoracoplasty for tuberculosis in 1944. Multiple complications followed a coronary artery bypass graft in October 1991 (a). In January 1992, the patient developed a relentless fever and the sputum was positive for *M. tuberculosis*. On the film of January 1992 (b), lucencies in the left upper lobe represent necrotic foci from which bronchogenic spread occurred (arrow).

B. EXTRAPULMONARY

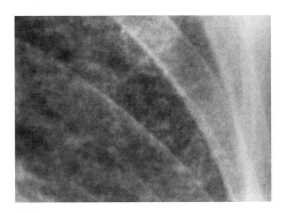

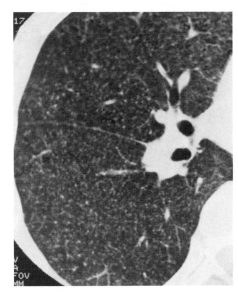

16a   16b

Figure 10-16a,b A 43-year-old male with multiple abdominal fistulae and abscesses as a result of a gunshot wound. One year following the initial injury, he developed miliary lesions in the lung. Bronchoscopy demonstrated caseating granulomas, *M. tuberculosis* was grown from the lungs, and multiple abscesses were visualized in the abdomen. Miliary lesions are seen on a chest radiograph (a), and to better advantage on computed tomography (b).

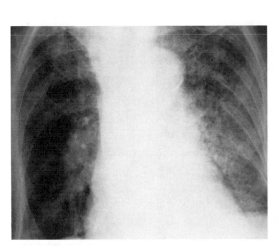

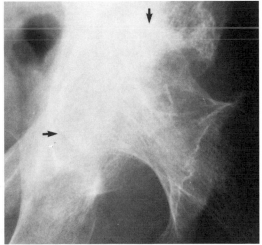

17a   17b

Figure 10-17a,b A 50-year-old female with a history of congestive heart failure and hip pain who was treated with steroids. The chest radiograph initially was thought to suggest congestive heart failure (a). However, typical miliary lesions are noted throughout both lungs. Such miliary spread may occur either in primary or reactivation tuberculosis. The left hip film demonstrates narrowing and destruction of the joint space (arrows) (b). Lack of marginal erosions of the joint are unusual. Aspiration of the hip demonstrated *M. tuberculosis*. Presumably, the steroids led to the breakdown of preexisting tuberculous foci.

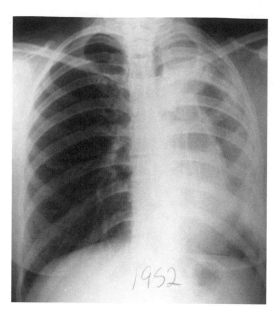

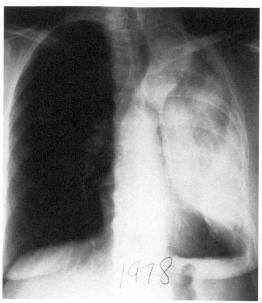

18a **18b**

Figure 10-18a,b Progressive fibrothorax. A fibrothorax resulting from a tuberculous empyema is shown with progressive contraction and calcification over 26 years. Computed tomography, may demonstrate fluid within areas of the "fibrothorax". Viable organisms may be present as well, predisposing to reinfection.

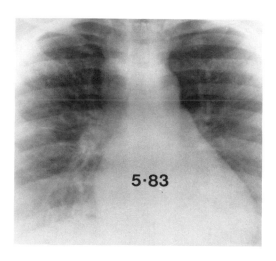

19a

Figure 10-19a–d A 35-year-old female with a cough. A chest radiograph in May 1983 demonstrates paratracheal adenopathy on the right (a). A barium swallow shows ulceration of the esophagus with extravasation of contrast at the level of the subcarinal lymph nodes (arrows)(b,c). Follow-up in October demonstrates healing with a residual esophageal diverticulum (arrows) (d). Fistulization occurred from erosion of tuberculous lymph nodes into the esophagus.

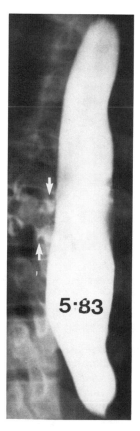

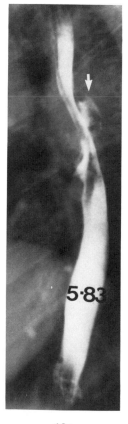

19b **19c**

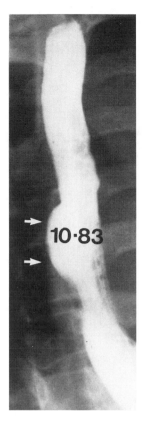

19d

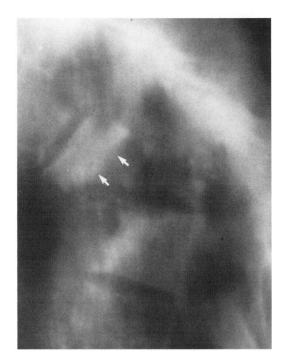

20a

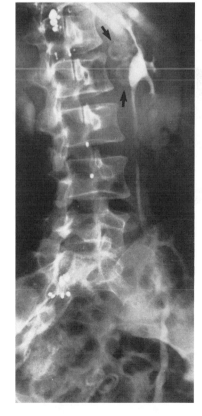

20b

Figure 10-20a,b Tuberculosis of the spine and cavitary tuberculosis of kidney: destruction of the inferior portion of an upper thoracic vertebral body and complete destruction of the vertebral body below resulted in a gibbus deformity (a). Usually, the initial infection results from hematogenous spread. Spread from one vertebral body to the next may occur across the disc space or beneath the anterior and posterior longitudinal ligaments. The cavitary lesions in the kidney (arrows) are filled with debris (b). Stricture formation may occur with healing, and careful follow-up with intravenous pyelography is warranted to avoid obstruction. (Photo courtesy of Arthur Rosenfield, M.D.)

III. HEALING

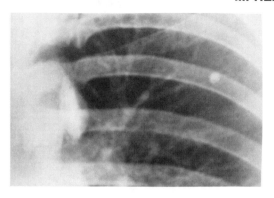

Figure 10-21   Formation of Ranke complex: calcified nodule associated with a calcified mediastinal lymph node.

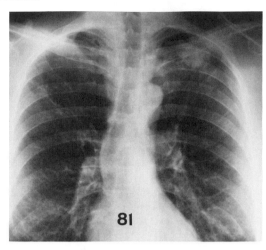

22a

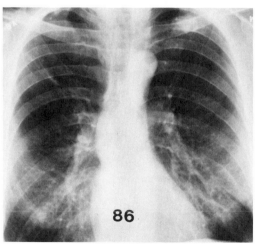

22b

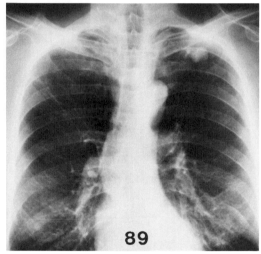

22c

Figure 10-22a–c   Tuberculoma formation in a 40-year-old male: a 1981 radiograph shows a poorly marginated opacity in the left upper lobe and some scarring (stable over several years) in the right upper lobe (a). *M. tuberculosis* was grown on culture. Films in 1986 (b) and 1989 (c) demonstrate contraction of the left upper lobe opacity with increasing density to form a smooth lobulated mass, typical of a tuberculoma. At autopsy, tuberculomas may contain viable organisms.

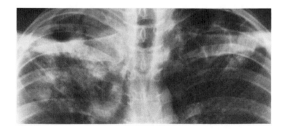

Figure 10-23   Biapical cavities as well as nodules in a 39-year-old alcoholic male. Complete resolution occurred after 1 year of therapy.

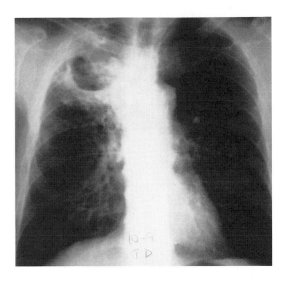
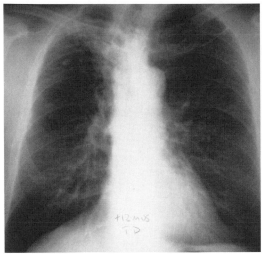

24a   **24b**

Figure 10-24a,b Healing with cavity closure: a large cavity in the right upper lobe seen in October has an air fluid level (a). Note the calcified nodule in the left perihilar region. Twelve months following treatment, the cavity has closed with right upper lobe volume loss and residual apical nodular opacities (b). In cavitary tuberculosis, air fluid levels are slightly unusual, but do occur. Cavities may or may not close completely. Radiographic stability for 6 months must be documented to describe "inactive" tuberculosis.

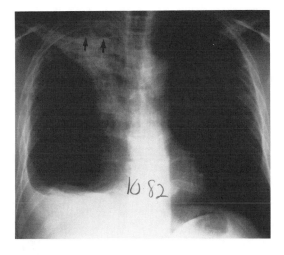
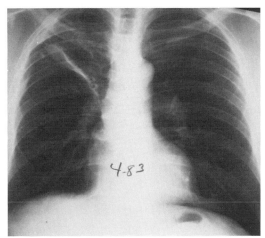

25a   **25b**

Figure 10-25a,b Healing of cavitary disease: the right upper lobe infiltrate with multiple lucencies representing cavities is seen in association with a pleural effusion (a). Considerable resolution was demonstrated 6 months later with clearing of the pleural effusion and volume loss of the right upper lobe (b).

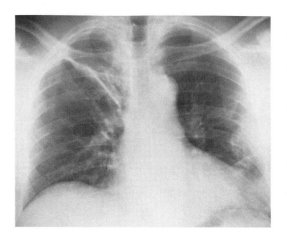

26a

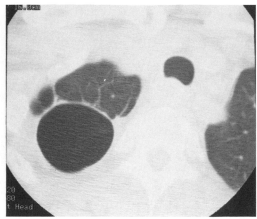

26b

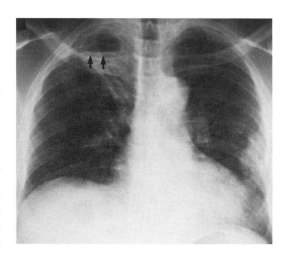

Figure 10-26a–c A 55-year-old male alcoholic with cavitary tuberculosis diagnosed in October 1982 (a) that healed with contraction and residual cystic spaces by April 1983 (b). He presented in December 1992 with weakness, seizures, and vomiting. A posteroanterior chest radiograph demonstrates an air fluid level in the right upper lobe (c). Although tuberculosis was suspected, it was not found at bronchoscopy and the infiltrate healed with antibiotic therapy. This demonstrates that air fluid levels may occur in preexisting spaces and do not necessarily reflect necrosis with cavitation, as would be seen in active tuberculosis.

26c

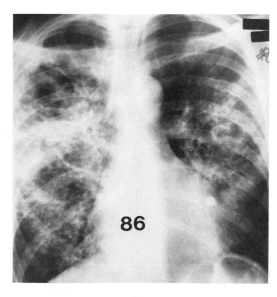

Figure 10-27a–c A 32-year-old male with active tuberculosis and a positive sputum smear. Over a 2-year period, healing occurs with progressive destruction of the parenchyma and extensive bullous formation in the right lung. Minimal nodular changes are seen on the left.

27a

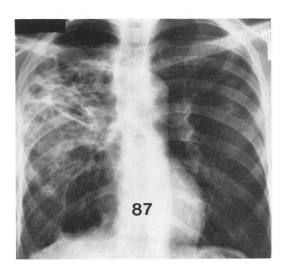

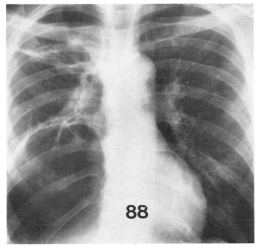

27b

27c

IV. TUBERCULOSIS OR CANCER?

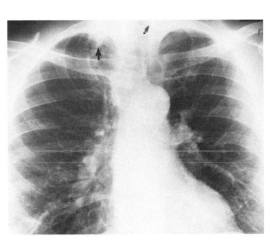

28a

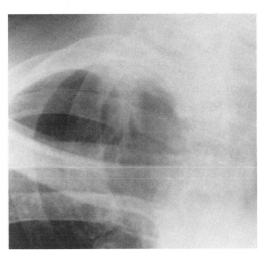

28b

Figure 10-28a,b A 60-year-old male with a 50 pack-year smoking history and an apical density at the right apex. The skin test was negative and old films were not available. The irregular margins of this lesion are highly suspicious for a neoplasm, but at resection, the lesion proved to be tuberculous.

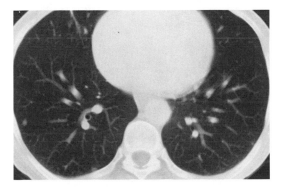

Figure 10-29 A 54-year-old male nonsmoker who had computed tomography of the lung performed to evaluate the pulmonary hilum. The hilum is shown to be normal, but nodular opacities are noted peripherally at both bases. These are too small to evaluate for density using the computed tomography phantom technique because they are less than 4 mm in size. At surgery, multiple subpleural nodules were found that were nonnecrotic granulomas. A lymph node resected at the same time was culture positive for *M. tuberculosis*.

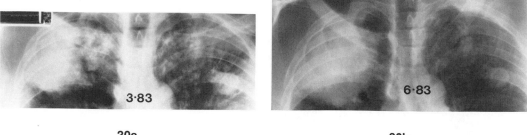

30a   30b

Figure 10-30a,b A 50-year-old male with a cough and weight loss. His sputum was positive on culture for *M. tuberculosis*. A large mass in the right upper lobe was found to be an adenocarcinoma on needle biopsy (a). A film in June demonstrates some resolution of the tuberculous foci, but progression of neoplasm (b). Presumably, these are concurrent problems rather than a scar carcinoma in association with long standing tuberculosis.

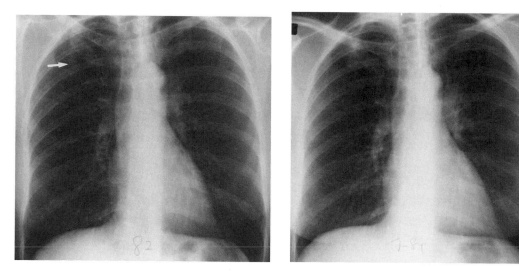

31a   31b

Figure 10-31a–c A 44-year-old white female with a history of incomplete treatment for tuberculosis. The patient was followed for several years, and a growing mass was resected and proved to be an adenocarcinoma. Multiple granulomas were noted in the specimen as well. The patient had a 40 pack-year smoking history, but stopped 6 years before entry into the clinic. Adenocarcinoma is the most frequently associated "scar" carcinoma, but other cell types have been reported as well. It is important when evaluating serial films to compare films widely separated in time (e.g., 2 years) if they are available. Subtle progressive changes over repeated short intervals (e.g., 3 to 6 months) may be overlooked, as happened to this patient over a 6-year period.

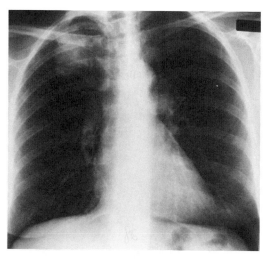

31c

V. TUBERCULOSIS AND NON-HIV-RELATED IMMUNOSUPPRESSION

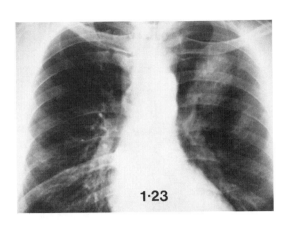

32a

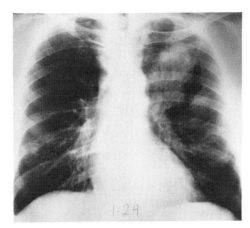

32b

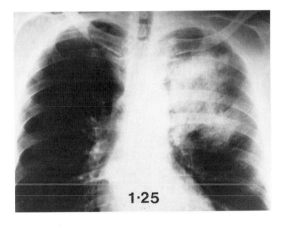

1·25

32c

Figure 10-32a–c A 67-year-old male with fever and chronic myelogenous leukemia. Over 3 days, aggressive opacification of the left upper lobe was noted. Sputum smear and culture were positive for *M. tuberculosis*. Rapid progression may be related to immunosuppression.

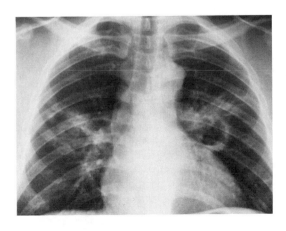

Figure 10-33 A 50-year-old male with Wegener's granulomatosis who was completing 1 year of treatment with full doses of cyclophosphamide. He presented with a fever and nasal stuffiness. Recurrence of Wegener's granulomatosis has not been reported once complete remission has occurred in a patient on full doses of chemotherapy. In this case, there was no evidence of relapse, and another cause of cavitary disease was sought. Although tuberculosis is very unusual in patients with Wegener's granulomatosis, the bronchoscopy was positive for *M. tuberculosis*.

VI. HIV-RELATED TUBERCULOSIS

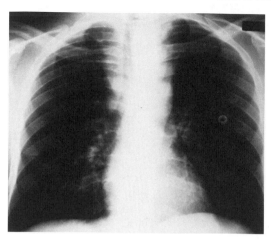

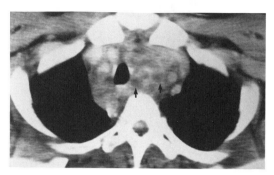

34a   34b

Figure 10-34a,b An intravenous drug abuser, who is HIV positive, with a 3 month history of fever and a mass in the neck. Mediastinal widening extending into the neck with deviation of the trachea to the right is seen on a chest radiograph (a). Computed tomography demonstrates multiple enlarged lymph nodes with low density centers (arrows) (b). *M. tuberculosis* was obtained at mediastinoscopy. Thoracic adenopathy is not a feature of AIDS-related complex, and an infectious or neoplastic cause should be sought to explain the adenopathy.

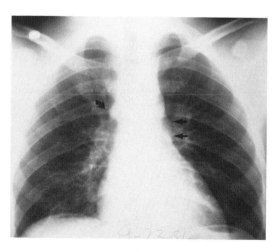

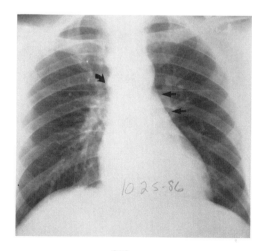

35a   35b

Figure 10-35a–c A 27-year-old HIV-negative intravenous drug abuser, on peritoneal dialysis for 1 year, who presented with fevers. A chest radiograph from September 23, 1986 shows free intraperitoneal air, as well as azygos (curved arrow) and aortopulmonary adenopathy (arrow) (a). Empiric therapy for tuberculosis ensued for 6 weeks but was discontinued when cultures were negative. The chest radiograph from October 25, 1986 demonstrates regression of the aortopulmonary and azygos adenopathy (arrows) (b). A routine chest radiograph from May 11, 1987 demonstrates a mediastinal mass, and the patient was noted to be HIV positive at the same time (c). Thoracotomy demonstrated *M. tuberculosis* of the mediastinal nodes. Adenopathy is far more common in patients with tuberculosis who are HIV positive than those who are HIV negative. Careful comparison with a baseline radiograph is mandatory, as the adenopathy may be subtle. Tuberculosis may be the first manifestation of AIDS. (Photo courtesy Ernest Moritz, M.D.)

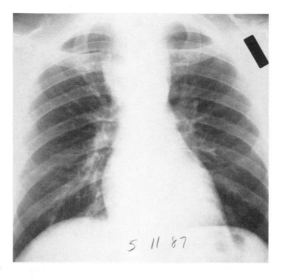

35c

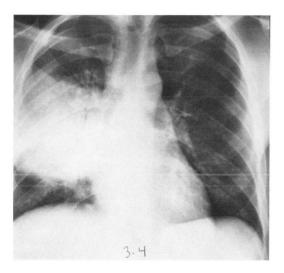

36a

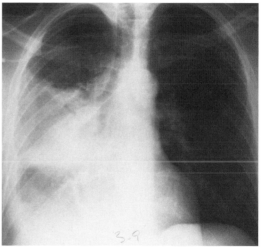

36b

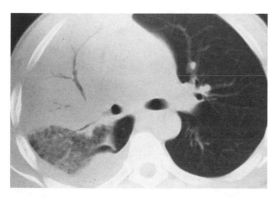

36c

Figure 10-36a–c A 37-year-old HIV-positive male intravenous drug abuser with a fever and cough. Six months before admission, he had been diagnosed with tuberculosis, but he discontinued therapy after 4 months. There is consolidation of the right upper lobe with bulging of the fissure, as well as paratracheal adenopathy (a). A pleural effusion developed in 5 days (b). Computed tomography demonstrates dense consolidation with a bulging fissure, a pleural effusion, and spread to the right lower lobe (c). The sputum was positive for *M. tuberculosis*. Tuberculosis can be very aggressive in immunocompromised patients, particularly those with low CD4 counts. The infiltrate with a bulging fissure is more typical of staphylococcal and gram-negative organisms.

226

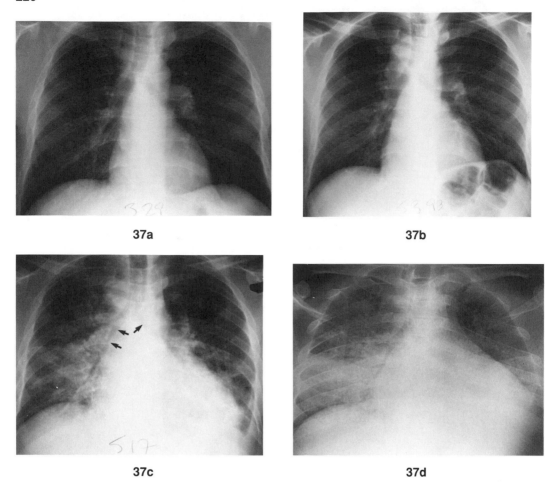

37a

37b

37c

37d

Figure 10-37a–d A 29-year-old intravenous drug abuser with AIDS and a CD4 count of 53 who presented with a fever and cough. A film of March 29 (a) demonstrates some hilar adenopathy that has progressed to include paratracheal adenopathy by May 3 (b). The film of May 17 demonstrates an impressive increase in the mediastinal and hilar adenopathy with narrowing of the bronchus intermedius as well as the left main stem bronchus (arrows) (c). Diffuse parenchymal infiltrates developed rapidly as well (d). After 12 days, the admission sputum culture was positive for *M. tuberculosis*. The sputum became positive on smear when the parenchymal infiltrates appeared. Rapid clearing resulted after 2-1/2 weeks of therapy, and the patient never required intubation. This is an example of extremely rapid progression of both lymphadenopathy and parenchymal infiltration in an immunocompromised patient. This patient typifies what once was called "galloping consumption".

Figure 10-38a–c A 28-year-old HIV-positive female, presenting with cough, fever, abdominal pain, and back pain. Blood cultures were positive for *M. tuberculosis*, and miliary dissemination occurred, followed by ARDS, shown here with three consecutive daily chest radiographs (a–c). Bronchoscopy following intubation demonstrated AFB on smear. Although unusual, tuberculosis is a well-known cause of ARDS.

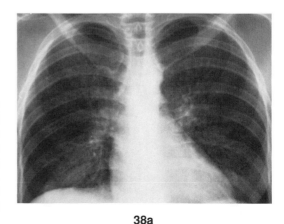

38a

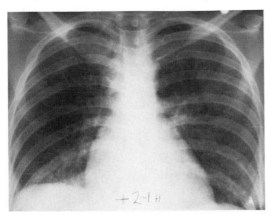

38b

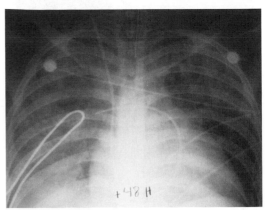

38c

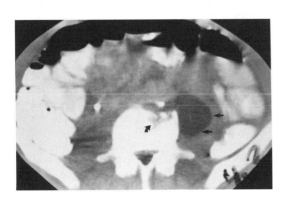

39a

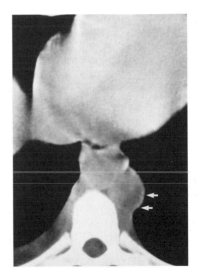

39b

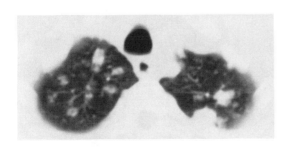

39c

Figure 10-39a–c A 32-year-old HIV-positive male with a history of intravenous drug abuse, who presented with abdominal pain and was found to have a perforated duodenal ulcer. Computed tomography demonstrates destruction of a vertebral body (curved arrow), with a paraspinal fluid collection (arrow) (a). Similar fluid collections were noted elsewhere in the abdomen. Drainage of the paraspinal collection demonstrated *M. tuberculosis*. Mediastinal computed tomography shows a paravertebral mass extending superiorly from the abdomen, representing a tuberculous abscess (arrow) (b). Chest computed tomography shows parenchymal involvement as well (c).

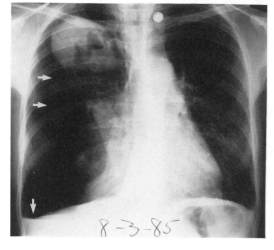

40a

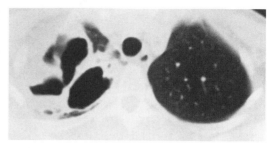

40b

Figure 10-40a–c A 27-year-old HIV-positive female who is an intravenous drug abuser and presented with a 1 month history of a cough and fever, followed by the sudden onset of right sided chest pain. A hydropneumothorax is demonstrated (arrows) (a). A sharply marginated mass with multiple air fluid levels is seen in the right upper lobe (a). Extensive cavitation ensued (b), and multiple smaller cavitary lesions were noted on computed tomography (c). Resection of the abscess showed *Pneumocystis carinii* on silver stain, and cultures grew *M. tuberculosis*, *M. avium* complex (MAC), *Klebsiella*, and *Enterobacter*. A portion of a resected rib showed necrotizing granulomas in the marrow. This patient responded well to therapy, but died 3 months later with a severe electrolyte disturbance. The chest radiograph during that admission showed no infiltrates.

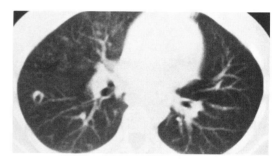

40c

VII. ATYPICAL MYCOBACTERIOSIS: HIV- AND NON-HIV-RELATED

A. HIV-RELATED

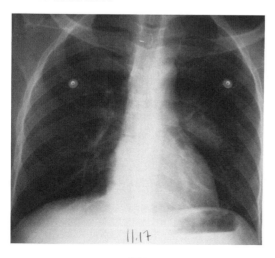

41a

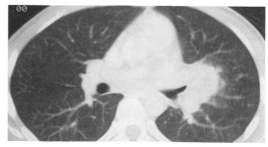

41b

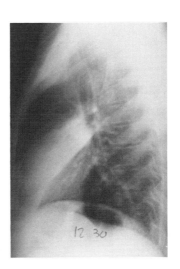

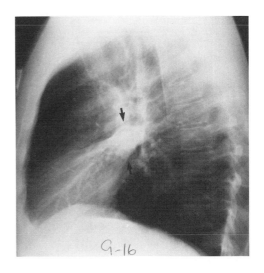

41c

41d

Figure 10-41a–d A 36-year-old HIV-positive male with left hilar adenopathy, seen on chest radiography (a) and computed tomography (b), followed by lingular consolidation (c,d). At bronchoscopy, an endobronchial mass was found that occluded the lingular bronchus. This was AFB positive on smear and MAC was cultured.

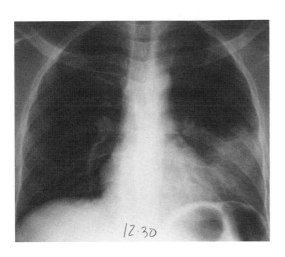

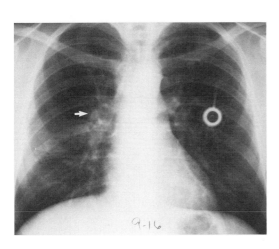

42a

42b

Figure 10-42a–e A 33-year-old HIV-positive male with progressive middle lobe consolidation (a–c) that resulted in complete collapse of the middle lobe (d,e). Adenopathy can be appreciated (arrows) (a,b). Bronchoscopy yielded *M. kansasii*. This is much less frequent than MAC. Consolidation with atelectasis should suggest endobronchial disease and, in the HIV population, mycobacterial disease should be considered strongly.

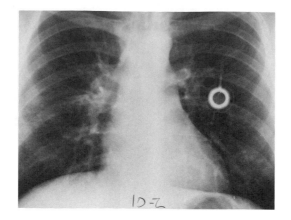

42c

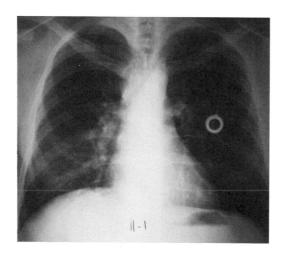

42d

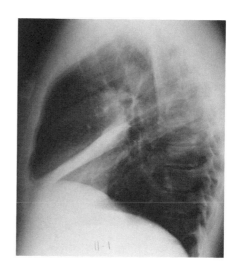

42e

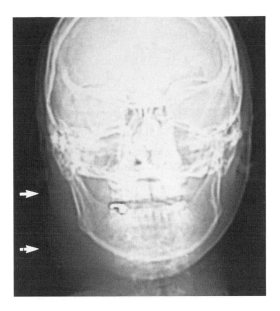 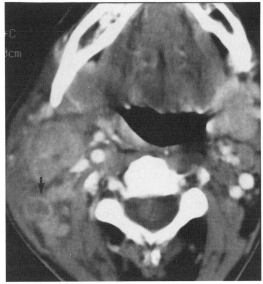

43a   **43b**

Figure 10-43a,b   A 37-year-old male with AIDS and a CD4 count of 16 who presented with a fever and neck swelling. A digitized radiograph shows massive swelling in the right neck (a) and computed tomography shows large nodes with low-density central areas typical of tuberculous lymphadenitis (arrow) (b). Culture of the biopsied node was positive for MAC.

B. NON-HIV-RELATED

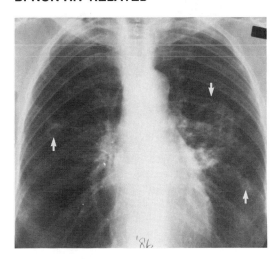 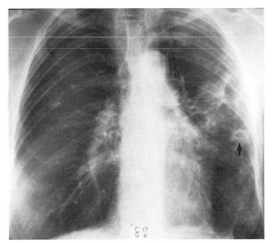

44a   **44b**

Figure 10-44a–c   A 71-year-old female with a history of whooping cough as a child. This was followed by multiple episodes of pneumonia. Bronchiectasis was diagnosed on bronchography in 1977 and, when required, intermittent antibiotics were administered for infection. MAC was seen in increasing concentration in the sputum with the onset of hemoptysis in 1986. A chest radiograph shows cavitary lesions of various sizes in the right and left lungs (a). Over 2 years, the largest cavity on the left has contracted and a new cavity is noted below this (arrow) (b). After 4 years of chemotherapy, the sputum finally became negative and the chest radiograph stabilized (c). Bronchiectasis may be a predisposing factor for infections with atypical mycobacteria.

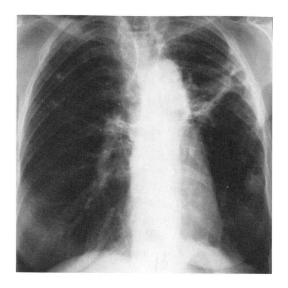

44c

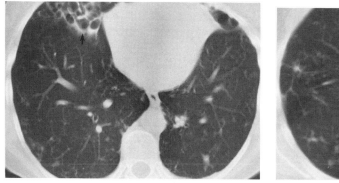

45a

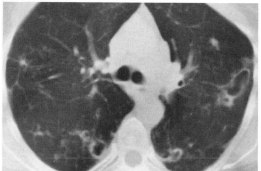

45b

Figure 10-45a,b A 54-year-old female with a history of recurrent pneumonias following an episode of whooping cough as a child. She presented with mild hemoptysis and a positive PPD. In 1992 her sputum was positive for acid-fast bacilli which initially were identified by probe as *M. tuberculosis,* then biochemically as *M. xenopi,* and finally as a relatively new mycobacterium, *M. celatum.* (for more information on this species, please refer to Chapter 9, this volume). Computed tomography demonstrates an area of cystic bronchiectasis in the right middle lobe (arrow) (a). Elsewhere are cavities of varying sizes, some being irregularly shaped (b). Smaller cavitary lesions were present on a computed tomographic examination 7 years previously.

VIII. LOOK ALIKES

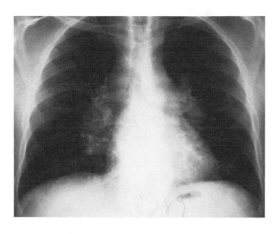

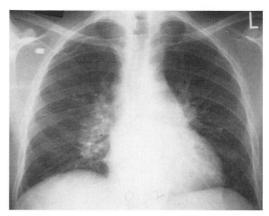

46a   46b

Figure 10-46a,b   A 48-year-old HIV-positive male with a history of intravenous drug abuse who presented with a septic groin. A chest radiograph demonstrates extensive bilateral hilar and paratracheal adenopathy (a). A chest radiograph performed 2 years earlier demonstrates that the adenopathy is stable (b). Stable adenopathy is not a feature of tuberculous adenopathy or of HIV disease. A transbronchial biopsy showed noncaseating granulomas compatible with sarcoidosis.

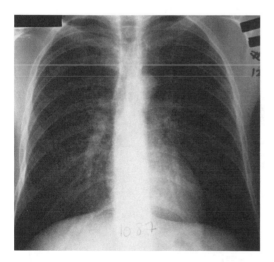

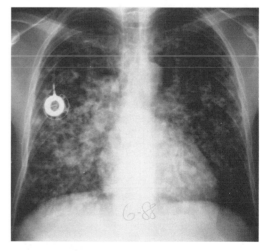

47a   47b

Figure 10-47a,b   A 24-year-old HIV-positive Puerto Rican male who presented with fevers. A chest radiograph from October 1987 demonstrates typical miliary lesions that are the result of histoplasmosis, and not tuberculosis (a). Histoplasmosis is endemic in Puerto Rico and this radiograph is thought to represent endogenous reinfection. The patient responded transiently to antifungal therapy but eventually relapsed (b).

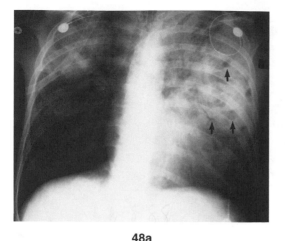

48a

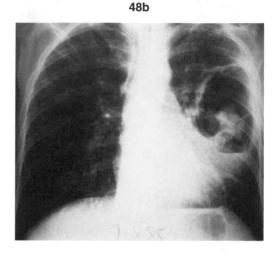

48b

Figure 10-48a–c A 53-year-old HIV-positive male who presented with a fever. Bilateral consolidation is noted, but there also are areas of lucency (arrows) within the consolidated left lung, suggesting cavitation and necrosis (a). Computed tomography shows extensive cavitation with sloughing of lung on the left (b). A chest radiograph from July 8 demonstrates a large cavity with a central mass (c). This gradually resolved and represents pulmonary gangrene. In this instance, *S. pneumoniae* was obtained. Gangrene most frequently results from *Klebsiella*, and less commonly from *S. pneumoniae* infection. Occasionally, tuberculosis will produce a similar appearance.

48c

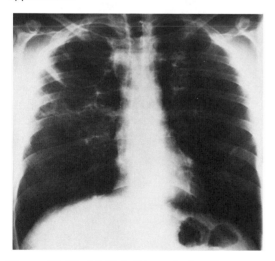

Figure 10-49 Multiple thin-walled cystic spaces that are the residua of a previous *Pneumocystis carinii* infection. These may rupture to produce pneumothoraces. The thin walls are fairly smooth and should not be confused with the cavities of mycobacterial disease.

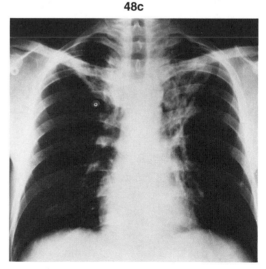

Figure 10-50 Atypical distribution of *P. carinii* pneumonia which occurs in patients who are on inhaled pentamidine. This appearance may mimic tuberculosis due to its upper lobe distribution, but the history of prophylactic pentamidine therapy should raise the possibility that this is *P. carinii* pneumonia.

ACKNOWLEDGMENTS

Thanks to Mr. Michael Brown for photography and to Ms. Louise Leader for preparation of the manuscript.

Chapter 11

Chemotherapeutic Agents for Mycobacterial Infections

Michael H. Cynamon, M.D. and Sally P. Klemens, M.D.

CONTENTS

0-8493-4825-0/94/$0.00+$.50
© 1994 by CRC Press, Inc.

I. INTRODUCTION

Chemotherapy for mycobacterial disease began in the late 1940s with the introduction of streptomycin (SM). Rifampin (RIF), the most recent major new therapeutic innovation, was developed in the late 1960s. During the past quarter century there has been little progress in the identification and development of new antituberculosis drugs. Development of new and better agents has been a low priority in developed countries. In addition, the realities of the marketplace have not provided incentives to the pharmaceutical industry to pursue research in this area. In spite of the regrettable lack of research support in the area of mycobacterial disease in general, and of tuberculosis in particular, dramatic improvements in the chemotherapy of tuberculosis have taken place.

Early in the chemotherapy era it became apparent that emergence of resistance during monotherapy could be circumvented with combination therapy. Isoniazid (INH), streptomycin (SM), and *p*-aminosalicylic acid (PAS) in combination were used in 18- to 24-month regimens. Ethambutol (EMB) subsequently replaced PAS, and RIF replaced SM. Supervised intermittent therapy and short-course therapy were found to be effective strategies in large clinical trials supported by the British Medical Research Council. INH combined with RIF for 9 months or INH, RIF, and pyrazinamide (PZA)

Table 11-1 **Antituberculosis agents**

Agent	Mechanism of Action	Mechanism(s) of Resistance
Isoniazid	Inhibits mycolic acid synthesis	Inactivation of catalase-peroxidase gene (*katG*); probable mutation of target enzyme
Ethionamide	Inhibits mycolic acid synthesis	Probable mutation of target enzyme
Pyrazinamide	Unknown	Decreased pyrazinamidase activity; probable mutation of target enzyme
Rifampin	Inhibits DNA-dependent RNA-polymerase; suppresses initiation of chain formation	Mutation of target enzyme (β-subunit)
Ethambutol	Inhibits arabinogalactan synthesis	Probable mutation of target enzyme
Aminoglycoside	Binding to the 30 S ribosomal subunit; inhibits protein synthesis	Reduced affinity for drug by ribosome; reduced transport into cell
Quinolone	Inhibits DNA gyrase	Probable mutation of target enzyme

for 2 months followed by INH and RIF for 4 months were established as effective short-course regimens. Shorter course regimens likely will require new agents rather than newer combinations.

There has been less study of regimens for the treatment of multidrug resistant tuberculosis (MDRTB), particularly when resistance to INH, RIF, EMB, and SM is coexistent. Resistance to the so-called primary agents is emerging slowly throughout the world. This was not felt to be a problem in the United States until outbreaks of MDRTB in HIV-infected patients occurred in several urban areas in this country.[1,2] These events refocused attention on tuberculosis as a contemporary public health problem here and abroad. There is presently an appreciation of the potential problems of MDRTB associated with a perception that new agents are required to combat the emergence of drug resistance. Several promising agents may emerge during this period. If we are not to repeat the mistakes of the past, continued emphasis on intermittent supervised or directly observed therapy will be necessary.

Development of new agents for the treatment of slow growing mycobacteria is difficult because of the long treatment regimens, the use of multidrug therapy, and the need to evaluate relapse rates following the completion of therapy. In addition, there are uncertainties related to the preclinical evaluation of candidate agents. It is unclear whether *in*

vitro susceptibility testing coupled with knowledge of pharmacokinetic parameters can predict how an agent will perform in the murine tuberculosis model or in human disease. The murine tuberculosis model may not accurately forecast efficacy in human disease. Additional study of both *in vitro* susceptibility testing and the murine tuberculosis model is needed to validate their ability to predict efficacy in human disease. This is particularly true with regard to organisms judged to be "resistant" to various agents *in vitro*.[3]

II. ISONIAZID, PYRAZINAMIDE, AND ETHIONAMIDE

A. ISONIAZID

Chorine reported that nicotinamide had antituberculous activity in a murine model of tuberculosis.[4] Subsequent examination of nicotinamide analogs yielded INH[5] and PZA.[6,7]

INH, ethionamide (ETA), and PZA are analogs of nicotinamide. The mechanisms of action for these agents have not been clearly established (Table 11-1). INH is thought to inhibit mycolic acid synthesis.[8-11] Other mechanisms of action have been proposed for INH, including action as an antimetabolite for NAD[12] or pyridoxal phosphate.[13] The mechanism of resistance to INH was thought to be related to decreased uptake,[14] however, recent studies by Quemard et al.[8] suggest that resistance may

Table 11-2 **Antimicrobial agents used to treat tuberculosis in adults[a]**

Agent	Daily Dose	Peak Serum Level (μg/ml)	Dose That Corresponds to Peak Serum Level	Maximum Daily Dose	MIC Range in μg/ml (Reference)
Isoniazid	5 mg/kg	3–5	300 mg	300 mg	0.1–0.2(132)
Ethionamide	0.5–1g	20	1 g	1 g	2.5–10 (133)
Pyrazinamide	15–30 mg/kg	30–40	1.5 g	2 g	6.25–50(134)
Rifampin	10 mg/kg	4–32	600 mg	600 mg	0.1–0.5(135)
Rifabutin	5–10 mg/kg	0.49	300 mg	600 mg	0.04–0.08(136)
Ethambutol	15–25 mg/kg	2–5	25 mg/kg	2.5 g	0.5–2 (137)
Streptomycin	15 mg/kg	25–50	1 g	1 g	0.25–2 (138)
Kanamycin	15 mg/kg	22	7.5 mg/kg	1 g	1.5–3 (139)
Amikacin	15 mg/kg	33	7.5 mg/kg	1 g	0.5–1 (139)
		55	15 mg/kg		
Capreomycin	15 mg/kg	20–47	1 g	1 g	1.25–2.4 (139)
Cycloserine	0.5–1 g	10	250 mg	1 g	6.25–25 (140)
Ciprofloxacin	1–1.5 g	3.4–5.4	1 g	1.5 g	0.12–2 (81)
Ofloxacin	400–800 mg	2.9–5.6	400 mg	800 mg	0.12–2 (81)
PAS	150 mg/kg	41–68	4 g	12 g	1–10 (141)

[a] Data abstracted from References 86, 130, 131, as well as from references cited above and in the text.

not be due to a difference in drug uptake or the level of peroxidase activity. They found decreased mycolic acid synthesis in cell extracts from INH-resistant *M. aurum* as compared to INH-sensitive *M. aurum*. Cole et al. recently reported characterization of an *M. tuberculosis* gene, *katG*, encoding both catalase and peroxidase activity.[15] This gene restored sensitivity to INH in a resistant mutant of *M. smegmatis*. Furthermore, deletion of *katG* from the chromosome was associated with INH resistance in two patient isolates of *M. tuberculosis*. INH may function as a prodrug that is activated by *katG*.

INH is thought to be bactericidal against actively growing tubercle bacilli. This agent is active against *M. tuberculosis* complex. It has variable *in vitro* activity against nontuberculous mycobacteria, perhaps being active most reliably against *M. kansasii*. It is not active *in vitro* against *M. avium* complex or clinically important rapid growers.

1. Absorption, Distribution, and Elimination

INH is well absorbed following oral dosing achieving serum concentrations between 3 and 5 μg/ml (Table 11-2) 1–2 h after a 300 mg dose.[16] Serum concentrations in rapid acetylators are 20–50% of those in slow acetylators. INH is distributed into all body tissues and fluids including CSF. It is minimally bound to plasma proteins, crosses the placenta readily, and achieves levels in milk comparable to those in maternal serum.

INH is metabolized in the liver to acetylisoniazid, which subsequently is transformed to the mono- and diacetylhydrazine, isonicotinic acid, and isonicotinyl glycine.[16] Approximately 75–95% of the INH is excreted in the urine over 24 h as INH and its metabolites (predominately acetylisoniazid and isonicotinic acid).[16] INH can be administered safely at its usual dose to individuals with a serum creatinine less than 12 mg/dl.[17] It also may be administered intramuscularly or intravenously.

2. Adverse Effects

Excretion of pyridoxine is enhanced by isoniazid, resulting in decreased serum pyridoxine levels. Pyridoxine deficiency can manifest itself as peripheral neuropathy, which usually is preceded by paresthesia of the hands and feet. This effect occurs in approximately 20% of patients, particularly those who are malnourished, alcoholics, or have diabetes mellitus. Although as little as 6 mg/day of pyridoxine is effective in preventing peripheral neuropathy, 25 or 50 mg/day often is given concurrently with INH. Other manifestations of nervous system toxicity that occur rarely are convulsions, optic neuritis, toxic encephalopathy, muscle twitching, ataxia, tinnitus, dizziness, euphoria, memory impairment, and toxic psychosis.

Hepatic dysfunction, manifested by modest increases (less than threefold) in serum AST (SGOT) and ALT (SGPT) occurs in approximately 20% of patients on INH during the initial 4 to 8 weeks of therapy. Patients should be carefully monitored monthly for symptoms of hepatitis (anorexia, malaise, fatigue, nausea, and jaundice). The incidence of INH-associated hepatitis is age related. It is rare in patients less than 20 years old, occurs in 0.3% of patients 20–34 years old, increases to 1.2% for patients 35–49 years old, and occurs in 2.3% of those individuals older than 50 years of age.[18] Continuation of INH after the appearance of symptoms of hepatic dysfunction increases the severity of hepatic injury and has led to death from fulminant hepatitis in some individuals.[19,20] The mechanism of INH-associated hepatitis has not been clarified.[21] INH should not be given to patients with acute liver disease or with a history of previous INH-associated hepatitis.

INH has been associated with dryness of the mouth, epigastric distress, tinnitus, urinary retention, and methemoglobinemia. Although uncommon, INH also has been associated with a "lupus-like" syndrome consisting of fever, rash, and arthralgias. INH can be used safely to treat clinical tuberculosis during pregnancy. Preventive therapy usually can be initiated during the postpartum period.

Overdose of INH (usually greater than 1.5 g) may lead to coma, severe intractable seizures, metabolic acidosis, and hyperglycemia. The seizures are thought to result from decreased γ-aminobutyric acid concentrations due to inhibition of CNS pyridoxal-5-phosphate activity by INH. Seizures do not respond well to diazepam or phenobarbital, however, pyridoxine hydrochloride intravenously (comparable to dose of INH ingested) has been effective in treating INH-induced seizures.

3. Drug Interactions

INH therapy has been associated with increased serum levels of carbamazepine and symptoms of carbamazepine toxicity (ataxia, headache, vomiting, blurred vision, drowsiness, and confusion). The interaction is thought to result from INH-induced inhibition of the hepatic metabolism of carbamazepine. If INH and carbamazepine are used concurrently, serum concentrations of the anticonvulsant should be monitored. INH inhibits hepatic metabolism of phenytoin resulting in toxicity in some patients. Patients receiving both INH and phenytoin should be observed for development of phenytoin toxicity. Usually, the dose of phenytoin is reduced where it is administered concomitantly with INH.

B. PYRAZINAMIDE

PZA has a narrow spectrum of activity. It is active against *M. tuberculosis* but is not active against *M. bovis* (a closely related member of *M. tuberculosis*

complex) or nontuberculous mycobacteria. The mechanism of action of PZA is not known. PZA is converted to pyrazinoic acid by nicotinamidase intracellularly.[22] Some PZA-resistant isolates of *M. tuberculosis* and isolates of *M. bovis* have markedly reduced levels of nicotinamidase activity. Therefore, a mutation in this enzyme may be one mechanism of resistance. It is likely that PZA is a prodrug of pyrazinoic acid since pyrazinoate esters have been shown to circumvent PZA resistance *in vitro*.[23] PZA is thought to be bacteriostatic. It is unclear whether it inhibits primarily intracellular or extracellular organisms.[24] This agent's clinical importance increasingly has been recognized since its use facilitated 6-month chemotherapy regimens.[25]

1. Absorption, Distribution, and Elimination

PZA is well absorbed within 1 to 2 h after oral administration achieving serum levels between 30 and 40 μg/ml following a 1.5-g dose.[26] It is distributed into body tissues and fluids including the cerebrospinal fluid (CSF). PZA is approximately 50% bound to plasma proteins. Serum pyrazinoic acid levels peak several hours later than PZA and exceed that of the parent drug. PZA is hydrolyzed primarily in the liver to pyrazinoic acid followed by hydroxylation to 5-hydroxypyrazinoic acid.[27] A small fraction of PZA is excreted in the urine; however, approximately one-third of the dose is excreted as pyrazinoic acid.[26]

2. Adverse Effects

Transient elevation of serum transaminases, jaundice, hepatitis, fever, anorexia, malaise, and hepatic tenderness are the most common adverse effects of PZA. Liver toxicity is thought to be dose related and was reported to occur in approximately 15% of patients receiving 3 g per day with jaundice occurring in 3%.[28] The incidence of drug-induced hepatotoxicity in patients receiving 25–35 mg/kg of PZA is less than 5%.

Pyrazinoic acid competes with uric acid for renal tubular excretion frequently leading to hyperuricemia and, occasionally, episodes of acute gout. Rash, arthralgias, vomiting, dysuria, and photosensitivity rarely have been associated with PZA therapy. This agent should be used cautiously in patients with diabetes mellitus because management of diabetes may become difficult.

3. Drug Interactions

No data are available on drug interactions with PZA.

C. ETHIONAMIDE

Thioisonicotinamide was synthesized in 1952. It was found to be active against *M. tuberculosis in vitro* and in a murine model of tuberculosis, however, it was not effective in human tuberculosis.[29] Ethionamide (ETA), the α-ethyl derivative of thioisonicotinamide, subsequently was synthesized and found to have improved activity.[30] The mechanism of action of ETA is thought to be inhibition of mycolic acid synthesis.[31,32] There is no cross-resistance, therefore ETA and INH are likely to have different targets in the mycolic acid synthetic pathway. The mechanism of resistance to ETA is not known.

1. Absorption, Distribution, and Elimination

Peak serum levels of ETA after a 250 mg oral dose is approximately 1.8 μg/ml.[33] The serum $t_{1/2}$ is between 2 and 3 h.[33] This agent is thought to be widely distributed achieving levels comparable to that of serum in various body fluids. The predominant metabolite of ETA is a sulfoxide; a methyl derivative also is found to a lesser extent.[33] The sulfoxide transformation appears to occur in the liver. A small percentage (less than 1%) of ETA is excreted unchanged in the urine.

2. Adverse Effects

The most frequent side effects of ETA are anorexia, nausea, vomiting, diarrhea, and gastrointestinal discomfort.[34] These effects may be managed by changing the time of drug administration or decreasing the dosage. Antiemetics often can ameliorate nausea and vomiting, however, discontinuation of ETA may be necessary. A metallic taste, likely related to the sulfur, sometimes has been noted. Postural hypotension, depression, and drowsiness have been observed. Additional side effects include convulsions, peripheral neuropathy, olfactory disturbances, diplopia, blurred vision, dizziness, paresthesias, headache, tremors, and hallucinations.

Transient elevation of serum bilirubin, AST (SGOT), and ALT (SGPT) has occurred in patients taking ETA. Hepatitis has been reported to occur and usually is reversible after ETA is discontinued. Rash, stomatitis, photosensitivity, thrombocytopenia, purpura, and goiter (with and without hypothyroidism) have rarely been associated with use of ETA. In addition, hypoglycemia, gynecomastia, menorrhagia, joint pain, and acne have been reported. ETA should be used cautiously in patients with diabetes mellitus because management of diabetes may become difficult. ETA should be avoided in patients with severe hepatic dysfunction. The safety of ETA during pregnancy has not been established.

3. Drug Interactions

Seizures associated with cycloserine use may be aggravated by concurrent use of ETA.

III. RIFAMYCINS

A. RIFAMPICIN (RIFAMPIN)

In the 1950s, Lepetit Laboratories in Italy recognized a new class of antimicrobials called rifamycins. One of the original compounds, rifamycin B, was isolated from an organism belonging to the genus *Streptomyces*, later reclassified as *Nocardia mediterranei*. Subsequent chemical modifications to the original compounds resulted in agents with increased antibacterial activity, rifamycin SV and rifamycin B diethylamide. Rifampin (RIF), 3-4-(4-methylpiperazinyl-iminomethylidene)-rifamycin SV, was synthesized in 1965.

RIF is an important agent in the treatment of tuberculosis, leprosy, and diseases caused by the nontuberculous mycobacteria. RIF has good *in vitro* and *in vivo* activity against *M. tuberculosis, M. kansasii,* and *M. marinum*.[35,36] It has modest *in vitro* and *in vivo* activity against *M. avium* complex[37-39] and poor activity against the rapid growers *M. fortuitum* and *M. chelonae*.[36,40]

The mechanism of action of RIF appears to be inhibition of the β-subunit of DNA-dependent RNA polymerase.[31,41] RIF is considered to be bactericidal and is active against both intracellular and extracellular *M. tuberculosis*. Its use in combination with isoniazid in treatment regimens for tuberculosis allowed the shortening of duration of therapy from 18–24 months to 6–9 months. The mechanism of resistance to RIF has not been demonstrated in mycobacteria, however, it is likely to be spontaneous mutation of the target enzyme.

1. Absorption, Distribution, and Elimination

RIF is well absorbed from the gastrointestinal tract, although the presence of food decreases absorption. A single 600 mg dose in fasting patients results in peak serum concentrations between 8 and 12 μg/ml at 2 h after administration (range of 1–4 h).[42] RIF penetrates tissues well and reaches effective concentrations both in tuberculous cavities and in cerebrospinal fluid in the setting of inflamed meninges. RIF crosses the placenta, but no adverse fetal effects have been proved.[43]

RIF is deacetylated in the liver and enters the bile, where there is subsequent enterohepatic circulation. RIF induces its own hepatic metabolism over time, however, the deacetylated metabolite retains antimycobacterial activity. Both RIF and the deacetylated metabolite are excreted in the urine.

RIF is not cleared appreciably by either peritoneal dialysis or hemodialysis. It should be given in standard doses to patients with renal failure.

2. Adverse Effects

Patients should be advised that RIF is widely distributed in bodily fluids and will impart an intense orange-red color to urine, sweat, saliva, and tears; soft contact lenses may be permanently discolored. Otherwise, the most common side effects are rash (seen in 1%), fever (seen in 1%), and nausea or vomiting. Transient abnormalities in liver function have been reported, but severe hepatotoxicity due to RIF is infrequent.[35] The occurrence of severe toxicity may increase with underlying liver disease and concomitant use of isoniazid. Thrombocytopenia also has been described with RIF use.

Intermittent administration of higher doses of RIF has been associated with immunologically mediated reactions, such as anemia, thrombocytopenia, leukopenia, acute renal failure, and a "flu-like" syndrome consisting of chills, fever, myalgias, arthralgias, and gastrointestinal upset. These reactions occur mostly in persons receiving a dosage of 15 mg/kg or greater and are rare at the recommended daily or twice-weekly dose.

3. Drug Interactions

RIF is a potent inducer of hepatic microsomal enzymes. Its use may result in decreased activity of warfarin derivatives, oral contraceptives, sulfonylureas, corticosteroids, digoxin, methadone, barbiturates, phenytoin, ketoconazole, fluconazole, β-adrenergic blocking agents, verapamil, cyclosporine, and theophylline.[35,44,45] When RIF and methadone are used concurrently, methadone doses must be increased at least 50% over baseline doses. In addition, methadone may need to be administered in divided doses when used with RIF. Because of induced alterations in steroid metabolism, breakthrough bleeding and pregnancy have been reported with concurrent use of RIF and oral contraceptive agents. An alternative method of contraception is recommended during therapy with an RIF-containing regimen.

When RIF is taken with *p*-aminosalicylic acid, serum RIF levels may decrease. It is recommended that these two agents be dosed at least 8 h apart.

B. RIFABUTIN

Rifabutin (ansamycin), a semisynthetic derivative of rifamycin S, belongs to the spiropiperdylrifamycins. Rifabutin is more active than RIF *in vitro* against *M. tuberculosis*, *M. kansasii*, *M. marinum*, *M. xenopi*, *M. haemophilum,* and *M. avium* complex.[37,39,46,47] Cross-resistance to rifabutin is incomplete for RIF-resistant isolates of *M. tuberculosis* and *M. avium* complex.[46,47] The mechanism of action of rifabutin is similar to that of RIF.

1. Absorption, Distribution, and Elimination

Rifabutin is incompletely absorbed from the gastrointestinal tract, with bioavailability ranging from 12 to 20%.[48] A peak serum concentration of less than 1 μg/ml is achieved 2 to 3 h after a single 600 mg oral dose.[48] Rifabutin is taken up by tissues and the level achieved in lung is approximately 5- to 10-fold higher than that in serum.[46] Elimination occurs through both the liver and kidney. There appear to be two major metabolites, 31-OH rifabutin and 25-deacetyl rifabutin.[49] The terminal $t_{1/2}$ ranges from 12 to 18 h, making it suitable for intermittent administration.

2. Adverse Effects

Rifabutin has been used as part of multidrug regimens for the treatment of RIF-resistant tuberculosis,[50,51] for treatment of pulmonary *M. avium* complex disease,[52] and for disseminated *M. avium* complex infections in persons with acquired immune deficiency syndrome.[53,54] The efficacy of these regimens and of rifabutin in particular is not clear. Rifabutin also has been used as single agent therapy in a placebo-controlled study of prevention of disseminated *M. avium* complex infection in persons with underlying HIV infection and profound immune compromise. Rifabutin appears to be generally well tolerated, with a side effect profile similar to that of RIF (rash, pruritus, fever, and gastrointestinal distress).[49]

3. Drug Interactions

Insufficient data are available to comment on drug interactions with rifabutin, however, induction of hepatic microsomal enzymes and autoinduction of its own metabolism occurs with RBT,[55] but may be less than that seen with RIF. The interaction between RBT and methadone may be less than that seen with RIF; however, additional study is needed before recommendations can be made. RBT reduces the area under the zidovudine concentration–time curve by 20–30%; however, the clinical significance of this interaction is not clear. There currently is no recommendation to alter the zidovudine dose because of this reported interaction. Preliminary data supplied by Adria Pharmaceuticals suggest no significant interaction between RBT and didanosine or RBT and fluconazole.

C. RIFAPENTINE

Rifapentine is 3-(4-cyclopentylpiperazinyliminomethyl)-rifamycin SV. Its activity *in vitro* is superior to that of RIF against isolates of *M. tuberculosis* and *M. avium* complex.[37,47,56,57] It also has enhanced activity compared to RIF in murine models of infection due to these mycobacterial species.[38,58]

1. Absorption, Distribution, and Elimination

Administration of 300–600 mg oral dose of rifapentine yielded peak serum levels of 11–14 µg/ml with a half-life of 14–24 h.[46,59] Unlike RIF, absorption seems to be enhanced following administration after a meal. Few data are available with regard to the distribution, metabolism, and elimination of rifapentine.

2. Adverse Effects

There is limited clinical experience with rifapentine in humans with mycobacterial infections.

3. Drug Interactions

No data are available on drug interactions with rifapentine.

IV. ETHAMBUTOL

Ethambutol hydrochloride is a synthetic agent that was developed from *N,N′*-diisopropylethylenediamine, which was found to be active against *M. tuberculosis* in a screening program.[60] The *d*-enantiomer of ethambutol is approximately 200 times more active than the *ℓ*-enantiomer. Ethambutol is active against *M. tuberculosis*, *M. kansasii*, *M. avium* complex, and some other nontuberculous mycobacteria. Ethambutol inhibits the introduction of D-arabinose into arabinogalactan.[61,62] The mechanism of resistance to ethambutol has not been firmly established, however, resistance likely is due to mutation of the target enzyme.[63] Ethambutol is thought to be "weakly" bactericidal and is active against actively growing organisms.

A. ABSORPTION, DISTRIBUTION, AND ELIMINATION

Ethambutol is rapidly absorbed from the gut with a bioavailability of approximately 80% of administered dose.[64] Peak serum levels 2–4 h after oral doses of 25 or 12.5 mg/kg were 4–5 and 2 µg/ml, respectively.[64] Lee et al. measured a mean peak serum level of 4 µg/ml after a 15 mg/kg oral dose.[65]

Ethambutol appears to have a large volume of distribution, which in part is due to active uptake of drug by erythrocytes. Plasma protein binding is between 20 and 30%.[66] Ethambutol crosses the placenta. It is present in breast milk at levels comparable to that in serum.

The $t_{1/2}$ is between 3 and 4 h in patients with normal renal function. Ethambutol is primarily eliminated by the kidneys in part by active tubular secretion.[64,65] Hepatic metabolism (oxidation to an aldehyde intermediate that is converted to the dicarboxylic acid) accounts for approximately 20% of the total body clearance of ethambutol. Approximately 50% of an oral dose of the drug is excreted unchanged in the urine, and 8–15% is excreted as inactive metabolites. Approximately 20% of the initial dose is excreted in the feces as unchanged drug. Accumulation of drug has been observed in patients with decreased renal function.

B. ADVERSE EFFECTS

Ethambutol has been well tolerated at the usual daily dose of 15 mg/kg.[67] Its most important toxicity is retrobulbar neuritis, which can present with decreased visual acuity, constriction of visual fields, central and peripheral scotomas, or loss of red-green color discrimination. Optic neuritis appears to be related to dose and duration of therapy, being quite unusual at 15 mg/kg/day. Visual acuity should be measured with a Snellen eye chart prior to and during therapy.

Subjective visual symptoms may occur before or concurrent with decreased visual acuity, therefore, patients should be asked periodically about blurred vision and other visual symptoms. Each eye should be tested separately since changes in visual acuity may be unilateral or bilateral. Ocular toxicity, when detected early, usually is reversible during a period of weeks to months after ethambutol is discontinued. Recovery of visual function can take a year or more. Rarely the dysfunction is not reversible. Ethambutol should be used only when visual acuity can be monitored.

Dermatitis, pruritus, headache, malaise, dizziness, fever, mental confusion, disorientation, joint pain, GI discomfort, abdominal pain, nausea, vomiting, anorexia, and rarely anaphylactoid reactions have been associated with use of ethambutol. Peripheral neuropathy infrequently has been reported. Elevated serum uric acid levels (in approximately 50% of patients) and the occurrence of acute gout occasionally have been associated with ethambutol.[68]

Although ethambutol is teratogenic in animals in high doses, it has not been reported to produce fetal abnormalities during human pregnancy.

C. DRUG INTERACTIONS

There have been no significant drug interactions reported for EMB.

V. AMINOGLYCOSIDES (AMINOGLYCOSIDIC AMINOCYCLITOLS): STREPTOMYCIN, KANAMYCIN, AND AMIKACIN

Aminoglycosides contain one or two amino sugars linked to an aminocyclitol nucleus. Streptidine is the nucleus of streptomycin, and 2-deoxystreptamine is the nucleus of kanamycin and amikacin. The aminoglycosides are bactericidal and are thought to inhibit protein synthesis by binding to the 30 S ribosomal subunit. They are effective against extracellular mycobacteria. Resistance to an aminoglycoside may result from decreased cell wall permeability, alteration of the ribosomal binding site, or aminoglycoside-modifying enzymes (acetylation, adenylation, or phosphorylation). The latter mechanism (usually plasmid mediated) frequently is present in gram-positive and gram-negative bacteria. Cross-resistance between kanamycin (amikacin) and streptomycin in mycobacteria has not been reported.[69] Cross-resistance occurs between kanamycin and amikacin in *M. tuberculosis* isolates, therefore aminoglycoside-modifying enzymes are not likely to be involved in these organisms.[70]

A. ABSORPTION, DISTRIBUTION, AND ELIMINATION

The aminoglycosides are well absorbed after parenteral (intramuscular or intravenous) administration. They are poorly absorbed from the gut. These agents usually are given in divided doses for the therapy of bacterial infections, however, they should be used in a single daily dose for the treatment of infections caused by slow-growing mycobacteria. Following an intramuscular (im) dose, peak plasma levels usually are achieved within 0.5–2 h and measurable levels may be present for 8–12 h or longer.

Aminoglycosides are widely distributed into body fluids (extracellular fluids) and are minimally protein bound. They diffuse poorly and unpredictably into the CSF even in patients with meningeal inflammation, achieving levels less than 50% of the serum level. Aminoglycosides accumulate in body tissues and are slowly released after therapy is discontinued. Aminoglycosides cross the placenta and reach levels in fetal serum of 16–50% of that in maternal serum.

The $t_{1/2}$ of aminoglycosides usually is 2–4 h. The serum levels and the $t_{1/2}$ are higher and longer, respectively, in patients with decreased renal function. These agents are not metabolized and are excreted predominantly by glomerular filtration. Particular caution must be used in monitoring renal function in elderly patients who start out with age-related decreases in GFR. The majority of a single parenteral dose of an aminoglycoside is excreted within 24 h in the urine. Aminoglycosides can be removed by hemodialysis and, to a lesser extent, by peritoneal dialysis.

B. ADVERSE EFFECTS

Eighth cranial nerve toxicity may occur as a result of aminoglycoside therapy. Streptomycin usually is associated with vestibular symptoms such as dizziness, ataxia, vertigo, and nystagmus. Kanamycin and amikacin usually are associated with auditory symptoms such as hearing loss (decreased high-frequency perception detectable by audiometric testing occurs prior to middle frequency impairment), tinnitus, or roaring in ears. Auditory nerve damage may be irreversible.

Aminoglycoside-induced nephropathy may be associated with elevation of BUN and serum creatinine, with decreased creatinine clearance due to tubular necrosis. Nonoliguric azotemia is the common form, with oliguria occurring rarely. Nephropathy is generally reversible after discontinuation of drugs, however, dialysis is sometimes necessary. Streptomycin is thought to be less nephrotoxic than kanamycin or amikacin at usual doses.

Headache, tremor, lethargy, paresthesia, peripheral neuropathy, arachnoiditis, encephalopathy, and acute brain syndrome rarely have been associated with aminoglycoside therapy. Optic neuritis has also been associated with use of aminoglycosides. Hypersensitivity reactions including rash, urticaria, stomatitis, pruritus, fever, generalized burning, and eosinophilia have been associated with aminoglycoside therapy. Anaphylaxis and transient agranulocytosis have occurred rarely. Cross-allergenicity occurs among the aminoglycosides.

Less frequent adverse effects such as nausea, vomiting, anemia, granulocytopenia, thrombocytopenia, tachycardia, arthralgia, hepatic necrosis, myocarditis, transient elevation of hepatic enzymes, and serum bilirubin have been associated with use of aminoglycosides.

Ototoxicity and nephrotoxicity are more likely to occur in elderly patients (due to decreased creatinine clearance), dehydrated patients, patients with preexisting renal impairment, or patients concurrently receiving other nephrotoxic and/or ototoxic agents. Aminoglycoside therapy should be accompanied by periodic assessment of renal function and eighth cranial nerve function. During antimycobacterial therapy monitoring serum levels is more useful to ensure that appropriate therapeutic levels are achieved rather than to predict nephrotoxicity.

C. DRUG INTERACTIONS

The concurrent use of other agents with nephrotoxic potential should be avoided.

VI. CAPREOMYCIN SULFATE

Capreomycin is a polypeptide derived from *Streptomyces capreolus*. It is a complex of capreomycin IA, IB, IIA, and IIB. The chemical structures of these components have not been defined. Capreomycin is thought to be bacteriostatic and to inhibit protein synthesis. Resistance to this agent develops in a step-wise manner *in vitro*. "Partial" cross-resistance between capreomycin and kanamycin has been observed.

A. ABSORPTION, DISTRIBUTION, AND ELIMINATION

Capreomycin is given im due to poor absorption from the gut. One gram of capreomycin im yields peak serum levels between 20 and 47 µg/ml at 1–2 h and approximately 10 µg/ml at 6 h. It is not known how this agent is distributed in body tissue or fluids, nor whether it crosses the placenta. The $t_{1/2}$ of capreomycin is 4–6 h. In patients with decreased renal function the serum levels are higher and the $t_{1/2}$ is prolonged. It is excreted in the urine predominantly by glomerular filtration without metabolic transformation. Approximately 57% of a 1-g dose is excreted in the urine within 24 h.

B. ADVERSE EFFECTS

Renal dysfunction associated with increased BUN and serum creatinine results from tubular necrosis. Renal dysfunction usually is reversible after discontinuation of capreomycin. Renal function should be monitored carefully particularly in those patients at increased risk (i.e., elderly patients, patients with preexisting renal dysfunction, and patients receiving other potentially nephrotoxic drugs). Hypokalemia, hypocalcemia, hypomagnesemia, and alkalosis may occur secondary to renal tubular dysfunction.

Capreomycin therapy can result in auditory and vestibular dysfunction secondary to eighth nerve injury. Hearing loss usually is reversible. Headache, tinnitus, and vertigo associated with capreomycin have been reported.

Capreomycin can cause pain, induration, and sterile abscesses at injection sites. Eosinophilia occurs frequently in patients on daily therapy and usually resolves when the frequency is reduced to less than three times per week. Leukocytosis, leukopenia, and thrombocytopenia have been associated with this agent. In addition, hypersensitivity reactions (rash, urticaria, and photosensitivity) have been reported.

Dosage reduction based on creatinine clearance is necessary for patients with decreased renal function.[71] Dosage adjustments are designed to achieve a mean steady-state capreomycin level of 10 µg/ml.[71]

C. DRUG INTERACTIONS

No data are available on drug interactions with CAP. The concurrent use of other agents with nephrotoxic potential should be avoided.

VII. CYCLOSERINE

Cycloserine is derived from *Streptomyces orchidaceus* and also has been synthesized. It is an analog of D-alanine. Cycloserine inhibits cell wall synthesis by blocking alanine racemase and D-alanine-D-alanine synthetase. These components are needed for synthesis of peptidoglycan, which is an essential part of bacterial cell walls.[72] Primary and acquired resistance to cycloserine has been demonstrated in human disease. The mechanism of resistance to cycloserine in mycobacteria has not been determined. *Streptococcus* mutants selected for resistance to cycloserine had increased levels of alanine racemase and D-alanine-D-alanine synthetase.[73]

A. ABSORPTION, DISTRIBUTION, AND ELIMINATION

After oral administration, approximately 70–90% of the cycloserine is absorbed from the gut. Peak levels of 8–20 µg/ml occur within 2–4 h after a 250-mg dose.[74]

Cycloserine is widely distributed in body fluids and tissues in concentrations approximately equal to that in the serum. The CSF level of cycloserine is reported to be 80–100% of the serum level in patients with inflamed meninges and 50–80% of the serum level in patients with uninflamed meninges. This agent is not bound to plasma proteins. Cycloserine crosses the placenta and is present in breast milk.

The serum $t_{1/2}$ is approximately 10 h in patients with normal renal function. Approximately 65% of an oral dose of cycloserine appears unchanged in the urine after glomerular filtration. Most of the remaining 35% is metabolized to unknown products. Serum levels of cycloserine are greater and the $t_{1/2}$ is longer in patients with compromised renal function.

B. ADVERSE EFFECTS

Nervous system symptoms appear to be related to doses of cycloserine greater than 500 mg per day. Drowsiness, somnolence, dizziness, headache, lethargy, depression, tremor, dysarthria, hyperreflexia, anxiety, vertigo, confusion and disorientation with loss of memory, paresis, clonic seizures, convulsions, and coma have been associated with use of this drug. Alcohol appears to increase the occurrence of seizures. Psychosis with suicidal behavior, personality changes, hyperirritability, and aggression has occurred in patients treated with cycloserine. Nervous system effects are thought to be reduced when the serum levels of cycloserine are below 30 µg/ml. Pyridoxine hydrochloride (100 mg daily) may ameliorate the CNS toxicity of cycloserine. Anticonvulsants and sedatives may be useful for convulsions, anxiety, or tremor.

Hypersensitivity reactions (rash or photosensitivity) rarely have been associated with this agent.

Renal, hepatic, and hematologic parameters should be monitored while patients are receiving cycloserine.

C. DRUG INTERACTIONS

Concurrent use of ethionamide has been reported to potentiate neurotoxicity of cycloserine.

Cycloserine inhibits hepatic metabolism of phenytoin; therefore serum levels of phenytoin should be monitored and evidence of phenytoin intoxication should be looked for in patients treated concurrently with these agents.

VIII. *p*-AMINOSALICYLIC ACID

p-Aminosalicyclic acid (PAS), a weakly bacteriostatic agent, currently is available only from the Centers for Disease Control and Prevention. Recent outbreaks of multidrug-resistant tuberculosis have provided a stimulus to resume manufacturing this agent, and it likely will be marketed in the near future.

A. ABSORPTION, DISTRIBUTION, AND ELIMINATION

PAS is well absorbed from the gastrointestinal tract and is widely distributed throughout the body except the central nervous system. Oral dosing of 4 and 12 g of PAS produces peak serum concentrations of 70–80 and 130–210 µg/ml, respectively.[42] Serum $t_{1/2}$ of PAS is approximately 1 h. The drug is rapidly metabolized in the intestinal mucosa and liver via acetylation and conjugation. The predominant mode of elimination is by the kidneys, primarily as the acetylated or glycine-conjugated metabolites. Dosage reduction is necessary in patients with renal failure.

B. ADVERSE EFFECTS

Side effects of PAS include a high frequency of gastrointestinal intolerance (nausea, vomiting, and diarrhea), hypersensitivity reactions, and, infrequently, hepatitis.[35] Other rare side effects include hypoprothrombinemia, thrombocytopenia, goiter, and a "lupus-like" syndrome.[75] The sodium salt (PAS is available either as a sodium or calcium salt) may be contraindicated in patients who require sodium restriction. PAS may precipitate acute hemolytic anemia in persons who are deficient in glucose-6-phosphate dehydrogenase.

C. DRUG INTERACTIONS

PAS reduces the rate of acetylation of INH; however, the effect is not clinically significant. Probenecid inhibits renal excretion of PAS and increases serum levels of PAS. Diphenhydramine impairs GI absorption of PAS. Certain PAS preparations (granule formulations that contain bentonite) may interfere with the absorption of RIF, resulting in decreased serum RIF concentrations. It is recommended that these two agents be dosed 8–12 h apart.

IX. THIACETAZONE

Thiacetazone currently is not available in the United States; therefore many practitioners are not familiar with this agent. In many developing countries, thiacetazone is included in a conventional regimen in combination with INH and SM.[76] A recent study by Heifets et al. employed the BACTEC methodology to evaluate the activity of thiacetazone against *M. tuberculosis* and *M. avium*.[77] Although the bactericidal activity against either species was low, the inhibitory levels for *M. tuberculosis* ($n = 14$) and for *M. avium* ($n = 68$) were 0.08–1.2 and 0.02–0.15 µg/ml, respectively.

A. ABSORPTION, DISTRIBUTION, AND ELIMINATION

Thiacetazone has not been well studied from a pharmacokinetic standpoint. It appears to be well absorbed from the gastrointestinal tract, with peak serum levels reported between 4 and 5 h after administration.[78] Peak serum levels are in the range of 1–4 µg/ml following a 150-mg oral dose.[42,78] Two potential metabolites have been identified, *p*-aminobenzaldehyde-thiosemicarbazone and *p*-acetylaminobenzoic acid, although the metabolic fate of thiacetazone has not been clearly delineated.[42,78] Approximately 20% of the drug is excreted unchanged in the urine.

B. ADVERSE EFFECTS

Minor side effects of thiacetazone include anorexia or gastrointestinal distress in up to 10%, flushing or transient rash, dizziness, headache, and drowsiness. Serious side effects include severe cutaneous reactions, agranulocytosis, hepatotoxicity, and deafness.[79] Hypersensitivity reactions may be more severe in individuals who are seropositive for the human immunodeficiency virus.[80]

C. DRUG INTERACTIONS

Thiacetazone may potentiate the vestibular toxicity of SM. Severe liver damage has been reported in patients receiving INH and thiacetazone concurrently, although the contribution of each individual agent is not clear.

X. FLUOROQUINOLONES

A. CIPROFLOXACIN

The quinolone class of antimicrobials includes several groups of heterocyclic carbonic acid derivatives. These agents are related structurally to nalidixic acid. The mechanism of action of the quinolones is inhibition of DNA gyrase, an enzyme essential for maintenance of DNA superhelical twists. One mechanism of resistance to fluoroquinolones appears to be alteration in subunit A of DNA gyrase, although this has not been demonstrated as yet for mycobacteria.

The newer quinolones have significant advantages in pharmacokinetics and tissue penetration compared with the parent compounds, although development of clinical resistance remains a problem.

Ciprofloxacin is active *in vitro* against *M. tuberculosis* with MICs in the range of 0.125–2.0 µg/ml.[81,82] Activity also has been reported *in vitro* against *M. malmoense, M. fortuitum,* and *M. kansasii.* Clinical experience with ciprofloxacin therapy in patients with mycobacterial infections is limited.[40,83] MICs for *M. avium* complex are less favorable and range from 1 to 16 µg/ml,[81,84] however, ciprofloxacin has been included as part of multidrug regimens for the treatment of disseminated *M. avium* complex infection in persons with AIDS.[85]

1. Absorption, Distribution, and Elimination

Ciprofloxacin hydrochloride is rapidly and well absorbed from the gastrointestinal tract. The rate of absorption is slowed in the presence of food. Magnesium-, aluminum-, or calcium-containing antacids will decrease the bioavailability of ciprofloxacin. Peak serum concentrations are generally attained within 0.5–2 h after oral administration. Peak serum concentrations following 500 and 1,000 mg oral doses are 1.6–2.9 and 3.4–5.4 µg/ml, respectively. Ciprofloxacin is widely distributed into body tissues, and tissue levels typically exceed that seen in serum. The exception is penetration into the cerebrospinal fluid, where levels may only be 6–10% of peak serum concentrations. Ciprofloxacin crosses the placenta and is distributed into breast milk.

The elimination half-life in adults with normal renal function is 3–5 h. In persons with impaired renal function, serum concentrations are higher and the half-life is prolonged. Ciprofloxacin is metabolized in the liver yielding at least four metabolites, some of which retain antibacterial activity. Ciprofloxacin and its metabolites are excreted in urine and feces.

2. Adverse Effects

Ciprofloxacin generally is well tolerated, but side effects include gastrointestinal distress (nausea, vomiting, diarrhea, and abdominal pain) in 2–10% of patients.[86] Headache, restlessness, and neuropsychiatric symptoms (phobia, depersonalization, anxiety, depression, manic reactions, and psychosis) have been reported but occur in only 1–2% of patients. Some of the neuropsychiatric side effects may be related to the fact that ciprofloxacin, like other fluoroquinolones, is a GABA inhibitor. Rash occurs in 1–4% of patients. Severe hypersensitivity reactions have been described. Crystalluria, cylinduria, hematuria, and transient liver function abnormalities are infrequent adverse effects. Arthropathy is noted in juvenile animals receiving ciprofloxacin. Therefore this agent should not be used in children or adolescents.

3. Drug Interactions

Antacids containing magnesium, aluminum, or calcium can decrease absorption of ciprofloxacin. Antacids should not be administered within 4 h of ciprofloxacin dosing. Probenecid interferes with renal tubular secretion of ciprofloxacin and may result in increased serum concentration and prolonged half-life. Concomitant administration of ciprofloxacin and theophylline derivatives may result in higher theophylline concentrations and subsequent toxicity.[87] Concomitant administration of ciprofloxacin and warfarin derivatives may result in a prolonged prothrombin time, perhaps due to displacement of warfarin from plasma proteins.[88]

B. OFLOXACIN

Ofloxacin is active against *M. tuberculosis,* with MICs in the range of 0.3–2.5 µg/ml.[89,90] Ofloxacin has been evaluated in a clinical study of 19 "treatment-failure" cases of cavitary pulmonary tuberculosis. The study evaluated the activity of ofloxacin (300 mg per day for 6–8 months) in combination with the patients' previous "ineffective" regimen; thus, the study was considered, in effect, to evaluate the use of ofloxacin alone.[91] Conversion of sputum to negative occurred in 5 of 19 patients, with a decline in the number of recoverable bacilli in the majority of the remaining patients. In a subsequent uncontrolled trial of ofloxacin in the treatment of multidrug-resistant tuberculosis, 10 of 17 patients responded.[50] Ofloxacin is active *in vitro* against *M. bovis* and *M. fortuitum* but has limited activity against *M. avium* complex and *M. chelonae*.

1. Absorption, Distribution, and Elimination

Absorption of ofloxacin is rapid and nearly complete with oral bioavailability of 85–100%. Peak serum concentration are reached within 0.5–2 h. Peak serum concentrations following 200 and 400 mg doses are 1.5–2.7 and 2.9–5.6 µg/ml, respectively. Ofloxacin is widely distributed into body tissues, and peak concentrations in cerebrospinal fluid are 28–87% that of serum levels. Ofloxacin crosses the placenta and is present in breast milk.

The elimination half-life in adults with normal renal function ranges from 4 to 8 h. Ofloxacin will reach higher serum levels and exhibit a prolonged half-life in patients with decreased creatinine clearance. Less than 10% of a single dose of ofloxacin is metabolized. The majority of drug is excreted unchanged in the urine, the remainder is excreted as metabolites in the urine or feces.

2. Adverse Effects

The side effect profile for ofloxacin is similar to that of ciprofloxacin. Gastrointestinal distress has been reported in 3–10% of patients. CNS symptoms, including drowsiness, cognitive changes, depression, and euphoria, can be seen in 1–3% of patients. Rash, arthropathy, and transient liver function abnormalities have been reported. Crystalluria has not been demonstrated in animal studies.

3. Drug Interactions

Ingestion of antacids, multivitamins, and mineral supplements containing divalent or trivalent cations may decrease absorption of ofloxacin. Interaction between ofloxacin and theophylline derivatives may be less than that seen with ciprofloxacin; however, plasma theophylline concentrations should be monitored if ofloxacin is used concurrently.

C. NEWER FLUOROQUINOLONES

Two promising newer quinolones under development are sparfloxacin and levofloxacin. MICs for sparfloxacin (AT-4140) against *M. tuberculosis* are one or two dilutions lower than that of either ciprofloxacin or ofloxacin.[92] The activity of sparfloxacin 50–100 mg/kg in a murine model of tuberculosis was on the same order as that of the standard dose of isoniazid (25 mg/kg) used in mouse studies and was more active than ofloxacin 300 mg/kg.[92] Phase I studies of sparfloxacin in humans show peak serum concentrations after oral doses of 200 and 400 mg of 0.65 and 1.39 µg/ml, respectively, with elimination half-life on the order of 16 h.[93]

Ofloxacin occurs as a racemic mixture of two isoenantiomers. Levofloxacin, the ℓ-isomer, is more active *in vitro* and *in vivo* against gram-positive and gram-negative organisms than ofloxacin. It appears to be better tolerated than the racemic mixture.[94,95] Early studies of levofloxacin in a murine model of tuberculosis show greater than a 2-fold improvement in activity compared with ofloxacin.[96] Insufficient human data are available to provide pharmacokinetic parameters.

XI. CLOFAZIMINE

Clofazimine has been in use since 1962 for the treatment of leprosy. It is a substituted iminophenazine dye with the chemical name 3-(*p*-chloroanilino)-10-(*p*-chlorophenyl)-2,10-dihydro-2-(isopropylimino)phenazine. Clofazimine has activity *in vivo* in the mouse foot-pad model of *M. leprae* infection and is used in combination drug therapy for multibacillary leprosy.[97]

Clofazimine has promising *in vitro* activity against *M. tuberculosis*, with MICs in the range of 0.1–10 µg/ml, depending on the pH of the media. Clofazimine has activity in murine and guinea pig models of tuberculosis, but had neither therapeutic nor prophylactic activity in a rhesus monkey model of infection.[98] Interspecies differences in peak serum levels may help explain the observed variation in activity. Recently, clofazimine activity in a murine model of drug-resistant tuberculosis was reported.[3] Assessment of its activity in human disease is necessary to determine whether clofazimine has a role as an antituberculosis agent.

Clofazimine has activity *in vitro* and *in vivo* against *M. avium* complex and has been used in multidrug regimens for the treatment of *M. avium* complex infection in persons with AIDS.[54]

The mechanism of action of clofazimine is not well understood, but may involve inhibition of the template function of the DNA strand, thus resulting in growth inhibition.[97]

A. ABSORPTION, DISTRIBUTION, AND ELIMINATION

Clofazimine is absorbed slowly and incompletely from the gastrointestinal tract. Bioavailability of the commercial preparation (microcrystalline suspension in an oil-wax base) approximates 70%. After a single 200 mg oral dose in fed subjects, peak serum concentrations average 0.41 µg/ml, with a prolonged time (8–12 h) to reach maximum concentrations.[99] Clofazimine distributes into fatty tissues and is taken up by macrophages. It crosses the placenta and is distributed into breast milk.

Few data are available regarding the metabolism of clofazimine. Three urinary metabolites have been identified, but the overall metabolic fate of clofazimine and its metabolites is not known.

Elimination characteristics of clofazimine are interesting and seem to correspond to a two-phase elimination. The initial elimination half-life is 7–10 days, followed by a much longer elimination half-life of approximately 70 days as the drug is released slowly from tissues.[99] The effects of peritoneal dialysis and hemodialysis on clofazimine levels are not known.

B. ADVERSE EFFECTS

The most frequently reported side effects include discoloration of the skin and abdominal pain. Red-brown discoloration of the skin and conjunctiva occurs in the majority of patients and may last several years after discontinuation of the drug. Other bodily fluids, such as sweat, tears, sputum, and feces, also may be discolored. Additional skin conditions, such as xeroderma, pruritus, and exfoliative dermatitis, occur as well. Corneal discoloration and maculopathy have been reported.

Gastrointestinal side effects include abdominal pain, nausea, anorexia, diarrhea, and weight loss. Irritation of the GI tract and deposition of clofazimine crystals have been implicated in these reactions.

C. DRUG INTERACTIONS

Reduction in the rate of absorption of rifampin has been described with clofazimine, although overall bioavailability of rifampin was not affected significantly.

XII. MACROLIDES

Erythromycin is produced by *Streptomyces erythraeus* and belongs to the macrolide group of antimicrobial agents. The mechanism of action of the macrolides appears to be inhibition of protein synthesis by reversible binding to the 50 S ribosomal subunit. Erythromycin has limited activity against mycobacteria and is used only in infections caused by susceptible strains of *M. chelonae*.[40]

A. CLARITHROMYCIN

Clarithromycin differs structurally from erythromycin only by the methylation of a hydroxyl group at position 6 of the lactone ring. The presence of the methyl group minimizes the acid-catalyzed degradation to the inactive hemiketal and spiroketal products, which may mitigate the adverse gastrointestinal effects seen with erythromycin. Clarithromycin has activity *in vitro* and *in vivo* against *M. kansasii*, *M. fortuitum*, *M. chelonae*, *M. leprae*, and *M. avium* complex with MICs generally less than 2 µg/ml against these spe-

cies.[84,100,101] It has promising activity for the treatment of disseminated *M. avium* complex infection in persons with AIDS.[102] MICs against *M. tuberculosis* are not as favorable, and currently, clarithromycin is not considered a useful agent against this species.

1. Absorption, Distribution, and Elimination

Clarithromycin is absorbed rapidly from the gastrointestinal tract; its absorption exceeds that of erythromycin. Bioavailability is on the order of 50–55%. Administration with food may delay the rate but not the overall extent of absorption. There is rapid first-pass metabolism to 14-hydroxyclarithromycin, which retains antimicrobial activity. Peak serum concentrations of 2.1 µg/ml are achieved following a single 400 mg dose of clarithromycin,[103] but much higher tissue concentrations are reached. The extent of penetration into CSF is not known.

Clarithromycin is eliminated both by renal and nonrenal means. Elimination half-life following a single 250 mg dose is approximately 4 h, with approximately 38% of the dose excreted in urine and 40% excreted in feces. The serum half-life is prolonged in patients with renal failure and dosage reduction may be required. Moderate to severe hepatic impairment reduces formation of the 14-hydroxy metabolite, but is accompanied by increased renal clearance of the parent drug. Dosage modification is necessary only when concurrent hepatic and renal impairment is present.

2. Adverse Effects

The overall incidence of side effects with clarithromycin is similar to or lower than that with erythromycin. Diarrhea, nausea, and abdominal discomfort are reported in 2–3% of patients taking the drug. Hepatomegaly, elevation of liver function tests, headache, reversible hypoacusis, pruritus, and rash have been reported. Safety and efficacy of clarithromycin have not been established for children less than 12 years old.

3. Drug Interactions

Use of clarithromycin in patients who are receiving theophylline may result in an increase in serum theophylline concentrations. Serum theophylline concentrations should be monitored closely if these agents are used concurrently.

Peak serum concentrations of zidovudine are reduced when clarithromycin is used concurrently, but the clinical significance of this finding is uncertain.

B. AZITHROMYCIN

Azithromycin is an azalide antibiotic that differs from erythromycin chemically by a methyl-substituted nitrogen in the macrolide ring. Azithromycin has *in vitro* and *in vivo* activity against *M. avium* complex and *M. kansasii*, although MICs are several-fold higher than those of clarithromycin.[104-106] Azithromycin has promising activity for the treatment of disseminated *M. avium* complex infection in persons with AIDS.[107]

1. Absorption, Distribution, and Elimination

Bioavailability of azithromycin is approximately 40% after a single oral dose. Peak serum concentration following a 500-mg oral dose is 0.4 μg/ml. The serum half-life after a single 500-mg dose is 11–14 h. High tissue concentrations are achieved, particularly in liver and spleen.[108]

2. Adverse Effects

Profile of adverse effects seen with azithromycin is similar to that with clarithromycin.[109]

3. Drug Interactions

As with clarithromycin, serum theophylline concentration should be monitored if azithromycin and theophylline are used concurrently.

C. ROXITHROMYCIN

Roxithromycin (RU 28965, Hoechst Roussel) is a 14-membered ring structure modified at the C-9 position. Roxithromycin has activity *in vitro* against *M. tuberculosis*, *M. avium* complex, and the rapidly growing mycobacteria.[106,110,111] The MIC_{90} against isolates of *M. tuberculosis* in one series (*n* = 199) was 4 μg/ml.[110] Activity of roxithromycin has been reported against *M. leprae* in the mouse footpad model;[112] however, its activity *in vivo* against other mycobacteria has not been reported.

1. Absorption, Distribution, and Elimination

Roxithromycin is well absorbed from the gastrointestinal tract with bioavailability ranging from 72 to 85%. A peak serum concentration of 5.7 μg/ml is obtained after a single 150-mg dose.[109] Roxithromycin achieves higher serum levels than either clarithromycin or azithromycin, but is similarly concentrated within tissues. Serum half-life of a single 150-mg dose is 10.5 h.[109]

2. Adverse Effects

Gastrointestinal distress is less frequent than with erythromycin, but diarrhea, abdominal pain, and nausea have been reported in approximately 3% of adults taking roxithromycin at 150 mg orally twice a day in Phase I and Phase II clinical trials. Dermatologic reactions such as pruritis, rash, and urticaria are infrequent. Central nervous system side effects such as dizziness, tinnitus, vertigo, and headache occur infrequently.

The peak serum concentration, area under the concentration–time curve, and serum half-life are increased in the presence of renal insufficiency. The dosing interval should be double for patients with creatinine clearances less than 15 ml/min.[113]

3. Drug Interactions

Preliminary data suggest that roxithromycin may exert less of an effect than erythromycin on theophylline clearance; however, serum theophylline concentrations should be monitored if roxithromycin is used comcomitantly with theophylline.

XIII. β-LACTAMS

β-Lactams have *in vitro* activity against slow growing and rapid growing mycobacteria. Amoxicillin/clavulanate and other β-lactam/β-lactamase inhibitor combinations have been reported to have activity *in vitro* against *M. tuberculosis*,[114,115] however, clinical efficacy or convincing activity in a murine infection model has not been demonstrated. Cefoxitin, cefmetazole, and imipenem have *in vitro* activity against *M. fortuitum*.[116-118] Cefoxitin was less active against *M. chelonae* subsp. *chelonae*.[117] Cefoxitin has been used for treatment of pulmonary and nonpulmonary infections caused by rapid growers.[119] Imipenem and cefmetazole were more active than cefoxitin against *M. fortuitum*, and imipenem was the only β-lactam active against *M. chelonae* subsp. *chelonae*.[118] The pharmacology of the β-lactams has been well summarized previously.[86]

XIV. SULFONAMIDES

The *in vitro* activity of sulfonamides against rapid growers has been evaluated extensively.[117] *M. fortuitum* isolates are susceptible to sulfonamides, however, *M. chelonae* isolates usually are resistant to the sulfonamides.[117,120] Trimethoprim is not active against *M. fortuitum* or *M. chelonae* isolates when used alone, nor is there enhanced activity when combined with sulfamethoxazole. Wallace et al. has reported *in vitro* activity of sulfonamides against *M. kansasii* and a good clinical response to sulfonamide-containing regimens in *M. kansasii*-infected patients.[121] The *in vitro* activity of sulfonamides against other nontuberculous mycobacteria has not been evaluated adequately, however, they have been found to have *in vitro* activity against *M. marinum* and *M. scrofulaceum* isolates.[120] Testing of *M. avium* complex isolates *in vitro* with sulfisoxazole has yielded variable results.[122,123]

XV. TETRACYCLINES

Tetracycline and its derivatives minocycline and doxycycline have modest *in vitro* activity against *M. fortuitum* and *M. chelonae*.[124,125] These agents have not been found to be particularly active against *M. tuberculosis* and other slow growing mycobacteria with the exception of *M. leprae*.[126,127] Tetracyclines presently do not have a role in treatment of disease caused by *M. tuberculosis*.

XVI. FUTURE PROSPECTS

The revival of interest in mycobacterial infections is due in part to the emergence of multidrug-resistant *M. tuberculosis* and the frequent occurrence of disseminated *M. avium* complex infection in patients with advanced HIV infection. New agents can be developed by modification of current agents, by screening existing chemical libraries, by evaluating natural products, and perhaps by targeting specific biochemical pathways with sophisticated molecular biological techniques. Agents that will facilitate ultra-short-course treatment for tuberculosis and preventive therapy are desirable. Agents with efficacy against multidrug-resistant tuberculosis also are needed.

Immunomodulators are not likely to have clinical application for the treatment of tuberculosis. Liposome-encapsulated antimicrobial agents have been demonstrated to have enhanced activity compared to nonencapsulated drugs in macrophage culture[128] as well as in murine models of mycobacterial disease.[129] This novel drug delivery system is unlikely to be clinically practical unless the candidate product has exceptional activity and can be utilized intermittently on a once or twice a week dosing schedule.

Analogs of currently used agents with enhanced activity can be synthesized as our understanding of the common mechanisms of resistance is increased.[23] The quinolones remain the most promising class of new antituberculosis agents. The macrolides are another fertile group for chemical manipulation, based on their exciting activity against *M. avium* complex.

At the present time it is not known whether ultra-short-course regimens (2 or 3 months duration) would be achievable with currently active agents. Ultra-short-course therapy is a desirable goal for the mycobacterial therapeutic research and development agenda.

REFERENCES

1. Fischl, M. A., Uttamchandiani, R. B., Daikos, G. L., Poblete, R. B., Moreno, J. N., Reyes, R. R., Boota, A. M., Thompson, L. M., Cleary, T. J., Lai, S., An outbreak of tuberculosis caused by mutliple-drug resistant tubercle bacilli among patients with HIV infection, *Ann. Intern. Med.,* 117, 177, 1992.

2. Centers for Disease Control, Nosocomial transmission of multi-drug resistant tuberculosis among HIV-infected persons — Florida and New York, 1988–1991, *MMWR,* 40, 585, 1991.

3. Cynamon, M. H., DeStefano, M. S., Klemens, S. P., Therapy of multidrug resistant tuberculosis (MDR-TB): lessons from mice, *Program Abstr. World Congr. Tuberc.,* Bethesda, MD, November 16–19, 1992, 29.

4. Chorine, M. V., Action of nicotinamide on bacilli of the species mycobacterium, *C.R. Hebd. Seances Acad. Sci.,* 220, 150, 1945.

5. Fox, H. H., The chemical attack on tuberculosis, *Trans. N. Y. Acad. Sci.,* 15, 234, 1953.

6. Kushner, S., Dalalian, H., Sanjurjo, J. L., Bach, F. L., Safir, S. R., Smith, V. L., Williams, J. H., Experimental chemotherapy of tuberculosis II, *J. Am. Chem. Soc.,* 74, 3617, 1952.

7. Solotorovsky, M., Gregory, F. J., Ironson, E. J., Bugie, E. J., O'Neill, R. C., Pfister, K., Pyrazinoic acid amide — An agent active against experimental murine tuberculosis, *Proc. Soc. Exp. Biol. Med.,* 79, 563, 1952.

8. Quemard, A., Lacave, C., Lancelle, G., Isoniazid inhibition of mycolic acid synthesis by cell extracts of sensitive and resistant strains of *Mycobacterium aurum, Antimicrob. Agents Chemother.,* 35, 1035, 1991.

9. Davidson, L. A., Takayama, K., Isoniazid inhibition of the synthesis of monounsaturated long-chain fatty acids in *Mycobacterium tuberculosis* H37Ra, *Antimicrob. Agents Chemother.,* 16, 104, 1979

10. Takayama, K., Wang, L., David, H. L., Effect of isoniazid on the *in vivo* mycolic acid synthesis, cell growth, and viability of *Mycobacterium tuberculosis, Antimicrob. Agents Chemother.,* 2, 29, 1972

11. Winder, F. G., Collins, P. B., Inhibition by isoniazid of synthesis of mycolic acids in *Mycobacterium tuberculosis, J. Gen. Microbiol.,* 63, 41 1970.

12. Iwainsky, H., INH-mode of action, in *Antituberculosis Drugs,* Bartmann, K., Ed., Springer-Verlag, Berlin, 1988, 476.

13. Krishna Murti, C. R., Isonicotinic acid hydrazide, in *Antibiotics,* Vol. III, Corcoran, J. W., Hahn, F. E., Eds., Springer-Verlag, Berlin, 1975, 623.

14. Youatt, J., A review of the action of isoniazid, *Am. Rev. Resp. Dis.,* 99, 729, 1969.

15. Zhang, Y., Heym, B., Allen, B., Young, D., Cole, S., The catalase-peroxidase gene and isoniazid resistance of *Mycobacterium tuberculosis, Nature (London),* 358, 591, 1992.

16. Weber, W. W., Hein, D. W., Clinical pharmacokinetics of isoniazid, *Clin. Pharmacokinet.,* 4, 410, 1979.

17. Bowersox, D. W., Winterbauer, R. H., Steward, G. L., Orme, B., Barron, E., Isoniazid dosage in patients with renal failure, *N. Engl. J. Med.,* 84, 1973.

18. Public Health Service, U.S. Department of Health, Education, and Welfare, Isoniazid-associated hepatitis: summary of the report of the Tuberculosis Advisory Committee and special consultants to the Director, Center for Disease Control, *MMWR,* 23, 97, 1974.

19. Garibaldi, R. A., Drusin, R. E., Ferebee, S. H., Gregg, M. B., Isoniazid-associated hepatitis, Report of an outbreak, *Am. Rev. Resp. Dis.,* 106, 357, 1972.

20. Maddrey, W. C., Boitnoit, J. K., Isoniazid hepatitis, *Ann. Intern. Med.,* 79,1, 1973.

21. Mitchell, J. R., Zimmerman, H. J., Ishak, K. G., Thorgeirsson, U. P., Timbrell, J. A., Snodgrass, W. R., Nelson, S. D., Isoniazid liver injury: clinical spectrum, pathology, and probable pathogenesis, *Ann. Intern. Med.,* 84, 181, 1976.

22. Konno, L., Feldmann, F. M., McDermott, W., Pyrazinamide susceptibility and amidase activity of tubercle bacilli, *Am. Rev. Resp. Dis.,* 95, 461, 1967.

23. Cynamon, M. H., Klemens, S. P., Chou, T.-S., Gimi, R. H., Welch, J. T., Antimycobacterial activity of a series of pyrazinoic acid esters, *J. Med. Chem.,* 35, 1212, 1992.

24. Mitchison, D. A., The Garrod Lecture: Understanding the chemotherapy of tuberculosis-current problems, *J. Antimicrob. Chemother.,* 29, 477, 1992.

25. Grosset, J. H., Present status of chemotherapy for tuberculosis, *Rev. Infect. Dis.,* 11 (Suppl. 2), S347, 1989.

26. Ellard, G. A., Absorption, metabolism and excretion of pyrazinamide in man, *Tubercle,* 50, 144, 1969.

27. Weiner, I. M., Tinker, J. P., Pharmacology of pyrazinamide: Metabolic and renal function studies related to the mechanism of drug-induced urate retention, *J. Pharmacol. Exp. Ther.,* 180, 411, 1972.

28. McDermott, W., Ormond, L., Muschenheim, C., Deuschle, K., McCune, R. M., Tompsett, R., Pyrazinamide-isoniazid in tuberculosis, *Am. Rev. Tuberc.,* 69, 319, 1954.

29. Veterans Hospital (Madison, Wisconsin), Thioisonicotinamides, *Quart. Prog. Rep. V.A. Chem. Tuberc.,* 10, 44, 1955.

30. Rist, N., Grumbach, F., Liberman, D., Experiments on the antituberculous activity of alpha-ethyl-thionicotinamide, *Am. Rev. Tuberc.,* 79, 1, 1959.

31. Winder, F. G., Mode of action of the antimycobacterial agents and associated aspects of the molecular biology of the mycobacteria, in *The Biology of Mycobacteria,* Vol. 1, Ratledge, C., Stanford, J., Eds., Academic Press, New York, 1982, 353.

32. Quemard, A., Lancelle, G., Lacave C., Mycolic acid synthesis: a target for ethionamide in mycobacteria?, *Antimicrob. Agents Chemother.,* 36, 1316, 1992.

33. Jenner, P. J., Ellard, G. A., Gruer, P. J. K., Aber, V. R., A comparison of the blood levels and urinary excretion of ethionamide and prothionamide in man, *J. Antimicrob. Chemother.,* 13, 267, 1984.

34. Girling, D. J., Adverse effects of antituberculosis drugs, *Drugs,* 23, 56, 1982.

35. Perez-Stable, E. J., Hopewell, P. C., Current tuberculosis treatment regimens, in *Clinics in Chest Medicine,* Vol. 10, Snider, D. E., Jr., Ed., W.B. Saunders, Philadelphia, 1989, 323.

36. Wolinsky, E., Mycobacterial diseases other than tuberculosis, *Clin. Infect. Dis.,* 15, 1, 1992.

37. Cynamon, M. H., Comparative *in vitro* activities of MDL 473, rifampin and ansamycin against *Mycobacterium intracellulare, Antimicrob. Agents Chemother.,* 28, 440, 1985.

38. Klemens, S. P., Cynamon, M. H., Activity of rifapentine against *Mycobacterium avium* infection in beige mice, *J. Antimicrob. Chemother.,* 29, 555, 1992.

39. Saito, H., Sato, K., Tomioka, H., Comparative *in vitro* and *in vivo* activity of rifabutin and rifampicin against *Mycobacterium avium* complex, *Tubercle,* 69, 187, 1988.

40. Wallace, R. J., Jr., The clinical presentation, diagnosis and therapy of cutaneous and pulmonary infections due to the rapid growing mycobacteria, *M. fortuitum* and *M. chelonae,* in *Clinics in Chest Medicine,* Vol. 10, Snider, D. E., Jr., Ed., W.B. Saunders Co., Philadelphia, 1989, 419.

41. Kono, K., Oizumi, K., Oka, S., Mode of action of rifampin in mycobacteria. II. Biosynthetic studies on the inhibitors of ribonucleic acid polymerase of *Mycobacterium bovis* BCG by rifampin and uptake of rifampin-^{14}C by *Mycobacterium phlei, Am. Rev. Resp. Dis.,* 107, 1006, 1973.

42. Peloquin, C. A., Antituberculosis drugs: Pharmacokinetics, in *Drug Suspectibility in the Chemotherapy of Mycobacterial Infections,* Heifets, L. B., Ed., CRC Press, Boca Raton, FL, 1991, 61.

43. Snider, D., Pregnancy and tuberculosis, *Chest,* 86 (Suppl.), 10S, 1984.

44. Van Scoy, R. E., Wilkowske, C. J., Antituberculous agents, *Mayo Clin. Proc.,* 67, 179, 1992.

45. Borcherding, S. M., Baciewicz, A. M., Self, T. H., Update on rifampin drug interactions II, *Arch. Intern. Med.,* 152, 711, 1992.

46. Traxler, P., Vischer, W. A., Zak, O., New rifamycins, *Drugs Future,* 13, 845, 1988.

47. Dickinson, J. M., Mitchison, D. A., *In vitro* activity of new rifamycins against rifampicin-resistant *M. tuberculosis* and MAIS-complex mycobacteria, *Tubercle,* 68, 177, 1987.

48. Skinner, M. H., Hsieh, M., Torseth, J., Pauloin, D., Bhatia, G., Harkonen, S., Merigan, T. C., Blaschke, T. F., Pharmacokinetics of rifabutin, *Antimicrob. Agents Chemother.,* 33, 1237, 1989.

49. Battaglia, R., Pianezzola, E., Salgarollo, G., Zini, G., Benedetti, M. S., Absorption, disposition, and preliminary metabolic pathway of ^{14}C-rifabutin in animals and man, *J. Antimicrob. Chemother.,* 26, 813, 1990.

50. Hong Kong Chest Service/British Medical Research Council, A controlled study of rifabutin and an uncontrolled study of ofloxacin in the retreatment of patients with pulmonary tuberculosis resistant to isoniazid, streptomycin and rifampicin, *Tuberc. Lung Dis.,* 73, 59, 1992.

51. Chan, S. L., Yew, W. W., Ma, W. K., Girling, D. J., Aber, V. R., Flemingham, D., Allen, B. W., Mitchison, D. A., The early bactericidal activity of rifabutin measured by sputum viable counts in Hong Kong patients with pulmonary tuberculosis, *Tuberc. Lung Dis.,* 73, 33, 1992.

52. O'Brien, R. J., Geiter, L. J., Lyle, M. A., Rifabutin (ansamycin LM 427) for the treatment of pulmonary *Mycobacterium avium* complex, *Am. Rev. Resp. Dis.,* 141, 841, 1990.

53. Agins, B. D., Berman, D. S., Spicehandler, D., El-Sadr, W., Simberkoff, M. S., Rahal, J. J., Effect of combined therapy with ansamycin, clofazimine, ethambutol, and isoniazid for *Mycobacterium avium* infection in patients with AIDS, *J. Infect. Dis.,* 159, 784, 1989.

54. Dautzenberg, B., Truffot, C., Mignon, A., Rozenbaum, W., Katlama, C., Perrone, C., Parrot, R., Grosset, J., Rifabutin in combination with clofazimine, isoniazid and ethambutol in the treatment of AIDS patients with infections due to opportunist mycobacteria, *Tubercle,* 72, 168, 1991.

55. Strolin Benedetti, M., Efthymiopoulos, C., Sassella, D., Moro, E., Repetto, M., Autoinduction of rifabutin metabolism in man, *Xenobiotica,* 20, 1113, 1990.

56. Dickinson, J. M., Mitchison, D. A., *In vitro* properties of rifapentine (MDL 473) relevant to its use in intermittent chemotherapy of tuberculosis, *Tubercle,* 68, 113, 1987.

57. Heifets, L. B., Lindholm-Levy, P. J., Flory, M. A., Bactericidal activity *in vitro* of various rifamycins against *Mycobacterium avium* and *Mycobacterium tuberculosis*, *Am. Rev. Resp. Dis.,* 141, 626, 1990.

58. Dhillon, J., Dickinson, J. M., Guy, J. A., Ng, T. K., Mitchison, D. A., Activity of two long-acting rifamycins, rifapentine and FCE 22807, in experimental murine tuberculosis, *Tuberc. Lung Dis.,* 73, 116, 1992.

59. Birmingham, A. T., Coleman, A. J., L'e Orme, M., Park, B. K., Pearson, N. J., Short, A. H., Southgate, P. J., Antibacterial activity in serum and urine following oral administration in man of DL 473 (a cyclopentyl derivative of rifampicin), *Br. J. Clin. Pharmacol.,* 6, 455P, 1978.

60. Thomas, J. P., Baughn, C. O., Wilkinson, R. G., Shepard, R. G., A new synthetic compound with antituberculous activity in mice: Ethambutol (dextro-2-2'-(ethylenediimino)-di-1-butanol), *Am. Rev. Resp. Dis.,* 83, 891, 1961.

61. Takayama, K., Armstrong, E. L., Kunugi, K. A., Kilburn, J. D., Inhibition by ethambutol of mycolic acid transfer into the cell wall of *Mycobacterium smegmatis*, *Antimicrob. Agents Chemother.,* 16, 240, 1979.

62. Kilburn, J. O., Takayama, K., Effects of ethambutol on accumulation and secretion of trehalose mycolates and free mycolic acid in *Mycobacterium smegmatis*, *Antimicrob. Agents Chemother.,* 20, 401, 1981.

63. Stanley, A., Belisle, J. T., Brennan, P. J., Inamine, J. M., Identification and characterization of *Mycobacterium avium* genes which confer resistance to ethambutol, Frontiers in Mycobacteriology: *M. avium*, The Modern Epidemic, Abstr. 68, Vail, CO, October 1992.

64. Place, V. A., Peets, E. A., Buyske, D. A., Little, R. R., Metabolic and special studies of ethambutol in normal volunteers and tuberculosis patients, *Ann. N. Y. Acad. Sci.,* 135, 775, 1966.

65. Lee, C. S., Brater, D. C., Gambertoglio, J. G., Benet, L. Z., Disposition kinetics of ethambutol in man, *J. Pharmacokin. Biopharm.,* 8, 335, 1980.

66. Lee, C. S., Gambertoglio, J. G., Brater, D. C., Benet, L. Z., Kinetics of oral ethambutol in the normal subject, *Clin. Pharmacol. Ther.,* 22, 615, 1977.

67. Doster, B., Murray, F. J., Newman, R., Woolpert, S. F., Ethambutol in the initial treatment of pulmonary tuberculosis, *Am. Rev. Resp. Dis.,* 107, 177, 1973.

68. Postlethwaite, A. E., Bartel, A. G., Kelley, W. N., Hyperuricemia due to ethambutol, *N. Engl. J. Med.,* 286, 761, 1972.

69. Hoffner, S. E., Kallenius, G., Susceptibility of streptomycin-resistant *Mycobacterium tuberculosis* strains to amikacin, *Eur. J. Clin. Microbiol. Infect. Dis.,* 7, 188, 1988.

70. Allen, B. W., Mitchison, D. A., Chan, Y. C., Yew, W. W., Allan, W. G., Girling, D. J., Amikacin in the treatment of pulmonary tuberculosis, *Tubercle,* 64, 111, 1983.

71. Physicians Desk Reference: PDR, Medical Economics Co., Oradell, NJ, 1990, 1203.

72. Neuhaus, F. C., D-cycloserine and D-carbamyl-D-serine, in *Antibiotics,* Vol. I, Gottlieb, D., Shaw, P. D., Eds., Springer-Verlag, New York, 1967, 40.

73. Reitz, R., Slade, H. D., Neuhaus, F. C., On the biochemical basis of D-cycloserine resistance, *Fed. Proc.,* Abstr. 25, 344, 1966.

74. Nair, K. G. S., Epstein, I. G., Baron, H., Mulinos, M. G., Absorption, distribution, and excretion of cycloserine in man, *Antibiot. Ann.,* 1955, 136.

75. Masel, M. A., A lupus-like reaction to antituberculous drugs, *Med. J. Aust.,* 2, 738, 1967.

76. Hopewell, P. C., Sanchez-Hernandez, M., Baron, R. B., Ganter, B., Operational evaluation of treatment of tuberculosis: results of a "standard" 12-month regimen in Peru, *Am. Rev. Resp. Dis.,* 129, 439, 1984.

77. Heifets, L. B., Lindholm-Levy, P. J., Flory, M., Thiacetazone: *In vitro* activity against *Mycobacterium avium* and *M. tuberculosis, Tubercle,* 71, 287, 1990.

78. Ellard, G. A., Dickinson, J. M., Gammon, P. T., Mitchison, D. A., Serum concentrations and antituberculosis activity of thiacetazone, *Tubercle,* 55, 41, 1974.

79. Miller, A. B., Fox, W., Tall, R., An international co-operative investigation into thiacetazone (thioacetazone) side effects, *Tubercle,* 47, 33, 1966.

80. Nunn, P., Kibuga, D., Gathua, S., Brindle, R., Imalingat, A., Wasunna, K., Lucas, S., Gilks, C., Omwega, M., Were, J., Cutaneous hypersensitivity reactions due to thiacetazone in HIV-1 seropositive patients treated for tuberculosis, *Lancet,* 337, 627, 1991.

81. Heifets, L. B., Lindholm-Levy, P. J., Bacteriostatic and bactericidal activity of ciprofloxacin and ofloxacin against *Mycobacterium tuberculosis* and *Mycobacterium avium* complex, *Tubercle,* 68, 267, 1987.

82. Van Caekenberghe, D., Comparative *in-vitro* activities of ten fluoroquinolones and fusidic acid against *Mycobacterium* spp., *J. Antimicrob. Chemother.,* 26, 381, 1990.

83. Kahana, L. M., Spino, M., Ciprofloxacin in patients with mycobacterial infections: experience in 15 patients, *DICP,* 25, 919, 1991.

84. Gorzynski, E. A., Gutman, S. I., Allen, W., Comparative antimycobacterial activities of difloxacin, temafloxacin, enoxacin, pefloxacin, reference fluoroquinolones, and a new macrolide, clarithromycin, *Antimicrob. Agents Chemother.,* 33, 591, 1989.

85. Chiu, J., Nussbaum, J., Bozzette, S., Tilles, J. G., Young, L. S., Leedom, J., Heseltine, P. N. R., McCutchan, J. A., The California Collaborative Treatment Group, Treatment of disseminated *Mycobacterium avium* complex infection in AIDS with amikacin, ethambutol, rifampin and ciprofloxacin, *Ann. Intern. Med.,* 113, 358, 1990.

86. McEvoy, G. K., Ed., Anti-infective agents, in *American Hospital Formulary Service Drug Information,* American Society of Hospital Pharmacists, Inc., Bethesda, MD, 1992.

87. Janknegt, R., Drug interactions with quinolones, *J. Antimicrob. Chemother.,* 26 (Suppl. D), 7, 1990.

88. Jolson, H. M., Tanner, L. A., Green, L., Grasela, T. H., Jr., Adverse reaction reporting of interaction between warfarin and fluoroquinolones, *Arch. Intern. Med.,* 151, 1003, 1991.

89. Truffot-Pernot, C., Ji, B., Grosset, J., Activities of pefloxacin and ofloxacin against mycobacteria: *in vitro* and mouse experiments, *Tubercle,* 72, 57, 1991.

90. Tomioka, H., Sato, K., Saito, H., Comparative *in vitro* and *in vivo* activity of fleroxacin and ofloxacin against various mycobacteria, *Tubercle,* 72, 176, 1991.

91. Taukamura, M., Nakamura, E., Yoshii, S., Amano, H., Therapeutic effect of a new antibacterial substance ofloxacin (DL 8280) on pulmonary tuberculosis, *Am. Rev. Resp. Dis.,* 131, 352, 1985.

92. Ji, B., Truffot-Pernot, C., Grosset, J., In vitro and *in vivo* activities of sparfloxacin (AT-4140) against *Mycobacterium tuberculosis, Tubercle,* 72, 181, 1991.

93. Kanamura, M., Nakashima, M., Uematsu, T., Takikuchi, T., Pharmacokinetics and safety of a new quinolone, AT-4140, in healthy volunteers, *Program Abstr. 28th Intersci. Conf. Antimicrob. Agents Chemother.,* Abstr., 1490, 1988.

94. Fu, K. P., Lafredo, S. C., Locodo, J., Isaacson, D., Tobia, A. J., *In vivo* antibacterial activity of a L-isomer of ofloxacin (L-ofloxacin; DR-3355), an active isomer of racemic ofloxacin (OFL) in murine infection models, *Program Abstr. 31st Intersci. Conf. Antimicrob. Agents Chemother.*, Abstr., 1202, 1991.

95. Kawada, Y., Aso, Y., Kamidono, S., Ohmori, H., Kumazawa, J., Comparative study of DR-3355 and ofloxacin in complicated urinary tract infections, *Program Abstr. 31st Intersci. Conf. Antimicrob. Agents Chemother.*, Abstr., 884, 1991.

96. Klemens, S. P., Cynamon, M. H., unpublished data.

97. Garrelts, J. C., Clofazimine: a review of its use in leprosy and *Mycobacterium avium* complex infections, *DICP*, 25, 525, 1991.

98. Schmidt, L. H., Observations on the prophylactic and therapeutic activities of 2-(*p*-chloranilino)-5-(*p*-chlorophenyl)-3,5-dihydro-3-(isopropylimino)phenazine (B.663), *Bull. Int. Union Tuberc.*, 30, 316, 1959.

99. Holdiness, M. R., Clinical pharmacokinetics of clofazimine: a review, *Clin. Pharmacokinet.*, 16, 74, 1989.

100. Heifets, L. B., Lindholm-Levy, P. J., Comstock, R. D., Clarithromycin minimal inhibitory and bactericidal concentrations against *Mycobacterium avium*, *Am. Rev. Resp. Dis.*, 145, 856, 1991.

101. Klemens, S. P., Cynamon, M. H., Activity of clarithromycin against *Mycobacterium avium* complex infection in beige mice, *Antimicrob. Agents Chemother.*, 36, 2413, 1992.

102. Dautzenberg, B., Truffot, C., Legris, S., Meyohas, M.-C., Berlie, H. C., Mercat, A., Chevret, S., Grosset, J., Activity of clarithromycin against *Mycobacterium avium* infections in patients with the acquired immune deficiency syndrome, *Am. Rev. Resp. Dis.*, 144, 564, 1991.

103. Kirst, H. A., Sides, G. D., New directions for macrolide antibiotics: Pharmacokinetics and clinical efficacy, *Antimicrob. Agents Chemother.*, 33, 1419, 1989.

104. Kirst, H. A., Sides, G. D., New directions for macrolide antibiotics: structural modifications and *in vitro* activity, *Antimicrob. Agents Chemother.*, 33, 1413, 1989.

105. Cynamon, M. H., Klemens, S. P., Activity of azithromycin against *Mycobacterium avium* infection in beige mice, *Antimicrob. Agents Chemother.*, 36, 1611, 1992.

106. Naik, S., Ruk, R., *In vitro* activities of several new macrolide antibiotics against *Mycobacterium avium* complex, *Antimicrob. Agents Chemother.*, 33, 1614, 1989.

107. Young, S. L, Wiviott, L., Wu, M., Kolonoski, P., Bolan, R., Inderlied, C. B., Azithromycin for treatment of *Mycobacterium avium-intracellulare* complex infection in patients with AIDS, *Lancet*, 388, 1107, 1991.

108. Girard, A. E, Girard, D., English, A. R., Gootz, T. D., Cimochowksi, C. R., Faiella, J. A., Haskell, S. L., Retsema, J. A., Pharmacokinetics and *in vivo* studies with azithromycin (CP-62, 993), a new macrolide with an extended half-life and excellent tissue distribution, *Antimicrob. Agents Chemother.*, 31, 1948, 1987.

109. Bahal, N., Nahata, M. C., The new macrolides: Azithromycin, clarithromycin, dirithromycin, and roxithromycin, *Ann. Pharm.*, 26, 46, 1992.

110. Casal, M., Gutierrez, J., Gonzalez, J., Ruiz, P., *In vitro* susceptibility of *Mycobacterium tuberculosis* to a new macrolide antibiotic: RU-28965, *Tubercle*, 63, 141, 1987.

111. Brown, B. A., Wallace, R. J., Jr., Onyi, G. O., De Rosas, V., Wallace, R. J., III, Activities of four macrolides including clarithromycin, against *Mycobacterium fortuitum, Mycobacterium chelonae,* and *M. chelonae*-like organism, *Antimicrob. Agents Chemother.*, 36, 180, 1992.

112. Gelber, R. A., Siu, P., Tsang, M., Murray, L. P., Activities of various macrolide antibiotics against *Mycobacterium leprae* infection in mice, *Antimicrob. Agents Chemother.*, 35, 760, 1991.

113. Halstenson, C. E., Opsahl, J. A., Schwenk, M. H., Kovarid, J. M., Puri, S. K., Matzke, G. R., Disposition of roxithromycin in patients with normal and severely impaired renal function, *Antimicrob. Agents Chemother.*, 34, 385, 1990.

114. Wong, C. S., Palmer, G. S., Cynamon, M. H., *In vitro* susceptibility of *Mycobacterium tuberculosis, Mycobacterium bovis,* and *Mycobacterium kansasii* to amoxicillin and ticarcillin in combination with clavulanic acid, *J. Antimicrob. Chemother.*, 22, 863, 1988.

115. Sorg, T. B., Cynamon, M. H., Comparison of four β-lactamase inhibitors in combination with ampicillin against *Mycobacterium tuberculosis*, *J. Antimicrob. Chemother.*, 19, 59, 1987.

116. Cynamon, M. H., Palmer, G. S., *In vitro* susceptibility of *Mycobacterium fortuitum* to N-formimidoyl thienamycin and several cephamycins, *Antimicrob. Agents Chemother.*, 22, 1079, 1982.

117. Swenson, J. M., Wallace, R. J., Jr., Silcox, V. A., Thornsberry, C., Antimicrobial susceptibility of five subgroups of *Mycobacterium fortuitum* and *Mycobacterium chelonae*, *Antimcrob. Agents Chemother.*, 28, 807, 1985.

118. Wallace, R. J., Jr., Brown, B. A., Onyi, G. O., Susceptibilities of *Mycobacterium fortuitum* biovar. fortuitum and the two subgroups of *Mycobacterium chelonae* to imipenem, cefmetazole, cefoxitin and amoxicillin-clavulanic acid, *Antimicrob. Agents Chemother.*, 35, 773, 1991.

119. Wallace, R. J., Jr., Swenson, J. M., Silcox, V. A., Bullen, M. G., Treatment of nonpulmonary infections due to *Mycobacterium fortuitum* and *Mycobacterium chelonei* on the basis of *in vitro* susceptibilities, *J. Infect. Dis.*, 152, 500, 1985.

120. Wallace, R. J., Jr., Wiss, K., Bushby, M. B., Hollowell, D. C., *In vitro* activity of trimethoprim and sulfamethoxazole against the nontuberculous mycobacteria, *Rev. Infect. Dis.*, 4, 326, 1982.

121. Ahn, C. H., Wallace, R. J., Jr., Steele, L. C., Sulfonamide containing regimens for disease caused by rifampin-resistant *Mycobacterium kansasii*, *Am. Rev. Resp. Dis.*, 135, 10, 1987.

122. Berlin, O. G. W., Clancy, M. N., Bruckner, D. A., *In vitro* susceptibility of sulfisoxazole against *Mycobacterium avium* complex, in *Program Abstr. 28th Intersci. Conf. Antimicrob. Agents Chemother.*, Abstr. 1227, 1988.

123. Davis, C. E., Jr., Carpenter, J. L., Trevino, S., *In vitro* susceptibility of *Mycobacterium avium* complex to antibacterial agents, *Diagn. Microbiol. Infect. Dis.*, 8, 149, 1987.

124. Swenson, J. M., Wallace, R. J., Jr., Silcox, V. A., Thornsberry, C., Antimicrobial susceptibility of five subgroups of *Mycobacterium fortuitum* and *Mycobacterium chelonae*, *Antimicrob. Agents Chemother.*, 28, 807, 1985.

125. Wallace, R. J., Jr., Dalovisio, J. R., Pankey, G. A., Disk diffusion testing of susceptibility of *Mycobacterium fortuitum* and *Mycobacterium chelonei* to antibacterial agents, *Antimicrob. Agents Chemother.*, 16, 611, 1979.

126. Gelber, R. H., Activity of minocycline in *Mycobacterium leprae*-infected mice, *J. Infect. Dis.*, 156, 236, 1987.

127. Ji, B., Perani, E. G., Grosset, J. H., Effectiveness of clarithromycin and minocyline alone and in combination against experimental *Mycobacterium leprae* infection in mice, *Antimicrob. Agents Chemother.*, 35, 579, 1991.

128. Majumdar, S., Flasher, D., Friend, D. S., Nassos, P., Yajko, D., Hadley, W. K., Duzgunes, N., Efficacies of liposome-encapsulated streptomycin and ciprofloxacin against *Mycobacterium avium. M. intracellular* complex infections in human peripheral blood monocyte/macrophages, *Antimicrob. Agents Chemother.*, 36, 2808, 1992.

129. Cynamon, M. H., Klemens, S. P., Swenson, C. E., TLCG-65 in combination with other agents in the therapy of *Mycobacterium avium* infection in beige mice, *J. Antimicrob. Chemother.*, 29, 693, 1992.

130. Maller, R., Isaksson, B., Nilsson, L., Soren, L., A study of amikacin given once versus twice daily in serious infection, *J. Antimicrob. Chemother.*, 22, 75, 1988.

131. Holdiness, M. R., Clinical pharmacokinetics of the antituberculosis drugs, *Clin. Pharmacokinet.*, 9, 108, 1984.

132. Heifets, L. B., Lindholm-Levy, P. J., Flory, M., Comparison of bacteriostatic and bactericidal activity of isoniazid and ethionamide against *M. avium* and *M. tuberculosis*, *Am. Rev. Resp. Dis.*, 143, 268, 1991.

133. Heifets, L. B., Antituberculosis drugs: Antimicrobial activity *in vitro*, in *Drug Susceptibility in the Chemotherapy of Mycobacterial Infections*, Heifets, L. B. Ed., CRC Press Inc., Boca Raton, FL, 1991, 20.

134. Salfinger, M., Heifets, L., Determination of pyrazinamide MICs for *Mycobacterium tuberculosis* at different pHs by the radiometric method, *Antimicrob. Agents Chemother.*, 32, 1002, 1988.

135. Trnka, L., Rifampicin (RMP), in *Antituberculosis Drugs*, Bartmann, K., Ed., Springer-Verlag, Berlin, 1988, 205.

136. Heifets, L. B., Iseman, M. D., Determination of *in vitro* susceptibility of mycobacteria to ansamycin, *Am. Rev. Resp. Dis.*, 132, 710, 1985.

137. Otten, H., Ethambutol (EMB), in *Antituberculosis Drugs*, Bartmann, K., Ed., Springer-Verlag, Berlin, 1988, 197.

138. Suo, J., Chang, C.-E., Lin, T. P., Heifets, L. B., Minimal inhibitory concentrations of isoniazid, rifampin, ethambutol, and streptomycin against *M. tuberculosis* strains isolated before treatment of patients in Taiwan, *Am. Rev. Resp. Dis.*, 138, 999, 1988.

139. Heifets, L. B., MIC as a quantitative measurement of the susceptibility of *M. avium* strains to seven antituberculosis drugs, *Antimicrob. Agents Chemother.*, 32, 113, 1988.

140. Otten, H., Cycloserine (CS), and terizidone (TZ), in *Antituberculosis Drugs*, Bartmann, K., Ed., Springer-Verlag, Berlin, 1988, 158.

141. Trnka, L., Mison, P., *p*-Aminosalicylic acid (PAS), in *Antituberculosis Drugs*, Bartmann, K., Ed., Springer-Verlag, Berlin, 1988, 51.

Drug Resistance

Marian Goble, M.D.

CONTENTS

0-8493-4825-0/94/$0.00+$.50
© 1994 by CRC Press, Inc.

I. BACKGROUND

The thrust of treatment programs for tuberculosis is to avoid treatment failure and to prevent the emergence of drug-resistant strains. Nevertheless, drug-resistant tuberculosis remains a problem and appears to be increasing in prevalence and in complexity.[1]

A. HISTORICAL

Early in the antibiotic era, streptomycin, given as a single agent, was shown to be highly effective in producing clinical, roentgenographic, and bacteriologic improvement in patients with serious illness from tuberculosis. Frequently the improvement was short lived and patients relapsed with tubercle bacilli resistant to streptomycin.[2] Subsequently, with the development of new antituberculosis medications, resistance of tubercle bacilli to any effective drug could be induced if that drug was used as a single agent.[3,4] It was discovered that properly administered multiple drug therapy prevented the emergence of drug resistance.[5,6] Until it was understood that patients required prolonged multiple drug therapy for tuberculosis, inadequate regimens were prescribed commonly. Drug-resistant disease followed, most commonly to isoniazid and/or streptomycin.

New drugs were developed. Specific regimens for drug-resistant tuberculosis were studied over the years. Earlier studies[7-13] involved the use of pyrazinamide, cycloserine, p-aminosalicylate (PAS), ethionamide, kanamycin, and viomycin (viomycin no longer is available in the United States, but is of interest because of common cross-resistance with capreomycin). Later, as ethambutol, capreomycin, and rifampin became available, regimens including these drugs also were studied in retreatment situations.[14,15] Although some reports were not based on carefully controlled studies with uniform criteria, results suggest that in using drugs to which the bacilli were susceptible, three drugs in the regimens gave better results than two drugs.[7,11,16,17]

In several studies outside the United States, retreatment regimens of pyrazinamide, cycloserine, and ethionamide were given to patients with tuberculosis resistant to isoniazid, PAS, and streptomycin; a successful outcome was reported in 90% of cases.[7,11,12] In a developing nation where isoniazid, streptomycin, and thiacetazone (an antituberculosis drug that never became commercially available in the United States) had been standard therapy for tuberculosis, patients who had experienced treatment failure were retreated with a regimen including pyrazinamide and PAS; results were acceptable.[18,19]

At the National Jewish Center in Denver, CO[20] prior to 1971, a regimen of kanamycin, ethionamide, and pyrazinamide was given to 108 patients with tubercle bacilli resistant to isoniazid and streptomycin; a successful outcome occurred in 92% of these patients. A similar group of 164 patients was treated with capreomycin or viomycin in place of kanamycin, with either ethambutol or rifampin replacing one of the oral drugs; similar results were achieved, provided the organisms were susceptible to the drugs chosen. For 36 patients, cycloserine or PAS was among the drugs selected; a successful outcome occurred in 78%. Because of the limited number of drugs that were effective when taken orally, one injectable medication usually was included in these regimens, along with two oral drugs.

Most of the patients with drug-resistant tuberculosis were isolated cases who had acquired drug resistance because of inadequate treatment or noncompliance. Prior to 1990, in the United States, only occasional clusters of drug-resistant cases were reported.[21-26] The incidence of drug resistance in the United States remained stable for many years.[27-33] In the late 1980s the overall incidence of tuberculosis started to increase. Persons infected with the human immunodeficiency virus, if exposed to tuberculosis, were unusually vulnerable to developing active (rather than latent) disease. Socioeconomic conditions favored overcrowding in poorly ventilated facilities. Tuberculosis programs had suffered prior cutbacks, in some instances, so that increasing numbers of patients received inadequate therapy. Although some inadequately treated patients continued to have drug-susceptible tuberculosis, others developed drug-resistant disease in situations favoring spread of the disease to other persons. In the early 1990s increasing outbreaks of drug-resistant tuberculosis have been reported.[34-46]

B. MECHANISMS[47,48]

In the process of multiplication of *M. tuberculosis*, mutations having resistance to any drug occur at a fairly predictable rate.[49] Mutants resistant to rifampin have a probable incidence of 1 in 10^8; mutants resistant to isoniazid, streptomycin, ethambutol, kanamycin, or PAS have a probability of 1 in 10^6; mutants resistant to ethionamide, capreomycin, cycloserine, or thiacetazone occur at a rate of about 1 in 10^3 tubercle bacilli.[50] This resistance occurs despite the absence of antibiotic exposure. Exposure to a single antituberculosis medication selects for drug resistance by killing or suppressing susceptible bacilli and leaving the resistant bacilli unaffected and free to multiply. Natural resistance to more than one drug (that is, multiple drug resistance due to spontaneously occurring mutations) is very unlikely, suggesting that the mutations to various drugs are unlinked genetically. Other mechanisms of resistance have been proposed.[51-55]

1. Primary Resistance

Primary resistance refers to drug resistance of the bacilli from a patient who has never received treatment, who presumably has contracted his or her infection from an index case with drug-resistant tubercle bacilli. Initial resistance is another term used to include drug-resistant bacilli from patients with no prior treatment, or with no known prior treatment, with antituberculosis chemotherapy.

2. Secondary Resistance

Secondary, or acquired resistance, refers to resistance of the bacilli after exposure to the antimicrobial agent, the mutant bacilli having been selected for survival. A patient with untreated cavitary tuberculosis has on the order of 1 in 10^8 tubercle bacilli in the cavity.[47,48] Since mutations to isoniazid resistance occurs at a frequency of 1 in 10^6, an infection with 10^8 bacilli would include approximately 10^2 that are resistant to isoniazid. If the patient is treated with isoniazid by itself, almost all the bacilli would be killed, but those few remaining would be isoniazid resistant. At the time of the reduction in the number of the isoniazid-susceptible bacilli, the patient may improve clinically, roentgenographically, and even bacteriologically. The bacterial count may become very low, even low enough that the bacilli no longer are detectable by usual bacteriologic tests. However, if the host defenses are unable to control the resistant bacilli, they multiply and become the predominant organisms as the infection progresses; the patient then has isoniazid-resistant tuberculosis. A decrease in the numbers of bacilli, followed by an increase associated with the emergence of drug resistance, is called the "fall and rise" phenomenon.[47]

Sometimes the host defenses control the drug-resistant bacilli temporarily and these persisting living drug-resistant bacilli remain dormant. However, if the balance between the host's defenses and the bacilli changes, and the drug-resistant persisters[54,55] later multiply aggressively, the patient will relapse with drug-resistant tuberculosis. Inadequate therapy may result in treatment failure or relapse with secondary or acquired drug resistance. This inadequate therapy may result from inappropriate prescription, such as the use of a single effective agent or because of the patient's noncompliance with the prescribed regimen.[56]

3. Multidrug Resistance

The occurrence of multidrug-resistant tuberculosis is favored by inappropriate management of tuberculosis. In the presence of tuberculosis already resistant to a single drug, therapy with that drug is ineffective. If one other single drug is included in the regimen, or added to the regimen, this is equivalent to monotherapy with the potentially effective second drug. Emergence of resistance to this second drug is to be anticipated, superimposed on the previously existing resistance to the first drug.[57]

4. Cross-Resistance[47,58]

Cross-resistance between streptomycin and kanamycin or capreomycin is unusual, between

kanamycin and capreomycin is fairly frequent,[59] and between kanamycin and amikacin is frequent. Cross-resistance between thiacetazone (a drug not available in the United States, but used in developing nations) and ethionamide and between isoniazid and ethionamide has been reported.[60,61] Cross-resistance between the quinolones and between rifamycin derivatives also occurs.

C. PREVALENCE OF DRUG RESISTANCE[27,32,62-64]

See Chapter 1 (this volume) for a discussion of prevalence.

II. PREVENTION OF DRUG RESISTANCE[65-68]

A. APPROPRIATE THERAPEUTIC REGIMENS

There is no known way to prevent nature's mutations to resistance. However, thoughtful treatment of tuberculosis can minimize significantly the selection of these drug-resistant mutants as the predominant population in patients being treated for the first time and in patients undergoing retreatment. Applying an effective and efficient tuberculosis treatment program is followed ultimately by a decrease in the prevalence of drug resistance.[69-71]

1. Initial Treatment

It is well accepted practice to employ more than one drug in therapy of disease due to *M. tuberculosis* (see Chapter 6, this volume). By using two effective antimicrobial drugs, the mutants resistant to drug A are controlled by drug B, and the drug-resistant mutants to drug B are controlled by drug A.[72] Two drug therapy with agents such as isoniazid and rifampin works well *if* the bacterial population is susceptible to both drugs. However, sometimes the tubercle bacilli are resistant to one of the drugs chosen. This resistance may be unsuspected, and not documented until the susceptibility studies are reported, often belatedly. Meanwhile, the patient is receiving therapy with only one effective drug. If the bacterial population is large, mutants will emerge that are resistant to the drug that has been working, in addition to the inherited resistance of these same organisms to the originally ineffective drug. These multiply-resistant tubercle bacilli will become the predominant strain in the infection. This scenario of compounding the problem of drug resistance can be prevented if a sufficient number of effective antimycobacterial drugs are given from the start. Accordingly, the American Thoracic Society recommends that patients being treated for the first time be started on isoniazid, rifampin, pyrazinamide, and either ethambutol or streptomycin, until the results of susceptibility tests of their bacilli are known, unless there is little possibility of primary resistance to isoniazid.[73] Overtreatment in the early phase of therapy is preferable to undertreatment that favors the emergence of multidrug resistance.

2. Retreatment

The patient's history, especially regarding prior antituberculosis chemotherapy, and the susceptibility of the tubercle bacilli he or she is harboring should be evaluated fully before starting treatment. After the susceptibility of the organism is known, it is important to prescribe at least three previously unused drugs to which the patient's strain of *M. tuberculosis* is susceptible. In this way the likelihood of selecting mutants resistant to the drugs in the new regimen is minimized. *A single drug should never be added to a failing regimen.*

B. ASSURANCE OF ADHERENCE[74-77]

A regimen is effective only if it is taken appropriately. If a patient takes only part of the drugs prescribed, either by taking a reduced (ineffective) dose, or by omitting one or more drugs, there is danger of resistance emerging. Nonadherence is known to lead to treatment failure and to drug resistance. If a patient with a history of treatment failure associated with prior nonadherence is being considered for retreatment, it is unwise to add new drugs until the compliance issue is dealt with. If the patient does not follow the new regimen, the patient may destroy the potential effectiveness of the additional drugs and render himself or herself essentially untreatable. For further discussion on adherence issues refer to Chapter 14 (this volume).

C. PREVENTION OF TUBERCULOUS DISEASE AMONG THOSE EXPOSED TO A PATIENT WITH ACTIVE DRUG-RESISTANT TUBERCULOSIS

Early in the chemotherapy era, transmission of tuberculosis from a drug-resistant index case was questioned. More recently, evidence for such transmission of drug-resistant tuberculosis has been substantiated.[39,40,43,78-81]

1. Environmental Measures[82,83]

See Chapter 3 (this volume) for a discussion of environmental measures.

2. BCG

Bacillus Calmette–Guérin (BCG) vaccine may be appropriate for tuberculin-negative contacts unavoidably exposed to a patient with multidrug-resistant tuberculosis (see Chapters 8 and 15, this volume).

3. Chemotherapeutic Regimens[67]

See Chapter 13 (this volume) for a discussion of chemotherapeutic regimens.

III. RECOGNITION AND EVALUATION

A. PERSONS AT RISK

Overall, the recent incidence of drug resistance among patients with tuberculosis in the United States is estimated at 8–14%;[32,65] accordingly, drug resistance should be a consideration in any patient. However, drug resistance is distributed unevenly throughout the United States. Large cities tend to have a high prevalence of drug resistance.[22,84-87] New York City[26,88-90] has an especially high prevalence. Certain groups of patients have a greater likelihood of harboring drug-resistant bacilli.

1. Previously Treated Patients

In a survey of specimens from 30 large health departments in the United States, 23% of strains of *M. tuberculosis* from unselected previously treated patients showed resistance to one or more drugs.[32] Pockets with even higher prevalence of drug resistance have been reported. Drug resistance was found less frequently among those who responded to a good regimen initially and later relapsed[91] than among those who initially had a poor regimen and failed to respond.[92]

2. Patients on Therapy But Not Responding

Ordinarily, a person on a good antituberculosis regimen should have sputum smears negative for acid-fast bacilli 2–3 months after the initiation of therapy. If sputum conversion does not occur, drug resistance should be suspected (also suspect nonadherence).

3. Nonadherent Patients[93]

By taking part of the prescribed therapy, drug-resistant bacilli can be selected for survival. However, if a patient is totally nonadherent and does not take any antituberculosis medicine, his tubercle bacilli will remain drug susceptible.

4. Persons from Developing Nations[56,94-96]

In countries with very limited resources, it may not be possible to furnish adequate drugs on a regular, predictable basis to impoverished patients with tuberculosis. The infrastructure may be inadequate to deliver and monitor therapy. Therefore, patients may receive medication irregularly, may take only one drug at a time, or may receive drugs in inadequate combinations. In some areas it is possible for patients to receive medicine for tuberculosis without a prescription, further promoting inadequate therapy and the emergence of drug resistance.

5. Immunocompromised Patients[37,39-41,43-45,97]

See Chapter 6 (this volume) for a discussion of immunocompromised patients. Patients infected with human immunodeficiency virus (HIV), especially those with the acquired immunodeficiency syndrome (AIDS), are at very high risk of developing active tuberculous disease (rather than latent infection alone) when exposed to an infectious case of drug-susceptible or -resistant tuberculosis. In regions where there is a significant probability of exposure to drug-resistant tuberculosis, treatment should be started promptly using sufficient medications to cover the possibility of both drug-susceptible and drug-resistant organisms. Drug-resistant disease requires appropriate, prompt, aggressive management in these patients.[98] Drug susceptibility studies certainly should be done. When the results of the susceptibility studies are known, treatment can be modified.

6. Household Contacts

Household contacts who have converted to tuberculin positive while exposed to a patient with infectious drug-resistant tuberculosis can be expected to be infected with the same strain as the index case. If these contacts subsequently develop disease, it is likely to be drug resistant with a pattern comparable to that of the index case at the time of transmission of infection.

7. Other Persons Likely to Be in Contact with Drug-Resistant Patients

a. Homeless Persons[99]

Homeless persons may have been present in a crowded, poorly ventilated shelter while a person with infectious drug-resistant disease was present in the facility.

b. Prisoners[39]

Prisoners similarly may have been exposed to drug-resistant tuberculosis in crowded, poorly ventilated facilities.

c. Persons in Medical Care Situations[37,39-45]

Persons in medical care situations may have been present when a patient with drug-resistant tuberculosis had contaminated the air he or she was breathing. The diagnosis of tuberculosis may not have been suspected. Precautions for airborne infection may have been omitted, exposing health care staff and possibly other patients to viable, airborne tubercle bacilli.

8. Patients with Conditions That Impair Delivery of Drugs to the Site of Infection

Patients who have undergone gastrectomy[100] or ileal bypass surgery may not absorb sufficient antituberculosis medications to cure their tuberculosis, but enough to select out drug-resistant mutants for survival.

Patients with tuberculosis involving extensively calcified pleura,[101] or very thick-walled cavities or heavily fibrotic areas, although absorbing their drugs properly, may have insufficient blood supply to the infected tissue site. The impaired circulation cannot deliver sufficient antimicrobial drugs to the infected tissue site to cure the tuberculosis. The extremely large number of organisms increases the likelihood of multidrug-resistant organisms. Also, variable penetration of antituberculosis medications may have the effect of monotherapy at the site of infection, thus selecting the resistant members of the bacterial population for survival.

B. HISTORY: EMPHASIS ON DETAILS OF PRIOR CHEMOTHERAPY

The usual medical history should be taken. In addition, it is important to question the patient about any of the above mentioned risk factors, and to follow through on any leads by finding out more details. History should include surgical procedures and collapse therapy for tuberculosis. History of antituberculosis chemotherapy is of paramount importance. Obtaining details in complex cases may be difficult, especially if the patient has been under the care of multiple providers, in multiple localities. Frequently it is necessary to contact the previous providers in order to obtain as complete a history as possible. Patients may not be reliable in presenting their histories, possibly due to lack of information, forgetfulness, or embarrassment regarding poor adherence. A complete and accurate medication history is essential; prior use of an antituberculosis drug, especially if it was used ineffectively, can compromise its usefulness in the regimen being proposed. In retreatment of patients with multidrug-resistant tuberculosis, the use of three antituberculosis drugs that the patient had not received before was predictive of a favorable outcome.[102] Medication history should include the following:

1. Drugs received, with dosages and dates.
2. How the drugs were added: one at a time (favoring selection for resistance), or several simultaneously.
3. Adherence with therapy.
4. Adverse reactions to medications.
5. Response to therapy, including bacteriological response. In cases where the patient has received more than one regimen, effort should be made to determine the response to each regimen employed.
6. In complex cases, a flow sheet can organize the important aspects of the drug history into a

PATIENT: Twenty year old female from
         a developing nation
         Cough, fever, night sweats, weight loss
         Extensive cavities left lung

ORGANISM: Mycobacterium tuberculosis

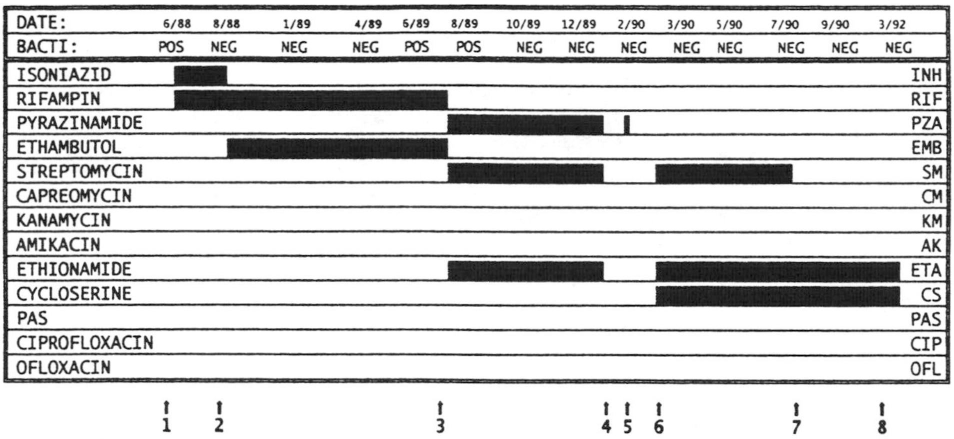

DATE:	6/88	8/88	1/89	4/89	6/89	8/89	10/89	12/89	2/90	3/90	5/90	7/90	9/90	3/92	
BACTI:	POS	NEG	NEG	NEG	POS	POS	NEG	NEG	NEG	NEG	NEG	NEG	NEG	NEG	
ISONIAZID															INH
RIFAMPIN															RIF
PYRAZINAMIDE															PZA
ETHAMBUTOL															EMB
STREPTOMYCIN															SM
CAPREOMYCIN															CM
KANAMYCIN															KM
AMIKACIN															AK
ETHIONAMIDE															ETA
CYCLOSERINE															CS
PAS															PAS
CIPROFLOXACIN															CIP
OFLOXACIN															OFL

         !   !   !   ! ! !   !   !
         1   2   3   4 5 6   7   8

1. INH and RIF started.
2. Pretreatment isolate reported resistant to INH; INH stopped; EMB started.
3. Resistance to INH and RIF reported; RIF and EMB stopped; PZA, SM, ETA started.
4. Liver enzymes six times normal; all drugs stopped.
5. Challenge dose of PZA.
6. SM, ETA, CS started.
7. SM stopped.
8. Therapy completed.

Figure 12-1 (Example 1) Patient with primary resistance to isoniazid was treated inappropriately with isoniazid and rifampin. Ethambutol was added as a single drug, inappropriately. Resistance to rifampin was acquired. Retreatment with pyrazinamide, streptomycin, and ethionamide was started. (The bacilli were susceptible to these previously unused drugs.) Liver function abnormalities developed; all drugs were stopped. Challenge with pyrazinamide was followed by liver function abnormalities. Streptomycin, ethionamide, and cycloserine were tolerated. Long-course chemotherapy was completed (see Figure 12-3 for details of management of liver function abnormalities).

C. CLINICAL MANIFESTATIONS

Clinical manifestations of drug-resistant tuberculosis are the same as for drug-susceptible tuberculosis. However, patients with acquired drug-resistant tuberculosis may have more pulmonary parenchymal scarring because of the chronicity of their disease. This may be associated with respiratory impairment. Patients with tuberculosis not responding to therapy in the expected manner should be evaluated or reevaluated for drug resistance. As in drug-susceptible disease, extrapulmonary tuberculosis is common among patients with AIDS and drug-resistant disease.

D. SUSCEPTIBILITY STUDIES[103-105]

Susceptibility testing and history of prior chemotherapy have been cornerstones in the detection and management of drug-resistant tuberculosis (see Chapter 4, this volume). The American Thoracic Society recommends that susceptibility studies be performed routinely on all positive cultures.[73] Susceptibility studies should be done in a reliable laboratory. In the earlier years of the chemotherapy era, the clinical relevance of susceptibility testing and the criteria for resistance of tubercle bacilli to various antituberculosis medications were debated.[52,106] Nonuniformity of drug resistance of tubercle bacilli from patients with chronic tuberculosis has been recognized.[47,107] At the National Jewish Center, during the 1960s and 1970s, retreatment regimens for isoniazid-resistant tuberculosis were based on in vitro susceptibility of the organisms to the drugs in the individually tailored regimens prescribed. In vitro susceptibility to three drugs in a regimen was predictive of a favorable outcome.[20] More recently, 134 previously treated cases of multidrug-resistant tuberculosis were reviewed at the National Jewish Center.[102] These patients were shedding tubercle bacilli resistant to an average of six drugs, including isoniazid and rifampin. Increasing numbers of drugs to which the bacilli were resistant was predictive of poor outcome. Surprisingly, in vitro susceptibility of the organisms to the drugs used in the new retreatment regimens was not necessarily predictive of outcome. The latter observation in this series of very complex cases is unexplained. This study does not negate the usefulness of in vitro susceptibility studies. However, it does indicate that the need persists for research in better methodology and in the application of the information obtained.

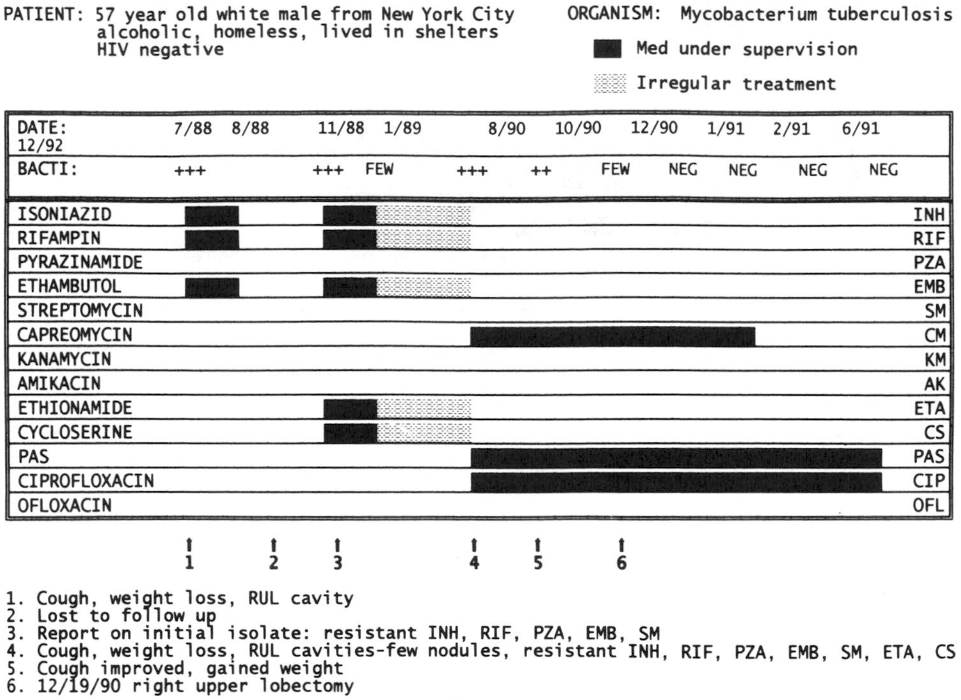

PATIENT: 57 year old white male from New York City   ORGANISM: Mycobacterium tuberculosis
alcoholic, homeless, lived in shelters
HIV negative

■ Med under supervision

▒ Irregular treatment

DATE: 12/92	7/88	8/88	11/88	1/89	8/90	10/90	12/90	1/91	2/91	6/91	
BACTI:	+++		+++	FEW	+++	++	FEW	NEG	NEG	NEG	NEG	
ISONIAZID											INH
RIFAMPIN											RIF
PYRAZINAMIDE											PZA
ETHAMBUTOL											EMB
STREPTOMYCIN											SM
CAPREOMYCIN											CM
KANAMYCIN											KM
AMIKACIN											AK
ETHIONAMIDE											ETA
CYCLOSERINE											CS
PAS											PAS
CIPROFLOXACIN											CIP
OFLOXACIN											OFL

↑1   ↑2   ↑3   ↑4   ↑5   ↑6

1. Cough, weight loss, RUL cavity
2. Lost to follow up
3. Report on initial isolate: resistant INH, RIF, PZA, EMB, SM
4. Cough, weight loss, RUL cavities-few nodules, resistant INH, RIF, PZA, EMB, SM, ETA, CS
5. Cough improved, gained weight
6. 12/19/90 right upper lobectomy

Figure 12-2 (Example 2) Patient with multidrug resistance was treated with isoniazid, rifampin, and ethambutol. He was noncompliant. Retreatment with isoniazid, rifampin, ethambutol, ethionamide, and cycloserine was started; compliance was poor. Additional drug resistance was acquired. He was retreated with capreomycin, PAS, and ciprofloxacin, under supervision. The bacilli in his sputum diminished. Adjunctive right upper lobectomy was followed by culture conversion to negative. Long-term supervised chemotherapy was continued for an additional 2 years.

that the need persists for research in better methodology and in the application of the information obtained.

Where multidrug resistance is likely, isolates should be sent to a reference laboratory experienced in the testing of drugs that are used less commonly. Results of susceptibility studies serve as a guide for determining therapy for patients with newly diagnosed tuberculosis and for patients with long-standing disease. Methods of reporting may vary from one laboratory to another. If there is any uncertainty about the interpretation of the test results, it is essential to communicate with the laboratory performing the test or with their clinical consultants.

IV. TREATMENT

Tuberculosis resistant to one or more drugs is treated with multiple other drugs to which the bacilli are susceptible.[20,108,109] If the patient has received prior medications for tuberculosis and the regimen has failed, the drugs employed in the failing regimen cannot be relied upon to have full efficacy.[110] The new regimen should contain at least three antitu-

berculosis agents, especially in the early phase of therapy. Drugs and dosages are listed in Table 12-1. Although selection of a regimen of first line drugs is desirable, the usefulness of these drugs in patients with drug-resistant disease is limited. They are the drugs to which the organisms are most likely to be resistant.

A. FIRST LINE AND SECOND LINE DRUGS

The first line drugs, also known as primary or standard drugs, are those recommended for the treatment of newly diagnosed tuberculosis. The drugs considered first line do not always remain the same, and are related to the historical and geographic context. In the United States in the 1990s, they are the drugs applicable to short-course (6–9 months) chemotherapy. They include isoniazid, rifampin, pyrazinamide, ethambutol, and streptomycin. The other antituberculosis medications are considered second line, secondary, or reserve drugs.

In the 1960s, pyrazinamide was considered a second line drug. It was used effectively during the entire course of therapy in patients being retreated, but was considered too hepatotoxic for routine use.

Table 12-1 **Drugs, dosage, and monitoring**

Drugs[a]	Dosage[b]	Monitoring/Comments[c]
Isoniazid	300–600 mg po daily	SGOT monthly and give with pyridoxine 50 mg if using larger dose
Rifampin	600 mg po daily	SGOT and bilirubin monthly; single dose on empty stomach (2 h before or after eating)
Ethambutol	25 mg/kg until culture negative; then 15 mg/kg po daily	Visual acuity and color vision monthly
Pyrazinamide	30–40 mg/kg po daily	SGOT and uric acid monthly; may split dose initially to improve tolerance; then single daily dose
Ethionamide	500–1000 mg po daily	SGOT monthly; may split dose or give at bedtime to improve tolerance
Cycloserine	500–1000 mg po daily	Serum drug levels weekly until stable; give with pyridoxine 50–200 mg
p-Aminosalicylate (PAS)	10–12 g po daily	SGOT monthly; may split dose or give at bedtime to improve tolerance
Streptomycin, capreomycin, kanamycin, or amikacin	15 mg/kg im 5 days weekly until culture negative; then 3 times weekly	Creatinine, electrolytes, audiometry at least monthly; observe for problems with balance
Ofloxacin	400–800 mg po daily	Antacids, sucralfate, calcium, iron, and zinc decrease absorption; efficacy of ofloxacin for TB needs further documentation
Ciprofloxacin	750–1500 mg po daily	Antacids, sucralfate, calcium, iron, and zinc decrease absorption; efficacy of ciprofloxacin for TB needs further documentation
Clofazimine	100–300 mg daily	Efficacy unproven

[a] Oral drugs (and injectable drugs) are listed in the order of preference; use two oral drugs and one injectable drug that the patient has not received previously and to which the bacilli are susceptible.

[b] Dosages suggested for drug-resistant tuberculosis may not apply to drug-susceptible disease.

[c] On multidrug therapy, monitor complete blood count every 1–3 months. For more complete information on side effects see Chapter 11 (this volume).

Ethionamide, although effective, always has been a reserve drug because it is difficult to tolerate in therapeutic dosages. Cycloserine is another secondary drug; it is associated with frequent central nervous system toxicity and has a small window between the therapeutic and toxic dose. PAS was employed as a first line drug in the 1950s and 1960s. Because of frequent gastrointestinal side effects, and because of lesser efficacy, PAS lost its position as a first line drug when ethambutol and rifampin became available. Among the drugs that must be given parenterally because of poor gastrointestinal absorption, capreomycin was approved for long-term use in tuberculosis. It has remained a second line drug, used as a substitute for streptomycin. Kanamycin, although not officially approved for long-term use in tuberculosis, has been used effectively for several decades as a second line drug in retreatment. Similarly, amikacin is being used as a secondary drug. In some developing nations, thiacetazone (an inexpensive drug not available in the United States) is used as a standard drug, along with isoniazid and streptomycin.

B. PROGRAM APPROACH
1. Situations Suitable for a Program Approach

In regions where the prevalence of drug resistance is high, it may be advisable to treat all newly diagnosed tuberculosis patients with a regimen designed to be effective against both drug-susceptible and drug-resistant tubercle bacilli. This presupposes knowledge of the susceptibility patterns of the tuberculosis cases in the community. It is essential to survey for drug resistance periodically. It also is important to know which regimen or regimens have been used commonly in the community, and what the treatment practices have been.[69] Resistance is likely to be directed against drugs used in the community, especially if the drugs have been employed in inadequate or unsupervised regimens.

By administering a regimen likely to be effective against both drug-susceptible and drug-resistant disease, the patient can be spared the wait for the results of susceptibility studies before starting effective therapy.[110] Immediate initiation of therapy is especially important in patients with immunodeficiency and in patients who are ill with rapidly progressive tuberculosis.[98]

2. Examples

In localities where isoniazid and streptomycin resistance is prevalent, a reasonable approach is to begin all patients on a regimen of isoniazid, rifampin, ethambutol, and pyrazinamide.[111] This is excellent therapy for patients with drug-susceptible disease. After susceptibility is documented, ethambutol is stopped; after 2 months of therapy pyrazinamide is stopped and the patient continues to receive isoniazid and rifampin to complete 6 months. The four drug regimen also provides good therapy for patients with isoniazid- and/or streptomycin-resistant bacilli. When the laboratory studies document resistance to isoniazid (with or without resistance to streptomycin) but susceptibility to rifampin and ethambutol, isoniazid can be stopped; pyrazinamide can be stopped after 2 months of therapy. Rifampin and ethambutol should be continued to complete at least 12 months either daily or intermittently.

Short-course and intermittent regimens, using various combinations of the primary drugs, have yielded varying results.[112-119] Excellent results have been reported[117] with short-course regimens involving the use of isoniazid, rifampin, pyrazinamide, plus either ethambutol or streptomycin, for the full 6-month period. The drugs were given either daily or three times weekly for tuberculosis, including disease resistant to isoniazid and/or streptomycin. Although the latter drugs were included in the study, they probably did not contribute to the efficacy of the regimens when resistance to them was present. These short-course regimens are applicable if the patient has received no prior therapy with rifampin nor pyrazinamide nor a third drug in the regimen, and the tubercle bacilli from the patient are fully susceptible to these drugs. Other regimens for drug ressistant tuberculosis, not consisting exclusively of first-line drugs, must be given daily for longer periods (see duration of this chapter). For dosages of drugs used in intermittent regimens, see Chapter 6 of this volume.

In sections of New York City,[98] outbreaks of tuberculosis resistant to isoniazid, rifampin, ethambutol, pyrazinamide, streptomycin, and ethionamide have been reported. Initial treatment regimens employing six drugs may be appropriate, aiming to provide adequate antimicrobial coverage while awaiting the results of susceptibility studies on the patient's organisms. A regimen of isoniazid, rifampin, pyrazinamide, capreomycin, ciprofloxacin, and cycloserine has been proposed. The first three drugs give excellent coverage if the patient has a drug-susceptible strain; the latter three provide coverage for anticipated drug resistance. When the susceptibility studies have been reported, the regimen is adjusted appropriately. The potential for toxicity of such a regimen is high. However, the patient is likely to be spared the risk of acquiring resistance to additional drugs resulting from inadequate therapy during the waiting period.

C. INDIVIDUALLY TAILORED APPROACH[20,110,120-124]

A standard regimen, or "program approach," is not applicable to all situations. Many patients require a regimen tailored to their particular circumstances.

1. Selection of Drugs

Patients who already have undergone several courses of therapy, and have been exposed to multiple antituberculosis medications, require individually prescribed regimens. These regimens should contain at least three[7,11,16,17] previously unused drugs to which the tubercle bacilli are susceptible. Thorough evaluation is essential (as described in the previous section). Frequently these patients are chronically ill, but generally do not have acute or urgent illness. Thus the benefit accrued by deferring treatment to obtain the necessary information on which to base rational therapy (that is, a detailed drug history and full susceptibility studies) outweighs the potential risk of waiting. There are relatively few drugs effective against *M. tuberculosis*. Because of drug resistance and suboptimal prior use, some of the drugs no longer are effective against their bacilli. Options for effective therapy are limited. These patients cannot afford another experience of treatment failure.

Sometimes a patient will have received adequately selected medications for a brief time, the drugs having been stopped simultaneously, but prematurely, at a time when the drug regimen was working. In such cases, a short duration of prior therapy is correlated with continuing *in vitro* susceptibility and continuing clinical efficacy of the drugs so used.[91] However, if previously used drugs were employed in a regimen that was failing, or in which the drugs had been added in inadequate combinations, those drugs cannot be depended on for efficacy, despite *in vitro* susceptibility.[125] Sometimes physicians have included isoniazid in a regimen where susceptibility tests have shown resistance to low concentrations, but sensitivity to higher concentrations of this drug. Impairment of efficacy is similar with low levels or high levels of resistance.[106] If any degree of resistance to isoniazid is found, isoniazid cannot be depended on as a major effective drug in the regimen.

Patient factors, such as preexisting medical conditions that may predispose to side effects, should be considered where possible in selecting specific drugs for the new retreatment regimen. For instance, patients with gastrointestinal problems are likely to have problems tolerating ethionamide; patients with prior hearing loss may develop significantly impaired hearing when treated with an aminoglycoside. Where possible, it is preferable to avoid drugs to which the patient is particularly likely to react, provided other drugs are capable of controlling the tuberculosis. The antituberculosis drugs currently available, along with their potential side effects, are discussed in Chapter 11 (this volume).

2. Examples

Example 1 (see Figure 12-1): A 20-year-old woman from a developing nation had been treated (inappropriately) with isoniazid and rifampin for cavitary tuberculosis. (Primary) isoniazid resistance of the initial isolate was reported belatedly and ethambutol was added as a single new drug (inappropriately). After a short period of improvement, including conversion to negative cultures, positive cultures again were reported (the fall and rise phenomenon), this time with resistance to both isoniazid and rifampin. The patient was referred for retreatment. Options among the oral drugs were pyrazinamide, ethionamide, cycloserine, and PAS; ethambutol was not considered a good option since it had been in use in a regimen that was ultimately failing. All of the injectable drugs were potentially effective. Streptomycin was chosen since it had not been used before, is slightly more effective, and is less expensive than the other parenteral drugs. Pyrazinamide and ethionamide were chosen because of slight superiority compared to the other available oral drugs; they were likely to be tolerated by this young patient. The regimen of streptomycin, pyrazinamide, and ethionamide was effective. The patient's sputum cultures converted to negative.

However, the patient developed liver function abnormalities during therapy (see Section V.B.1 and Figure 12-3). Either pyrazinamide or ethionamide could have caused the problem. All medications were stopped until the liver function tests stabilized at normal values. Pyrazinamide challenge

resulted in elevation of liver enzymes. Another drug had to be substituted for pyrazinamide. Available options were cycloserine and PAS. Because of the potential of PAS for producing gastrointestinal side effects that might enhance the gastrointestinal side effects of ethionamide, PAS seemed undesirable. Cycloserine was chosen, and was introduced with streptomycin uneventfully. (The replacement of pyrazinamide with a single drug was appropriate in this case in which the patient's disease was responding to therapy. This is not the same as adding a single drug to a *failing* regimen). Small doses of ethionamide produced no abnormalities in the liver function tests. Therefore the patient received full dosage of ethionamide along with cycloserine and streptomycin. The oral drugs were continued for an additional 2 years. Streptomycin was stopped after 5 months on the revised regimen. The patient continued to have negative cultures.

Example 2 (see Figure 12-2): A 57-year-old homeless alcoholic man from New York City had been started on what appeared to be a reasonable regimen of isoniazid, rifampin, and ethambutol for extensive cavitary tuberculosis. His initial isolate later was reported to be resistant to isoniazid, rifampin, pyrazinamide, ethambutol, and streptomycin. Two new drugs, ethionamide and cycloserine, were added to the regimen. This might have salvaged the situation if the bacterial count had been low and if the patient had cooperated with therapy. The patient took his treatment irregularly and developed resistance to these drugs also. He was referred for retreatment with tubercle bacilli resistant to isoniazid, rifampin, pyrazinamide, ethambutol, streptomycin, ethionamide, and cycloserine. Among the oral drugs, the only choices for a new effective regimen were PAS and ciprofloxacin or ofloxacin. Among the injectable antibiotics, capreomycin, kanamycin, and amikacin were potentially effective. Capreomycin was chosen because of its lesser toxicity; it was given in combination with PAS and ciprofloxacin. This was believed to be a weak regimen for a patient with extensive disease, but no further medical options were available. Since the tuberculosis was fairly well localized, the option of adjunctive pulmonary resection was pursued. At the time of surgery, sputum smears were negative and few tubercle bacilli were present on sputum cultures. The right upper lobe was resected without complications. All smears and cultures were negative postoperatively. Therapy with multiple drugs was continued for 2 years beyond culture conversion.

3. Duration of Therapy

Regimens based on drugs other than rifampin must be given for prolonged periods. In cases of rifampin

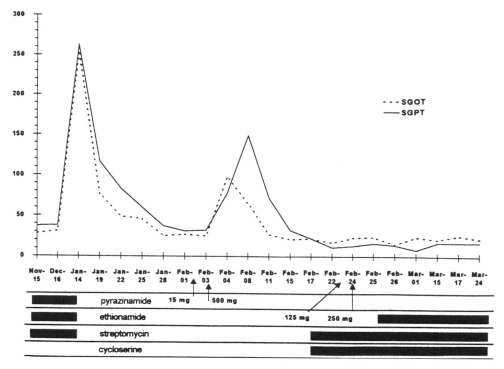

Figure 12-3 Management of drug-related liver function abnormalities. The patient had been receiving pyrazinamide, ethionamide, and streptomycin. After 4 months of therapy, the SGOT (AST) rose to 6 times the upper limit of normal (normal 8–40). Either pyrazinamide or ethionamide could have produced the abnormality. All drugs were stopped. Liver function tests returned to normal gradually. The patient was rechallenged with pyrazinamide, 15 mg, with no change in SGOT or SGPT (ALT). The next day, she was rechallenged with pyrazinamide 500 mg, followed by elevation of the serum enzymes. Medications were withheld until the enzymes became normal. Streptomycin and cycloserine were introduced without problem. Ethionamide 125 mg, then, the next day, 250 mg, was given with no increase in the enzymes. The full dosage of ethionamide was tolerated, along with streptomycin and cycloserine (see also Figure 12-1 and Section IV.C.2).

resistance with isoniazid susceptibility, isoniazid and ethambutol (with streptomycin for the first one to three months) should be continued to complete eighteen months. When resistance to both isoniazid and rifampin is present, at least two drugs should be continued for 2 years beyond culture conversion. The third drug, usually an injectable drug, is stopped 4–6 months after the first of a series of negative cultures. The date of culture conversion is suggested as a marker for timing the duration of treatment so that patients with slow responses (probably associated with more refractory disease) will be given longer courses of therapy. Patients with acquired drug resistance already have demonstrated their ability to fail to respond to treatment, or to respond and later relapse. Giving them a prolonged course of therapy seems prudent. Studies done before the availability of rifampin suggest that 18–24 months of chemotherapy was associated with lower relapse rates than shorter regimens.[126-128] Accordingly, patients who, because of drug resistance, cannot benefit from rifampin require prolonged therapy. A possible exception to this

is a regimen of streptomycin, pyrazinamide, and isoniazid given daily or three times weekly for 9 months. Under study conditions this 9-month regimen was effective against drug susceptible tuberculosis.[128a] Since rifampin was not included in the regimen, one might infer that the regimen would be effective against tuberculosis resistant to rifampin but susceptible to the other drugs.[128a]

D. MULTIDRUG-RESISTANT TUBERCULOSIS

At the National Jewish Center, the current practice is to tailor regimens based on history of no prior use of a given drug, along with full *in vitro* susceptibility to that drug.[121] A recent review[102] showed a successful outcome in 65% of 134 patients who had *M. tuberculosis* resistant to a median of six drugs, including isoniazid and rifampin, and who previously had received a median of six drugs. These patients were treated in the era before AIDS had become a widespread problem. They received a median of four drugs in their new regimens.

Many of these patients did not have an ideal regimen available to them. Employing more than three drugs when the selected drugs did not appear to have promise of maximal efficacy may have salvaged some patients; however, the results were not as good as those achieved when three optimal antituberculosis drugs were available. Some patients did not have two potentially effective oral drugs for their regimens. Two injectable medications (usually kanamycin and capreomycin) and one oral antituberculosis drug were given. Limited (unpublished) data suggest that although toxicity was not doubled, efficacy was diminished when compared to regimens employing one injectable and two oral drugs. At another institution, medical treatment of patients resistant to multiple drugs, including isoniazid and rifampin, was effective for 34 of 102 patients.[129] In both of these series, adjunctive surgery salvaged a few additional patients.

E. PATIENTS INFECTED WITH HIV

Patients with immune deficiency and drug-resistant disease, including those with AIDS, are treated with multiple drug therapy in a manner similar to patients with drug-resistant disease and a normal immune system. They should be treated at least as long as other patients with drug-resistant disease; it is not known whether they require longer treatment.

F. EXTRAPULMONARY TUBERCULOSIS

Experience in managing drug-resistant extrapulmonary tuberculosis is limited. Because bacterial counts are low in most extrapulmonary sites, spontaneous mutation of bacilli to resistance and subsequent selection of these resistant bacilli for survival are unlikely. Thus acquired resistance in extrapulmonary tuberculosis has not been a major problem. However, primary drug resistance has increased in some regions. In these areas, immunocompromised patients who have been infected with resistant bacilli and who have a high incidence of extrapulmonary disease are causing an increased incidence of drug resistance in extrapulmonary tuberculosis. Treatment is recommended with regimens selected in the same manner as for drug-resistant pulmonary tuberculosis. Specific studies on the treatment of drug-resistant extrapulmonary tuberculosis are needed. For management of problems related to site of infection, see Chapter 7 (this volume).

G. OTHER MEDICATIONS

In recent years, ciprofloxacin and ofloxacin have been added to the therapeutic armamentarium against tuberculosis. Laboratory tests of susceptibility and of achievable serum concentrations look favorable;[130] limited reports of clinical experience are encouraging.[131-134] Until further information from clinical trials with these drugs for tuberculosis becomes available, it seems reasonable to refrain from depending on them where more traditional drugs are likely to be effective. However, drug resistance or prior ineffective use may have blunted the efficacy of multiple other drugs. An adequate new regimen may not be possible using only traditional drugs. In these cases, ofloxacin or ciprofloxacin may be used as one of three new drugs in the regimen. When a three-drug regimen includes cycloserine or PAS (and probably has marginal efficacy), ofloxacin or ciprofloxacin may be added as a fourth drug. Since ofloxacin and ciprofloxacin are structurally similar, employing more than one of them simultaneously is not advised.

Rifabutin (ansamycin, LM427) has become available recently, but has not been approved for use in tuberculosis. It has been used as an investigational drug for treating multidrug-resistant tuberculosis.[135-137] Cross-resistance with rifampin is common.[138] However, if the bacilli are resistant to rifampin only at low concentrations, they may remain susceptible to rifabutin. Reports of clinical efficacy have been conflicting. At the National Jewish Center, a small series of patients was treated with rifabutin in multidrug regimens for pulmonary tuberculosis due to drug-resistant *M. tuberculosis*. These patients did not have good therapeutic options. At least transient benefit occurred if the tubercle bacilli were susceptible to rifabutin. Rifabutin appeared to contribute to improvement, making some patients better candidates for surgical resection, with ultimate control of their very refractory disease.[139]

Clofazimine,[140] a drug employed extensively in treating leprosy, has been used in the management of patients with multidrug-resistant tuberculosis for whom therapeutic options were limited. Since many variables and adverse factors were present in this group of patients, the independent effect of this drug was impossible to determine. Clofazimine certainly was not outstanding in its efficacy against *M. tuberculosis* in these clinical situations, despite favorable *in vitro* susceptibility. Its role in the treatment of tuberculosis has yet to be determined.

H. CHILDREN AND PREGNANT WOMEN

See Chapter 8 (this volume) for a discussion of tuberculosis in children and pregnant women.

I. MONITORING
1. Efficacy

A favorable response of patients, especially complex multidrug-resistant cases, to regimens for drug-resistant tuberculosis is less predictable than the response of drug-susceptible cases to appropriate therapy. Therefore, careful monitoring of response is appropriate.

a. Reversal of Infectiousness

It is unwise to assume that a patient with drug-resistant tuberculosis is noninfectious because he or she has received a given duration of therapy, such as 2 weeks. Reversal of infectiousness must be documented by sputum smears and cultures. The consequences of exposure to a patient with drug-resistant tuberculosis must be considered (see also Chapter 3, this volume).

A suggested schedule for obtaining bacteriology is as follows:

1. Sputum smear and culture every 2 weeks until three consecutively negative cultures have been documented.
2. Sputum smear and culture every 2 months for the next 2 years.
3. Sputum smear and culture twice yearly for the following 2 years.
4. Bacteriology should be reevaluated if the patient has symptoms suggestive of active tuberculosis.

A patient with a positive sputum smear should be considered potentially infectious and kept in isolation. A patient with drug-resistant pulmonary tuberculosis is likely to represent minimal risk of contagion when he or she no longer is coughing and has two or three consecutively negative sputum smears. However, a series of two or three *cultures* with a final report of negative should be the criterion for release from restriction of contact. While awaiting documentation of culture conversion, the patient should avoid prolonged close contact with other persons in enclosed poorly ventilated places. He or she should not have any contact with infants or immunocompromised patients, who are particularly susceptible to tuberculosis and are at increased risk of developing very serious forms of tuberculosis.

Culture conversion occurs an average of 2 months[20] after the initiation of therapy when patients are on good regimens for drug-resistant tuberculosis. If a patient continues to have positive smears or cultures more than 3 months after starting a new regimen, the efficacy of the regimen should be questioned; treatment may be failing with the emergence of resistance to additional drugs. The patient should be reevaluated. Adherence with the regimen must be reassessed; drug dosages and timing, serum drug levels and possible drug interactions should be checked. Susceptibility studies should be done on a current specimen.

b. Chest X-Rays

Chest X-rays, although important, are not reliable indicators of treatment failure or relapse.

c. Clinical Response

As in drug-susceptible tuberculosis, clinical response in drug-resistant tuberculosis frequently is observed long before bacteriological control of the disease has been accomplished. Symptoms such as cough, fever, and night sweats tend to respond to effective treatment for drug-resistant tuberculosis. However, side effects of the medications may prevent weight gain and an improved feeling of well being.

2. Serum Drug Levels[141]

Strict attention must be paid to accurate documentation of times of dosing and times of blood drawings. If other medications interfere with the assay, these should be omitted for a sufficient time to avoid this confounding factor. The measurement of serum drug levels should be performed by a laboratory with sufficient experience and quality control in the techniques. The physician should consult with the laboratory regarding the optimal time to draw blood levels, so that the results will be interpretable. Consultation regarding pharmacokinetic data can maximize the benefits of the proper study of serum drug levels. These services most likely are available at referral centers specializing in the management of drug-resistant tuberculosis.

Monitoring of serum drug levels is especially indicated in the following circumstances:

1. Patients with acquired immune deficiency, since they may not absorb their medications properly.
2. Patients with gastrointestinal problems that may impair absorption, such as prior gastrectomy or ileal bypass.
3. Patients with reduced renal clearance (trough levels of drugs cleared by the kidneys are especially important).
4. Patients who have not improved on a regimen that should have been effective, despite documented adherence.
5. Cycloserine use: a drug with a narrow therapeutic window between effective and toxic doses.

3. Side Effects

Side effects (see also Chapter 11, this volume) are likely to occur from the medications used for treatment of tuberculosis that is resistant to the more commonly used drugs.[20,142-145] Therefore, clinical and laboratory monitoring should be done systematically, and should be in keeping with the anticipated adverse effects of the drugs employed (see Table 12-1). Frequent observation of the patient is essential.

V. MANAGEMENT OF ADVERSE DRUG EFFECTS

A. FACTORS TO CONSIDER
1. Type and Seriousness of the Reaction

If the reaction is life threatening, the offending drug must be discontinued. If it is unclear which drug in the regimen is responsible for the life threatening reaction, all drugs must be stopped. Reactions that are uncomfortable or even damaging may not warrant stopping of medication when put into the context of the whole clinical situation.

2. Seriousness of the Patient's Illness

The seriousness of the patient's illness and its implications for the life and the long-term quality of life (including long-term isolation of the patient if the tuberculosis is not controlled) must be balanced against the seriousness of the adverse effects of the medications.

3. Timing

The time when the adverse effects of medications occur may influence the way the reaction is managed. Modifying therapy by stopping one or more drugs, either temporarily or permanently, is likely to have a more dire effect on outcome if done early in the course of a regimen.

4. Options for Replacement Therapy

In multidrug-resistant tuberculosis, few drugs are useful for a given patient. Some drugs have become ineffective due to drug resistance. If a drug is lost because of side effects, therapeutic options are limited further. Accordingly, the continuation of medications in the face of side effects that would be entirely unacceptable under more favorable circumstances may be justified where there are no reasonable, effective alternatives.

5. Remaining Regimen

When a medication must be stopped, one must look at the remaining regimen. The altered regimen may not contain sufficient drugs to control the infection and to protect against the development of further drug resistance. It may be preferable to stop all medications pending the introduction of a new regimen.

B. SPECIFIC PROBLEMS

For problems related to first line drugs, see Chapter 11 (this volume).

1. Liver Toxicity

Liver function abnormalities are detected by performing blood tests of liver function regularly (generally monthly), and repeating these tests if symptoms of hepatitis develop. Clinically significant elevations of serum transaminase may occur with or without symptoms where the patient has been receiving either pyrazinamide or ethionamide. If the routine monthly SGOT (AST) is more than twice the upper limit of normal, weekly, rather than monthly rechecks are advised. SGPT (ALT) and the bilirubin should be tested also. Other causes of liver function abnormality should be evaluated. It may be possible to continue the potentially hepatotoxic medications, with close monitoring, if the enzyme levels in the serum stabilize at less than three times the upper limit of normal. If the serum enzymes continue to rise, all hepatotoxic medications must be stopped when the SGOT is about five times the upper limit of normal. Usually, at this level, the bilirubin is not elevated.

Frequently, where pyrazinamide or ethionamide toxicity occurs, the SGOT and SGPT continue to rise for a week or two (sometimes more) despite removing all hepatotoxic agents from the regimen. Then the serum enzymes gradually come down over a course of weeks. The enzymes may take months to return to normal if the elevation is severe. As the serum enzymes approach normal, sometimes they vacillate for a time, before stabilizing at normal levels. If the bilirubin becomes elevated, it is likely to normalize before the enzymes. Although some physicians use alkaline phosphatase and GGT levels as a guide to toxicity, this author has found them elevated in many patients with drug-resistant tuberculosis without other signs suggestive of drug-induced liver toxicity (see also Section V.C).

2. Renal Toxicity

Kidney function abnormalities can develop where the aminoglycosides (amikacin, kanamycin, and streptomycin), or the polypeptide antibiotic capreomycin are used. Renal dysfunction frequently is manifested by a gradual increase in the serum creatinine, without accompanying symptoms. When progressive decrease in renal function occurs, the potential benefit of the drug, as opposed to the risk it is presenting, must be reevaluated. Premature discontinuation of the drug may be the only reasonable option. However, the severity of the tuberculosis, the time of occurrence of the toxicity, and the absence of other therapeutic options may suggest that continuing the offending drug is in the best interest of the patient. Cautious modification of dosing and close monitoring of serum drug levels and creatinine may allow continuation of the injectable medication without posing an unacceptable risk.

3. Severe Central Nervous System Toxicity

Psychosis, severe depression, or convulsions associated with cycloserine mandates discontinuation of this drug. These side effects usually are associated with excessive serum levels of cycloserine. Blood for serum drug levels should be drawn at the time of the reaction. Generally, cycloserine should not be reintroduced after a severe reaction. Pyridoxine always should be given with cycloserine,[146] to decrease the likelihood of serious side effects.

4. Severe Allergic Reactions

In cases of anaphylaxis, severe skin rashes, or suspected drug fever, the offending drug must be stopped. Because of uncertainty about which drug caused the problem, all medications may need to be stopped. The patient must be treated for the immediate problem, such as giving epinephrine for anaphylaxis or antihistamines for pruritic symptoms. Corticosteroids sometimes are necessary to save the life of the patient or to prevent undue morbidity; however, since they may exacerbate uncontrolled infection, their use should be avoided if possible. The risk–benefit ratio must always be considered with as much certainty as possible.

5. Toxicity to the Eighth Cranial Nerve

Eighth cranial nerve toxicity from amikacin, kanamycin, streptomycin, or capreomycin is not fatal but is likely to be permanent.

a. Vestibular

Damage to the vestibular branch may occur with or without damage to the auditory branch, and damage to the auditory branch may or may not be associated with vestibular damage. If a patient on aminoglycosides or capreomycin experiences slight balance disturbance or vertigo shortly after the injection, the experience may be transient and benign. However, caution is advised, since these minor symptoms may be the prodrome of a more serious and permanent vestibular abnormality. The patient may not be willing to endure vertigo or impairment of mobility, even in the face of serious tuberculosis, thus demanding the decision to stop the offending agent, possibly prematurely. If a patient does develop a significant balance disturbance, physical therapy may help the patient to compensate.

b. Auditory

Auditory damage generally comes on gradually, involves the high frequencies initially, and, with time, gradually affects the frequencies related to understanding speech. When the routine audiogram shows high frequency loss, the patient may be asymptomatic, or may have a feeling of fullness in the ears, or may experience tinnitus. If the offending medication is stopped at this point, chances are the damage will remain at that level, but slight improvement may follow. The damage is likely to progress and persist if the offending drug is continued. Worsening after stopping the offending drug has been reported, but this is unusual. Patients vary in the sensitivity of their eighth nerves to the adverse effects of medications. Occasional patients experience rapid hearing loss or rapid loss of vestibular function on minimal doses of aminoglycosides. More commonly, the problem progresses gradually, over the course of months.

In dealing with patients suffering hearing loss from their medication, it is important to be straightforward with the patient concerning the potential for permanent damage. Also, the patient must understand the importance of the toxic medicine in the long-term control of his or her tuberculosis. A patient may survive with hearing impairment (although with curtailment in quality of life). However, the tuberculosis may be fatal, if not brought under control, or may interfere more significantly with life quality. If continuing the aminoglycoside or polypeptide is indicated for the tuberculosis, the patient's informed input is helpful. In practice, patients generally opt for continuing the medication, realizing their predicament. If the hearing continues to deteriorate, the situation is reviewed with the patient again. Of course, if it is possible to decrease the dose or to stop the offending medicine without compromising the effectiveness of the regimen, this is done, and further toxicity is curtailed. Sometimes it may be possible, provided efficacy is equivalent in the given case, to substitute capreomycin, which is likely to be somewhat less ototoxic, for kanamycin or amikacin, and thus potentially slow down further hearing deterioration (see also Section V.A).

6. Ocular Toxicity

Visual loss associated with ethambutol is more likely to occur at the higher doses used in drug-resistant disease. If a patient has visual loss, usually manifested by decreased vision over a period of days to weeks (as opposed to presbyopia that occurs over months to years) or has color discrimination changes or visual field disturbances, ethambutol toxicity is likely. The drug must be stopped and ophthalmologic evaluation obtained. If ethambutol is causing the visual problem and the drug is continued, the loss may progress rapidly to blindness. Usually, after the drug is stopped, vision will return. It may take many months if impairment is advanced. Few cases have not had return of vision. Although a few patients have received ethambutol again after having recovered from ethambutol ocular toxicity, this practice is not recommended.

7. Minor Mental and Neurological Changes

Cycloserine administration commonly is associated with minor mental changes, including forgetfulness, sadness, euphoria, nervousness, and impairment of concentration or of coordination. If the patient feels that he or she is in control of his or her life, reassurance is appropriate, along with careful monitoring of behavior and of serum drug levels. Minor tremors may be benign; if progressive, dosage may have to be reduced or the drug discontinued. The optimal dosage of cycloserine is difficult to predict. Serum drug levels should be monitored routinely, every 1 to 2 weeks, in the first month or two of therapy, until stabilized. At the National Jewish Center, a 2-h level of 25–30 µg/ml is considered desirable. The serum drug levels should be repeated if the patient has increasing psychological or neurological symptoms. Dosage adjustment may be necessary. If symptoms continue to escalate, cycloserine must be stopped. Ordinarily, the serious side effects, such as psychoses or convulsions, do not occur unless the serum level of the drug is excessive. There are a few patients, however, who develop serious problems with subtherapeutic serum levels. Cycloserine cannot be used in such patients. Patients receiving cycloserine should be cautioned that the drug may interfere with their ability to operate a motor vehicle.

Caffeine-like effects from ciprofloxacin or ofloxacin can be made more tolerable by giving the drug early in the day.

8. Minor Cutaneous Reactions

Cutaneous reactions may occur in association with any of the antituberculosis medications. When a patient develops a minimal, localized rash, a few hives, or slight itching, close observation, with or without the use of an antihistamine, is a reasonable course of action. However, if the reaction is moderately severe, or if a mild reaction progresses, stopping medication is recommended. Often it is not possible to tell which medicine is responsible for the reaction; it may be necessary to stop all drugs, while waiting for the reaction to clear (see also Section V.C).

9. Gastrointestinal Problems

Anorexia, nausea, vomiting, abdominal pain or burning, bloating, loose stools, and bad taste in the mouth make a patient feel miserable but usually are not sufficient to warrant discontinuation of medication. These problems very frequently are associated with ethionamide and PAS and, with lesser frequency, with other antituberculosis medications. Sometimes these problems can be avoided by introducing ethionamide and PAS gradually, over the course of a few days. (Prolonged periods on subtherapeutic doses should be avoided.) When a patient experiences gastrointestinal symptoms it is essential to check for more serious associated problems, such as hepatic dysfunction, that may be induced by these medications.

Once liver damage has been ruled out, palliative therapy may be given. The patient should be reassured that his or her symptoms, although very distressing, are not life threatening. When a patient recognizes the seriousness of the underlying disease and its threat to life or to long-term well being, he or she may be willing to endure minor discomfort from the medicines. The problem of perverted sense of taste may be masked by lemon drops, mints, or licorice; however, the benefit is transient. Drugs causing nausea or other gastrointestinal distress may be tolerated with food (provided this does not significantly impair absorption of the drug), or at bedtime, allowing the patient to sleep off the noxious side effect. Sometimes the dosage may be split without reducing efficacy.

Frequently, however, the symptoms are severe enough that the patient cannot be expected to deal with them without some pharmacologic help. Antacids may be helpful. (These must not be given within 2 h of the quinolones.) Antiemetics often will work, given on an as-needed basis if the nausea is occasional, but given regularly to prevent chronic nausea. Antiemetics may themselves be potentially hepatotoxic; liver function should be evaluated before starting them and during their use. Sometimes experimentation is necessary before arriving at the best antiemetic for a given patient. Persistence is important. Metoclopramide is helpful for some patients, either with or without an antiemetic. Patients with pain or burning may require ranitidine or cimetidine. The polypharmacy should be reevaluated periodically, since sometimes the original side effects will have run their course, making the extra drugs superfluous. Unfortunately, often the medicines given to relieve symptoms must be continued as long as the offending antituberculosis drugs are given in their full amounts.

10. Musculoskeletal Problems

Serum uric acid almost invariably is elevated when pyrazinamide is used in prolonged high dosage. Usually increasing hydration is the only treatment needed. For the occasional patient who develops clinical gout, pyrazinamide may be stopped temporarily and the gout treated. After the gout is under control, allopurinol may be added. The pyrazinamide may then be reintroduced.

Inflammation of the fascia with pain and restriction of motion of the hands and shoulders sometimes develops during ethionamide therapy.[147] Physical therapy may help maintain range of motion, making it feasible to delay having to stop the drug.

11. Endocrine Problems

Hypothyroidism occasionally may develop when a patient is receiving either ethionamide or PAS. When these two drugs are used simultaneously, hypothyroidism develops frequently. It is treated by thyroid replacement; stopping the offending drugs is not necessary. Thyroid function and replacement therapy should be reassessed when the patient has completed antituberculosis therapy. Gynecomastia, impotence, menstrual disturbances, and hair loss sometimes occur, especially with ethionamide. Empathy and reassurance that the problems are drug related and are unlikely to be permanent may help make these problems more tolerable.

12. Electrolyte Problems

Loss of electrolytes, especially magnesium and potassium, is frequent in patients receiving capreomycin or the aminoglycosides, but generally is not a cause to stop the drug. Potassium can be replaced orally, if tolerated. If significant hypomagnesemia is present, parenteral replacement is advised. Low serum potassium may not respond to potassium replacement in the presence of low serum magnesium until the hypomagnesemia has been corrected. The patient may not recognize symptoms of low serum electrolytes. However, weakness that may have been attributed to other factors may improve after normalization of the electrolytes. The potential for cardiac problems associated with electrolyte abnormalities should be appreciated.

13. Local Problems with Injections

Tenderness of injection sites may be alleviated by moist heat, exercise, massage, and ultrasound therapy (1.5 W/cm^2 for 5 min over each area immediately after the injection).[148] Intravenous administration of medication may be appropriate in some instances.

C. REINTRODUCING MEDICATIONS AFTER DRUG REACTIONS
1. Wait for the Reaction to Clear

Following liver toxicity, several consecutive normal results of liver function tests should be evident. In the case of allergic reactions, the skin should have cleared completely. The patient should be in stable condition before attempting to reintroduce medications.

If these reactions have not cleared completely, the target organs may be especially sensitive. Introducing medications that may not have caused a problem at a less vulnerable time may precipitate a reaction. Also, if a reaction has only partially cleared, it may be difficult to differentiate the ups and downs of the original reaction from the effect of the drug being introduced.

After a serious reaction, the waiting period before reintroducing medicines should be prolonged. Extreme caution should be observed when medications are reintroduced. Where an adverse reaction has been especially severe, one should avoid reintroducing the drugs that were present in the regimen at the time of the reaction, if possible. When a patient has tuberculosis in the usual chronic form, the disease is not likely to progress significantly during the waiting period. When a patient has aggressive tuberculosis, the omission of medications while awaiting resolution of a drug reaction may lead to the deterioration or the demise of the patient. However, the prompt introduction of a potentially toxic medication also could have dire consequences. Decision making in these circumstances is exceedingly difficult.

2. Plan a Strategy

Evaluate the options for an effective regimen, considering the likelihood that at least one drug from the former regimen must be excluded. All drugs likely to have efficacy should be considered, including drugs with potential for side effects that are not apt to be immediately life threatening. With the listed principles in mind, determine the safest way an effective regimen can be introduced in the least amount of time.

3. Reintroduce One Drug at a Time

When reintroducing drugs present in the regimen at the time of the reaction, do so one at a time, to clarify which drug is responsible if a reaction should recur. Whereas the original adverse event may have taken a long time to emerge, the same reaction is likely to recur within a day or two after the offending medication is reintroduced.

4. Prevent the Emergence of Additional Drug Resistance

Recognize that a long period of time may be needed to safely introduce previously used drugs. Plan a sequence of introduction that will provide adequate antimycobacterial coverage as promptly as possible, to prevent the emergence of additional drug resistance.[149] Sometimes medications deemed undesirable for extended use may be introduced temporarily to provide adequate coverage while gradually adding the medications planned for the longer term regimen. These "extra" drugs may be discontinued when the patient is tolerating adequate doses of the proposed long-term regimen.

5. Substitutions

Substitute one drug for the drug causing the adverse reaction if the reaction occurs within the first month of therapy or if the reaction occurs after the patient clearly is showing a favorable response to therapy. However, if there is some question of possible failure of the regimen the patient had been receiving, two new drugs should be substituted for the one lost due to toxicity.

6. Reintroduce Drugs Cautiously

After a reaction affecting the liver, reintroduce suspected hepatotoxic drugs in a step-wise manner, starting with a low dose and increasing daily for 3 days. Check liver function tests before each dose. If stable, the drug challenge can proceed. When the patient is on the full regimen, liver function tests should be repeated at least every 1–2 weeks for the next month, to ensure stability (see example in Figure 12-3).

A desensitizing schedule should be used if drugs in the former regimen are reintroduced after a skin reaction or drug fever. Emergency measures should be available immediately during desensitization. Suspected drugs may be reintroduced one at a time on a desensitization schedule. Varying schedules have been proposed; the essential ingredients in all of them are caution, close observation of the patient, immediate availability of emergency intervention (epinephrine and airway management), and incremental dosing, starting at very minute doses of the suspected drug. Complete blood count, serum creatinine and liver enzymes should be monitored, along with close clinical observation. If the allergic reaction was particularly severe, it is wiser to avoid reintroducing the offending drug. However, when no reasonable substitute is available, very cautious desensitization, starting with a very tiny dose, may make reintroduction of an effective regimen possible. Careful monitoring, under some circumstances, may require an intensive care unit setting. Desensitization can be done most safely under the care of an allergist in a hospital specializing in the management of difficult cases of tuberculosis.

VI. SURGERY

A. HISTORICAL

Surgical resection of residual pulmonary lesions was performed frequently in the early years of the chemotherapy era when physicians were unsure of the long-term benefits of chemotherapy. Surgical therapy largely was abandoned when the efficacy of medical therapy was documented. With good multidrug regimens the outcome of chemotherapy was at least 90% successful, and little additional benefit could be expected by subjecting the patient to the risk of surgery. However, in cases of tuberculosis resistant to multiple drugs, or when serious drug reactions limit the use of effective medications, poorer results of medical treatment are anticipated; the option of surgery is more attractive.[50,150-153]

B. FACTORS TO CONSIDER
1. Localization of Disease

The patient's disease must be sufficiently well localized to make resection feasible. Precise localization with computed tomography is helpful, since on routine X-ray views some areas of disease may be obscured by overlying markings. A ventilation-perfusion scan is helpful in evaluating the functional status of various areas of the lungs. Since, in the pathogenesis of tuberculosis, blood vessels may be destroyed, nonfunctional lung tissue in the distribution of the involved vessel may be present despite a benign appearance on X-ray. Leaving poorly vascularized tissue adjacent to the resected area may lead to poor healing. The perfusion status of the opposite lung may influence the decision whether to operate.

2. Condition of the Patient

The patient's general condition and lung function must be such that the potential risk of the procedure is not prohibitive. The criteria for operability in high-risk pulmonary resective surgery have been reviewed recently.[154] An estimate of the residual lung function following resection should show a predicted postpneumonectomy FEV_1 value of greater than 0.8 liters. However, in dire circumstances, the clinician may have to accept a slightly lower number.

3. Optimal Timing

Timing of the surgical procedure is critical. Complications of a complete or partial lung resection are reduced when the patient's infection is under good control and the sputum cultures are consistently negative. For patients who are on such poor regimens that culture conversion seems unlikely, surgery is best performed when the semiquantitative count of tubercle bacilli is at its anticipated nadir; that is, if the "fall and rise phenomenon" is in process, do the surgery after the "fall" and before the "rise." Judgment is necessary, and experience is helpful in estimating the preferred time for surgery.

4. Experience of the Surgical Team

The problems of distortion of anatomy, massive pleural adhesions, and destruction of tissue planes make surgery for tuberculosis very difficult. The patient should be given the benefit of a surgical team experienced with the problems involved.

5. Antituberculosis Chemotherapy

Medications should be continued in the perioperative period and for 2 years beyond culture conversion to manage the inevitable residual bacilli. Occasionally a second surgical procedure is necessary if there is a significant lesion in the contralateral lung and the patient can withstand bilateral resections. Where the amount of residual disease is small and no cavities are left behind, the bacillary load is likely to be small. The few remaining tubercle bacilli are likely to be controlled by medications that may not have been effective against a more massive bacterial burden.

VII. PROBLEMS IN THE MANAGEMENT OF DRUG-RESISTANT TUBERCULOSIS

A. NEED FOR RESOURCES AND EXPERIENCED PERSONNEL

The treatment of drug-resistant tuberculosis, especially multidrug-resistant disease, is time consuming, resource intensive, and fraught with risks. Adequate resources and experienced personnel are highly desirable in helping patients with drug-resistant tuberculosis toward recovery. In complex cases, it is possible to squander the last opportunity for the patient to undergo effective therapy by treating under less than ideal circumstances. It is recommended that such patients be referred to a center specializing in the management of difficult drug-resistant cases before all reasonable treatment options have been used up.

Hospitalization frequently is required during the initiation of therapy, in view of the complexity of the regimens, the toxicity of the drugs, and the need for close monitoring of the patient. Isolation facilities within the hospital are essential (see Chapter 3, this volume).

Psychological support often is needed to help the patients cope with their chronic illness. Repeated teaching is helpful; some patients respond and become more cooperative with their treatment; some do not. Ancillary services such as physical therapy, occupational therapy, and recreational therapy are important in enhancing the quality of life of these chronically ill patients.

B. TREATMENT FAILURES

Patients with multidrug-resistant tuberculosis, although sometimes salvageable by aggressive therapy, have high failure (35%) and relapse (14%) rates, according to a recent analysis from the National Jewish Center.[102] These patients are returned to the community with the recommendation of "home isolation." Some patients are conscientious and knowledgeable, and have homes with sufficient space and ventilation, along with means for delivery of food and other necessities. In such cases home isolation presents minimal hazard. When these prerequisites are not met, individuals with refractory drug-resistant tuberculosis are potential problems in the community. At the time of this writing the problem has not been solved. Reopening of sanatoria, in a limited way, may afford a place for some of these individuals.

Continuing partially effective therapy sometimes reduces symptoms, such as cough, and sometimes reduces the number of bacilli in the sputum. Until new drugs become available, the prospects for these patients are grim.

New drug development has been scant. Ofloxacin and ciprofloxacin have been introduced recently, and show promise of effectiveness. Rifabutin has been used in clinical trials; reports of clinical efficacy in tuberculosis have been conflicting (see also Section IV.G). Amoxicillin/clavulanate has been used anecdotally.[155] Sparfloxacin shows promise by laboratory tests.[156] Older therapies, such as therapeutic pneumoperitoneum, have been revived, but appear to be of very limited value. Surgical resection, as an adjunct to chemotherapy, has salvaged some patients. However, multiple drug therapy, appropriately prescribed and administered, remains the cornerstone of therapy for tuberculosis.

New drugs must be developed, and as they are developed, must be used appropriately, according to known principles of multidrug therapy. If a new drug is used as monotherapy, or if a new drug is used as a single effective agent added to a failing regimen, acquisition of resistance to the new drug is predictable. It is hoped that new drugs will be developed; it is also hoped that the new drugs will be used appropriately to reduce, rather than enhance, the problem of drug resistance.

REFERENCES

1. Snider, D. E., Roper, W. L., The new tuberculosis [editorial; comment], *N. Engl. J. Med.*, 326, 703, 1992.
2. Wolinsky, E., Reginster, A., Steenken, W., Drug-resistant tubercle bacilli in patients under treatment with streptomycin, *Am. Rev. Tuberc.*, 58, 335, 1948.
3. Wallace, A. T., Stewart, S. M., Turbbull, F. A. W., Crofton, J. W., Isoniazid resistance in patients with pulmonary tuberculosis treated on isoniazid alone, *Tubercle*, 35, 164, 1954.
4. American Thoracic Society, Ethambutol in the treatment of tuberculosis. A statement by the committee on therapy, *Am. Rev. Resp. Dis.*, 98, 320, 1968.
5. American Trudeau Society, Current status of drug therapy in tuberculosis, *Am. Rev. Tuberc.*, 61, 436, 1950.
6. Kass, I., Russell, W. F., Heaton, A., Miyamoto, T., Middlebrook, G., Dressler, S. H., Changing concepts in the treatment of pulmonary tuberculosis, *Ann. Intern. Med.*, 47, 744, 1957.
7. Jancik, E., Zelenka, M., Tousek, J., Makova, M., Chemotherapy for patients with cultures resistant to streptomycin, isoniazid and PAS, *Tubercle*, 44, 443, 1963.

8. Fischer, D. A., Lester, W., Dye, W. E., Moulding, T. S., Re-treatment of patients with isoniazid-resistant tuberculosis. Analysis and follow-up of 146 cases, *Am. Rev. Resp. Dis.*, 97, 392, 1968.

9. Fischer, D. A., Kass, I., Dye, W. E., Lester, W., Treatment of Isoniazid-resistant tuberculosis, *Antimicrobial Agents and Chemotherapy, Proceedings of the of 4th Interscience Conference on Antimicrobial Agents and Chemotherapy,* American Society for Microbiology, New York, 1964, 699.

10. Somner, A. R., Brace, A. A., Ethionamide, pyrazinamide and cycloserine used successfully in the treatment of chronic pulmonary tuberculosis, *Tubercle*, 43, 345, 1962.

11. Tousek, J., Jancik, E., Zelenka, M., Jancikova-Makova, M., The results of treatment in patients with cultures resistant to streptomycin, isoniazid and PAS: a five-year follow-up, *Tubercle*, 48, 27, 1967.

12. Zierski, M., Treatment of patients with cultures resistant to the primary anti-tuberculosis drugs, *Tubercle*, 45, 96, 1964.

13. Zierski, M., Zachara, A., Late results in re-treatment of patients with pulmonary tuberculosis, *Tubercle*, 51, 172, 1970.

14. Davidson, P. T., Goble, M., Lester, W., The antituberculosis efficacy of rifampin in 136 patients, *Chest,* 61, 574, 1972.

15. Vall-Spinosa, A., Lester, W., Moulding, T., Davidson, P. T., Rifampin in the treatment of drug-resistant *Mycobacterium tuberculosis* infections, *N. Engl. J. Med.*, 283, 616, 1970.

16. Fox, W., Changing concepts in the chemotherapy of pulmonary tuberculosis: the John Barnwell lecture, *Am. Rev. Resp. Dis.*, 97, 767, 1968.

17. International Union Against Tuberculosis, A comparison of regimens of ethionamide, pyrazinamide and cycloserine in re-treatment of patients with pulmonary tuberculosis, *Bull. Int. Union Tuberc.*, 42, 7, 1969.

18. East African/British Medical Research Councils, Streptomycin plus PAS plus pyrazinamide in the retreatment of pulmonary tuberculosis in East Africa, *Tubercle*, 52, 191, 1971.

19. Study by East African and British Medical Research Councils, Streptomycin plus PAS plus pyrazinamide in the retreatment of pulmonary tuberculosis in East Africa: second report, *Tubercle*, 54, 283, 1973.

20. Lester, W., Treatment of drug-resistant tuberculosis, *Dis. Month*, April 1, 1971.

21. Centers for Disease Control, Multi-drug-resistant tuberculosis — North Carolina, *MMWR*, 35, 785, 1987.

22. Schiffman, P. L., Ashkar, B., Bishop, M., Cleary, M. G., Drug-resistant tuberculosis in a large southern California hospital, *Am. Rev. Resp. Dis.*, 116, 821, 1977.

23. Reves, R., Blakey, D., Snider, D. E., Farer, L. S., Transmission of multiple drug-resistant tuberculosis: report of a school and community outbreak, *Am. Epidemiol.*, 113:4, 423, 1981.

24. Carpenter, J. L., Obnibene, A. J., Gorby, E. W., Neimes, R. E., Koch, J. R., Perkins, W. L., Antituberculosis drug resistance in South Texas, *Am. Rev. Resp. Dis.*, 128, 1055, 1983.

25. Steiner, P., Rao, M., Mitchell, M., Steiner, M., Primary drug-resistant tuberculosis in children: Emergence of primary drug-resistant strains of *M. tuberculosis* to rifampin, *Am. Rev. Resp. Dis.*, 134, 446, 1986.

26. Steiner, P., Roa, M., Victoria, M. S., Hunt, J., Steiner, M., A continuing study of primary drug-resistant tuberculosis among children observed at the Kings County Hospital Medical Center between the years 1961 and 1980, *Am. Rev. Resp. Dis.*, 128, 425, 1983.

27. Horne, N. W., Drug resistant-tuberculosis: a review of the world situation, *Tubercle* (Suppl.), 50, 2, 1968.

28. Doster, B., Caras, G., Snider, D. E., Jr., A continuing survey of primary drug resistance in tuberculosis, 1961 to 1968, *Am. Rev. Resp. Dis.*, 113, 419, 1976.

29. Hobby, G. L., Johnson, P. M., Boytar-Papirnyik, V., Primary drug resistance: a continuing study of drug resistance in tuberculosis in a veteran population in the United States — September 1962 to September 1971, *Transact. 31st VA Armed Forces Pul. Conf.*, 1972, 36.

30. Hobby, G. L., Johnson, P. M., Boytar-Papirnyik, V., Primary drug resistance: a continuing study of drug resistance in tuberculosis in a veteran population within the United States. X. September 1970 to September 1973, *Am. Rev. Resp. Dis.*, 110, 95, 1974.

31. Kopanoff, D. E., Kilburn, J. O., Glassroth, J. L., Snider, D. E., Farer, L. S., Good, R. C., A continuing survey of tuberculosis primary drug resistance in the United States, March 1975 to November 1977. A U. S. Public Health Service cooperative study, *Am. Rev. Resp. Dis.*, 118, 835, 1978.

32. Cauthen, G. M., Kilburn, J. O., Kelly, G. D., Good, R. C., Resistance to antituberculosis drugs in patients with and without prior treatment; survey of 31 state and large city laboratories, 1982–1986, *Am. Rev. Resp. Dis.*, 137(Suppl.), 260, 1988.

33. Snider, D. E., Cauthen, G. M., Farer, L. S., Kelly, G. D., Kilburn, J. O., Good, R. C., Dooley, S. W., Drug-resistant tuberculosis [letter], *Am. Rev. Resp. Dis.*, 144, 732, 1991.

34. Brudney, K., Dobkin, J., Resurgent tuberculosis in New York City: human immunodeficiency virus, homelessness, and the decline of tuberculosis control programs, *Am. Rev. Resp. Dis.*, 144, 745, 1991.

35. Reichman, L. B., The U-shaped curve of concern [editorial], *Am. Rev. Resp. Dis.*, 144, 741, 1991.

36. Centers for Disease Control, Outbreak of multidrug-resistant tuberculosis in Texas, California, and Pennsylvania, *MMWR*, 39, 369, 1990.

37. Centers for Disease Control, Nosocomial transmission of multidrug-resistant tuberculosis to health-care workers and HIV-infected patients in an urban hospital — Florida, *MMWR*, 39, 718, 1990.

38. Centers for Disease Control, Transmission of multidrug-resistant tuberculosis from an HIV positive client in a residential substance-abuse facility — Michigan, *MMWR*, 40(8), 129, 1991.

39. Centers for Disease Control, Transmission of multidrug-resistant tuberculosis among immunocompromised persons in a correctional system — New York, 1991, *MMWR*, 41(28), 507, 1992.

40. Centers for Disease Control, Nosocomial transmission of multidrug-resistant tuberculosis among HIV-infected persons — Florida and New York, 1988–1991, *MMWR*, 40, 585, 1991.

41. Pitchenik, A. E., Burr, J., Laufer, M., Miller, G., Cacciatore, R., Bigler, W. J., Witte, J. J., Cleary, T., Outbreaks of drug-resistant tuberculosis at AIDS center [letter], *Lancet*, 336, 440, 1990.

42. Calder, R. A., Duclos, P., Wilder, M. H., Pryor, V. L., Scheel, W. J., *Mycobacterium tuberculosis* transmission in a health clinic, *Bull. Int. Union Tuberc. Lung Dis.*, 66, 103, 1991.

43. Edlin, B. R., Tokars, J. I., Grieco, M. H., Crawford, J. T., Williams, J., Sordillo, E. M., Ong, K. R., Castro, K. G., et al., An outbreak of multidrug-resistant tuberculosis among hospitalized patients with the acquired immunodeficiency syndrome, *N. Engl. J. Med.*, 326, 1514, 1992.

44. Fischl, M. A., Uttamchandani, R. B., Daikos, G. L., Poblete, R. B., Moreno, J. N., Reyes, R. R., Boota, A. M., Thompson, L. M., et al., An outbreak of tuberculosis caused by multiple-drug-resistant tubercle bacilli among patients with HIV infection, *Ann. Intern. Med.*, 117, 177, 1992.

45. Pearson, M. L., Jereb, J. A., Frieden, T. R., Crawford, J. T., Davis, B. J., Dooley, S. W., Jarvis, W.R., Nosocomial transmission of multidrug-resistant *Mycobacterium tuberculosis*. A risk to patients and health care workers, *Ann. Intern. Med.*, 117, 191, 1992.

46. Busillo, C. P., Lessnau, K., Sanjana, V., Soumakis, S., Davidson, M., Mullen, M. P., Talavera, W., Multidrug resistant *Mycobacterium tuberculosis* in patients with human immunodeficiency virus infection, *Chest*, 102, 797, 1992.

47. Canetti, G., The J. Burns Amberson lecture: Present aspects of bacterial resistance in tuberculosis, *Am. Rev. Resp. Dis.*, 92, 687, 1965.

48. Canetti, G., *The Tubercle Bacillus in the Pulmonary Lesion of Man; Histobacteriology and Its Bearing on the Therapy of Pulmonary Tuberculosis*, Springer, New York, 1955.

49. David, H. L., Probability distribution of drug-resistant mutants in unselected populations of *Mycobacterium tuberculosis*, *Appl. Microbiol.*, 20, 810, 1970.

50. Shimao, T., Drug resistance in tuberculosis control, *Tubercle*, 68(2) (Suppl.), 5, 1987.

51. Pollock, M. R., Drug resistance and mechanisms for its development, *Br. Med. Bull.*, 16, 16, 1960.

52. International Union Against Tuberculosis, The clinical significance of bacterial resistance: a symposium held in Paris on September 20, 1957, *Bull. Int. Union Tuberc.*, 27, 215, 1957.

53. Schmidt, L. H., Grover, A. A., Hoffmann, R., Rehm, J., Sullivan, R., The emergence of isoniazid-sensitive bacilli in monkeys inoculated with isoniazid-resistant strains, *Transact. 17th VA Armed Forces Conf. Chemo.*, 264, 1958.

54. McDermott, W., Microbial persistence (The Alpha Kappa Kappa lecture), *Yale J. Biol. Med.*, 30, 257, 1958.

55. McDermott, W., The J. Burns Amberson lecture — The chemotherapy of tuberculosis, *Am. Rev. Resp. Dis.*, 86, 323, 1962.

56. Hershfield, E. S., Drug resistance _ response to Dr. Shimao, *Tubercle*, 68(Suppl.), 17, 1987.

57. Tripathy, S. P., Menon, N. K., Mitchison, D. A., Narayana, A. L. S., Somasundaram, P. A., Scott, H., Velu, S., Response to treatment with isoniazid plus PAS of tuberculosis patients with primary isoniazid resistance, *Tubercle*, 50, 257, 1969.

58. Winder, F. G., Mode of action of the antimycobacterial agents and associated aspects of the molecular biology of mycobacteria, in *Biology of the Mycobacteria*, Vol. 1, Ratledge, C., Stanford, J., Eds., Academic Press, London, 1982, chap. 8.

59. Tsukamura, M., Yamamoto, M., Hayashi, M., Noda, Y., Torii, T., Further studies on cross resistance in *Mycobacterium tuberculosis*, with special reference to streptomycin, kanamycin, and viomycin resistance, *Am. Rev. Resp. Dis.*, 85, 426, 1962.

60. Tsukamura, M., Cross-resistance of tubercle bacilli, *Kekkaku*, 52, 47, 1977.

61. Lefford, M. J., The ethionamide sensitivity of East African strains of *Mycobacterium tuberculosis* resistant to thiacetazone, *Tubercle*, 50, 7, 1969.

62. Kleeberg, H. H., Boshoff, M. S., *World Atlas of Initial Drug Resistance*, Prepared for the Scientific Committee on Bacteriology and Immunology of the International Union Against Tuberculosis, Paris, 1980.

63. Kleeberg, H. H, Olivier, M., *World Atlas of Initial Drug Resistance*, 2nd rev. ed., S. Africa Medical Research Council, Pretoria, 1984.

64. Meissner, G., Primary drug resistance of the tubercle bacillus: bacteriology, therapeutic and epidemiological aspects, *Bull. Int. Union Tuberc.*, 32(2), 15, 1962.

65. Centers for Disease Control, National action plan to combat multidrug-resistant tuberculosis, *MMWR*, 41, 5, 1992.

66. Centers for Disease Control, Meeting the challenge of multidrug-resistant tuberculosis: summary of a conference, *MMWR*, 41, 51, 1992.

67. Centers for Disease Control, Management of persons exposed to multidrug-resistant tuberculosis, *MMWR*, 41, 61, 1992.

68. Grzybowski, S., Cost of tuberculosis control, *Tubercle*, 68(Suppl.), 33, 1987.

69. Boulahbal, F., Khaled, S., Tazir, M., The interest of follow-up of resistance of the tubercle bacillus in the evaluation of a programme, *Bull. Int. Union Tuberc. Lung Dis.*, 64, 23, 1989.

70. Weyer, K., Primary and acquired drug resistance in adult black tuberculosis patients in South Africa, *Am. Rev. Resp. Dis.*, 143(4) (Suppl.), A121, 1991.

71. Kim, S. J., Hong, Y. P., Drug resistance of *Mycobacterium tuberculosis* in Korea, *Tubercle Lung Dis.*, 73, 219, 1992.

72. Cohn, M. L., Middlebrook, G., Russell, W. F., Combined drug treatment of tuberculosis. I. Prevention of emergence of mutant populations of tubercle bacilli resistant to both streptomycin and isoniazid *in vitro*, *J. Clin. Invest.*, 38, 1349, 1959.

73. American Thoracic Society, Control of tuberculosis in the United States, *Am. Rev. Resp. Dis.*, 146, 1623, 1992.

74. Addington, W.W., Patient compliance: the most serious remaining problem in the control of tuberculosis in the United States, *Chest*, 76(Suppl.), 741, 1979.

75. Chaulet, P., Compliance with anti-tuberculosis chemotherapy in developing countries, *Tubercle*, 68(Suppl.), 19, 1987.

76. Reichman, L. B., Compliance in developed nations, *Tubercle*, 68(Suppl.), 25, 1987.

77. Sbarbaro, J. A., Compliance: Inducements and enforcement, *Chest*, 76(Suppl.), 750, 1979.

78. Snider, D. E., Kelly, G. D., Thompson, N. J., Kilburn, Good, R. C., Infectiousness and pathogenicity of drug resistant *Mycobacterium tuberculosis*, *Am. Rev. Resp. Dis.*, 123(Suppl.), 254, 1981.

79. Snider, D. E., Kelley, G. D., Cuathen, G. M., Thompson, N. J., Kilburn, J. O., Infection and disease among contacts of tuberculosis cases with drug-resistant and drug-susceptible bacilli, *Am. Rev. Resp. Dis.*, 132, 125, 1985.

80. Dooley, S. W., Castro, K. G., Hutton, M. D., Mullan, R. J., Polder, J. A., Snider, D. E., Jr., Guidelines for preventing the transmission of tuberculosis in health-care settings, with special focus on HIV-related issues, *MMWR*, 39, 1, 1990.

81. Dooley, S. W., Jarvis, W. R., Martone, W. J., Snider, D. E., Jr., Multi-drug resistant tuberculosis [editorial; comment], *Ann. Intern. Med.*, 117, 257, 1992.

82. Nardell, E. A., Multidrug-resistant tuberculosis [letter], *N. Engl. J. Med.*, 327, 1174, 1992.

83. Nardell, E. A., Nosocomial tuberculosis in the AIDS era: strategies for interrupting transmission in developing countries, *Bull. Int. Union Tuberc. Lung Dis.*, 66, 107, 1991.

84. Ben-Dov, I., Mason, G. R., Drug resistant tuberculosis in southern California: trends 1969 to 1984, *Am. Rev. Resp. Dis.*, 135, 1307, 1987.

85. Barnes, P. F., The influence of epidemiologic factors on drug resistance rates in tuberculosis, *Am. Rev. Resp. Dis.*, 136, 325, 1987.

86. Riley, L. W., Arathoon, E., Loverde, V. D., The epidemiologic patterns of drug-resistant *Mycobacterium tuberculosis*: a community-based study, *Am. Rev. Resp. Dis.*, 139, 1282, 1989.

87. Areas, A., Chaparala, B., Martin, H. K., Muthuswamy, P., Serai, L., Drug resistant tuberculosis at Cook County Hospital, *Am. Rev. Resp. Dis.*, 139(Suppl.), A315, 1989.

88. Chawla, P. K., Klapper, P. J., Kamholz, S. L., Pollack, A. H., Heurich, A. E., Drug resistant tuberculosis in an urban population including patients at risk for human immunodeficiency virus infection, *Am. Rev. Resp. Dis.,* 146, 280, 1992.

89. Jacobs, M., Hussain, E., D'Amato, R. F., Incidence of drug resistant *Mycobacterium tuberculosis* in a New York City medical center, *Am. Rev. Resp. Dis.,* 145(Suppl.), A101, 1992.

90. Frieden, T. R., Sterling, T., Pablos-Mendez, A., Kilburn, J. O., Cauthen, G. M., Dooley, S. W., The emergence of drug-resistant tuberculosis in New York City, *N. Engl. J. Med.,* 328, 521, 1993.

91. Suwanogool, S., Smith, S. M., Smith, L. G., Eng, R., Drug-resistance encountered in the retreatment of *Mycobacterium tuberculosis* infections, *J. Chronic Dis.,* 37(12), 925, 1984.

92. Costello, H. D., Caras, G. J., Snider, D. E., Jr., Drug resistance among previously treated tuberculosis patients, a brief report, *Am. Rev. Resp. Dis.,* 121, 313, 1980.

93. Matthews, J. I., Rajput, M. A., Neimus, R., Drug resistant tuberculosis in south Texas, *Chest,* 92(2) (Suppl.), 145S, 1987.

94. Byrd, R. B., Fish, D. E., Roethe, R. A., Glover, J. N., Wooster, L. D., Tuberculosis in oriental immigrants: a study in military dependents, *Chest,* 76, 136, 1979.

95. Aitken, M. L., Sparks, R., Anderson, K., Albert, R. K., Predictors of drug resistant *Mycobacterium tuberculosis,* *Am. Rev. Resp. Dis.,* 130, 831, 1984.

96. Nolan, C. M., Elarth, A. M., Tuberculosis in a cohort of Southeast Asian refugees, a five year study, *Am. Rev. Resp. Dis.,* 137, 805, 1988.

97. Lessnau, K., Talavera, W., Busillo, C., Sanjana, V., Soumakis, S., Davidson, M., Mullen, M., Multi-drug resistant *Mycobacterium tuberculosis* in patients with human immunodeficiency virus infection, *Am. Rev. Resp. Dis.,* 145(Suppl.), A815, 1992.

98. Fischl, M. A., Daikos, G. L., Uttamchandani, G. L., Poblete, R. B., Moreno, J. N., Reyes, R. R., Boota, A. M., Thompson, L. M., et al., Clinical presentation and outcome of patients with HIV infection and tuberculosis caused by multiple-drug-resistant bacilli, *Ann. Intern. Med.,* 117, 184, 1992.

99. Pablos-Mendez, A., Raviglione, M. C., Battan, R., Ramos-Zuniga, R., Drug-resistant tuberculosis among the homeless in New York City, *N. Y. State J. Med.,* 90, 351, 1990.

100. Welsh, C. H., Drug-resistant tuberculosis after gastrectomy. Double jeopardy?, *Chest,* 99, 245, 1991.

101. Iseman, M. D., Madsen, L. A., Chronic tuberculous empyema with bronchopleural fistula resulting in treatment failure and progressive drug resistance, *Chest,* 100, 124, 1991.

102. Goble, M., Iseman, M. D., Madsen, L. A., Waite, D., Ackerson, L., Horsburgh, C. R., Jr., Treatment of 171 patients with pulmonary tuberculosis resistant to isoniazid and rifampin, *N. Engl. J. Med.,* 328, 527, 1993.

103. Heifets, L. B., Drug susceptibility in the management of chemotherapy of tuberculosis, in *Drug Susceptibility in the Chemotherapy of Mycobacterial Infections,* Heifets, L. B., Ed., CRC Press, Boca Raton, FL, 1991, chap. 3.

104. Heifets, L. B., Qualitative and quantitative drug-susceptibility tests in mycobacteriology, *Am. Rev. Resp. Dis.,* 137(5), 1217, 1988.

105. McClatchy, J. K., Antimycobacterial drugs: Mechanisms of action, drug resistance, susceptibility testing, and assays of activity in biological fluids, in *Antibiotics in Laboratory Medicine,* Lorian, V., Ed., Williams & Wilkins, Baltimore, 1985, 181.

106. Stewart, S. M., Crofton, J. W., The clinical significance of low degrees drug resistance in pulmonary tuberculosis, *Am. Rev. Resp. Dis.,* 89, 811, 1964.

107. Wang, C., Lou, Y., A study of the ununiformity of drug resistance of tubercle bacilli from patients with chronic pulmonary tuberculosis, *Am. Rev. Resp. Dis.,* 141(4) (Suppl.), A448, 1990.

108. International Union Against Tuberculosis, Antituberculosis regimens of chemotherapy — Recommendations from the committee on treatment of the International Union Against Tuberculosis, *Bull. Int. Union Tuberc. Lung Dis.,* 63, 60, 1988.

109. Moulding, T. S., Davidson, P. T., Goble, M., The treatment of tuberculosis, *Sem. Resp. Med.,* 2, 215, 1981.

110. Crofton, J., The prevention and management of drug-resistant tuberculosis, *Bull. Int. Union Tuberc.,* 62, 6, 1987.

111. Davidson, P. T., Drug resistance and the selection of therapy for tuberculosis [editorial], *Am. Rev. Resp. Dis.,* 136, 255, 1987.

112. Hong Kong Tuberculosis Treatment Services/ Brompton Hospital/British Medical Research Council, A controlled clinical trial of daily and intermittent regimens of rifampicin plus ethambutol in the retreatment of patients with pulmonary tuberculosis in Hong Kong, *Tubercle,* 55, 1, 1974.

113. Poland National Research Institute, A comparative study of daily followed by twice or once weekly regimes of ethambutol and rifampicin in the retreatment of patients with pulmonary tuberculosis: second report, *Tubercle,* 57, 105, 1976.

114. Zierski, M., Prospects of retreatment of chronic resistant pulmonary tuberculosis patients. A critical review, *Lung,* 154, 91, 1977.

115. Mitchison, D. A., Nunn, A. J., Influence of initial drug resistance on the response to short-course chemotherapy of pulmonary tuberculosis, *Am. Rev. Resp. Dis.,* 133, 423, 1986.

116. Swai, O. B., Aluoch, J., Githui, W. A., Thiong'o, R., Edwards, E. A., Controlled clinical trial of a regimen of two durations for the treatment of isoniazid resistant pulmonary tuberculosis, *Tubercle,* 69, 5, 1988.

117. Hong Kong Chest Service/British Medical Research Council, Controlled trial of four thrice-weekly regimens and a daily regimen all given for 6 months for pulmonary tuberculosis, *Lancet,* 1, 171, 1981.

118. Hong, Y. P., Kim, S. C., Chang, S. C., Kim, S. J., Jin, B. W., Park, C. D., Comparison of a daily and three intermittent retreatment regimens for pulmonary tuberculosis administered under programme conditions, *Tubercle,* 69, 241, 1988.

119. Hong Kong Chest Service/British Medical Research Council, Controlled trial of 2, 4 and 6 months of pyrazinamide in 6-month, three-times-weekly regimens for smear-positive tuberculosis, including an assessment of a combined preparation of isoniazid, rifampin, and pyrazinamide. Results at 30 months, *Am. Rev. Resp. Dis.,* 143, 700, 1991.

120. Donath, J., Chitkara, R. K., Drug-resistant tuberculosis; a tactical approach to therapy, *J. Resp. Dis.,* 9, 73, 1988.

121. Goble, M., Drug-resistant tuberculosis, *Sem. Resp. Infect.,* 1, 220, 1986.

122. Iseman, M. D., Goble, M., Treatment of tuberculosis, *Adv. Intern. Med.,* 33, 253, 1988.

123. Iseman, M. D., Madsen, L. A., Drug-resistant tuberculosis, *Clin. Chest Med.,* 10, 341, 1989.

124. McDonald, R. J., Memon, A. M., Reichman, L. B., Successful supervised ambulatory management of tuberculosis treatment failures, *Ann. Intern. Med.,* 96, 297, 1982.

125. Crofton, J., Treatment of patients with drug-resistance in economically developed countries, *Tubercle,* 50, 65, 1969.

126. Crofton, J., Douglas, A., Treatment of pulmonary tuberculosis, in *Respiratory Diseases,* F. A. Davis, Philadelphia, 1969, chap. 14.

127. Medical Research Council report by their Tuberculosis Chemotherapy Trials Committee, Long-term chemotherapy in the treatment of chronic pulmonary tuberculosis with cavitation, *Tubercle,* 43, 201, 1962.

128. Crofton, J., Tuberculosis undefeated, *Br. Med. J.,* 2, 679, 1960.

128a. Hong Kong Chest Service/British Medical Research Council,, Controlled trial of 6-month and 9-month regimens of daily and intermittent streptomycin plus isoniazid plus pyrazinamide for pulmonary tuberculosis in Hong Kong. the results up to 30 months, *Am. Rev. Respir. Dis.,* 115, 727, 1977.

129. Gonzalez-Montaner, L. J., Dambrosi, A. O., Abbate, E. H., Treatment and results of multiple resistance pulmonary tuberculosis, *Am. Rev. Resp. Dis.,* 141:4, A450, 1990.

130. Chen, C., Shih, J., Lindholm-Levy, P. J., Heifets, L. B., Minimal inhibitory concentrations of rifabutin, ciprofloxacin, and ofloxacin against tuberculosis isolated before treatment of patients in Taiwan, *Am. Rev. Resp. Dis.,* 140, 987, 1989.

131. Kahana, L. M., Spino, O., Ciprofloxacin in patients with mycobacterial infections: experience in 15 patients, *DICP,* 25, 919, 1991.

132. Tsukamura, M., Nakamura, E., Yoshii, S., Amano, H., Therapeutic effect of a new antibacterial substance ofloxacin (DL8280) on pulmonary tuberculosis, *Am. Rev. Resp. Dis.,* 131, 352, 1985.

133. Yew, W. W., Kwan, S. Y., Ma, W. K., Khin, M. A., Chau, P. Y., In-vitro activity of ofloxacin against *Mycobacterium tuberculosis* and its clinical efficacy in multiply resistant pulmonary tuberculosis, *J. Antimicrob. Chemother.,* 26, 227, 1990.

134. Stocks, J. S., Wallace, R. J., Preliminary data on the safety and efficacy of drug regimens containing ofloxacin in the therapy of multiple drug resistant mycobacterial infections, *Am. Rev. Resp. Dis.,* 135(Suppl.), A136, 1987.

135. Lyle, M. A., O'Brien, R. J., Rifabutin (ansamycin LM427) for the treatment of rifampin resistant tuberculosis, *Am. Rev. Resp. Dis.,* 139(4) (Suppl.), A316, 1989.

136. O'Brien, R. J., Lyle, M. A., Snider, D. E., Jr., Rifabutin (ansamycin LM 427): a new rifamycin-S derivative for the treatment of mycobacterial diseases, *Rev. Infect. Dis.,* 9, 519, 1987.

137. Pretet, S., Lebeaut, A., Parrot, R., Truffot, C., Grosset, J., Dinh-Xuan, A. T., Combined chemotherapy including rifabutin for rifampicin and isoniazid resistant pulmonary tuberculosis, *Eur. Resp. J.,* 5, 680, 1992.

138. Heifets, L. B., Lindholm-Levy, P. J., Iseman, M. D., Rifabutine: minimal inhibitory and bactericidal concentrations for *Mycobacterium tuberculosis*, *Am. Rev. Resp. Dis.*, 137, 719, 1988.

139. Madsen, L., Goble, M., Iseman, M., Ansamycin (LM 427) in the retreatment of drug-resistant tuberculosis, *Am. Rev. Resp. Dis.*, 133(Suppl.), A206, 1986.

140. Donaldson, R., Wallace, A., Drug-resistant pulmonary tuberculosis treated with ethambutol, a rifamycin and a riminophenazine (B663), *Br. J. Dis. Chest*, 64, 161, 1970.

141. Peloquin, C. A., Antituberculosis drugs: Pharmacokinetics, in *Drug Susceptibility in the Chemotherapy of Mycobacterial Infections*, Heifets, L. B., Ed., CRC Press, Boca Raton, FL, 1991, chap. 2.

142. Moulding, T., Davidson, P. T., Tuberculosis II: toxicity and intolerance to antituberculosis drugs, *Drug Ther.*, February, 41, 1974.

143. Gonzalez-Montaner, L. J., Dambrosi, A., Manassero, M., Dambrosi, V. Y. M., Adverse effects of antituberculosis drugs causing changes in treatment, *Tubercle*, 63, 291, 1982.

144. Hajjaj, M., Xie, H. J., Enarson, D. A., Allen, E. A., Grzybowski, S., Serious drug toxicity in tuberculosis treatment programs, *Am. Rev. Resp. Dis.*, 141, A441, 1990.

145. Johnston, R. F., Hopewell, P. C., Chemotherapy of pulmonary tuberculosis, *Ann. Inter. Med.*, 70, 359, 1969.

146. Matsui, M. S., Rozovski, S. J., Drug-nutrient interactions, *Clin. Ther.*, 4, 423, 1982.

147. Seaman, J. M., Goble, M., Madsen, L., Steigerwald, J. C., Fasciitis and polyarthritis during antituberculosis treatment, *Arthritis Rheum.*, 28, 1179, 1985.

148. Casewitt, C., Ultrasound for relief of painful injection sites, *Clin. Manage.*, 4, 50, 1983.

149. Horne, N. W., Grant, I. W. B., Development of drug resistance to isoniazid during desensitization: a report of two cases, *Tubercle*, 44, 180, 1963.

150. Hui, K. K. L., Mary-Aquines, Sr., Surgery for first line drug-resistant tuberculosis, *Dis. Chest*, 49, 57, 1966.

151. Iseman, M. D., Madsen, L., Goble, M., Pomerantz, M., Surgical intervention in the treatment of pulmonary disease caused by drug-resistant *Mycobacterium tuberculosis*, *Am. Rev. Resp. Dis.*, 141, 623, 1990.

152. Mahmoudi, A., Iseman, M. D., Surgical intervention in the treatment of drug-resistant tuberculosis: update and extended follow-up, *Am. Rev. Resp. Dis.*, 145(Suppl.), A816, 1992.

153. Muthuswamy, P., Chechani, V., Baker, W., Surgical management of pulmonary tuberculosis, *Am. Rev. Resp. Dis.*, 145(Suppl.), A816, 1992.

154. Zibrak, J. D., O'Donnell, C. R., Marton, K., Indications for pulmonary function testing, *Ann. Intern. Med.*, 112, 763, 1990.

155. Nadler, J. P., Berger, J., Nord, J. A., Cofsky, R., Saxena, M., Amoxicillin-clavulanic acid for treating drug-resistant *Mycobacterium tuberculosis*, *Chest*, 99(4), 1025, 1991.

156. Ji, B., Truffot-Pernot, C., Grosset, J., *In vitro* and *in vivo* activity of sparfloxacin (AT-4140) against *Mycobacterium tuberculosis*, *Tubercle*, 72, 181, 1991.

Chapter 13

Skin Testing and Chemoprophylaxis

Lloyd N. Friedman, M.D.

CONTENTS

0-8493-4825-0/94/$0.00+$.50
© 1994 by CRC Press, Inc.

I. PURIFIED PROTEIN DERIVATIVE (PPD)

Tuberculin PPD is a purified protein derivative prepared from culture filtrates of *Mycobacterium tuberculosis*. It is employed in skin testing to detect persons infected with *M. tuberculosis*. PPD-S, lot number 49608, prepared in 1939 by Siebert and Glenn,[1] was adopted in 1951 by the World Health Organization Expert Committee on Biologic Standardization as the international standard for tuberculin PPD.[2] The international unit, also known as the tuberculin unit (TU), is the biologic activity represented by 0.00002 mg of PPD-S. PPD-S was used for comparison testing in the formulation of all commercially prepared PPD for use in the United States.[3,4]

II. PREPARATION OF PPD

There are two basic methods of PPD preparation: the ammonium sulfate and the trichloroacetic acid precipitation methods. In both cases, the PPD is prepared by growing large amounts of *M. tuberculosis* in liquid culture, steaming for 3 h at 100°C to sterilize, and then filtering. The filtrate undergoes a series of precipitation, washing, buffering, and centrifugation steps until it becomes the concentrated stock solution. The ammonium sulfate precipitation method results in a PPD with a higher protein and polysaccharide percentage, whereas the trichloroacetic acid precipitation method results in a PPD with higher percentage of nucleic acids.[2] PPD-S was formulated with the ammonium sulfate precipitation method. The commercially available Aplisol[R] brand (Parke-Davis) also was formulated by the ammonium sulfate method, whereas Tubersol[R] (Connaught) was formulated by the trichloroacetic acid method. For a given strength, the commercially available PPD brands are assumed to be equal in potency and in the ability to detect tuberculous infection. The preparation of old tuberculin (OT), which rarely is used, is similar to the above preparation without the precipitation and centrifugation steps.

The standard strength of PPD for skin testing is 5 TU, which is the biologic equivalent of 0.0001 mg of PPD-S. One TU is one-fifth and 250 TU is 50 times the concentration of 5 TU, but this is not reflected to the same degree in their biologic equivalencies. PPD RT-23 is a standard tuberculin in use in countries other than the United States, and 2 TU is biologically equivalent to 5 TU of PPD-S.[5]

III. SKIN TEST PLACEMENT AND REACTIONS

A. PLACEMENT

The Mantoux test has been standardized as the intradermal placement of 0.1 ml (5 TU) of PPD into the volar, or, rarely, the dorsal surface of the forearm. A 27-gauge short beveled needle is the favored instrument of delivery. Interpretation of the test is performed within 48–72 h. Induration is assessed by palpation, inspection, or both, and is measured in the transverse direction only.[3,4,6,7] Other techniques, such as the ballpoint pen method, have been used with some success.[8,9] Regardless of the technique, proficiency at skin test measurement occurs only after proper training and experience.[10,11]

The following reactions have been described after intradermal PPD administration: immediate hypersensitivity and Arthus reactions; retest phenomenon (early, altered, or accelerated reaction); cutaneous basophil hypersensitivity (i.e., Jones–Mote reactivity); and delayed-type hypersensitivity (DTH).

B. REACTIONS
1. Early Reactions

The early reactions, i.e., the Arthus reaction and immediate hypersensitivity reaction, occur to one or more of the components of tuberculin. The Arthus reaction is an IgG immune complex reaction peaking in 2–6 h with erythema, edema, hemorrhage, and necrosis. Immediate hypersensitivity is an IgE-mediated reaction with the rapid development of a wheal and flare that usually resolves by 24 h.[6] With 250 TU, the reaction may peak in 24 h and resolve slowly.[12] In a study by Tarlo et al., immediate hypersensitivity occurred to an injection of 5 TU of PPD in 76 (2.3%) of 3,248 patients who underwent tuberculin skin tests, only 3 of whom also had a DTH response.[13] Prior exposure to tuberculin was not a prerequisite for this reaction, as 28% of those evaluated had had no previous exposure to tuberculin.

2. Retest Phenomenon

The retest phenomenon is a reproducible phenomenon described in past literature.[11,12,14-16] It is a form of local hypersensitivity where a tuberculin injection placed at the site of a previous tuberculin test may induce a markedly accelerated reaction that begins usually within 3 h, peaks at 12–24 h, and resolves by 48 h. It may occur as an early and more pronounced component of the usual tuberculin reaction in a tuberculin-positive individual, and is a reproducible phenomenon.[14,16] A well-controlled study of the retest phenomenon was conducted by the World Health Organization Tuberculosis Research Office on 216 unvaccinated PPD-positive individuals.[16] Repeat tests were applied on both arms 3 months after initial testing and, on average, the reaction at the retest site was 13 mm larger than the control site at 6 h, and reached a peak much earlier. The rate of vesiculation at 24 h was 30% vs. 5% of controls. Although the retest site consistently reached a maximum induration that was approximately 4 mm greater than the control site, the induration was equivalent at 3 days, and less at 6 days. The study found no appreciable retest phenomenon with 5 TU in 14 PPD-negative individuals, but Duboczy et al. showed that it did occur, although to a lesser degree, with higher doses of tuberculin in PPD-negative individuals.[12,15] Persistence of the phenomenon has been reported as long as 12 years after a test.[12] It is not thought to be related to the Arthus reaction, and is thought to be closely allied to delayed-type hypersensitivity.[17]

3. Cutaneous Basophil Hypersensitivity

Cutaneous basophil hypersensitivity or Jones–Mote reactivity is thought to be a form of delayed-type hypersensitivity with a prominent infiltrate of basophils.[18,19] The pure form is not seen in humans. In guinea pigs, the sensitivity usually is transient (2–4 weeks) and the reaction is less indurated and more erythematous than the typical tuberculin reaction. The onset of the reaction is within 4–6 h after injection and is maximal at 18–24 h.[18] The phenomenon is transferred by lymphocytes and probably represents a response to true infection. It has been stated that it does not play an important role in PPD interpretation,[3] but there has been only one study addressing this issue in humans, and the results showed a prominent basophilic response in 5 (56%) of 9 tuberculin-positive persons biopsied after PPD administration.[20] This phenomenon is thought to be not separate from, but part of, the delayed-type hypersensitivity response to tuberculin. It has not been described as a reaction to tuberculin in nonsensitized individuals.

4. Delayed-Type Hypersensitivity

The delayed-type hypersensitivity reaction is the classic reaction to tuberculin and usually begins within 4–6 h, is maximal at 48–72 h, and subsides over a few days.[21] In some cases, especially in the elderly, the peak is delayed and may be maximal at 7 days. Slutkin et al. showed that a 7-day reading could add an additional 5% to the number of persons who reacted to tuberculin in his study.[22] In general, the reaction is indurated with erythema, and may have necrosis or vesiculation. It is dependent on cell-mediated immunity and is transferrable by T lymphocytes, but not by serum antibodies. A special fibrin gel network is the essential component that allows induration rather than edema alone to occur. It has been shown in recent studies that the etiology of induration in delayed-type hypersensitivity is not simply the accumulation of cells and fluid in the skin, which can occur with any type of insult, but is related to the deposition of a special fibrin gel network

that can trap and hold significant amounts of fluid, protein, and cells, so that a relatively pronounced border is present in the skin.[21] Support for this concept may be found in a study of eight patients with afibrinogenemia who had no induration, but had normal kinetics, intensity of erythema, and diameter during the delayed-type hypersensitivity response to a variety of skin test antigens.[23]

Due to the possibility of several types of reactions, Duboczy recommends that for the most accurate reading, an assessment of the reaction be made at 24 and 48 h.[12] For practical purposes, a patient should return for a reading once only, but should be questioned about the course of the reaction.

C. MULTIPLE PUNCTURE TESTS

Tuberculosis skin tests have been administered with multiple puncture techniques employing both old tuberculin and PPD, but these techniques should not be used to guide treatment decisions, unless there is vesiculation. Vesiculation is considered a positive reaction, and it is the only reaction that may be interpreted. In 3 studies, the multiple puncture test, in comparison with the Mantoux test, did not achieve 100% sensitivity, even where the antigen was PPD and the cutting point was 1 mm.[23a,23b,23c] The range in these 3 studies was 96 to 99% sensitivity; the specificity was poor. Although, in general, a completely negative PPD multiple puncture test without any erythema or induration usually indicates that the Mantoux will be negative, this never has been proven. Multiple puncture tests never should be used in adults, and, although they are easy to place in infants and small children, Starke has stated that the intradermal Mantoux is the only test that should be used (see Chapter 8, this volume). He also states that multiple puncture tests are absolutely contraindicated in infants or children who have had the BCG vaccine, are close contacts of infectious cases, are ill, or are in high risk groups.

D. FALSE-POSITIVE TESTS

The greatest concern with false-positive tests centers on the incidence of cross-reactivity with atypical mycobacteria. The mode for the diameter of induration in persons infected with tuberculosis appears to be at 16–17 mm,[3] with means in various groups ranging from 12.8 to 18.8 mm.[4] The mean induration to PPD-S after exposure to nontuberculous mycobacteria has been estimated to be 8 mm with very few reactions at 15 mm.[24] Therefore a cutting point of 15 mm of induration will eliminate cross-reactivity almost completely, but will decrease sensitivity. A cutting point of 5 mm will yield much more cross-reactivity, but will

Table 13-1 **Factors causing decreased ability to respond to tuberculin**[a]

Factors related to the person being tested
    Infections
            Viral (measles, mumps, chicken pox)
            Bacterial (typhoid fever, brucellosis, typhus, leprosy, pertussis, overwhelming
               tuberculosis, tuberculous pleurisy)
            Fungal (South American blastomycosis)
    Live virus vaccinations (measles, mumps, polio)
    Metabolic derangements (chronic renal failure)
    Nutritional factors (severe protein depletion)
    Diseases affecting lymphoid organs (Hodgkin's disease, lymphoma, chronic lymphocytic
     leukemia, sarcoidosis)
    Drugs (corticosteroids and other immunosuppressive agents)
    Age (newborns, elderly patients with "waned" sensitivity)
    Recent or overwhelming infection with *M. tuberculosis*
    Stress (surgery, burns, mental illness, graft-versus-host reactions)
Factors related to the tuberculin used
    Improper storage (exposure to light and heat)
    Improper dilutions
    Chemical denaturation
    Contamination
    Adsorption (partially controlled by adding Tween® 80)
Factors related to the method of administration
    Injection of too little antigen
    Delayed administration after drawing into syringe
    Injection too deep
Factors related to reading the test and recording results
    Inexperienced reader
    Conscious or unconscious bias
    Error in recording

[a] From American Thoracic Society/Centers for Disease Control.[6]

enhance the sensitivity markedly.[3] The cutting point in a particular region of the country may be modified by knowledge of the prevalence of atypical mycobacteria versus the prevalence of tuberculosis disease in that region.[6]

E. BOOSTER PHENOMENON

Any PPD-reactive individual may lose skin test reactivity,[25] and persons over 55 years of age are particularly susceptible to this loss.[6,26] The booster phenomenon refers to the ability of a negative tuberculin skin test to reactivate the immune response in a previously infected person and cause a subsequent skin test to become positive.[27] PPD in standard doses cannot cause systemic sensitization. Thus, a boosted skin test represents true infection. The elderly in nursing homes, who require yearly skin test screening, are particularly prone to this phenomenon.[26,28] The prevalence of the booster phenomenon has been reported as high as 15% in elderly persons with an initially negative PPD.[22] If a second test is placed 1 year after the first in a PPD-negative individual who has a history of tuberculous infection, it might appear as if the individual is a new convertor. Therefore,

all individuals undergoing repeated yearly skin tests should anticipate a two-step procedure,[6] as well as all individuals with diminished immune responses. In persons whose first test is read negative, a second test should be performed 1 week after placement of the first test. The reading of the second test is the final result.

A third sequential skin test also has been shown to add to the overall rate of tuberculin positivity. Gordin et al. showed that of 1726 elderly persons, 477 (28%) were positive to a first test, 158 (9%) were positive to a second test, and 67 (4%) were positive to a third test.[29] However, at this time, three-step testing is not recommended due to problems with the reproducibility, and therefore validity, of boosted reactions that are less than 15 mm in diameter.[30]

F. ANERGY

False negative tests may be due to a host of causes (Table 13-1). An addition to Table 13-1 should be clotting function abnormalities such as those found in persons with congenital afibrinogenemia, disseminated intravascular coagulation, hepatic failure, or in persons on anticoagulants such as

Table 13-2 **Indications for skin test screening**[a]

1. Persons with signs and/or symptoms suggestive of tuberculous disease
2. Recent contacts of persons known or suspected to have tuberculosis
3. Persons with undiagnosed upper lobe fibrotic lesions
4. Persons with HIV infection
5. Alcoholics and intravenous drug abusers
6. Persons with medical conditions known to increase the risk of disease if infection has occurred, i.e., silicosis, gastrectomy, jejunoileal bypass, weight at or below 90% of ideal body weight, chronic renal failure, diabetes mellitus, high dose corticosteroid treatment or other stronger immunosuppressive therapy, some hematologic disorders such as leukemia or lymphoma, other malignancies
7. Groups at high risk of infection with tuberculosis: foreign born persons from Asia, Africa, Latin America, Oceania, and certain Caribbean countries; medically underserved low-income populations including high-risk racial or ethnic minority populations (e.g., blacks, Hispanics, native Americans); residents of long-term care facilities (e.g., correctional institutions, mental institutions, and nursing homes)
8. Groups that would pose a significant risk to others if diseased: employees of health care facilities, schools, and child care facilities

[a] Adapted from American Thoracic Society/Centers for Disease Control,[6] American Thoracic Society,[37] and Centers for Disease Conrol.[38]

coumarin or heparin. The reduction or absence of induration is due to the lack of the special fibrin gel network mentioned earlier.

Even if none of these causes is present, 17.4 to 21.0% of patients with tuberculosis had less than 5 mm of induration response to 5 TU of PPD in 3 studies,[31-33] and 19.1 to 24.5% had less than 10 mm of induration in 3 studies.[31,32,34] Nash and Douglass found 49 (24.5%) of 200 patients with active pulmonary tuberculosis who had less than 10 mm of induration response to 5 TU of PPD, and 16 (8%) who also were negative to 250 TU PPD (<10 mm), with positive control antigens.[34] Rooney et al. showed that 16 (76%) of 21 tuberculosis patients with an initially negative response to PPD (with Tween[R]) became reactive (induration of 5 mm or greater) after 2 weeks of treatment and nutritional support.[32] There are several proposed pathophysiologic mechanisms of skin test anergy in otherwise healthy hosts with tuberculosis. These include the lack of available circulating lymphocytes due to disease elsewhere, desensitization by the antigenic load, the presence of an abnormally high number of T suppressor cells at the skin test site, or the presence of supressor adherent cells (see Chapter 2, this volume).

Anergy testing may be performed with injections of candida antigen, mumps antigen, trichophyton antigen, diluted tetanus toxoid, streptokinase/streptodornase antigen, or the multiple puncture Multitest[R] (tetanus toxoid antigen, diphtheria toxoid antigen, streptococcus antigen, old tuberculin, candida antigen, trichophyton antigen, proteus antigen, and a glycerine control). The Multitest[R] does not deliver a standard amount of antigen.

Furthermore, it does not contain mumps antigen. The Centers for Disease Control and Prevention recommend that at least two separate injectable antigens to which most healthy persons in the population would be sensitized, be used in anergy testing.[35] In one study that compared injections of tetanus toxoid, candida, mumps, and trichophyton in HIV-positive individuals, persons with more than 800 CD4 cells reacted most often to tetanus (88.5%), and those with 200 CD4 cells or less reacted most often to mumps (21.3%).[36] HIV-related anergy will be discussed below in Section VI.C.

IV. SCREENING

The American Thoracic Society (ATS) and the Centers for Disease Control (CDC) along with the American Academy of Pediatrics and the Infectious Disease Society of America recently published indications for tuberculosis screening with tuberculin skin testing.[6,37,38] These indications may be found in Table 13-2. In addition to the recent attention to screening in HIV-positive individuals, the CDC has focused specifically on screening in at-risk minority populations,[39] homeless persons,[40] migrant farm workers,[41] and foreign-born persons entering the United States.[42] Although not listed, potential organ donors also should be screened because of the risk to a recipient that a dormant infection in an organ might pose.

Other groups, not mentioned specifically, that have been reported to have an increased risk of exposure or have an increased association with tuberculosis include pulmonary fellows,[43] other physicians and medical students,[44] and certain HLA phenotypes.[45]

Table 13-3 **Infection and treatment**[a]

Induration	Groups in Whom Infection Is Presumed to Be Present at the Specified Degree of Induration	Treatment[b]
<5 mm	Adolescents and children who are close contacts	Treat until 12 weeks after last exposure, at which time skin test is repeated
≥5 mm	Close contacts	Treat all ages for 6–12 months
	HIV+, or unknown status at risk	Treat all ages for 12 months
	Upper lobe fibrotic lesion	Treat all ages for 12 months if not previously treated. Four months of multidrug chemotherapy also is acceptable
≥10 mm	Silicosis	Treat all ages for 12 months if not previously treated. Four months of multidrug chemotherapy also is acceptable
	High incidence or risk to others (see Table 13-2: numbers 7 and 8, and text)	Treat age <35 for 6–12 months
	IVDA (HIV negative)	Treat all ages for 6–12 months
≥10 mm	Medical risk (see Table 13-2: number 6, and text; exclude silicosis, which now is considered separately, see above)	Treat all ages for 6–12 months (12 months in persons who are immunocompromised)
≥15 mm[c]	Low risk	Treat age <35 for 6–12 months
10 mm increase over a 2-year period for age <35, or skin test induration ≥10 mm in a person <4 years of age, regardless of previous test results	Recent convertor	Treat for 6–12 months; treat for 9 months in infants and children
15 mm increase over a 2-year period for age ≥35[c]	Recent convertor	Treat for 6–12 months

[a] Adapted from American Thoracic Society,[37] Centers for Disease Control,[48] and American Thoracic Society/Centers for Disease Control.[49]

[b] Isoniazid 300 mg per day, or 15 mg/kg, up to 900 mg, twice weekly.

[c] The degree of induration that is accepted as a positive result may be modified based on regional factors such as the risk of atypical mycobacterial infections and the risk of actual tuberculous infection. In areas where the risk of actual tuberculous infection far exceeds the risk of atypical infection, such as New York City, the degree of induration that is accepted as positive should be 10 mm (see text for details).

In addition, pet dogs and cats in close contact with a tuberculous case should be screened. Although there have been no reported cases of transmission from pet to human, it certainly is possible that this might occur, as organisms have been recovered from laryngeal swabs of pet dogs, and fulminant lung lesions have been documented. Dogs react well to tuberculin and cats do not, but skin testing is not considered reliable in either and a chest radiograph should be performed. Preventive therapy in exposed nondiseased animals is recommended by some regardless of skin test status. Treatment of disease is very successful with current regimens.[46,47]

V. INTERPRETATION

Once these individuals have been screened, those with a positive test based on the cutting points listed in Table 13-3 should be questioned and examined for signs and symptoms of tuberculosis and should have a chest radiograph performed.

The new cutting points for PPD positivity in terms of induration are based on the probability of exposure to tuberculous vs. nontuberculous mycobacteria, as well as the relative risk and morbidity of developing tuberculosis once exposed. Therefore one accepts a lesser degree of induration in groups not exposed to atypical mycobacteria, in groups more likely to have been exposed or more likely to spread typical tuberculosis, and in groups at high medical and socioeconomic risk. The groups assumed to be infected with *M. tuberculosis* for the specified degree of induration, who may require chemoprophylaxis, are noted in Table 13-3.[6,37,48,49]

Vesiculation indicates that the test is positive regardless of the degree of induration or the method of placement (i.e., multiple puncture or intradermal). Treatment should be administered accordingly.

Other factors that may merit specific consideration at 10 mm but are not mentioned specifically in the official statements are radiation therapy to the lung,[50,51] alcoholism,[52] and collagen vascular diseases such as systemic lupus erythematosus,[53] although it is difficult to separate the immunosuppressive effects of treatment from the actual disease. It should be noted that the actual effect of these risk factors on the subsequent development of tuberculosis in PPD-positive individuals has never been studied in a controlled fashion.

VI. CHEMOPROPHYLAXIS

Strictly speaking, the therapy we call "chemoprophylaxis" is actually treatment of infection.[54] The burden of organisms in tuberculous infection is low, and thus the development of resistance is not a major problem. Therefore, single-drug therapy with isoniazid represents an adequate course, and combination therapy might be even more effective. To truly eradicate tuberculosis worldwide, we must make an attempt to treat tuberculous infection, much the same way that we attempt to eradicate the treponeme in the "dormant" phase of syphilis. Safer and more potent drugs, as well as shorter durations of therapy, will be crucial aspects of this attempt. The term "chemoprophylaxis" should be reserved for the initial treatment after exposure to tuberculosis. It represents an attempt to prevent tuberculosis from infecting the individual, which is part of the purpose for beginning therapy immediately in exposed children and adolescents. However, for the purposes of this chapter, the term "chemoprophylaxis" will be used in the standard fashion.

The current recommendations for chemoprophylactic treatment are found in Table 13-3, adapted from the recommendations of the ATS and CDC.[37,48,49] Twelve months of isoniazid, 300 mg per day, is recommended for tuberculin-positive individuals who are HIV positive or have stable fibrotic lesions or silicosis. Other groups should receive a minimum of 6 months of therapy, although 1 year with compliance is preferable. The groups with no risk factors and groups who have a high incidence of disease should not be treated past 35 years of age. For high-risk individuals who are likely to be noncompliant, directly observed isoniazid given twice a week in a dose of 15 mg/kg should be considered, up to a total of 900 mg per dose.[48,49] Four months of multidrug therapy is an alternative mode of therapy for PPD-positive individuals with fibrotic or silicotic lesions. This will be addressed further below.

Persons with a history of tuberculous disease who were not treated with an adequate course of chemotherapy and do not have active disease presently should receive 1 year of isoniazid. This includes persons treated with surgical techniques before the introduction of adequate chemotherapeutic regimens.

The decision to treat these presumed tuberculous infections with isoniazid should be based on the ability of isoniazid to reduce the rate of development of active disease, and the relative benefit of this reduction versus the risk of isoniazid hepatitis. The reduction in active cases has been shown clearly for infected close contacts and persons with fibrotic lesions (see later). However, strong data for other groups are lacking, and they are represented by merit of their association with an increased incidence of tuberculous disease. Foreign-born individuals have an increased risk of previous exposure to tuberculosis but not necessarily an increased risk of development of tuberculosis once infected. The medical risk groups contain subsets almost surely at increased risk, but these have not been studied in a well-controlled fashion and have not been shown clearly to obtain the same benefit from isoniazid prophylaxis as other groups. Some of the pertinent data follow.

A. CLOSE CONTACTS AND RECENT CONVERTORS

The American Thoracic Society and the Centers for Disease Control and Prevention recommend that children and adolescents who have been close contacts of infectious persons within the past 3 months and have negative skin tests should receive isoniazid until at least 12 weeks after the last contact with the infectious source, at which time the skin test should be repeated.[48,49] If the repeat skin test is positive (5 mm or greater), therapy should be continued. These youngsters are at high risk for developing both infection and disease, and the opportunity to eradicate the organism at this stage, or to prevent infection, is one that should not be missed. Prophylaxis of HIV-positive anergic close contacts is addressed in the section on anergic HIV-positive individuals.

Before the acquired immunodeficiency syndrome (AIDS) crisis, the highest rate of development of disease from infection was in new-convertor, close contacts. In the United States Public Health Service (USPHS) trials, Ferebee found that there were 867 household contacts who were initially negative and converted to positive (5 mm or greater) within the first year.[54] Of those, 17 (2.0%) developed tuberculosis during the first year and 32 (3.7%) developed tuberculosis during the first 10 years (see Table 13-4). This rate of disease was higher than in those who initially were skin test positive at 10 mm. Experimental data to support the immediate use of isoniazid may be found in studies of guinea pigs inoculated intraperitoneally with high doses of tuberculous organisms and treated immediately with isoniazid to prevent skin test conversion or facilitate skin test reversion.[55] Clinical studies also have addressed reversion rates. Grzybowski and Allen showed the rate of reversion to be 22% in a young treated population (0 to 19 years).[56] Dahlstrom et al. found a 15% reversion rate in children on isoniazid for 1 year vs. a 3.6% reversion rate in controls.[57] In the USPHS trial, there were an equivalent amount of reverters in the placebo group (6.5%) and the isoniazid group (7.9%), suggesting little effect of isoniazid on the early eradication of organisms.[54] However, Houk et al., in a well-designed study, showed a dramatic, 89%, reversion rate in 179 naval personnel on isoniazid.[58] They showed clearly that this effect was related to the speed with which chemoprophylaxis was initiated after infection, with 100% reversion rates in persons started within 3 months, with most reversions occurring after only 3 months of therapy. There were no reversions in controls known to be PPD positive for at least 1 year. This study was important because the infections occurred aboard a ship with one primary source case, and allowed for relatively accurate timing of exposure and infection.

Close contacts who already have converted their skin tests (i.e., 5 mm or greater) also are at high risk for the development of tuberculosis disease, with the highest rate in the first year. Ferebee, in a review of chemoprophylaxis trials, described the rate of development of disease in the first year to be between 0.6 and 7.5% of those infected,[54] with a 75% reduction in new cases by the second year. Data from the USPHS trials of household contacts show that the risk of disease in the United States appears to be less than that in other countries. This may be explained by the increased intensity and duration of exposure of persons in developing countries. In fact, Grzybowski et al. have shown that persons exposed to a high bacillary load not only are at greater risk for developing infection, but also are at greater risk of developing disease once infected.[59]

The USPHS trials evaluated 27,847 household contacts of persons with active tuberculosis.[54] Subjects were randomized to isoniazid or placebo. Data for the convertors are presented in Table 13-4. As mentioned earlier, those persons who converted at 5 mm by the end of the first year of observation were at the highest risk for developing tuberculosis. Initial reactions of 10 mm or more were next highest, followed by initial reactions of 5 mm or more, and less than 10 mm. Overall, the reduction of risk with isoniazid prophylaxis was 60–70%, but it varied widely between groups. The group of household contacts who took at least 80% of their pills for a period of at least 10 months enjoyed a 68% reduction in cases of tuberculosis over a 10-year period (88% during the treatment year and 60% in posttreatment years). These data show clearly the increased risk of development of tuberculosis in close contacts, even at 5 mm induration, and support the use of isoniazid prophylaxis in close contacts at this level of induration. The protective effect of isoniazid is thought to continue even after the therapy ceases.[60]

The category of "recent convertors" comprises those persons with a positive skin test who are not known close contacts and who had a negative skin test within the preceding 2 years. They are not considered to be at the same high risk as are close contacts. Their initial inoculum probably is smaller, and the time of exposure usually is remote in comparison with close contacts. Therefore the cutting point for treatment in this group is an increase of 10 mm or greater for those less than 35 years old, and an increase of 15 mm or greater for those 35 years of age and older. However, serious consideration should be given to the use of 10 mm in all persons who live in high-risk areas, as noted above.

Infants and children less than 4 years old are considered positive if their skin test induration is 10 mm or greater because of their high risk of fulminant disease and the assumption that they probably are recent convertors.

B. FIBROTIC LESIONS AND SILICOSIS
1. Fibrotic Lesions
Stable upper lobe fibrotic lesions associated with a positive PPD (i.e., 5 mm or greater) are assumed to be tubercular and are at increased risk for reactivation. Persons with such lesions have been shown to benefit from isoniazid prophylaxis. The largest study involved 27,830 persons from Eastern Europe and

was performed by the International Union Against Tuberculosis.[61] The entry criteria included a PPD skin test reaction larger than 5 mm with a radiograph that showed "well delineated lesions of probable tuberculous origin, usually in the upper half of the lung, which had been stable during the year prior to entry."[62] There were four treatment groups: placebo, 12 weeks of isoniazid, 24 weeks of isoniazid, and 52 weeks of isoniazid. Lesions were categorized in 67% of persons as less than 2 cm², and in 30% of persons as 2 cm² or greater. Active tuberculosis was defined as a culture-positive case. The rate of development of tuberculosis in the placebo group during the first year was 0.4%, and during the first 5 years was 1.4%. Persons receiving 12 weeks of isoniazid showed a 21% reduction in cases, those receiving 24 weeks showed a 65% reduction, and those receiving 52 weeks showed a 75% reduction. However, when these data were analyzed for those who actually completed treatment, persons on 24 weeks of treatment showed a 69% reduction and those on 52 weeks of treatment showed a 93% reduction. Lesion size also appeared to influence outcome. Lesions 2 cm² or larger reactivated at a greater frequency and clearly benefited additionally from a full 52-week course of isoniazid. Compliant patients with lesions less than 2 cm² also benefited from a full 52-week course of therapy.

Snider et al., in their cost-effective analysis of the International Union Against Tuberculosis fibrotic lesion study, showed that a 24-week regimen was, overall, the most cost-effective choice for fibrotic lesions.[63] However, this study was based on all entrants, including noncompleters of therapy. The Centers for Disease Control[48] recommended a full year of isoniazid therapy for fibrotic lesions, probably due to the additional benefit gained for persons with larger lesions, and persons who were compliant with therapy.

Other studies also have shown the benefit of treating fibrotic lesions. Falk and Fuchs, in a Veteran's Administration Cooperative Study, found administration of isoniazid to be beneficial for persons with fibrotic lesions who had not been previously treated, but not beneficial for those who had been previously treated.[64] Katz et al. also found isoniazid to be beneficial.[65] Grzybowski et al. had success with isoniazid prophylaxis, and even greater success with isoniazid plus PAS.[66] Prolongation of therapy beyond 1 year did not appear to improve results.

Ferebee reviewed the USPHS data on 1 year of isoniazid prophylaxis for fibrotic lesions in three groups: persons in whom inactive untreated fibrotic lesions were discovered, persons in whom previously active tuberculosis had never been treated, and persons in whom previously active tuberculosis had been treated.[54] For the first group of untreated never-active fibrotic lesions, the rate of reactivation during the first year was 1.9% and the rate over 5 years was 6.9%, with a 63% overall reduction noted with isoniazid prophylaxis. For the second group of previously active but untreated cases, the rate of reactivation during the first year was 1.4%, and the rate over 5 years was 4.9%, with a 51% reduction noted with isoniazid prophylaxis. For the third group of previously treated, previously active tuberculosis, the rate of reactivation during the first year was 1.2%, and the rate over 5 years was 3.3%, with only a 17% reduction noted with isoniazid prophylaxis.

These data show clearly the benefit of prophylaxis in inactive untreated fibrotic lesions, as well as in old untreated tuberculosis, and support the use of 1 year of prophylactic isoniazid. There is little benefit in the use of prophylactic isoniazid in persons who were treated previously.

The latest recommendations suggest that fibrotic lesions in persons with tuberculous infection be treated with 4 months of multidrug therapy as outlined in Chapter 6 (this volume). This is based on the fact that initially one may not be able to distinguish between active and inactive disease, and, thus, it would not be unreasonable to start a patient on multidrug chemotherapy. After 2 months of therapy, when the cultures are reported negative, an additional 2 months of therapy would complete the recommended course of therapy for smear-negative, culture-negative pulmonary tuberculosis,[49] which is thought to be equivalent to or better than 1 year of isoniazid prophylaxis. In fact, any time an infiltrate is presumed to be tuberculous in a skin test-positive individual, and standard therapy for tuberculosis is started, that therapy should be continued for a total of 4 months in persons who meet the criteria for prophylaxis, even if the etiology of the infiltrate is proven to be nonmycobacterial.[49] This 4-month regimen in such individuals will serve as prophylaxis. In areas where the rate of primary isoniazid resistance is less than 4%, 4 months of isoniazid and rifampin therapy is considered adequate.[49]

2. Silicosis

A similar rationale as that noted for fibrotic lesions applies to the treatment of tuberculin-positive (i.e., induration at 10 mm or greater) individuals with silicosis. Persons with silicosis appear to be at greatly increased risk for the development of tuberculosis. There are numerous cross-sectional and retrospective studies that show an increased rate of tuberculosis in silicotics (as high as 43% in a past study).[67] More recently, Burke et al. demonstrated

Table 13-4   **Risk of tuberculosis in close contacts: percentage reduction with isoniazid**[a]

Induration	N	Risk of TB (First Year) [N (%)]	Risk of TB (10 Years) [N (%)]
5–9 mm			
Placebo	1616	8 (0.5)	31 (1.9)
Isoniazid	1716	3 (0.2)	18 (1.0)
Reduction (%)		65	45
≥10 mm			
Placebo	4992	61 (1.2)	147 (2.9)
Isoniazid	4852	12 (0.2)	57 (1.2)
Reduction (%)		80	60
<5 mm initially ≥5 mm at 1 year			
Placebo	867	17 (2.0)	32 (3.7)
Isoniazid	694	4 (0.6)	10 (1.4)
Reduction (%)		71	61

[a] Adapted from Ferebee.[54]

that tuberculosis case-finding remained very effective among silicotic individuals. In their study in Oklahoma of former miners older than 50 years of age, 8 (1.1%/year) of 367 persons developed culture-positive tuberculosis over a period of 2 years. Approximately one-third of the study group was silicotic.[68] Paul, in a 10-year survey in Rhodesian copper miners, showed that there was a 26-fold increase in tuberculosis in silicotic (2.89% per year) vs. nonsilicotic (0.11% per year) miners.[69] Westerholm et al. similarly have shown, in a 10-year retrospective survey of miners and foundry workers, a 33-fold increase in tuberculosis in silicotic cases (0.41% per year) vs. exposed miners without silicosis (0.012% per year).[70] There are conflicts concerning the benefit of isoniazid prophylaxis, but in one unpublished study there was a 50% reduction in tuberculosis in silicotics with the use of isoniazid vs. placebo.[67] Another study[71] showed a 93% reduction in cases, but it was flawed seriously by the inclusion of persons who already have been shown clearly to benefit from prophylaxis, i.e., new convertors, old untreated tuberculosis, and close contacts of diseased persons. There was no separation of these cases in the analysis. However, in view of the extent of the association of tuberculosis and silicosis, the experimental evidence that shows the potentiation of tuberculous growth by silica,[72] and the studies that suggest that isoniazid may be beneficial, 12 months of chemoprophylaxis is recommended in cases of tuberculous infection in silicotics. As noted with fibrotic lesions, it may be difficult to distinguish between active and inactive disease in tuberculous-infected individuals with silicosis. Thus, 4 months

of multidrug chemotherapy in such individuals who are shown to be culture negative is not an unreasonable alternative,[49] and the process is treated as if it were smear-negative, culture-negative pulmonary tuberculosis (see Table 6-4 in Chapter 6 of this volume). In areas where the rate of primary isoniazid resistance is less than 4%, 4 months of isoniazid and rifampin therapy is considered adequate.[49]

C. HIV-INFECTED INDIVIDUALS AND UNTESTED HIGH-RISK INDIVIDUALS

HIV infection has been shown clearly to increase the risk of developing active tuberculosis. National registry matching showed that 4% of AIDS cases also appeared on the tuberculosis registries.[73] The most convincing study of risk was performed by Selwyn et al. on 513 intravenous drug abusers, without a history of tuberculosis, who were enrolled in methadone maintenance programs in The Bronx, New York City. Seven (14.3%) of 49 HIV-positive, PPD-positive subjects with induration of 10 mm or greater developed active tuberculosis over an average of 21 months of follow-up. The risk of reactivation was estimated to be 7.9% per year.[74] This is the largest yearly risk described in the United States in recent times. There was one case (0.6%) of tuberculosis in 166 HIV-positive, PPD-negative subjects, and there were no cases in 236 HIV-negative subjects. All seven cases of tuberculosis in the HIV-positive, PPD-positive group occurred among the 36 persons who did not receive isoniazid prophylaxis either before or during the study. Because of these data, and the fact that asymptomatic HIV-positive persons may have a less vigorous response to PPD, isoniazid is recommended for a period of 1 year in persons with a skin test reaction size of 5 mm or greater. Since that time, Moreno et al. studied 84 HIV-positive, PPD-positive (5 mm or greater) individuals in Spain who had not received isoniazid and found that there were 10.4 cases of tuberculosis per 100-person-years during a mean follow-up of 26 months.[74a] This contrasted with 5.4 cases of tuberculosis per 100-person-years in 151 HIV-positive, PPD-negative, nonanergic individuals. The use of isoniazid for 9 to 12 months during the study period was reviewed in 24 patients with previously positive PPDs and in 13 patients whose PPDs converted from negative to positive during the study period. There was only 1 (3.7%) case of tuberculosis in the 27 HIV-positive, PPD-positive patients who received isoniazid vs. 29 (31%) cases of tuberculosis in 94 HIV-positive, PPD-positive patients who did not receive isoniazid. Moreno et al. also studied an anergic HIV-positive subset that will be discussed later. Pape et al[74b] studied 38 HIV-positive, PPD-positive (5 mm or greater) patients treated with isoniazid for 1 year and showed that the incidence per 100-person-years of tuberculosis in the 38 isoniazid-treated patients vs. the 25 control patients was 1.7 vs. 10.0, respectively. The reduction in tuberculosis cases with isoniazid was 83%. These data support the use of isoniazid for 1 year and, at the current time, there are no well-controlled studies to support the use of isoniazid for more than 1 year.

The management of anergic HIV-positive individuals is more difficult. Jordan et al.[75] performed a decision analysis for HIV-positive anergic drug abusers and, with a very conservative model, showed that isoniazid was justified where the infection rate was greater than 11–17% in black females, and 3–8% in all other groups. Selwyn et al.,[76] in a later study, showed that tuberculosis developed in 5 (7.6%) of 68 HIV-positive, anergic subjects over a period of 31 months, or 6.6 cases per 100 person-years of follow-up (95% confidence interval, 2.1–15.3). None of 18 HIV-negative anergic subjects developed tuberculosis. Moreno et al. studied 112 anergic HIV-positive individuals and found 20 (18%) cases of active tuberculosis (12.4 cases per 100-person-years) during a mean follow-up of 26 months.[74a] This was equivalent to the rate in the HIV-positive, PPD-positive individuals (see above).

The new CDC recommendation states that preventive therapy should be considered for HIV-positive anergic persons who either are known contacts of infectious tuberculous patients or are persons from groups in which the prevalence of tuberculous infection (i.e., a positive skin test) is 10% or greater, which, in the United States, might include intravenous drug abusers, prisoners, homeless persons, migrant laborers, and persons born in countries in Asia, Africa, Latin America, Oceania, and certain Caribbean countries with high rates of tuberculosis.[35,49] Each city or state must document the skin test-positive rates of each of these groups in their region through intensive screening. One also might consider therapy in a person exposed in the past to an infectious family member, where the exposed individual was not skin tested and evaluated for prophylaxis subsequently. Extreme caution should be exercised where black and Hispanic females, especially those who are postpartum, are treated, and there are those who believe that the threshold of 10% should be raised in black females because of the higher incidence of isoniazid fatalities.[75]

D. HIV-NEGATIVE INTRAVENOUS DRUG ABUSERS (IVDA)

HIV-negative intravenous drug abusers specifically have been shown to have an increased prevalence of tuberculous infection and disease.[78] They have an increased risk of exposure to tuberculosis, and it has been implied that they have a higher risk of developing disease once infected,[48] although this has never been proven. They certainly are at risk for contracting the AIDS virus and, for the above reasons, are targeted for chemoprophylaxis at 10 mm of induration, regardless of age.

E. GROUPS WITH HIGH RISK OF EXPOSURE

Groups clearly at an increased risk for exposure are delineated earlier in the section on screening. There are abundant data to show that foreign-born persons,[42,79,80] migrant workers,[41] Blacks,[39,81,82] Hispanics,[39,83] native Americans and Inuits,[39,84,85] persons of low socioeconomic status,[40,86-89] prisoners,[90,91] the elderly in nursing homes,[28,92] and physicians and other hospital employees[43,44,93] have an increased prevalence of tuberculous disease. However, there are no controlled data to support the contention that any of these groups is at an increased risk of developing tuberculosis once infected, although there is evidence that Blacks may be more susceptible to the organism.[82] These persons at increased risk for exposure are targeted for prophylaxis at 10 mm induration primarily because the probability of true infection with *M. tuberculosis* is higher than that of the general population, and because the eradication of tuberculosis in the United States depends in a large part on the management of infection in these groups.

Foreign-born individuals have been targeted specifically due to the fact that 22% of all United States tuberculosis cases from 1986 to 1989 occurred in such persons. Furthermore, a majority of these cases occurred within 5 years of entrance into the United States.[42] Therefore assurance of screening and treatment programs for immigrants is a high priority.[52]

F. MEDICAL RISK FACTORS

The groups at medical risk are considered more susceptible to the development of tuberculosis once infected (i.e., skin test induration of 10 mm or greater). There are no well-designed large scale studies such as USPHS trials or the International Union Against Tuberculosis trial to substantiate this claim or to show the benefit of isoniazid use. However, there are smaller studies to suggest that these risk factors are valid, and there is little disagreement that certain conditions predispose infected persons to disease. These data will be discussed as follows. Silicosis, previously addressed in this section, now is handled separately (see Section VI.B.2).

1. Clinical Situations Associated with Substantial Rapid Weight Loss or Chronic Undernutrition

Infected persons with weight loss who are post-gastrectomy, have chronic peptic ulcer disease, have had intestinal bypass for obesity, have chronic malabsorption syndromes, are alcoholics, or have carcinomas of the oropharynx or upper gastrointestinal tract that prevent adequate nutritional intake, all are considered to be at risk for reactivation tuberculosis.

a. Chronic Peptic Ulcer Disease/ Postgastrectomy

Thorn et al. evaluated 955 patients with peptic ulcer disease who underwent gastrectomy and were followed for an average of 4 years.[94] A preoperative radiograph was performed in 809 persons, and was abnormal in 60. Eight of these 60 people with abnormal results were found to have active tuberculosis on entry, and an additional 14 developed active pulmonary tuberculosis after gastrectomy. Further analysis focused on 616 males who had normal preoperative radiographs, 14 (2.3%) of whom subsequently developed active pulmonary tuberculosis. The rate in this group was 0.57% per year, was three times more frequent in gastric ulcers than duodenal ulcers, and was five times more frequent than a comparison group selected from another study. The greatest risk factor was preoperative weight loss as a percentage of ideal body weight. Males at or above 95% of their standard weight had an annual rate of 0.12%, those between 85 and 95% had an annual rate of 0.4%, and those at or below 85% had an annual rate of 1.78%. There was no weight analysis of the patients who were discovered to have active tuberculosis before the operation. On the basis of these data, the authors concluded that the development of tuberculosis was due to severe or long-standing peptic ulcer disease and only secondarily to the effects of the operation. They stated that if the chest radiograph and weight were normal before surgery,

there was no increased risk of developing pulmonary tuberculosis.

Hanngren and Reizenstein reviewed data on 38 patients who developed pulmonary tuberculosis after gastrectomy and found that dumping syndrome with malabsorption and malnutrition was a significant risk factor.[95] Frucht et al., in their study and review, found that weight loss was a major factor, and that active tuberculosis worsened after gastrectomy, but that there was no definite proof that gastrectomy itself led to an increased risk of developing tuberculosis.[96] Numerous other authors have noted the association of gastrectomy and tuberculosis, but Snider points out that a high proportion of those persons studied were older men, alcoholics, or had a low weight/height ratio.[97] He concluded, though, that it is reasonable to use preventive therapy in infected postgastrectomy patients, especially those with weight loss or a malabsorption syndrome.

b. Intestinal Bypass Surgery

Jejunoileal bypass, an operation associated with profound weight loss, also is associated with the development of tuberculosis.[98] In one study, 4 (4%) of 100 patients developed tuberculosis during the first year after surgery.[99] This was a 60-fold increase over the rate in the general population, and others have reported from 27 to 63 times the risk over comparison populations.[98] Furthermore, the rate of extrapulmonary involvement exceeded 80%. Fortunately, it is an extremely rare association, and the operation largely has fallen out of favor.

c. Reduced Weight

Reduced weight, alone, has been mentioned in the past as an indication for prophylactic therapy. This may have been due to reviews of the literature emphasizing weight loss, malnutrition, and body build as risk factors for tuberculosis.[45,100] Snider originally recommended that 85% of ideal body weight be used as a cutoff point.[100] Edwards et al. attributed a 1.5- to 3-fold increase in tuberculosis risk to skin test-positive persons at or below 90% of ideal body weight.[101] However, currently, reduced weight alone, without other risk factors or evidence of malnutrition, is not an indication for prophylactic therapy.

2. Diabetes

Diabetes and tuberculosis have had a very strong historical association.[102] Various studies have shown the strength of this association, but none has evaluated the risk of developing disease once infected. Oscarsson and Silwer noted a fourfold increase in tuberculosis among diabetics in Sweden, with an added risk for younger diabetics or those with severe diabetes.[103] Root found that tuberculosis was 13 to 16 times more common in persons with diabetes who were less than 20 years of age.[102] In 1946, Boucot, in a survey in Philadelphia of 3106 diabetics, estimated an overall twofold increase in the prevalence of tuberculosis in diabetics over the general population.[104] The overall incidence of active tuberculosis was 2.6%. It was higher in diabetics less than 40 years of age (5.3%), and much higher in diabetics less than 40 years of age who had had diabetes for longer than 10 years (17%).

The comparison was not as dramatic in autopsy studies. In 1934, Root summarized the data from numerous autopsy studies and found the incidence of tuberculosis in diabetics to be 28.4%, or 1.2 times that of the general population.[102] Similarly, Kessler, in 1971, analyzed mortality data in 10,066 diabetic patients seen at the Joslin Clinic from 1931 to 1959 and found that tuberculosis contributed to or was a cause of death in 26 (0.26%) patients, or 1.5 times the rate in nondiabetics.[105]

In an analysis of 145 relapses of tuberculosis in New York City in 1967, diabetes was found to be the second most important risk factor and was present in 12 (8.3%) of cases.[106]

Rose et al. performed a decision analysis to assess the utility of isoniazid prophylaxis in PPD-positive diabetics.[107] They estimated the risk of disease to be 1.5 times that of the general infected population based on Kessler's data, and varied the risk from one to fourfold in the sensitivity analysis. They found isoniazid to be beneficial for all persons, but that it added only a few days to the life expectancy. The decision to use isoniazid was considered to be a "toss-up."

More data are necessary to make an informed decision about the prophylaxis of diabetic patients. In the interim, it is probably safe to say that of all diabetics, the younger insulin-dependent diabetics with positive skin tests are at highest risk for the development of tuberculosis, especially those who are controlled poorly.

3. Chronic Renal Failure/Dialysis

Dialysis centers have reported increased rates of tuberculosis, varying from 0.12 to 3% per year.[108-114] In one study, 7 (28%) of 26 patients on chronic dialysis in South Africa developed tuberculosis over a 14-month screening period.[115] The cases may involve extrapulmonary sites in as many as 95% of cases,[114] and often develop insidiously. However many of the cases in these studies occurred in groups with other risk factors. In reviewing three reports from the United States, with a total of 23 cases, there were 6 Asians, 11 Blacks, 1 native American, 1 Hispanic, and 4 Whites.[108,111,112] A study from Canada showed that all tuberculosis in persons with chronic renal failure occurred in persons who had other risks, and that none occurred in white Canadians.[109] A study of 11 cases from a dialysis unit in the United Kingdom showed that all cases were derived from patients born in third-world countries.[110] The results found in these studies at least partially reflect the increased exposure and risk of disease due to causes other than chronic renal failure and dialysis. In fact, Freeman et al. from Iowa stated that no cases of tuberculosis occurred in 327 dialysis patients observed for variable lengths of time after 1964.[116] He stated that a policy of antituberculous prophylaxis was not warranted in his patients. However, a study from Japan in a reportedly homogeneous population showed a 6- to 16-fold increased risk.[114] Furthermore, Andrew et al. showed that the annual case rate of 0.58% per year in their group was four times greater than that of local Filipinos, the ethnic group with the highest rate of tuberculosis in San Francisco.[108] In addition, Cuss et al. stated that the rate of tuberculosis in Afro-Caribbeans and Asians in England was 70 times that of a matched population.[110]

These findings, along with the predominance of extrapulmonary tuberculosis in these studies, the difficulty in arriving at an early diagnosis, and the high death rates in some of these studies, support the use of isoniazid.

Isoniazid is removed by dialysis. Therefore, on dialysis days, persons on chemoprophylaxis should receive their isoniazid following dialysis.

4. Steroids/Immunosuppressives

There are no controlled trials to show that steroids alone predispose infected patients to develop tuberculosis. There are numerous descriptive studies but most are composed of cases where the patient's primary disease also caused immunosuppression (e.g., renal transplantation, systemic lupus erythematosus, rheumatoid arthritis, and sarcoidosis).[117-119] Of interest, in one study, 6 of the 14 cases were diagnosed 3–12 months after the steroids were discontinued.[119] There are two studies that show no risk, but both are limited by inadequate sample size and inadequate follow-up time.[120,121]

The best data on the timing of the immunosuppressive effect come from a study of 70 tuberculin reactors.[122] Each research subject was treated with 40 mg of prednisone per day in four divided doses and underwent a skin test every 72 h. Sixty-eight (97%) of 70 subjects reverted to negative after an average of 14 days. Reconversion to reactivity after the discontinuation of prednisone required an average of 6 days.

Schatz et al. suggested that a daily dose of 15 mg per day or greater was sufficient to cause anergy, although alternate-day dosing was thought to mitigate this effect. In their study, therapy was maintained for a mean of 5 years.[120] This study was limited in that patients read their own skin tests by drawing a circle around the induration, transferring it to tape, and mailing it on a postcard.

Millar and Horne suggested that immunosuppression was present in any person receiving more than 10 mg of prednisolone per day for a prolonged period of time.[118] In their study, immunosuppressive therapy lasted from 6 weeks to 10 years.

The ATS/CDC suggested that the lower limit of risk for tuberculosis begins where prednisone or its equivalent is used at a dose and duration of 15 mg per day for 2 weeks.[49] There are no data to show that this cumulative dose increases the risk of tuberculosis. Nonetheless, the data are more suggestive for doses of prednisone of 40 mg per day for 2 weeks, and certainly for long-term daily steroid use, and for any use of a stronger immunosuppressive agent such as a cancer chemotherapeutic agent or transplant antirejection therapy.

Furthermore, in cases where a patient is receiving a transplant, one must attempt to ascertain, where possible, the tuberculous status of the donor, as there have been reports of transfer of tuberculosis through transplanted organs that have presumably dormant infections.[123-126]

A full 12 months of prophylactic isoniazid therapy is recommended for persons who are immunosuppressed.[49]

5. Malignancy

Malignancies are associated with immunosuppression, weight loss, and the use of immunosuppressive chemotherapeutic agents. Kaplan et al. reviewed 201 cases at Memorial Hospital between 1950 and 1971 and found that the cancers could be divided into three risk groups for tuberculosis. The highest rates were in lung cancer, reticulum cell sarcoma, lymphosarcoma, and Hodgkin's disease, followed closely by head and neck cancer, stomach cancer, acute lymphocytic leukemia, and acute myelocytic leukemia, and lastly by breast, colon, and genitourinary cancer.[127] Another study has shown similar risks, but has ranked some of the cancers differently, giving most weight to head and neck cancer.[128] In both studies, the exposure and infection histories were not known, and the sample sizes were small. Nonetheless there is no dispute that cancer patients who are infected with tuberculosis are at an increased risk of developing active disease as their cancer progresses and their general health deteriorates, especially if their cancers

directly involve the immune system. Therefore, in patients with a positive skin test, isoniazid therapy is recommended for leukemias and lymphomas, and other cancers that affect the reticuloendothelial system, and "other malignancies," which include head and neck cancers, gastric cancers, probably lung cancer, and any cancer associated with profound weight loss and/or immunosuppression.

It also might be wise to use isoniazid prophylaxis in untreated PPD-positive individuals undergoing radiation therapy to the lung, although there are no data that address this issue directly.

A full 12 months of prophylactic isoniazid therapy is recommended in persons who are immunosuppressed.[49]

G. LOW-RISK INDIVIDUALS

Decision analyses have been performed for low-risk individuals with a skin test reading of 10 mm or greater. Taylor et al. and Tsevat et al. did not advocate isoniazid use in persons older than 20 years of age.[129,130] Rose et al. thought that there was sufficient data to support the use of isoniazid in persons up to 80 years of age, although there was an increased incidence of isoniazid hepatitis after 50 years of age.[131] Colice suggested that a policy of isoniazid prophylaxis would be beneficial where the isoniazid case-fatality rate was less than 1% or the tuberculosis case-fatality rate was greater than 6.7%.[132] Jordan et al. performed a decision analysis with specific consideration given to race and gender, due to the varied rates of isoniazid hepatitis and death in different demographic groups.[133] The results of the decision analysis showed that for low-risk reactors, isoniazid was favored for all 20 year olds, all 35 year olds except for black females, and no 50 year olds by a margin of 3–19 days of life; if total deaths were used as the end point, isoniazid was favored for all subgroups except for 50-year-old black females. For high-risk reactors, isoniazid was favored for all subgroups except 50-year-old black females by a margin of 1–44 days. Decisions favoring isoniazid prophylaxis were maintained until the tuberculosis case-fatality rate fell in some subgroups to 4–6%. However, the official recommendations have not changed with regard to the 35-year-old cutoff point.

Recently, the new cutting point in low-risk groups less than 35 years of age was raised to 15 mm,[48,49] especially in areas where there is a high prevalence of infection with atypical mycobacteria.[134] Decision analyses have not addressed specifically the issue of a 15-mm cutting point. However, it might be wise to continue with a cutting point of 10 mm in high-risk areas with a low prevalence of atypical mycobacteria, such as New York City.

VII. MONITORING CHEMOPROPHYLAXIS

Before beginning isoniazid, baseline liver function tests are recommended, but further blood testing in the absence of symptoms and risk factors for hepatitis is not recommended for those less than 35 years of age. For persons greater than 35 years of age, and in persons with preexisting liver disease or active alcoholism, transaminase levels should be obtained periodically along with close monitoring of symptoms. Always question for a history of previous isoniazid treatment and associated reactions, liver disease, other medications, alcohol abuse, evidence of, or risk factors for, peripheral neuropathy, such as might be the case in diabetics, and pregnancy. Pyridoxine at a dose of 25–50 mg daily is recommended in alcoholics, persons with malnutrition from a poor diet or malabsorption, and other persons at risk for peripheral neuropathy. All persons receiving isoniazid should be questioned in person or by telephone, at monthly intervals, about the presence of unexplained anorexia, nausea, vomiting, dark urine, icterus, rash, persistent extremity paresthesias, persistent fatigue, weakness, or fever for more than 3 days, and/or abdominal pain, especially in the right upper quadrant.[49] Isoniazid hepatitis usually is a subclinical chemical hepatitis. When symptoms appear, cessation of the drug is indicated and symptoms usually resolve. There have been idiosyncratic reactions with fulminant hepatic failure, but these are rare. Snider and Caras[135] recently searched multiple data sources to compile 177 isoniazid-related deaths that occurred between the years 1972 and 1988. During this period, there were an estimated 1,084,760 persons who started therapy, 655,867 of whom completed therapy. Of those who completed therapy, 23.2 per 100,000 died. Of 21 postpartum deaths, 8 (38%) were within 1 year of delivery. Isoniazid-completer deaths peaked in 1972 and 1973 at rates of 91.6 and 83.3 per 100,000, respectively, but was much lower during the last 4 years of the study: 7.7, 5.8, 14.0, and 7.1 per 100,000 for years 1985, 1986, 1987, and 1988, respectively. This may give us some reassurance about the dangers of isoniazid prophylaxis.

Hepatitis is an age-related phenomenon, and in a survey by Kopanoff et al., the criteria for hepatitis (usually greater than fivefold transaminase elevations) were met at the following rates: ages 0–20, 0%; ages 20–35, 0.3%; ages 35–50, 1.2%; and ages 50–65, 2.3%.[136] However, one should not be too secure about persons who are less than 20 years old because of a recent report of 8 patients who required liver transplants due to severe isoniazid-associated hepatitis, 3 of whom were less than 20 years old.[136a] The rate was 0.8% for those over 65 years of age, but Stead's rate of 4.4% is considered more accurate.[137] The death rate in the probable cases from the study by Kopanoff et al. was 7.6%, the majority occurring in black females.[136] Hepatitis tends to occur within the first few months of starting therapy. Minor elevations in transaminase levels may occur in 10–20% of persons and is not considered a contraindication to therapy. Fast acetylation no longer is thought to be a major factor in the development of hepatitis.[137a] Where there is close monitoring, most cases of hepatitis resolve with discontinuation of the drug. Alcoholics are at a higher risk for chemical hepatitis, but not necessarily for frank clinical hepatitis.[138] However, black and Hispanic females, especially pregnant and postpartum Hispanics, may be at increased risk for fulminant hepatitis for reasons that are unknown.[136,139,140] Monthly biochemical monitoring is recommended for postpubertal black and Hispanic females.[49]

Even in the absence of clinical hepatitis, strong consideration should be given to the discontinuation of isoniazid when the serum glutamic oxaloacetic transaminase or serum glutamic pyruvate transaminase is three to five times normal. Additional information on isoniazid maybe found in Chapter 11 (this volume).

VIII. RETREATMENT

Once a person has been treated either to prevent or cure tuberculous disease, there are no data to support retreatment with isoniazid should one of the high-risk medical conditions occur, although one should monitor closely persons with old tuberculosis who are profoundly immunosuppressed.

IX. SHORTER COURSES OF CHEMOPROPHYLAXIS

The ATS/CDC already have reduced the duration of chemoprophylaxis by using multidrug chemotherapy in persons with fibrotic lesions or silicosis.[49] There have been recommendations to decrease further the duration of chemoprophylaxis in other groups. On the basis of 2- to 3-month short-course four-drug therapy in Hong Kong in radiologically active, smear-negative, initially culture-negative, tuberculosis,[141] Grosset recommended study of a course of 2–3 months of isoniazid, rifampin, and pyrazinamide.[142] Currently, there are ongoing trials to study the use of 2 months of rifampin and pyrazinamide.

X. EXOGENOUS REINFECTION

Exogenous reinfection may occur in persons with waning immunity to tuberculosis. It is more likely that if immunity wanes, patients will be reinfected endogenously by their own organisms.[143] However, if the primary infection has been eradicated, or has been encapsulated with little or no contact with the immune system, and the PPD has reverted only to convert again with a new close exposure, isoniazid prophylaxis probably is wise. Such exogenous reinfection has been documented by Nardell et al. in four cases at a Boston shelter.[144] Furthermore, Small et al. recently reported four patients with advanced HIV infection and drug-sensitive tuberculosis who were reinfected with a new resistant strain (documented by RFLP) during therapy for active tuberculosis.[145]

XI. CONTACTS OF DRUG-RESISTANT CASES

Contacts of isoniazid-resistant cases will not benefit from isoniazid prophylaxis. The ATS/CDC recommends that such persons be treated with rifampin for 6 months with consideration given to adding ethambutol,[49] although some experts might prescribe a full 12 months of therapy.[146] If the source of contact is unclear, and isoniazid resistance is only suspected, isoniazid should be used.

The management of persons exposed to multidrug-resistant (MDR) tuberculosis is more difficult. Recent guidelines have been published by the CDC.[147] Close contacts, as well as casual contacts who are HIV positive, must receive prophylaxis. If the strain is not 100% isoniazid resistant, then isoniazid is the drug of choice. If it is 100% isoniazid resistant, but not 100% rifampin resistant, then rifampin is the drug of choice. If the strain is 100% resistant to both drugs, then the susceptibilities of the source case should be assessed and the following drug combinations may be considered: pyrazinamide and ethambutol, pyrazinamide and ciprofloxacin, pyrazinamide and ofloxacin, and other drugs such as streptomycin, kanamycin, amikacin, and capreomycin. p-Aminosalicylic acid, ethionamide, and cycloserine should not be considered because of the high risk–benefit ratio. Treatment should ensue for at least 6 months, and 12 months in immunocompromised patients. Consideration for beginning treatment in close contacts upon initial exposure, pending the 12-week skin test, also is advised. Therapy may be discontinued if the follow-up skin test is negative. More recent guidelines published by the American Thoracic Society and the Centers for Disease Control and Prevention suggest that ethambutol and pyrazinamide be administered for 6 months, but, if the organism is resistant to ethambutol, pyrazinamide and a quinolone should be used.[49]

It might be prudent to apply the most aggressive therapy to close contacts of MDR cases, regardless of skin test status. This potential epidemic must be controlled by attacking the organism at this early stage.

XII. PREGNANCY AND LACTATION

Women may be tested safely with tuberculin at any time during pregnancy. A reduction in cell-mediated immunity is noted during pregnancy but is not thought to interfere with skin testing.[148] In the past, prophylactic treatment was not recommended during pregnancy unless the patient was a recent convertor or was significantly immunosuppressed.[149] However, currently, if the pregnant woman is likely to have been infected recently or has a high-risk medical condition, especially HIV infection, she should be treated as soon as the infection is documented.[49] Breast-feeding during isoniazid administration is considered safe, if the child is not taking isoniazid also, as less than 20% of an infant's usual dose is consumed daily.[150] However, this decision must be individualized. For further information on these topics, please refer to Chapter 8 (this volume).

XIII. BACILLUS CALMETTE–GUÉRIN (BCG) VACCINATION AND SUBSEQUENT SKIN TESTING

The interpretation of the tuberculin skin test may be difficult in persons who have received BCG. Comstock et al. showed that 8–15 years after BCG vaccination (performed after the age of 5 years), 16% of persons had skin tests greater than 10 mm compared to 2% of controls.[151] Sepulveda et al.[152] showed that the mean tuberculin skin reaction in persons vaccinated three times and tested at least 5 years after the last vaccination correlated with the number of BCG scars: 2.3 mm for no scars, 6.7 mm for 1 scar, 10.9 mm for 2 scars, and 13.2 mm for 3 scars. Menzies et al.[153] evaluated tuberculin reactivity in 1511 school children and young adults in Montreal in whom BCG-V was administered 10–25 years earlier. Among 1041 persons vaccinated once in infancy, 7.9% had significant tuberculin reactions ($\geq$10 mm), and this was not different from controls when adjusted for socioeconomic factors. In subjects vaccinated at age 6 or above, the rate of significant skin test positivity was 25.5%, even 25 years after vaccination, whereas the rate in unvaccinated controls was 4.1%. However, it was also noted, somewhat unexpectedly, that skin test reactivity in persons vaccinated after infancy increased markedly from 11.7 to 28% as the interval from vaccination increased from 10 years to 17 or greater years. This was explained by the difference in age-related exposure rates, but this finding was not seen in the control group. One would expect BCG-related skin test reactivity to wane with time, and thus a concern is raised that the study group may have been more highly exposed to tuberculosis.

Most authorities believe that the BCG effect does not persist past 15 years, especially in persons who receive only one vaccination. It had been stated that if BCG was administered more than 10 years before the PPD skin test, it should not be allowed to influence the interpretation of the skin test.[154] Farer stated that for those persons vaccinated with BCG, the tuberculin test should be placed and the reaction should be interpreted in the usual way.[155] However, it would be wise to remember that BCG alone does cause positive skin tests in a finite percentage of persons, especially those recently vaccinated. The data of Sepulveda et al. and Menzies et al. suggest that skin test positivity may persist in persons vaccinated multiple times, or vaccinated after infancy. Until the ATS reviews this topic again, the current 1990 ATS statement asserts that "it is prudent to consider large reactions to 5 TU of PPD tuberculin in BCG-vaccinated persons as indicating infection with *M. tuberculosis*, especially among persons from countries with a high prevalence of tuberculosis."[6] See Chapter 15 of this volume for more information on BCG.

REFERENCES

1. Siebert, F. B., Glenn, J. T., Tuberculin purified protein derivative: Preparation and analysis of a large quantity for standard, *Am. Rev. Tuberc.*, 44, 9, 1941.
2. Landi, S., Production and standardization of tuberculin, in *The Mycobacteria: A Sourcebook*, Kubica, G. P., Wayne, L. G., Eds., Marcel Dekker, New York, 1984, 505.
3. Comstock, G. W., Daniel, T. M., Snider, D. E., Edwards, P. Q., Hopewell, P. C., Vandiveire, H. M., The tuberculin skin test, *Am. Rev. Resp. Dis.*, 124, 356, 1981.
4. Snider, D. E., The tuberculin skin test, *Am. Rev. Resp. Dis.*, 125, 108, 1982.
5. Guld, J., Bentzon, M. W., Bleiker, M. A., Griep, W. A., Magnusson, M., Waaler, H., Standardization of a new batch of purified tuberculin (PPD) intended for international use, *Bull. WHO*, 19, 845, 1958.
6. American Thoracic Society/Centers for Disease Control, Diagnostic standards and classification of tuberculosis, *Am. Rev. Resp. Dis.*, 142, 725, 1990.
7. Reichman, L. B., Tuberculin skin testing: the state of the art, *Chest*, 76, 764, 1979.
8. Jordan, T. J., Sunderam, G., Thomas, L., Reichman, L. B., Tuberculin reaction size measurement by the pen method compared to traditional palpation, *Chest*, 92, 234, 1987.
9. Sokal, J. E., Measurement of delayed skin-test responses, *N. Engl. J. Med.*, 293, 501, 1975.
10. Bearman, J. E., Kleinman, H., Glyer, V. V., LaCroix, O. M., A study of variability in tuberculin test reading, *Am. Rev. Resp. Dis.*, 90, 913, 1964.
11. Chaparas, S. D., Immunologically based diagnostic tests with tuberculin and other mycobacterial antigens, in *The Mycobacteria: A Sourcebook*, Kubica, G. P., Wayne, L. G., Eds., Marcel Dekker, New York, 1984, 195.
12. Duboczy, B. O., Two-reading technique for elimination of false readings in delayed type skin tests, *Am. Rev. Resp. Dis.*, 99, 961, 1969.
13. Tarlo, S. M., Day, J. H., Mann, P., Day, M. P., Immediate hypersensitivity to tuberculin: in vivo and in vitro studies, *Chest*, 71, 33, 1977.
14. Duboczy, B. O., Repeated tuberculin tests at the same site in tuberculin-positive patients, *Am. Rev. Resp. Dis.*, 90, 77, 1964.
15. Duboczy, B. O., Brown, B. T., Local sensitization to tuberculin, *Am. Rev. Resp. Dis.*, 84, 69, 1961.
16. WHO Tuberculosis Research Office, Repeated tuberculin tests in the same site, *Bull. WHO*, 12, 197, 1955.
17. Arnason, B. G., Waksman, B. H., The retest reaction in delayed sensitivity, *Lab. Invest.*, 12, 737, 1963.
18. Galli, S. J., Askenase P. W., Cutaneous basophil hypersensitivity, in *The Reticuloendothelial System*, Vol. 9, Phillips, S. M., Escobar, M. R., Eds., Plenum, New York, 1988, 321.
19. Lagrange, P. H., Cell-mediated immunity and delayed-type hypersensitivity, in *The Mycobacteria: A Sourcebook*, Kubica, G. P., Wayne, L. G., Eds., Marcel Dekker, New York, 1984, 681.
20. Askenase, P. W., Atwood, J. E., Basophils in tuberculin and "Jones-Mote" delayed reactions of humans, *J. Clin. Invest.*, 58, 1145, 1976.
21. Dvorak, H. F., Galli, S. J., Dvorak, A. M., Cellular and vascular manifestations of cell-mediated immunity, *Hum. Pathol.*, 17, 122, 1986.
22. Slutkin, G., Perez-Stable, E. J., Hopewell, P. C., Time course and boosting of tuberculin reactions in nursing home residents, *Am. Rev. Resp. Dis.*, 134, 1048, 1986.

23. Colvin, R. B., Mosesson, M. W., Dvorak, H. F., Delayed-type hypersensitivity skin reactions in congenital afibrinogenemia: lack of fibrin deposition and induration, *J. Clin. Invest.*, 63, 1302, 1979.

23a. Byrd, R. B., Gracey, D. R., Campbell, D. C., et al., The Mono-Vacc tuberculin skin test, *Dis. Chest.*, 56, 447, 1969.

23b. Catanzaro, A., Multiple puncture skin test and Mantoux test in southeast Asian refugees, *Chest*, 87, 346, 1985.

23c. Donaldson, J. C., Elliott, R. C., A study of co-positivity of three multipuncture techniques with intradermal PPD tuberculin, Am. Rev. Respir. Dis., 118, 843, 1978.

24. Edwards, P. Q., Edwards, L. B., Story of the tuberculin test: from an epidemiologic viewpoint, *Am. Rev. Resp. Dis.*, 81(Suppl.), 1, 1960.

25. Sutherland, I., Recent studies in the epidemiology of tuberculosis, based on the risk of being infected with tubercle bacilli, *Adv. Tuberc. Res.*, 19, 1, 1976.

26. Finucane, T. E., The American Geriatrics Society statement on two-step PPD testing for nursing home patients on admission, *J. Am. Geriatr. Soc.*, 36, 77, 1988.

27. Thompson, N. J., Glassroth, J. L., Snider, D. E., Farer, L. S., The booster phenomenon in serial tuberculin testing, *Am. Rev. Resp. Dis.*, 119, 587, 1979.

28. Centers for Disease Control, Prevention and control of tuberculosis in facilities providing long-term care to the elderly, *MMWR*, 39 (No. RR-10), 7, 1990.

29. Gordin, F. M., Perez-Stable, E. J., Flaherty, D., Reid, M. E., Schecter, G., Joe, L., Slutkin, G., Hopewell, P. G., Evaluation of a third sequential tuberculin skin test in a chronic care population, *Am. Rev. Resp. Dis.*, 137, 153, 1988.

30. Gordin, F. M., Perez-Stable, E. J., Reid, M., Schecter, G., Cosgriff, L., Flaherty, G., Hopewell, P. G., Stability of positive tuberculin tests: Are boosted reactions valid?, *Am. Rev. Resp. Dis.*, 144, 560, 1991.

31. Holden, M., Dubin, M. R., Diamond, P. H., Frequency of negative intermediate-strength tuberculin sensitivity in patients with active tuberculosis, *N. Engl. J. Med.*, 285, 1507, 1971.

32. Rooney, J. J., Crocco, J. A., Kramer, S., et al., Further observations on tuberculin reactions in active tuberculosis, *Am. J. Med.*, 60, 517, 1976.

33. McMurray, D. N., Echeverri, A., Cell-mediated immunity in anergic patients with pulmonary tuberculosis, *Am. Rev. Resp. Dis.*, 118, 827, 1978.

34. Nash, D. R., Douglass, J. E., Anergy in active pulmonary tuberculosis, *Chest*, 77, 32, 1980.

35. Centers for Disease Control, Purified protein derivative (PPD)-Tuberculin anergy and HIV infection: guidelines for anergy testing and management of anergic persons at risk of tuberculosis, *MMWR*, 40 (No. RR-5), 27, 1991.

36. Blatt, S. P., Hendrix, C. W., Butzin, C. A., Freeman, T. M., Delayed-type hypersensitivity skin testing predicts progression to AIDS in HIV-infected patients, *Ann. Intern. Med.*, 119, 177, 1993.

37. American Thoracic Society, American Academy of Pediatrics, Centers for Disease Control, and Infectious Disease Society of America, Control of tuberculosis in the United States, *Am. Rev. Resp. Dis.*, 146, 1623, 1992.

38. Centers for Disease Control, Screening for tuberculosis and tuberculous infection in high-risk populations: recommendations of the Advisory Committee for Elimination of Tuberculosis, *MMWR*, 39 (No. RR-8), 1, 1990.

39. Centers for Disease Control, Prevention and control of tuberculosis in U.S. communities with at-risk minority populations, *MMWR*, 41 (No. RR-5), 1, 1992.

40. Centers for Disease Control, Prevention and control of tuberculosis among homeless persons, *MMWR*, 41 (No. RR-5), 13, 1992.

41. Centers for Disease Control, Prevention and control of tuberculosis in migrant farm workers, *MMWR*, 41 (No. RR-10), 1, 1992.

42. Centers for Disease Control, Tuberculosis among foreign-born persons entering the United States: recommendations of the advisory committee for elimination of tuberculosis, *MMWR*, 39 (No. RR-18), 1, 1990.

43. Malasky, C., Jordan, T., Potulski, F., Reichman, L. B., Occupational tuberculous infections among pulmonary physicians in training, *Am. Rev. Resp. Dis.*, 142, 505, 1990.

44. Geiseler, P. J., Nelson, K. E., Crispen, R. G., Tuberculosis in physicians: a continuing problem, *Am. Rev. Resp. Dis.*, 133, 773, 1986.

45. Rieder, H. L., Cauthen, G. M., Comstock, G. W., Snider, D. E., Epidemiology of tuberculosis in the United States, *Epidemiol. Rev.*, 11, 79, 1989.

46. Green, C. E., Mycobacterial infections: Tuberculous mycobacterial infections, in *Infectious Diseases of the Dog and Cat*, Green, C. E., Ed., W. B. Saunders, Philadelphia, 1990, 558.

47. Snider, W. R., Tuberculosis in canine and feline populations: review of the literature, *Am. Rev. Resp. Dis.*, 104, 877, 1971.

48. Centers for Disease Control, The use of preventive therapy for tuberculous infection in the United States: recommendations of the Advisory Committee for Elimination of Tuberculosis, *MMWR*, 39 (No. RR-8), 9, 1990.

49. American Thoracic Society/Centers for Disease Control, Treatment of tuberculosis and tuberculosis infection in adults and children, *Am. J. Respir. Crit. Care Med.*, vol. 149, 1994.

50. Fulkerson, L. L., Perlmutter, G. S., Zack, M. B., Davis, D. O., Stein, E., Radiotherapy in chest malignant tumors associated with pulmonary tuberculosis, *Radiology*, 106, 645, 1973.

51. Bobrowitz, I. D., Elkin, M., Evans, J. C., Lin, A., Effect of direct irradiation on the course of pulmonary tuberculosis (using cancerocidal doses), *Dis. Chest*, 40, 397, 1961.

52. Friedman, L. N., Diagnostic standards and classification of tuberculosis (letter), *Am. Rev. Resp. Dis.*, 143, 895, 1991.

53. Feng, P. H., Tan, T. H., Tuberculosis in patients with systemic lupus erythematosus, *Ann. Rheum. Dis.*, 41, 11, 1982.

54. Ferebee, S. H., Controlled chemoprophylaxis trials in tuberculosis: a general review, *Adv. Tuberc. Res.*, 17, 28, 1970.

55. Bjerkedal, T., Palmer, C. E., Effect of isoniazid prophylaxis in experimental tuberculosis in guinea pigs: action of isoniazid in vivo, *Am. J. Hyg.*, 76, 89, 1962.

56. Grzybowski, S., Allen, E. A., The challenge of tuberculosis in decline: a study based on the epidemiology of tuberculosis in Ontario, Canada, *Am. Rev. Resp. Dis.*, 90, 707, 1964.

57. Dahlstrom, A. W., Wilson, J. L., Sedlacek B. B., The immediate effectiveness of isoniazid chemoprophylaxis as determined by the tuberculin test, *Dis. Chest*, 38, 599, 1960.

58. Houk, V. N., Kent, D. C., Sorensen, K., Baker, J. H., The eradication of tuberculosis infection by isoniazid chemoprophylaxis, *Arch. Environ. Health*, 16, 46, 1968.

59. Grzybowski, S., Barnett, G. D., Styblo, K., Contacts of cases of active pulmonary tuberculosis, *Bull. Int. Union Tuberc.*, 50, 90, 1975.

60. Comstock, G. W., Baum, C., Snider, D. E., Isoniazid prophylaxis among Alaskan Eskimos: a final report of the Bethel isoniazid studies, *Am. Rev. Resp. Dis.*, 119, 827, 1979.

61. International Union Against Tuberculosis Committee on Prophylaxis, Efficacy of various durations of isoniazid preventive therapy for tuberculosis: five years of follow-up in the IUAT trial, *Bull. WHO*, 60, 555, 1982.

62. Krebs, A., The IUAT trial on isoniazid preventive treatment in persons with fibrotic lung lesions, *Bull. Int. Union Tuberc.*, 51, 193, 1976.

63. Snider, D. E., Caras, G. J., Koplan, J. P., Preventive therapy with isoniazid: Cost-effectiveness of different durations of therapy, *J. Am. Med. Assoc.*, 255, 1579, 1986.

64. Falk, A., Fuchs, G. F., Prophylaxis with isoniazid in inactive tuberculosis: a Veterans Administration cooperative study XII, *Chest*, 73, 44, 1978.

65. Katz, J., Kunofsky, S., Damijonaitis, V., Lafleur, A., Caron, T., Effect of isoniazid upon the reactivation of inactive tuberculosis, *Am. Rev. Resp. Dis.*, 91, 345, 1965.

66. Grzybowski, S., Ashley, M. J., Pinkus, G., Chemoprophylaxis in inactive tuberculosis: Long-term evaluation of a Canadian trial, *Can. Med. Assoc. J.*, 114, 607, 1976.

67. Snider, D. E., The relationship between tuberculosis and silicosis, *Am. Rev. Resp. Dis.*, 118, 455, 1978.

68. Burke, R. M., Schwartz, L. P., Snider, D. E., The Ottawa county project: a report of a tuberculosis screening project in a small mining community, *Am. J. Public Health*, 69, 340, 1979.

69. Paul, R., Silicosis in northern Rhodesia copper miners, *Arch. Environ. Health*, 2, 96, 1961.

70. Westerholm, P., Ahlmark, A., Maasing, R., Segelberg, I., Silicosis and risk of lung cancer or tuberculosis: a cohort study, *Environ. Res.*, 41, 339, 1986.

71. Monaco, A., Antituberculous chemoprophylaxis in silicotics, *Bull. Int. Union Tuberc.*, 35, 51, 1964.

72. Allison, A. C., Hart, P. D., Potentiation by silica of the growth of *Mycobacterium tuberculosis* in macrophage cultures, *Br. J. Exp. Pathol.*, 49, 465, 1968.

73. Centers for Disease Control, Tuberculosis and human immunodeficiency virus infection: recommendations of the Advisory Committee for the Elimination of Tuberculosis, *MMWR*, 38, 236, 1989.

74. Selwyn, P. A., Hartel, D., Lewis, V. A., Schoenbaum, E. E., Vermund, S. H., Klein, R. S., Walker, A. T., Friedland, G. H., A prospective study of the risk of tuberculosis among intravenous drug users with human immunodeficiency virus infection, *N. Engl. J. Med.*, 320, 545, 1989.

74a. Moreno, S., Baraia-Etxaburu, J., Bouza, E., et al., Risk for developing tuberculosis among anergic patients infected with HIV, *Ann. Intern. Med.*, 119, 194, 1993.

74b. Pape, J. W., Jean, S. S., Ho, J. L., et al., Effect of isoniazid prophylaxis on incidence of active tuberculosis and progression of HIV infection, *Lancet*, 342, 268, 1993.

75. Jordan, T. J., Lewit, E. M., Montgomery, R. L., Reichman, L. B., Isoniazid as preventive therapy in HIV-infected intravenous drug abusers: a decision analysis, *J. Am. Med. Assoc.*, 265, 2987, 1991.

76. Selwyn, P. A., Sckell, B. M., Alcabes P., Friedland G. H., Klein, R. S., Schoenbaum, E. E., High risk of active tuberculosis in HIV-infected drug users with cutaneous anergy, *J. Am. Med. Assoc.*, 268, 504, 1992.

77. Deleted by author.

78. Reichman, L. B., Felton, C. P., Edsall, J. R., Drug dependence, a possible new risk factor for tuberculosis disease, *Arch. Intern. Med.*, 139, 337, 1979.

79. Nolan, C. M., Elarth, A. M., Tuberculosis in a cohort of southeast Asian refugees: a five-year surveillance study, *Am. Rev. Resp. Dis.*, 137, 805, 1988.

80. Powell, K. E., Meador, M. P., Farer, L. S., Foreign-born persons with tuberculosis in the United States, *Am. J. Public Health*, 71, 1223, 1981.

81. Centers for Disease Control, Tuberculosis in blacks — United States, *MMWR*, 36, 212, 1987.

82. Stead, W. W., Senner, J. W., Reddick, W. T., Lofgren, J. P., Racial differences in susceptibility to infection by Mycobacterium tuberculosis, *N. Engl. J. Med.*, 322, 422, 1990.

83. Centers for Disease Control, Tuberculosis among hispanics — United States, 1985, *MMWR*, 36, 568, 1987.

84. Centers for Disease Control, Tuberculosis among American Indians and Alaskan natives — United States, 1985, *MMWR*, 36, 493, 1987.

85. Rieder, H. L., Tuberculosis among American Indians of the contiguous United States, *Public Health Rep.*, 104, 653, 1989.

86. Centers for Disease Control, Tuberculosis control among homeless population, *MMWR*, 36, 259, 1987.

87. Friedman, L. N., Sullivan, G. M., Bevilaqua, R. P., Loscos, R., Tuberculosis screening in alcoholics and drug addicts, *Am. Rev. Resp. Dis.*, 136, 1188, 1987.

88. Reichman, L. B., O'Day, R., Tuberculous infection in a large urban population, *Am. Rev. Resp. Dis.*, 117, 705, 1978.

89. Schieffelbein, C. W., Snider, D. E., Tuberculosis control among homeless populations, *Arch. Intern. Med.*, 148, 1843, 1988.

90. Centers for Disease Control, Prevention and control of tuberculosis in correctional institutions: recommendations of the advisory committee for the elimination of tuberculosis, *MMWR*, 38, 313, 1989.

91. Snider, D. E., Hutton, M. D., Tuberculosis in correctional institutions (editorial), *J. Am. Med. Assoc.*, 261, 436, 1989.

92. Stead, W. W., Lofgren, J. P., Warren, E., Thomas, C., Tuberculosis as an endemic and nosocomial infection among the elderly in nursing homes, *N. Engl. J. Med.*, 312, 1483, 1985.

93. Haley, C. E., McDonald, R. C., Rossi, L., Jones, W. D., Haley, R. W., Luby, J. P., Tuberculosis epidemic among hospital personnel, *Infect. Control Hosp. Epidemiol.*, 10, 204, 1989.

94. Thorn, P. A., Brookes, V. S., Waterhouse, J. A. H., Peptic ulcer, partial gastrectomy, and pulmonary tuberculosis, *Br. J. Med.*, 1, 603, 1956.

95. Hanngren, A., Reizenstein, P., Studies in dumping syndrome, *Am. J. Dig. Dis.*, 14, 700, 1969.

96. Frucht, H., Kunkel, P., Spiro, H. M., Pulmonary tuberculosis following gastric resection, *Ann. Intern. Med.*, 46, 696, 1957.

97. Snider, D. E., Tuberculosis and gastrectomy, *Chest*, 87, 414, 1985.

98. Snider, D. E., Jejunoileal bypass for obesity: a risk factor for tuberculosis, *Chest*, 81, 531, 1982.

99. Bruce, R. M., Wise, L., Tuberculosis after jejunoileal bypass for obesity, *Ann. Intern. Med.*, 87, 574, 1977.

100. Snider, D. E., Tuberculosis and body build, *J. Am. Med. Assoc.*, 258, 3299, 1987.

101. Edwards, L. B., Livesay, V. T., Acquaviva, F. A., Palmer, C. E., Height, weight, tuberculous infection, and tuberculous disease, *Arch. Environ. Health*, 22, 106, 1971.

102. Root, H. F., The association of diabetes and tuberculosis: epidemiology, pathology, treatment and prognosis, *N. Engl. J. Med.*, 210, 1, 1934.

103. Oscarsson, P. N., Silwer, H., Incidence and coincidence of pulmonary tuberculosis among diabetics: search among diabetics in the county of Kristianstad, *Acta Med. Scand.*, 161 (Suppl. 335), 23, 1958.

104. Boucot, K. R., Tuberculosis among diabetics: The Philadelphia survey, *Am. Rev. Tuberc.*, 65(Suppl.), 1, 1952.

105. Kessler, I. I., Mortality experience of diabetic patients: a twenty-six year follow-up study, *Am. J. Med.*, 51, 715, 1971.

106. Edsall, J., Collins, J. G., Gray, J. A. C., The reactivation of tuberculosis in New York City in 1967, *Am. Rev. Resp. Dis.*, 102, 725, 1970.

107. Rose, D. N., Silver, A. L., Schechter, C. B., Tuberculosis chemoprophylaxis for diabetics: are the benefits of isoniazid worth the risk?, *Mt. Sinai J. Med.*, 52, 253, 1985.

108. Andrew, O. T., Schoenfeld, P. Y., Hopewell, P. C., Humphreys, M. H., Tuberculosis in patients with end-stage renal disease, *Am. J. Med.*, 68, 59, 1980.

109. Belcon, M. C., Smith, E. D. M., Kahana, L. M., Shimizu, A. G., Tuberculosis in dialysis patients, *Clin. Nephrol.*, 17, 14, 1982.

110. Cuss, F. M. C., Carmichael, D. J. S., Linington, A., Hulma, B., Tuberculosis in renal failure: a high incidence in patients born in the third world, *Clin. Nephrol.*, 25, 129, 1986.

111. Lundin, A. P., Adler, A. J., Berlyne, G. M., Friedman, E. A., Tuberculosis in patients undergoing maintenance hemodialysis, *Am. J. Med.*, 67, 597, 1979.

112. Pradhan, R. P., Katz, L. A., Nidus, B. D., Matalon, R., Eisenger, R. P., Tuberculosis in dialyzed patients, *J. Am. Med. Assoc.*, 229, 798, 1974.

113. Rutsky, E. A., Rostand, S. G., Mycobacteriosis in patients with chronic renal failure, *Arch. Intern. Med.*, 140, 57, 1980.

114. Sasaki, S., Takashi, A., Suenage, M., Tomura, S., Yoshiyama, N., Nakagawa, S., Shoji, T., Sasaoka, T., Takeuchi, J., Ten years' survey of dialysis-associated tuberculosis, *Nephron*, 24, 141, 1979.

115. Mitwalli, A., Tuberculosis in patients on maintenance dialysis, *Am. J. Kidney Dis.*, 18, 579, 1991.

116. Freeman, R. M., Newhouse, C. E., Lawton, R. L., Absence of tuberculosis in dialysis patients (letter), *J. Am. Med. Assoc.*, 233, 1356, 1975.

117. Haanaes, O. C., Bergmann, A., Tuberculosis emerging in patients treated with corticosteroids, *Eur. J. Resp. Dis.*, 64, 294, 1983.

118. Millar, J. W., Horne, N. W., Tuberculosis in immunosuppressed patients, *Lancet*, 2, 1176, 1979.

119. Sahn, S. A., Lakshminarayan, S., Tuberculosis after corticosteroid therapy, *Br. J. Dis. Chest*, 70, 195, 1976.

120. Schatz, M., Patterson, R., Kloner, R., Falk, J., The prevalence of tuberculosis and positive tuberculin skin tests in a steroid-treated asthmatic population, *Ann. Intern. Med.*, 84, 261, 1976.

121. Smyllie, H. C., Connolly, C. K., Incidence of serious complications of corticosteroid therapy in respiratory disease: a retrospective survey of patients in the Brompton Hospital, *Thorax*, 23, 571, 1968.

122. Bovornkitti, S., Kangsadal, P., Sathirapat, P., Oonsombatti, P., Reversion and reconversion rate of tuberculin skin reactions in correlation with the use of prednisone, *Dis. Chest*, 38, 51, 1960.

123. Carlsen, S. E., Bergin, C. J., Reactivation of tuberculosis in a donor lung after transplantation, *Am. J. Radiol.*, 154, 495, 1990.

124. Lakshminarayan, S., Sahn, S. A., Tuberculosis in a patient after renal transplantation, *Tubercle*, 54, 72, 1973.

125. Lenk, S., Oesterwitz, H., Scholz, D., Tuberculosis in cadaveric renal allograft recipients, *Eur. Urol.*, 14, 484, 1988.

126. Lloveras, J., Peterson, P. K., Simmons, R. L., Najarian, J. S., Mycobacterial infections in renal transplant recipients: seven cases and a review of the literature, *Arch. Intern. Med.*, 142, 888, 1982.

127. Kaplan, M. H., Armstrong, D., Rosen, P., Tuberculosis complicating neoplastic disease: a review of 201 cases, *Cancer*, 33, 850, 1974.

128. Feld, R. F., Bodey, G. P., Groschel, D., Mycobacteriosis in patients with malignant disease, *Arch. Intern. Med.*, 136, 67, 1976.

129. Taylor, W. C., Aronson, M. D., Delbanco, T. L., Should young adults with a positive tuberculin test take isoniazid?, *Ann. Intern. Med.*, 94, 808, 1981.

130. Tsevat, J., Taylor, W. C., Wong, J. B., Pauker, S. G., Isoniazid for the tuberculin reactor: Take it or leave it, *Am. Rev. Resp. Dis.*, 137, 215, 1988.

131. Rose, D. N., Schechter, C. B., Silver, A. L., The age threshold for isoniazid chemoprophylaxis: a decision analysis for low-risk tuberculin reactors, *J. Am. Med. Assoc.*, 256, 2709, 1986.

132. Colice, G. L., Decision analysis, public health policy, and isoniazid chemoprophylaxis for young adult tuberculin skin reactors, *Arch. Intern. Med.*, 150, 2517, 1990.

133. Jordan, T. J., Lewit, E. M., Reichman, L. B., Isoniazid preventive therapy for tuberculosis: decision analysis considering ethnicity and gender, *Am. Rev. Resp. Dis.*, 144, 1357, 1991.

134. Bass, J. B., Sanders, R. V., Kirkpatrick, M. B., Choosing an appropriate cutting point for conversion in annual tuberculin skin testing, *Am. Rev. Resp. Dis.*, 132, 379, 1985.

135. Snider, D. E., Caras, G. J., Isoniazid-associated hepatitis deaths: a review of available information, *Am. Rev. Resp. Dis.*, 145, 494, 1992.

136. Kopanoff, D. E., Snider, D. E., Caras, G. J., Isoniazid-related hepatitis: a U.S. Public Health Service surveillance study, *Am. Rev. Resp. Dis.*, 117, 991, 1978.

136a. Centers for Disease Control and Prevention, Severe isoniazid-associated hepatitis—New York, 1991–1993, *MMWR*, 42, 545, 1993.

137. Stead, W. W., To, T., Harrison, R. W., Abraham, J. H., Benefit-risk considerations in preventive treatment for tuberculosis in elderly persons, *Ann. Intern. Med.*, 107, 843, 1987.

137a. Gurumurthy, P., Krishnamurthy, M. S., Nazareth, O., et al., Lack of relationship between hepatic toxicity and acetylator phenotype in three thousand south Indian patients during treatment with isoniazid for tuberculosis, *Am. Rev. Respir. Dis.*, 129, 58, 1984.

138. Cross, F. S., Long, M. W., Banner, A. S., Snider, D. E., Rifampin-isoniazid therapy of alcoholic and nonalcoholic tuberculous patients in a U.S. Public Health Service cooperative trial, *Am. Rev. Resp. Dis.*, 122, 349, 1980.

139. Franks, A. L., Binkin, N. J., Snider, D. E., Rokaw, W. M., Isoniazid hepatitis among pregnant and postpartum hispanic patients, *Public Health Rep.*, 104, 151, 1989.

140. Moulding, T. S., Redeker, A. G., Kanel, G. C., Twenty isoniazid-associated deaths in one state, *Am. Rev. Resp. Dis.*, 140, 700, 1989.

141. Hong Kong Chest Service/Tuberculosis Research Centre, Madras/British Medical Research Council, A controlled trial of 2-month, 3-month, and 12-month regimens of chemotherapy for sputum-smear-negative pulmonary tuberculosis: results at 60 months, *Am. Rev. Resp. Dis.*, 130, 23, 1984.

142. Grosset, J. H., Present status of chemotherapy for tuberculosis, *Rev. Infect. Dis.*, 11(Suppl.), S347, 1989.

143. Stead, W. W., Pathogenesis of the sporadic case of tuberculosis, *N. Engl. J. Med.*, 277, 1008, 1967.

144. Nardell, E., McInnis, B., Thomas, B., Wiedhaas, S., Exogenous reinfection with tuberculosis in a shelter for the homeless, *N. Engl. J. Med.*, 315, 1570, 1986.

145. Small, P. M., Shafer, R. W., Hopewell, P. C., Singh, S. P., Murphy, M. J., Desmond, E., Sierra, M. F., Schoolnik, G. K., Exogenous reinfection with multidrug-resistant *Mycobacterium tuberculosis* in patients with advanced HIV infection, *N. Engl. J. Med.*, 328, 1137, 1993.

146. Koplan, J. P., Farer, L. S., Choice of preventive treatment for isoniazid-resistant tuberculous infection: use of decision analysis and the Delphi technique, *J. Am. Med. Assoc.*, 244, 2736, 1980.

147. Centers for Disease Control, Management of persons exposed to multidrug-resistant tuberculosis, *MMWR*, 41 (No. RR-11), 59, 1992.

148. Gillum, M. D., Make, D. G., Brief report: Tuberculin testing, BCG in pregnancy, *Infect. Control Hosp. Epidemiol.*, 9, 119, 1988.

149. Medchill, M. T., Gillum, M., Diagnosis and management of tuberculosis during pregnancy, *Obstet. Gynecol. Surv.*, 44, 81, 1989.

150. Snider, D., Pregnancy and tuberculosis, *Chest*, 86(Suppl.), 10S, 1984.

151. Comstock, G. W., Edwards, L. B., Nabangxang, H., Tuberculin sensitivity eight to fifteen years after BCG vaccination, *Am. Rev. Resp. Dis.*, 103, 572, 1971.

152. Sepulveda, R. L., Ferrer, X., Latrach, C., Sorensen, R. U., The influence of Calmette-Guérin bacillus immunization on the booster effect of tuberculin testing in healthy young adults, *Am. Rev. Resp. Dis.*, 142, 24, 1990.

153. Menzies, R., Vissandjee, B., Effect of bacille Calmette-Guérin vaccination on tuberculin reactivity, *Am. Rev. Resp. Dis.*, 145, 621, 1992.

154. Snider, D. E., Bacille Calmette-Guérin vaccinations and tuberculin skin tests, *J. Am. Med. Assoc.*, 253, 3438, 1985.

155. Farer, L. S., Prior BCG vaccination and PPD skin test, *J. Am. Med. Assoc.*, 250, 3106, 1983.

Chapter 14

Control of Tuberculosis

James L. Hadler, M.D., M.P.H.

CONTENTS

0-8493-4825-0/94/$0.00+$.50

I. INTRODUCTION

Methods to control the spread of tuberculosis are currently in a dynamic state. On the one hand, a national tuberculosis control strategy recently was developed in response to a call for its elimination in the United States early in the twenty-first century.[1] On the other hand, control of tuberculosis is threatened with two related but distinct new problems. The HIV epidemic has had a profound effect on tuberculosis incidence and transmission in the United States[2-7] and Africa[8-13] and, increasingly, many other parts of the world. The emergence and transmission of multidrug-resistant strains of *Mycobacterium tuberculosis*,[7,14-19] fueled by the HIV epidemic, are beginning to have an additional impact on the incidence of tuberculosis and its control strategies in the United States.[14,15]

The purpose of this chapter is to review basic principles of tuberculosis control as they relate to these and other tuberculosis control issues, and to outline and prioritize strategies for its control given the current epidemiology of tuberculosis in the United States. Throughout this chapter it is recognized that the ultimate responsibility for successful tuberculosis control in the United States lies with local, state, and federal officials. However, tuberculosis control cannot be achieved without the systematic efforts and participation of individual practitioners or without public interest and support.

II. PRINCIPLES OF TUBERCULOSIS CONTROL

For purposes of this discussion, tuberculosis control efforts can be broken into four major categories: (1) surveillance, (2) decreasing transmission from, and preventing the emergence of, drug-resistant disease among persons with infectious tuberculosis (case finding and case management), (3) prevention of development of infectious tuberculosis among persons with latent tuberculous infection (screening and preventive therapy), and (4) keeping uninfected persons from becoming infected with *M. tuberculosis*.

A. SURVEILLANCE

Surveillance is the collection of information that leads to the effective control of a disease. For effective tuberculosis control, there are a number of types of information that need to be systematically collected.

Foremost for any geographic area (e.g., city, county, state) is the determination of the incidence and epidemiology of tuberculosis in that area. This information becomes the basis to determine which groups should be targeted for case finding and tuberculin screening and to evaluate whether current efforts are effective in reducing group-specific incidence. Surveillance for incident disease generally is carried out through a combination of physician and laboratory reporting to local or state health departments with follow-up information about variables of concern. In the current era of HIV-related and multidrug-resistant tuberculosis, it has become increasingly important to get information on the HIV and drug susceptibility status of each reported case.[14,15] For institutions and occupational settings such as hospitals, correctional facilities, drug treatment programs, homeless shelters, and long-term care facilities that can expect to manage or be confronted with infectious tuberculosis cases, systematic periodic employee tuberculin screening programs may be the most effective surveillance tool to determine whether and where transmission is occurring.[2,20-24]

In addition to incidence measures of disease and infection, optimal tuberculosis control surveillance includes the collection of considerable information on the effectiveness of tuberculosis control activities. These include the effectiveness of case management (e.g., sputum conversion rates at set time intervals, treatment completion rates), the effectiveness of screening (e.g., the number and prevalence of latent tuberculous infections detected annually among target groups for screening, the percentage of them started on and completing preventive therapy), and, where appropriate, bacillus Calmette-Guérin (BCG) vaccination rates.

B. CASE MANAGEMENT

The single most important tuberculosis control principle is the minimization of potential for sustained transmission from persons with infectious tuberculosis and the minimization of their potential to develop drug resistance. Early identification of persons with pulmonary tuberculosis and prompt initiation of effective antituberculosis chemotherapy are essential to render a person noninfectious. To minimize the potential for relapse and development of drug resistance, it is necessary to ensure that each person started on therapy remains compliant with the recommended course of therapy until it is completed.

In the era of HIV-related and multidrug-resistant tuberculosis, the initial therapy must cover the possibility of drug resistance, and the duration of therapy may need to be extended. Individual physicians must report rapidly newly recognized cases of infectious tuberculosis to public health authorities so that efforts to ensure compliance can begin immediately. Increasingly, it appears that some form of supervised or directly observed therapy will become the standard for ensuring compliance in the United States.[25,26]

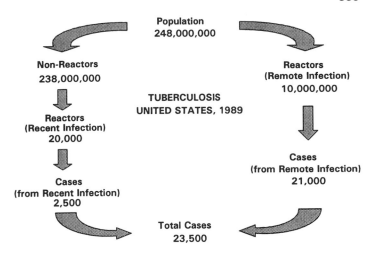

Figure 14-1 Epidemiology of tuberculosis and tuberculous infection, United States, 1989. (From CDC, Division of TB Elimination.[27])

C. SCREENING AND PREVENTIVE THERAPY

The second highest priority for tuberculosis control in the United States is to keep latently infected persons from developing infectious tuberculosis. It is estimated that approximately 90% of all incident cases of infectious tuberculosis in the United States arise from the reservoir of 5–6% of the population latently infected with *M. tuberculosis*:[22] only 10% currently arise from recently acquired infection (Figure 14-1). To the extent that the effective reservoir of latent infection can be reduced rapidly through tuberculin screening and preventive therapy efforts, there should be a corresponding immediate impact on incident tuberculosis. Because preventive therapy is the only tuberculosis control measure that acts to reduce the major source of current and immediate future infectious tuberculosis, its widespread use, more than any other tuberculosis control measure, has the potential immediately to impact tuberculosis incidence.[1,27]

HIV-related and multidrug-resistant tuberculosis play an important role in screening and preventive therapy strategies. Given that underlying HIV infection is now the strongest known predictor of development of infectious tuberculosis among persons with latent tuberculous infection,[2,28] screening efforts must be targeted toward the identification of persons with both HIV infection and latent tuberculosis. In addition, compliance with therapy for persons with HIV and tuberculous coinfection, given their extraordinary risk of development of tuberculosis, is of major public health concern. Public health authorities must know who has tuberculous and HIV coinfection to be able to ensure preventive therapy completion.

The impact of multidrug-resistant tuberculosis is more problematic. Where isoniazid resistance is common among persons presenting with tuberculosis for the first time, the effectiveness of preventive therapy may be correspondingly reduced unless efficacious alternatives are readily available or can be developed.[29]

The strategy of tuberculosis control through the widespread use of screening for latent infection and use of preventive therapy is not utilized in many parts of the world.[30-32] Barriers cited to its use include (1) limited resources and the need to focus first on case management, (2) lack of reliability of the tuberculin skin test for diagnosis of latent infection where BCG vaccine has been in widespread use, and (3) concern that widespread use of isoniazid as preventive therapy could either directly or indirectly promote development of isoniazid-resistant *M. tuberculosis*.

While it is a common concern that widespread use of isoniazid could promote emergence of drug-resistant strains, there is little direct evidence to suggest that this is happening in the United States where experience with preventive therapy is the greatest. For the first 20 years of use of isoniazid in the United States (1966–1986), no changes in drug-resistance patterns among persons diagnosed for the first time with tuberculosis were observed.[33-35] Anecdotal experience suggests that when active tuberculosis has been systematically ruled out before starting preventive therapy, subsequent emergence of drug-resistant disease is rare.[11] Although all of the factors behind the emergence of multidrug-resistant *M. tuberculosis* in the past few years in the United States are not yet known, it appears that the use of isoniazid preventive therapy has not been a factor. Investigation of outbreaks suggests that the main contributing factors have been inadequate case management of persons with drug-susceptible tuberculosis leading to acquired drug resistance, followed by transmission to persons with underlying immune deficiency who then rapidly develop initially drug-resistant disease and continue the cycle.[7,19,37-40] In parts of the world where primary isoniazid resistance is much more common than in the United States (e.g., in Southeast Asia), inadequate case management of initially drug-susceptible disease and widespread availability of isoniazid without prescription, permitting isoniazid monotherapy of disease, appear to underlie the problem.[36] Preventive therapy is not used. Thus, inability to ensure an adequate initial course of therapy (case management) in persons with drug-susceptible disease and transmission to persons without preexisting tuberculous infection appear to be the main sources of drug-resistant tuberculosis, not initial drug resistance in persons previously started on isoniazid-preventive therapy.

Given limited resources, the need for better case finding and case management in many parts of the world, and the unfortunate high potential for some persons with tuberculosis to find isoniazid and begin self-medication, it is unlikely that there will be a practical role for extensive use of preventive therapy as a major tuberculosis control strategy in those areas. However, as the HIV epidemic progresses and HIV-related tuberculosis becomes a major contributor to tuberculosis incidence, selective use of preventive therapy in persons with HIV infection may become an important adjunct tuberculosis control strategy. Studies have been initiated in several African countries to evaluate whether this approach is feasible and effective in reducing tuberculosis among the HIV infected.[41-43]

D. PREVENTION OF INFECTION

To a large extent, keeping persons without tuberculous infection from becoming infected is dependent on controlling emission of tubercle bacilli at their source: persons with active, infectious tuberculosis. However, to the extent that the potential for exposure is high (e.g., in some U.S. hospitals, in some countries) and the source is not always readily identified, strategies to directly reduce personal or group risk of exposure or to reduce risk of infection with exposure take on more importance. In particular, in the era of multidrug-resistant tuberculosis in which the potential to successfully treat latent tuberculous infection is uncertain, strategies for personal protection take on further importance.

Reduction of risk of exposure to tuberculosis can be achieved through use of means to reduce the number of suspended infectious droplet nuclei in any given closed space (e.g., dilution by frequent air exchange, ultraviolet light) or through the use of individual protection devices that filter out droplet nuclei from inhaled air. These strategies, which are covered in detail in Section IV of this chapter, and Chapter 3 of this volume, are practical only in selected institutional settings in which there is predictably high potential for individual or group exposure to persons with infectious tuberculo-

sis, e.g., hospitals continuously treating persons with tuberculosis or AIDS, bronchoscopy suites, some correctional institutions, and some homeless shelters.

Reduction of risk of development of latent or active tuberculous infection given any exposure to tubercle bacilli may be potentially reduced by the use of BCG vaccination. In spite of the questionable efficacy of the currently approved strains of BCG, the World Health Organization has recommended, and many countries in the world have depended on, BCG as a major component of their tuberculosis control strategy.[30] BCG is expected to benefit only persons who have not already been infected with *M. tuberculosis* and who are likely to be exposed in the future. There is no evidence that it affects subsequent disease incidence in persons latently infected. Its potential role in an overall tuberculosis control strategy is long range. It will result in a significant long-term decrease in tuberculosis only if the new tuberculous infection rate is high, vaccine coverage is high among groups likely to be exposed, and the strain used has high and long-term efficacy. In addition, widespread BCG use makes accurate interpretation of the tuberculin skin test more difficult. For these reasons, BCG vaccination has not been part of the U.S. tuberculosis control strategy.[44]

The emergence of multidrug-resistant tuberculosis in the United States, however, is causing the potential role of BCG vaccination in tuberculosis control efforts to be reevaluated. In particular, its use is being considered for health-care workers working in settings where exposure to multidrug-resistant strains is likely. There also has been discussion of its use in very high tuberculosis incidence areas of the United States where drug resistance is high, the incidence in children is high and increasing, and the likelihood of effective preventive therapy efforts seem low.[45] An additional limitation to its use in these settings is that BCG is contraindicated in persons with immune deficiency, and it is unclear whether BCG protection in a person with HIV infection will endure as CD4 counts fall.

Because BCG vaccines have not played a major role in the U.S. approach to tuberculosis control, they will not be discussed further in this chapter. They are discussed in more detail in Chapter 15 (this volume).

III. CURRENT STRATEGIES AND METHODS FOR TUBERCULOSIS CONTROL IN THE UNITED STATES

The preceding section broadly outlined basic tuberculosis control principles. In this section the strategies, methods, and roles of both public health and individual health-care providers to achieve these principles are described. In addition, tuberculosis control strategies and needs in special settings and situations are reviewed.

A. SURVEILLANCE
1. Measuring Disease Incidence

Since 1953 the Centers for Disease Control has been monitoring the occurrence of tuberculosis in the United States as a whole and in demographic subgroups through collection of standardized disease reporting from states. State and local health departments in turn have collected information in follow-up of reports of suspected tuberculosis cases from laboratories and health-care providers. This reporting system has been the main source of epidemiologic information on tuberculosis in the United States as presented in Chapter 1 (this volume). This information has been periodically supplemented by special time-limited data collection efforts by state and local health departments to gather additional information of interest through individual provider or patient contact. Variables for which supplemental information recently has been or is being collected at the state and national level have included occupation, alcohol and drug use, HIV infection status, and drug susceptibility.[46]

In response to the need to address both the recent increase in tuberculosis incidence in the United States and the emergence of multidrug-resistant tuberculosis, it has been recommended by several national advisory groups that routine surveillance for tuberculosis in the United States includes information on drug susceptibility, HIV status when known, and occupation of each reported case of tuberculosis.[14,15] Beginning in 1993, these new variables will be added to the national tuberculosis case surveillance system for all states. Table 14-1 lists variables for new tuberculosis cases that will be reported to the Centers for Disease Control.[47]

2. Measuring Prevalence of Drug Resistance

In the past, surveillance for drug resistance in the United States was done largely through special surveillance efforts by selected state and hospital-based laboratories.[33-35] This approach was limited by the facts that only a limited number of laboratories participated and that surveillance was focused on the incidence of primary drug resistance rather than all potentially infectious cases of tuberculosis. This system, which had been useful for determining nationwide trends in primary drug resistance, was discontinued in 1986 due to lack of funding.[35]

In the wake of recognition of the outbreaks of multidrug-resistant tuberculosis, a survey of drug susceptibility results collected by state health departments during January to March 1991 was done by the Centers for Disease Control. This showed an overall prevalence of resistance to both isoniazid and rifampicin of 3.1% in new cases nationally.[14,15] A separate 1991 survey in New York City showed that 7% of new cases had resistance to both drugs.[157]

Given the magnitude of the prevalence of drug-resistant tuberculosis in some parts of the United States and the demonstrated potential for its rapid amplification, several new surveillance efforts are planned. First, it has been recommended that initial isolates from all cases of tuberculosis be tested for susceptibility to first line antituberculosis drugs.[15] Second, the results of susceptibility testing from isolates tested at each state laboratory are now collected by electronic communication at the Centers for Disease Control. The latter system allows for real-time estimation of the current prevalence of drug resistance. However, it does not guarantee population representativeness, since only isolates tested by state health laboratories are included. Finally, no matter where susceptibility testing is performed, it has been recommended that each state health department collect such information on each newly diagnosed and relapsed case of tuberculosis and submit the information as part of a complete case report.[15] This system should enable detailed population-based evaluation of the epidemiology of drug resistance both at selected points in time and in an ongoing fashion.

3. Measuring Incidence of New Infection

There has been no systematic surveillance for incidence of new tuberculous infection in the United States. This is due in part to the fact that the periodic serial tuberculin testing required is impractical and logistically difficult to perform at the population level. However, surveillance for new infection has been an important tuberculosis control strategy and evaluation tool in institutional settings where there is a substantial potential for tuberculosis exposure. It has been a long-standing recommendation to screen employees periodically with tuberculin to determine institutional exposure potential, infection rates, and preventive therapy needs.[48]

In the current era in which tuberculosis exposure among the HIV infected can trigger outbreaks of disease with short incubation periods and high attack rates, determination of the incidence of infection takes on new importance. To prevent exposure of workers and patients to tuberculosis, especially HIV-infected health-care workers and patients to multidrug-resistant tuberculosis, hospitals increasingly are being required to have effec-

Table 14-1 **Epidemiologic and case management data elements: state and national tuberculosis case reporting, 1993**

Epidemiologic Elements

Sex	Country of origin
Race	Date of arrival in United States
Ethnic origin	Date of report
City of residence	Date counted
County of residence	

HIV Status[a,b]	Drug use in past year[a]
Homeless status[a]	Injecting
Institutional residence	Noninjecting
at time of diagnosis[a]	Excess alcohol
Correctional	Occupation[a]
Long-term care	

Case Management Elements

Previous diagnosis	Date therapy started
Site(s) of disease	Initial drug regimen
Smear/culture status	

Drug susceptibility[a]	Sputum conversion date[a]
Initial	Date therapy stopped[a]
Final	Reason therapy stopped[a]
Type of health-care provider[a,c]	Means of administration[a]
	Directly observed
	Self-administered

[a] Added to individual case reports beginning 1993.

[b] Options include negative, positive, indeterminate, refused, not offered, test done but results unknown, unknown.

[c] Options include health department, private/other, both

tive isolation facilities and procedures.[20,49] The only outcome measure that is readily obtainable to monitor the effectiveness of these costly changes is the incidence of new tuberculous infection among employees or, where possible, long-term residents. It may become necessary to have and rigorously enforce periodic employee tuberculin testing policies. Employee skin testing already has been used to evaluate the effectiveness of control measures implemented following recognition of multidrug-resistant tuberculosis outbreaks in several hospitals.[50-52] As part of the U.S. response to the recognition of extensive nosocomial multidrug-resistant tuberculosis outbreaks, there is a plan for the Centers for Disease Control to monitor nosocomial tuberculous infection rates systematically among a network of U.S. hospitals.[15]

4. Detection of Outbreaks

In the past there was no strategy to detect outbreaks of tuberculosis systematically. Given the recent recognition of many drug-sensitive and drug-resistant outbreaks of tuberculosis among HIV-infected persons, an increasing need has developed for sys-tematic surveillance to allow early recognition of such outbreaks so that intervention may occur.

There are several possible strategies for outbreak detection. One is recognition of high tuberculous infection rates among employees in institutions caring for substantial numbers of HIV-infected persons, and follow-up to determine infection or disease among HIV-infected clients who may have been exposed at the same time. This method depends on effective and systematic employee screening programs.

A second strategy for outbreak detection depends on collection of information from new HIV-related cases of tuberculosis about recent institutionalization (in hospitals, correctional settings, drug treatment programs, AIDS residences). To the extent that local and state health officials can get HIV-related information on new tuberculosis cases and interview them for recent potential institutional exposure, outbreaks may be detected early. As yet, this method is untried, but it has been recommended.[15]

A third possible strategy is an application of the restriction fragment-length polymorphism typing techniques. Such techniques have been used to confirm commonality of source in some of the multidrug-resistant tuberculosis outbreaks.[19,37] Currently, they are being used prospectively to evaluate isolates from the same geographic area to see if unsuspected clusters can be identified.[53,54]

5. Measuring the Effectiveness of Case Management

For several decades, tuberculosis control strategies in the United States have included the collection of information on the success of case management and selected screening and preventive therapy activities. These measures have provided guidance for program review and funding.

Case management measures in the United States have included documentation of sputum conversion rates by 3 months as an outcome measure of continuity and efficacy of therapy, and therapy continuity and completion rates at various points in time after its initiation. For U.S. cases diagnosed in 1990, 57% were documented to have converted from positive to negative sputum by 3 months, 81% were "continuous on therapy" for the first 6 months, and 76% completed therapy within 12 months of initiation. The national goal in each of these areas is 90%.[55] One factor contributing to the low sputum conversion rates is that many patients do not get systematic sputum monitoring once spontaneous cough and sputum production ends. If a negative culture was not documented before then, they are not counted as sputum converters, even though they may be asymptomatic and continuously taking therapy.

There currently is no published analysis of how case management measures vary between areas with recent increases in tuberculosis incidence compared to those with no increase, nor of what "threshold" correlates with subsequent emergence of significant problems. However, substantial and important differences are being seen in these measures between different areas of the country, in particular for those areas with recent sustained increases in tuberculosis incidence and/or higher levels of drug resistance. In particular, in New York City, which has the largest percentage increase in tuberculosis incidence in the United States in the past 5 years, and the highest percentage of cases with multidrug resistance, case management measures are among the lowest in the country. Only 56% of cases started on therapy in 1990 in New York City were documented to have been continuously on therapy for 6 months and 34% of all cases were declared lost to follow-up within this time period.[55] By contrast, more than 50% of states had a 6-month continuity of therapy index of 90% or greater and none had rates as low as in New York

City. Outside of New York City, only 4% of cases were declared "lost" in the first 6 months. In addition to New York, many large urban areas of the country have relatively low continuity of therapy indices, a warning sign of potentially similar problems to come. For example, in 1990, the 6-month continuity of therapy index was only 61% for Newark, 64% for Chicago, and 66% for Houston. In each, the increase in tuberculosis incidence from 1987 to 1991 (42.3, 5.7, and 11.1 cases per 100,000 population, respectively) has exceeded the overall national increase (1.1 cases per 100,000 population).[56,57]

Until recently, the 6-month continuity of therapy index was closely related to the percentage of those determined to have completed a course of therapy. If drug-resistant tuberculosis becomes increasingly more prevalent and more people are put on substantially longer courses of therapy, it may become increasingly important to use 12 month continuity figures and completion rates.

6. Measuring the Effectiveness of Screening and Prevention

National measures of the effectiveness of screening and prevention have focused largely on case-contact investigations. These measures have been both outcome and process oriented. One major outcome has been the number of cases of tuberculosis disease found among contacts. Process measures have included the number of latently infected contacts found and the percentages of them who are offered and complete a course of preventive therapy. From this information, it is possible to estimate the number of cases of tuberculosis that were prevented as a result of contact investigation. Contacts have been a focus because, until the HIV era, tuberculin-positive contacts of infectious tuberculosis cases had the highest predictable risk of developing infectious disease of any sizable, readily identifiable category of persons with latent tuberculous infection. Their investigation was and remains a major tuberculosis control priority.

In 1991, more than 85,000 persons were tuberculin tested as a result of contact investigation in the United States. Of these, 588 cases of active tuberculosis were found and 14,592 infected contacts began preventive therapy. In spite of these sizable numbers, there have been some disturbing changes in the past 5 years. Between 1987 and 1991, progressively fewer tuberculosis cases have had contacts identified. In 1987, the percentage of cases with contacts identified was 84%. By 1991, it was 74%. The percentage of identified contacts examined has gone from 92 to 90%, and the percentage of infected contacts less than 15 years of age who were started on preventive therapy has gone from 88 to 82%. Furthermore, the completion rate among this unquestionably at-risk contact group has slipped from 82 to 76%. The rates among other infected contacts show similar trends.[55] Why these regressive trends are occurring is not clear. However, it is possible that diminished resources, the increase in tuberculosis, and a new focus on preventing HIV-related and multidrug-resistant tuberculosis all are playing a role.

Recently, federal funding has supported systematic efforts to identify persons with HIV and latent tuberculous coinfection in drug treatment programs, correctional facilities, HIV counseling and testing sites, and sexually transmitted disease clinics. Data on the yield in identification of persons with coinfection and success in starting and completing a course of preventive therapy are only beginning to be available.[58] It is highly likely, however, that such measures will be used widely in the near future to evaluate the success of these new and high priority publicly funded efforts to screen for latent tuberculous infection and prevent development of infectious tuberculosis.

7. Respective Roles of Health-Care Providers and Public Health Agencies

Surveillance for tuberculosis cannot work effectively without substantial interaction between individual care providers and public health agencies.

To have an efficient surveillance system, individual care providers must (1) rapidly report to local and state public health authorities new and suspected cases of tuberculosis within 24–72 h of starting therapy, (2) assess the HIV and drug susceptibility status of each case,[2,15] (3) when requested, provide to public health authorities more detailed information on each reported case as outlined in Table 14-1, (4) regularly obtain follow-up sputum specimens to document conversion from positive to negative culture status on each case, and (5) immediately report to local public health authorities any case that is suspected of not taking therapy as prescribed.[1]

Public health agencies must in turn (1) promptly follow-up each case of newly reported tuberculosis to establish a relationship with the patient, to assess whether some form of supervised therapy is necessary, and to ensure that a thorough contact investigation is done, (2) maintain comprehensive data collection and analysis systems to ensure that complete surveillance information is collected on each newly reported case and the resulting data are analyzed, (3) establish and maintain the capacity to ensure that at least one isolate of *M. tuberculosis* on each newly active pulmonary case is tested for susceptibility to first line antituberculosis drugs, and (4) disseminate the results of tuberculosis surveillance to providers and the public on a regular basis.[1]

B. CASE FINDING AND CASE MANAGEMENT

Case finding and case management are at the core of tuberculosis control in the United States and worldwide. The three main goals of case finding and case management are to identify all infectious cases of tuberculosis, to rapidly render them noninfectious with appropriate initial therapy, and to keep them on therapy until cured so that they will not relapse and become infectious again or develop drug resistance. Of these three goals, the one that has been the focus of most public health attention, particularly in the United States, has been to keep patients on therapy until they are cured. Correspondingly, a major focus of this section is adherence to therapy.

1. Case Finding

Case finding has historically been an important tuberculosis control strategy in groups with a high tuberculosis prevalence. Methods have included population-based chest radiographic screening, initial symptom examination followed by sputum smear and/or chest radiograph,[30,32] and tuberculin skin testing followed by symptom and chest radiographic examination of all with significant reactions.

In the United States, the large population-based case finding strategy of the preantibiotic era has been largely abandoned. It is logistically difficult and not cost effective in most situations. However, there still are population subgroups, other than symptomatic patients seeking medical care, for which proactive case finding is potentially cost effective and is recommended.[20,21,23,24,59,60] In the United States these groups include (1) persons entering institutional settings in which persons at high risk of having tuberculosis are living, the environmental characteristics are conducive to transmission, and large numbers of susceptible persons are located (e.g., prisons and jails, health care facilities, and nursing homes), (2) contacts of infectious cases of tuberculosis, (3) homeless persons living in shelters, (4) migrant farm workers, and (5) persons entering the country with immigrant or refugee status.

The methods and frequency of attempts at case finding vary by group (Table 14-2). Where continued access to the groups is questionable and/or risk of active disease is high (jail entrants, homeless persons, migrant farm workers), screening methods should utilize initial symptom or radiologic evaluation. In groups for which prevalence of disease is likely to be lower (e.g., <1%) and especially if continued access for repeated screening and preventive therapy is likely (contacts, prison entrants, long term care residents), initial tuberculin skin testing should be performed.

Table 14-2   **Recommended tuberculosis case finding: candidate groups, methods, and frequency**

Group	Initial Screening Method	Frequency[a]
Contacts	Skin test and symptoms	Initial; 12 weeks
Jail[b] entrants	Symptoms or X-ray	Entry
Prison[c] entrants	Skin test and symptoms	Entry and annually
Long-term care entrants	Skin test and symptoms	Entry
Homeless	Symptoms and/or X-ray	As possible[d]
Migrant workers	Symptoms	As possible[d]
Immigrants and refugees	Chest X-ray and skin test	See note[e]
Admissions to hospitals	Skin test and symptoms	Entry

[a] Tuberculin and symptom screening should be repeated in all groups following exposure to a potentially infectious case.

[b] "Jail" refers to a holding institution for the detention of persons accused of criminal behavior, prior to the posting of bond and/or trial.

[c] "Prison" refers to an institution for the detention of persons who are sentenced.

[d] Should be initiated by local health agencies and repeated periodically as indicated by its productivity.

[e] All refugees and legal immigrants ≥15 years are required to have X-ray screening before entry. Some children <15 years are required to have tuberculin screening. All <35 years or with medical risk factors for tuberculosis should be tuberculin screened as soon after entry as possible.

The efficacy of case finding can be remarkably high in some subgroups. Based on recent screening at selected clinics and shelters, the prevalence of clinically active disease among the homeless has ranged as high as 1.6–6.8%, and the prevalence of latent infection from 18–57%.[23,61-64] Among migrant workers screened in 1988 in North Carolina, the prevalence of active tuberculosis was 0.5% in Hispanics and 3.5% in American blacks.[65] Among tuberculin positive contacts of active tuberculosis cases in 1990, 2.8% were found to have active disease.[55] Nonetheless, not all screening for active disease is so productive. Each geographic area needs to identify its own high risk groups and assess whether active case finding is indicated.

2. Choice of Therapy

Three main factors dictate choice of antituberculosis therapy: (1) the need to cover the potential for drug resistance, (2) the need to have a regimen that is of the shortest possible duration, and (3) cost.

In principle, it is recommended that a patient be started on a regimen containing at least two drugs to which the organism is likely to be susceptible. For most first time cases, this has meant a two- or three-drug regimen, the latter being a necessary initiation phase for the short-course 6- to 8-month regimens in general use in the United States and recommended by the USPHS and WHO.[66] However, given the emergence of multidrug-resistant tuberculosis in the United States, it now is nationally recommended that unless there is virtual certainty that a person has fully sensitive organisms, all first time tuberculosis cases should be started on a four-drug regimen to include isoniazid, rifampicin, pyrazinamide, and either ethambutol or streptomycin until the results of susceptibility tests are known.[25,67] This represents a major departure from pre-1992 recommendations and is intended to decrease the potential for institutional transmission from persons with organisms initially resistant to one or two drugs.

Shortening the course of antituberculosis treatment to make it easier to ensure a person completes treatment has been a major practical tuberculosis control research issue for decades. Highly efficacious regimens now exist that can be completed in as little as 6 months with as few as 62 doses of antituberculosis drugs.[68,69] The shortest course regimens generally require initiation of therapy with four drugs, including isoniazid, rifampicin, and pyrazinamide, with either ethambutol or streptomycin as the fourth drug. The same regimen that makes short-course treatment a possibility also covers the potential for single or even two-drug resistance. Thus, the best tuberculosis control strategy for the 1990s dictates initiation of at least four antituberculosis drugs in nearly all cases.

In some parts of the world, the cost of drugs has been a major concern. In particular, a standard WHO-recommended regimen in widespread use for either treatment from the outset or the continuation phase of an 8-month short-course regimen has been isoniazid and thiacetazone.[32] However, in the HIV era, use of thiacetazone is proving to be problematic. Not only do regimens using thiacetazone require a longer time to complete, but among HIV-infected cases, severe reactions, including death, are being observed with an unacceptable frequency, and higher relapse rates are being found than with the use of other regimens.[70,71] In one study of children, 13% of cases had fatal Stevens–Johnson syndrome-like reactions. In the same study, only 24% of HIV-positive children had a satisfactory response to treatment compared to 98% of those who were HIV negative.[71] Given its limitations, it appears that the role of thiacetazone in tuberculosis control worldwide will diminish greatly in the future.

3. Adherence to Therapy
a. Background
Achieving high rates of patient adherence to therapy has been identified repeatedly as a major obstacle to tuberculosis control in the United States.[72-78] Failure to achieve high adherence rates is a major factor underlying both the striking increase in tuberculosis in New York City[78] and in the emergence of drug resistance in the United States.[14]

In the absence of any systematic effort to ensure that patients with infectious tuberculosis will take antituberculosis medicines for at least 6 months, it can be expected that completion rates will be low and often less than 50%. For example, only 11% of tuberculosis cases in whom therapy was initiated as inpatients in Harlem Hospital Center in 1988 were shown to have completed therapy.[78] Even with some active follow-up systems in place, a number of U.S. cities were able to demonstrate only 50–70% completion rates.[55] Such low completion rates are inadequate either to ensure a decline in tuberculosis incidence or to prevent the emergence of drug resistance. It has been estimated that therapy completion rates of at least 70–85% are necessary to ensure a decline in tuberculosis incidence.[79]

Thus far, the problem of the emergence and spread of multidrug-resistant tuberculosis has been most prominent in areas of the country with less than 80% completion rates.[55] However, initiation of a problem requires only a single initially nonadherent case with the opportunity to expose many others. Correspondingly, it is critical that public health authorities and tuberculosis control programs take an aggressive role to ensure that each infectious case of tuberculosis receives a full and continuous course of treatment.[14,15]

There is a substantial medical literature on factors that affect a person's health-care seeking behavior and adherence to recommendations to take therapy for a long period of time.[80-84] There also have been a number of tuberculosis-specific studies of behavioral factors that influence whether a person with tuberculosis will complete a course of therapy.[85-94] The major conclusion to be drawn from a social and behavioral perspective is that adherence to antituberculosis therapy appears to be a complex interaction of a number of factors. These include the nature of patients and their understanding and beliefs regarding the importance of therapy, individual health-care providers and their commitment to meaningful involvement with the patient, and the nature of the health care delivery system (Table 14-3).[85,94]

The extent to which each of these factors can be influenced to improve treatment outcome has been studied minimally.[85] However, it has been demonstrated that passive tuberculosis clinic models in which the physician and health-care delivery system expect the patient to conform to their orders or configuration and in which little responsibility is taken for the patient's adherence to therapy do poorly when compared to more active models.[95-99] A comprehensive approach to the clinical aspects of tuberculosis control can be highly successful, even with a challenging clinic population, when individual clinicians are aware of their responsibility for each patient's adherence and the health-care delivery system is shaped, in part, around the needs of the tuberculosis patient.[95-97]

The rest of this section describes the specific case-management options that need to be considered to maximize the potential for continuous adherence to therapy.

b. Directly Observed/Supervised Therapy
A wide range of methods have been used to attempt to ensure high levels of adherence to therapy. These methods generally can be categorized into two groups: (1) those in which therapy is supervised or directly observed by a health-care worker or other observer, and (2) those that are intended to enhance adherence when the patient is self-administering medicines (Table 14-4).

Directly observed therapy (DOT) long has been recognized as a highly effective way to achieve adherence to therapy.[100] However, with the recognition of the failure of passive tuberculosis control efforts in New York City and the rapid emergence of multidrug-resistant tuberculosis, DOT quickly is becoming the treatment adjunct of choice for most tuberculosis patients in the United States.[25,26,78] Because of the increasing concern that even a single case of drug resistance could be rapidly amplified if many HIV-infected persons were exposed, the USPHS has recommended that most persons on antituberculosis therapy be on DOT.[25] New York City, the current epicenter of drug-resistant

Table 14-3 **Factors affecting adherence to therapy**

Patient Factors
1. Belief that treatment and its completion are important
2. Understanding of what is necessary to complete therapy
3. Degree to which taking medicines can be easily assimilated into daily life-style
4. Degree of support from community and health-care provider for taking medicine
5. Extent of perceived benefits of completing therapy
6. Belief that there must be a degree of control over therapy
7. Duration of therapy
8. Number of pills that must be taken daily
9. Personal cost
10. Side effects
11. Stability of life-style

Individual Provider Factors
1. Assumption of responsibility for completion of therapy
2. Assumption of responsibility to "educate" the patient
3. Assumption of responsibility for monitoring adherence
4. Extent of recognition of signs and symptoms of nonadherence
5. Extent to which the provider can prescribe simpler and shorter durations of therapy
6. Extent of ability to reduce time between last appointment reminder and any scheduled appointment

Clinic Factors
1. Accessibility of the clinic
   Distance from patient
   Cost of travel
   Cost of visit
   Convenient hours of operation
2. Ambience of health care
   Waiting times
   Cultural appropriateness including translating
   Staff attitudes
   Clinical setting
   Use of incentives (child care, free snacks)

tuberculosis in the United States, recently also has made this a programmatic goal.[26] These recommendations are based on the facts that (1) DOT provides immediate feedback on whether a patient is receiving prescribed therapy, (2) very high adherence rates have been achieved with DOT, and (3) DOT has proven to be highly cost effective when compared with hospitalization for retreatment and/or the consequences of acquired drug resistance.

DOT has been repeatedly demonstrated to achieve high adherence rates in therapeutic trials of twice-weekly therapy. In public health practice, success of DOT also has been well demonstrated. Although most states currently have limited outreach personnel and have used DOT only for patients who are felt likely or have proven to be nonadherent to self-administered therapy, success rates with DOT have been high. Most states report 95% 12-month completion rates in patients on DOT; rates are 5–20% higher than for those not initially on DOT.[101] In Mississippi, after having an outbreak of multidrug-resistant tuberculosis generated by a nonadherent case,[102,103] a statewide policy of starting all cases on DOT began in 1984 and was fully in place by 1986. Patients for whom it was feasible had to report at least twice weekly to tuberculosis clinics to get their medicines. Others received DOT at work, home, or other mutually convenient sites. More than 95% of new cases have been started on DOT. Twelve-month completion rates since 1986 have been greater than 90% compared to the 1990 national rate of 76%.[55,104] Although there was initial concern that some physicians and patients would be resistant to this policy, it was widely implemented with little resistance after it was promoted as "the way tuberculosis is treated."[105]

Table 14-4 **Strategies to ensure adherence to therapy**

1. Directly observed therapy
   The maximum benefits of DOT will occur when
   The supervisor is acceptable to patient
   Flexibility is used in selecting the place to give therapy (e.g., home, work, street)
   Twice-weekly therapy is used
   Inducements and incentives are used to ensure meetings
2. Self-administered therapy
   Patients started on self-administered therapy will do best when
   They are reported to local and state health departments
   They have a supportive family and physician
   They have periodic home visits
   Their pill-taking regimen is simple and associated with a daily activity
   Clinic visits and medicines are free or low cost
   Pills are given out in small quantities ($\leq$30 day supply)
   Clinic and/or home visits are scheduled at least monthly
   Preappointment reminders are used
3. Promptly identify potential nonadherence
   Clinicians need to use the following methods to promptly identify nonadherence so that it can
   be reported to public health agencies for immediate follow-up:
   Assess response to therapy
      Frequent symptom evaluation
      Frequent sputum smears and culture
   Use DOT whenever possible or
   Dispense medications in small quantities and closely monitor refills
   Count pills frequently: home visits, medication monitors
   Measure INH metabolites in urine

DOT generally is thought to be highly cost effective compared to self-administered alternatives.[68,78,100,106] While the cost for outreach to deliver therapy is not inconsequential, it is more than offset by savings in shorter initial hospital stays, and lower relapse, retreatment, rehospitalization, and drug resistance rates. Furthermore, the cost of outreach can be minimized by the use of twice-weekly regimens. Using twice-weekly regimens, as few as 62 meetings for DOT are necessary to complete a full course of treatment.[68]

DOT can be given in a variety of settings and by a variety of personnel. No single rigid model is necessary other than having a responsible person who is acceptable to the patient administer medicines and observe their ingestion on a daily, twice- or thrice-weekly basis at a site mutually agreed upon by both patient and observer. DOT has been given in clinic settings, in correctional institutions, in methadone and other drug treatment modalities, in the workplace, in schools, in homeless shelters, in the home, and on the street. Although DOT usually is provided by public health personnel such as outreach workers or clinic nurses, it also can be given by other trusted persons with regular predictable contact with the patient, e.g., nurses in drug treatment or occupational settings, teachers, social workers, and relatives.

Compliance with DOT sometimes can be a problem in settings in which the patient is not "captive," especially when the patient may be homeless and/or have substance abuse problems, may not predictably be in the same location at a given time, or may not agree on the importance of completing therapy. To maximize the potential for the person supervising the therapy and the patient to meet, incentives[94,107,108] or legal inducements[100] have been used successfully. Such incentives include free bus tokens, returnable cans and bottles, free meals, arrangements for housing and other social services, and small but meaningful gifts of use to the patient.[94,107-109] Legal inducements are discussed further in Section III.B.3.e.

c. Self-Administered Therapy

Traditionally, most patients have been managed initially with daily self-administered therapeutic regimens. Such regimens, if successful, are cheaper to administer than DOT and some physicians and patients prefer the implication of trust associated with them. However, as experience has shown, they are less reliable and more cumbersome when it comes to ensuring adherence to therapy.

Many of the factors that determine whether or not a patient will complete therapy (Table 14-3) can be influenced by the health-care provider and local public health authorities (Table 14-4). Of particular importance is that local health authorities know of each patient's diagnosis as soon as therapy is started. Reporting will enable them to become part of the "team" that lends educational and outreach support to the patient from the outset.[1]

Multiple studies have shown that in the majority of tuberculosis cases there is no single factor that will determine full adherence to therapy. An individual but comprehensive approach is needed for each patient.[85,94] Among the factors to which attention must be paid are patient education, provider and family support, and the establishment of simple and inexpensive pill-taking regimens. Patients need to know and understand why, what, how, and for how long they should take their antituberculosis therapy. This information may need to be reinforced repeatedly, in a culturally sensitive way, and with audiovisual aides.[85] Some patients may need guided practice and demonstration in pill ingestion.[94]

Supportive family, friends, and health-care providers are important to increase patient motivation.[85,94] Where support is lacking, some patients may need similar incentives to help with motivation as have been used to increase compliance with DOT.[90,94,107,108] Frequently scheduled clinic visits and/or home visits provide an opportunity for health-care providers to demonstrate interest as well as to monitor adherence to therapy. Minimizing clinic waits, providing bus tokens to get there, scheduling appointments at the patient's convenience, and assisting in getting help for the patient's other medical and social problems all can help to provide a supportive environment. Preappointment reminders, especially telephone calls, avoid potential embarrassment about missing or forgetting appointments and provide an opportunity to see if there are remediable obstacles to keeping an appointment.

Cost should not be a barrier to therapy for tuberculosis. Most public health departments provide antituberculosis therapy and clinic support free of charge to the patient. Patients should be aware of this option. Pill taking regimens should be as simple as possible and designed to minimize side effects. Combined drug preparations, where available, mean fewer pills. Regimens can be most easily remembered if associated with a daily activity (e.g., tooth brushing, eating). Medication side effects may be minimized by taking all pills at one time in the evening.[94]

For the patient for whom chronic nonadherence to self-administration of antituberculosis drugs is a problem, DOT should be considered.

d. Monitoring for Adherence

Methods to monitor adherence to therapy are listed in Table 14-4. Use of directly observed therapy is the optimal way to have prompt information on whether a patient is adhering to therapy. When an appointment is missed or a patient refuses to ingest pills, nonadherence is apparent immediately. Even with directly observed therapy, however, the potential exists for a patient to have unsuspected drug resistance or, rarely, to fake ingestion of therapy. Thus, it is also important to monitor the patient's response to therapy with follow-up sputum cultures and symptom evaluation, and if the response to therapy is poor, to consider testing for the presence of isoniazid metabolites in urine.[110-114]

Urine testing is the most practical direct measure of whether drugs are being ingested. At least two companies market practical test products.[94] Nonetheless, urine testing for isoniazid metabolites has some qualifications. The normal rate of isoniazid metabolism varies in different populations and the average time for its clearance from the urine can be as short as 4 h.[94,110-114] Thus, testing must be performed at an appropriate time interval following ingestion if it is to be reliable. In addition, some patients may not cooperate with urine testing.

For persons who are responsible for maintaining and ingesting their own antituberculosis drug supplies, two additional techniques have been used to monitor and reinforce adherence. These include (1) giving pills out in small amounts (≤30 day supply) and having the patient frequently return for refills, and (2) attempting periodically to determine whether pills are being consumed at the expected rate (home visits and pills counts, pill dispensers that record when pills are removed).[115-117] Dispensing isoniazid and other antituberculosis drugs in less than 30 day quantities has been a standard recommendation of the American Thoracic Society and the Centers for Disease Control to enable earlier recognition of side effects and nonadherence.[66,67] Monitoring adherence by noting a high frequency of clinic visits may not be adequate. Prediction of adherence to antituberculosis therapy based on patient reports of adherence, subjective assessment of behavior and personality traits, or by having patients bring back empty pill bottles has been shown to be less than completely reliable.[66,72,73,94,115] Thus, spot home visits for pill counts often have been used to supplement clinic observations. In addition, the widespread use of pill-dispensing devices that can automatically record when pills have been removed ("medication monitors") has been recommended.[117] Whether "medication monitors" will further enhance the early ability to predict which patients on self-administered therapy should be on directly observed therapy has not yet been evaluated.

Overall, there is no currently proven single, easy way to recognize nonadherent behavior other than by beginning all persons on directly observed therapy from the outset. Given that resources for directly observed therapy still are limited, many patients will be started on self-administered therapy and will need to be monitored individually via the variety of currently available methods.

e. Confinement/Quarantine

The emergence and rapid spread of multidrug-resistant tuberculosis in some urban areas has caused many to reexamine the potential role of the legal system to encourage adherence to therapy and/or minimize the potential of spread to others from persons who remain infectious for prolonged time periods. Unfortunately, there will be some patients for whom voluntary compliance with directly observed therapy will be a chronic problem, and some who will develop multidrug resistance and will not be expected to respond well to therapy. For these persons, a progressive course of legal alternatives should be available to minimize their potential to infect others and/or develop multidrug resistance.

Most states have laws that enable the courts to order directly observed therapy for persons not on therapy who are suspected of being infectious or who have stopped therapy before completing the recommended course. Such laws have been very useful in getting patients to comply with directly observed therapy and avoid the potential expense of institutional confinement.[100,118]

For those few cases where institutional confinement may be necessary to remove them from situations where the potential for transmission is high (e.g., homeless persons who do not cooperate with court-ordered directly observed therapy, persons with chronic multidrug-resistant tuberculosis who cannot be successfully managed or confined to their homes), suitable institutional settings in many states may no longer exist and need to be found.[106,119] Acute care hospitals are expensive and may not be equipped to successfully isolate persons who are chronically infectious. Many chronic disease hospitals do not have staff with sufficient training to manage patients with multidrug-resistant tuberculosis, especially those who may also be HIV infected and have substance abuse or mental health problems. Neither setting may have appropriate security to protect against patients who are determined to leave. At least one state has both identified an appropriate institutional setting and has demonstrated that, in some cases at least, institutional treatment of selected patients may be cost-effective.[118]

f. Respective Roles of Health-Care Providers and Public Health Agencies

To ensure appropriate therapeutic strategies and high completion rates, it is essential that clinicians and public health authorities collaborate on management of each case from the outset.[1,67] To initiate collaboration, clinicians and institutions should report suspect and confirmed cases of tuberculosis within 24–72 h of starting them on therapy, as required by law in every state. In addition, they need to update health departments regularly on the current treatment and clinical status of each patient and promptly notify them when patients under their care do not take therapy as prescribed or do not return for scheduled follow-up.

Public health authorities are responsible for ensuring that each patient is started and maintained throughout the treatment period on an appropriate and continuous course of therapy. To do this, it has been recommended that a specific health department employee be assigned to each tuberculosis case. This person should interview the patient and help develop the initial specific treatment and monitoring plan, including methods to be used to assess and ensure adherence (e.g., directly observed therapy).[1] This person should also be responsible for ensuring the education of the patient and continuity of therapy. Other health department responsibilities for case finding and management include provision of outreach services, maintenance of a record system to evaluate area-wide success with case management, provision of drugs and support of clinic services so that cost is not a barrier to patients receiving appropriate therapy, and institution of legal measures, should they become necessary, to ensure that all persons complete therapy in a timely manner.[1]

C. SCREENING AND PREVENTIVE THERAPY

Efforts to reduce the reservoir of latently infected persons who give rise to up to 90% of incident tuberculosis cases annually in the United States are second only to case management in importance as a tuberculosis control strategy.[1,67] To make best use of limited resources, it is essential that screening be targeted at persons who are potential candidates for preventive therapy, and who have a reasonable probability of completing therapy.[22,27] Currently, screening and preventive therapy are underutilized.[22,120,121] In one study to determine why tuberculosis is not prevented, it was found that although three-quarters of the tuberculosis patients surveyed had contact with a health-care provider within 5 years before the diagnosis of tuberculosis, less than one-third had been tuberculin tested, even though many had risk factors for tuberculosis.[120] Of those who had positive skin tests and other factors placing them at increased risk of disease, only 5% had been offered preventive therapy.

1. On Whom and Where to Perform Tuberculin Screening

In any given geographical area it is essential to know the epidemiology of incident tuberculosis cases to be able to plan potentially effective screening programs. There are some groups at particularly high risk, regardless of geographic area, toward which at least some screening efforts should be directed. Table 14-5 lists these groups and sites where screening programs should optimally be placed. In Chapter 13 (this volume) the rationale behind screening these groups and indications for preventive therapy are presented in detail.

a. HIV-Infected Persons and Intravenous Drug Users (IVDUs)

Given their extraordinarily high risk of disease once infected, intensive efforts are needed to identify persons with or at risk for tuberculous and HIV coinfection and get them to complete a course of therapy. Federal funding has been available since 1989 to support screening efforts in methadone maintenance drug treatment programs and in correctional settings where many IVDUs are incarcerated. In both, the opportunity exists to use directly observed therapy given by staff with regular client contact to ensure adherence to therapy. Early results from this initiative suggest that it is highly successful in identifying persons with coinfection and achieving completion of therapy.[58] Through 1991, 17% of those tested were found to be tuberculin positive; 1,998 persons had been started on preventive therapy and 84% completion rates were anticipated.

Other sites where HIV-infected persons can be expected to be found in higher than background prevalence include HIV counseling and testing sites, hospitals, other drug treatment modalities, and jails. Even if systematic skin testing programs were implemented in all, however, most provide only an opportunity for screening, not follow-up or DOT. There is the potential problem that it will be difficult to ensure continuity of therapy once persons with coinfection have been identified, especially for those who may have a history of drug abuse. At least one state has attempted to address this concern. HIV–tuberculous coinfection has become a reportable condition in Connecticut. Reported persons are monitored similarly to tuberculosis cases and directly observed therapy is offered to patients who are likely or have been proven to be nonadherent.[122]

Anergy screening panels have been used often to help interpret the tuberculin skin test in persons with HIV infection.[123] Their use in tuberculosis control efforts to find as many persons with coinfection as possible and begin them on therapy is somewhat limited at this time. Only two groups of HIV-infected persons who are found to be anergic are potentially candidates for a full course of preventive therapy: (1) contacts of known potentially infectious cases of pulmonary tuberculosis, and (2) persons whose risk of tuberculous infection is otherwise estimated to be ≥10% based on demographic or other factors.[123,124] Unless it is planned to begin anergic patients on preventive therapy, anergy testing, which may be costly and cumbersome, need not be a prerequisite to tuberculin screening efforts among HIV-infected groups. Given that most coinfected persons will react to tuberculin,[123] it remains prudent to use resources to identify them and to try to get them through a course of preventive therapy before focusing on anergy testing.

b. Contacts of Infectious Cases

Screening of close contacts of infectious cases has long been an effective tuberculosis control strategy. In 1990 in the United States, more than 21,000 infected contacts of cases of tuberculosis were identified, with most being started on and completing a course of preventive therapy. Tuberculous infection prevalence among identified contacts was higher than 20%. In addition, more than 500 cases of tuberculosis were identified and started on treatment before they would have been diagnosed otherwise.[55]

Several factors are critical in initiating a contact investigation.[67] These include timing of the investigation, potential infectiousness of the case, and places where the case has had the potential to transmit. In the HIV era, rapid initiation of contact investigations is crucial. Among immunosuppressed HIV-infected contacts, incubation periods of as short as 20 days from infection to overt disease have been observed. Initiation of investigation should take place as soon as there is a positive smear or other strong evidence that a patient has infectious tuberculosis. Correspondingly, as contacts are identified, appropriate counseling and HIV testing of contacts should occur if their HIV status is not already known.

Any patient with pulmonary tuberculosis should be considered potentially infectious. Patient factors that increase the likelihood of transmission to community and workplace contacts include smear positivity, positive sputum culture, presence of cavitation on chest X-ray, presence of cough, long duration of respiratory symptoms, and laryngeal involvement.[125,126] In hospital and health-care settings additional factors include the possibility that the patient was hospitalized for a period of time without appropriate isolation before being rendered noninfectious by therapy[18,19,37-39] and the possibility that cough-inducing (e.g., bronchoscopy) or other aerosol-generating procedures may have been performed.[127,128]

The sites where the patient has had indoor contact with others are also important to consider. In

Table 14-5 Potential sites and groups for tuberculin screening programs by risk group

Risk Group	Possible Screening Sites, Groups
HIV-infected and IVDUs	Correctional facilities, all admissions
	Drug treatment program admissions
	HIV specialty clinics, all clients
	HIV counseling and testing sites, all high-risk clients
	Hospitals, all at-risk admissions
	Jails, all admissions
Case contacts	Household, all
	Workplace, all close contacts
	"Recreational,"[a] all close contacts
	Institutional,[b] all close or high-risk contacts
Abnormal chest X-ray[c]	Radiology reading rooms, all CXRs
Medical risk factors	Hospitals, all admissions
	Physicians' offices, patients with risk factors
	Dialysis units, all clients
	Transplant units, all clients
	Oncology clinics, all clients
	Clinics specializing in autoimmune, or rheumatoid diseases, all on immunosuppressive therapy
Foreign-born and immigrants	After arrival to United States, all refugees and immigrants
	School and colleges, all entrants
	Selected occupational settings, all workers
High-risk urban residents and minorities	Selected hospitals, all admissions
	Physicians' offices
	Schools, entry and each mandated health assessment
	Selected occupational settings
Institutionalized	Correctional facilities, all admissions
	Long-term care facilities, all admissions
High-risk health-care workers	Acute care hospitals, all workers[d]
	Tuberculosis clinics, all workers
	HIV specialty clinics, all workers
	Correctional facilities, all workers
	Drug treatment programs, all workers
	Long-term care facilities, all workers
	Homeless shelters, all workers

[a] Includes contacts such as those in crack houses, bars (see text).

[b] Includes outpatient clinics specializing in the care of the HIV-infected or drug addicted, as well as hospital wards, residential correctional, long-term care and drug treatment programs.

[c] Screening in this case is for chest X-rays suggestive of old tuberculous scarring, not tuberculin screening.

[d] Some workers will need more frequent screening than others,e.g., those working with HIV-infected patients, in bronchoscopy rooms, with patients with undiagnosed pulmonary symptoms.

addition to household and workplace contacts, "recreational" contacts may have had sufficient exposure to cases for transmission to occur. Recently, transmission of tuberculosis among crack house contacts has been described,[129] and transmission to HIV-infected persons in a gay bar has been recognized.[130] "Home" increasingly includes homeless shelters, prison, and AIDS residences or other chronic care facilities. Many patients may have been seen in a variety of health-care settings for prolonged periods during which they were symptomatic before diagnosis.[131] In some of these settings, significant numbers of persons with HIV infection may be exposed.

Given that there may be many persons identified as contacts to any given case, it is critical to establish priorities for starting and ending a contact investigation. During the interview, a hierarchy of exposure among the identified contacts should be established. Those contacts with the most potential exposure to the index should be screened first. The investigation should end when there appears to be no evidence of transmission of tuberculous infection to contacts with progressively lesser levels of exposure (see also Chapter 1).

Because conversion of the tuberculin skin test can take up to 12 weeks after the infecting exposure occurs, it is essential to any contact investigation to repeat testing 10–12 weeks after contact with the source has been broken on those who were initially negative. As discussed in Chapter 13 (this volume), it is recommended that close contacts with an initial tuberculin skin test reaction of less than 5 mm of induration receive a chest radiograph and be considered for interim preventive therapy if the contact is a child. In addition, if circumstances suggest a high probability of infection, interim preventive therapy should also be considered for persons who are immunosuppressed (e.g., infected with HIV).[67]

c. Persons with Medical Conditions That Increase Tuberculosis Risk

Persons with medical conditions that increase tuberculosis risk, including those with abnormal chest X-rays, represent a diverse group. However, they all are candidates for preventive therapy if found to have tuberculous infection. Their common points of identification are usually clinical medical settings: specialty clinics, hospitals, or individual clinicians. Correspondingly, screening sites should be based where they receive medical care for their underlying medical conditions.

Baseline and periodic repeat tuberculin screening should be a routine in transplant, renal dialysis, and oncology units. Clinics specializing in the management of autoimmune conditions for which steroid or other immunosuppressive therapy commonly is used, and clinics specializing in management of silicosis, diabetes, and cancer, particularly hematologic cancers, should also have routine tuberculin screening protocols. Radiologists should be taught to provide routine chest radiographic readings that specifically address upper lobe fibrotic changes consistent with old tuberculosis and thus alert the clinician that the patient may be a candidate for preventive therapy.

Routine tuberculin screening of all admissions to hospitals also may be relatively productive in identifying latently infected persons with medical conditions that predispose to the development of tuberculosis. In a study of two urban Connecticut hospitals, more than 60% of admissions to general medical and surgical wards had conditions that would merit preventive therapy if they were found to be infected. Few persons in either hospital had been screened, including those with HIV infection.[132]

d. Persons Born in High-Incidence Countries

Tuberculin screening of persons born in high tuberculosis incidence countries, particularly those in Asia, Africa, Latin America, Oceania, and certain Caribbean countries, may be highly productive. The incidence of tuberculosis among this group has been estimated to be more than 10 times higher than that of the U.S. population as a whole,[60] and the prevalence of tuberculous infection as high as 50%. Given that most foreign born tuberculosis cases in the United States develop tuberculosis within 5 years of arrival and at least half are less than 35 years of age when they arrive,[4] screening should be targeted at younger age groups and recent arrivals.

Screening and preventive therapy programs have been supported for refugees entering the United States since the early 1980s. Similar programs have been recommended for immigrants, a group nearly 10 times the size of refugees.[60] States currently have the option to receive lists of all immigrants and ensure tuberculin screening shortly after arrival. Moreover, it has been recommended that programs be established throughout the United States to require tuberculin test screening at all school levels, including college for foreign-born students from high incidence countries entering school for the first time.[60] In addition, screening programs in occupational settings employing a high percentage of recent immigrants may be productive in identifying persons who are candidates for preventive therapy. Prior BCG vaccination is not a contraindication to tuberculin screening and use of preventive therapy.[67]

Screening programs in schools and stable occupational settings offer the opportunity to use directly observed therapy to ensure adherence to a complete course of therapy. Where possible, culturally sensitive outreach workers who speak the same language as new arrivals should be hired and trained to work with the persons responsible for giving directly observed therapy.[60] Such an approach in the refugee program has ensured higher preventive therapy completion rates than for the United States as a whole.

e. High-Risk Persons Who Are Medically Underserved

High-risk persons who are medically underserved tend to be characterized by poverty, but otherwise are a diverse group. In general they consist of geographically or race-ethnically defined population subgroups with a relatively high tuberculosis incidence. The high tuberculosis incidence is due in part to varying combinations of adverse social and economic factors, the HIV epidemic, and immigration of persons with tuberculous infection. There also may be a contribution from physician nonadherence to tuberculosis control recommendations and patient nonadherence in following prescribed recommended treatment regimens.[78,133] Correspondingly, each state or town needs to look at its tuberculosis epidemiology to identify who, if any, are the local high-risk groups.

Recommended sites for targeted screening programs also will be dependent on those targeted. It is recommended that broadly constituted local tuberculosis coalitions be built to review the underlying epidemiologic data. Planning, developing, and implementing screening programs should be a joint effort among the local health department, public and private community organizations, and health care providers.[133] At a minimum, screening and preventive therapy programs should be considered in local correctional facilities, drug treatment centers, long-term care facilities, and school settings. In all of these, directly observed preventive therapy is possible. With proper coordination of services, tuberculin screening also may be highly effective in hospitals, outpatient facilities, and homeless shelters, particularly if the latter have relatively stable populations.

f. Institutionalized Persons

A number of studies have shown that persons living in correctional facilities and in long-term care facilities, particularly nursing homes, are at considerably increased risk for tuberculosis compared to their noninstitutionalized counterparts,[21,24,134,135] and that preventive therapy can reduce that risk.[136,137] In both settings, the purpose of tuberculin screening is multifold: to help detect persons with active disease at the time of entry, to identify candidates for preventive therapy to lower the risk of disease occurrence within the institution, and to establish baseline skin test reactivity for future potential contact investigations. In addition, as discussed above, screening and preventive therapy efforts in correctional settings may play a highly contributory role in community tuberculosis control. Rates of tuberculin positivity in prisons have been found to be as high as 25% in Philadelphia, and average 18% in New York State.[138,139]

Tuberculin screening in these settings should be done at entry to the institution and again following exposure to a potentially infectious case of tuberculosis. In correctional settings with a high or increasing incidence of tuberculosis and a substantial percentage of HIV-infected inmates, annual screening programs for inmates may be productive. In addition to tuberculin screening, symptom and/or radiologic screening also may be warranted to rule out active disease at the time of admission. Many states have laws requiring some form of screening for tuberculosis in both settings.

g. High-Risk Health-Care Workers

Persons working in hospital settings in recent years have been shown to be at increased risk of acquiring tuberculous infection independent of the outbreaks associated with multidrug-resistant tuberculosis.[127,128,140-146] Workers in areas of hospitals where tuberculosis patients are apt to be seen before diagnosis (clinic waiting areas, emergency rooms), where HIV patients are congregated, and where sputum or abscess material may be aerosolized (bronchoscopy suites, sputum induction and aerosol treatment areas, autopsy rooms) are probably at the highest risk.[20] While specific ongoing risks generally cannot be quantitated, as many as a third of health care workers in high-risk areas have been known to convert their tuberculin test in a 1- to 2-year time period.[19,37,38] In spite of this, systematic skin testing programs are not in place or enforced in many institutions.[132,146,147]

Skin testing should be performed by the facility employee health service with testing done at initiation of employment and at least annually afterward.[20,67] Persons working in areas of particularly high risk should be tested more often. In addition to periodic screening, health care workers should be evaluated again if they have been exposed to a potentially infectious tuberculosis patient for whom recommended precautions were not taken.[20]

Because of their risk for rapid progression from infection to disease, HIV-infected health-care workers pose an additional concern, especially when they are exposed to multidrug-resistant tuberculosis. At present, management of exposure and infection is no different for them than for other health-care workers, other than recommending a longer course of preventive therapy.[20] However, specific guidelines are being developed that address the prevention of tuberculosis in immunosuppressed health-care workers and concerns raised by their potential to transmit to patients should they become infected with multidrug-resistant strains. Published guidelines are expected in 1993.[148] Preventive therapy for workers infected with multidrug-resistant tuberculosis is discussed in Chapter 13 (this volume).

2. Frequency of Screening

At a minimum, individuals for whom tuberculin screening is recommended should have at least one tuberculin test and have it recorded in a prominent place in an ongoing medical record. The frequency of repeat testing should be determined by the likelihood of exposure to infectious tuberculosis. This may require review or generation of local data and assistance of local public health officials in its interpretation.

Because the likelihood or consequences of continued exposure to tuberculosis is high for some high-risk persons, annual screening, at a minimum, is recommended for the following groups: persons with HIV infection and the staffs of TB clinics, health care facilities caring for HIV-infected patients, mycobacteriology laboratories, shelters for the homeless, substance abuse treatment centers, dialysis units, correctional institutions, and nursing homes.[67] Depending on local incidence and infection rates, annual testing also may be indicated for prisoners, persons repeatedly admitted to acute care hospitals, and children in high-risk populations, particularly those in medically underserved low-income groups. All persons should be retested if exposure to an infectious case occurs.

3. Adherence to Preventive Therapy

The main methods to maximize the potential for adherence to preventive therapy are the same as those used to get cases to adhere to therapy.

Directly observed preventive therapy should be used wherever possible. Given their extraordinary risk for development of tuberculosis, most persons with HIV–tuberculous coinfection should be placed on directly observed preventive therapy. Where required by state law, persons with coinfection should be reported to local and state public health departments so that close monitoring of patients can be done and outreach provided, including provision of directly observed therapy. Persons receiving preventive therapy in "captive" settings should also be receiving directly observed therapy wherever possible.[2,21,27,67] Such settings include correctional institutions, drug treatment programs that require at least twice-weekly interaction with the patient, and schools and occupational settings in which screening programs or contact investigations have been carried out. Where resources are particularly scarce and the need for directly observed preventive therapy exists, twice-weekly therapy should be used.[27]

For patients on self-administered therapy, dispensing a supply of medicines to last 30 days or less ensures that there will be at least monthly monitoring and reinforcement of the importance of completing therapy.[67] Dispensing medicines in 3 month supplies no longer is acceptable practice. Where possible, home visits for patient education and pill counts are helpful. Use of "medication monitors"[115-117] and testing of urine for isoniazid metabolites[110-114] may be helpful in determining whether particularly high-risk persons should be switched to directly observed preventive therapy.

Achieving high levels of patient motivation is particularly important when using preventive therapy. Patient education should address cultural concerns about taking preventive therapy and can often be done by trained workers of the same cultural background as the patient. Clinic visits should not be made cumbersome or unpleasant to the patient.

Waiting time should be minimized, hours of operation made as convenient as possible, and costs kept to a minimum. Enablers such as bus tokens and babysitting services may ensure that a patient gets to the clinic. Incentives such as food, clothes, and small rewards help some patients complete therapy.[67,85,94]

For patients who are found to be nonadherent, directly observed preventive therapy should be considered if other motivational methods have failed. The highest priority group for directly observed preventive therapy is those who are coinfected with HIV.

4. Role of Health-Care Providers, Institutions, and Public Health Agencies

The responsibility for the success of screening and preventive therapy is more diffuse than that for case finding and case management. However, it requires equal amounts of collaboration at the community level.

A substantial portion of the responsibility for success of tuberculin screening and preventive therapy efforts in the United States lies with individual health-care providers. Many persons in high risk groups are readily identifiable only to the individual provider, particularly those with medical factors that increase the risk of development of disease once a person has latent infection. Providers must be aware of indications for screening and preventive therapy and aggressively follow them. Lack of general application of preventive therapy will continue to slow efforts to progress toward tuberculosis elimination.[1]

Institutions also have a substantial role to play in tuberculin screening and preventive therapy efforts, particularly correctional institutions, drug treatment programs, hospitals, long-term care facilities, and schools. In each setting there is an opportunity not only to detect and control transmission within institutional confines, but to contribute to shrinking the effective reservoir of latent infection in the surrounding community. Each needs to have enforced policies and procedures to ensure that both high-risk staff and clients are screened and, as indicated, are started on preventive therapy. In addition, policies should encourage the administration of directly observed preventive therapy within the institution wherever feasible.

Public health agencies have a broad responsibility to oversee screening and preventive therapy efforts in the community.[22,27] They need to review surveillance data and provide guidelines for those who are at high risk and require screening. They must identify and work with institutions and health-care providers who provide services to high-risk populations and help them develop and institute appropriate screening programs. They should provide clinical and outreach support to help monitor persons started on preventive therapy and to ensure adherence. They are responsible for overseeing investigation of contacts of infectious tuberculosis cases. They should collect surveillance information to determine how well screening and preventive therapy efforts are working in each setting in which they have been initiated and to adjust screening recommendations where necessary.

D. SPECIAL SETTINGS

Tuberculosis transmission has been a threat in indoor settings where large numbers of persons at risk for infectious tuberculosis may be living. With the emergence of HIV-related tuberculosis and multidrug-resistant tuberculosis, three settings in particular have come to the fore: hospitals, correctional institutions, and homeless shelters. In each of these settings, environmental as well as human source control measures need to be considered, and special surveillance efforts are needed to determine the ongoing risk of transmission.

1. Hospitals

Hospitals to which persons with tuberculosis may be admitted need to have their own systematic tuberculosis control programs. These programs need to be based on a broad approach to tuberculosis control with attention paid to (1) prevention of the generation of infectious airborne particles by early identification and effective treatment of persons with tuberculous infection and active tuberculosis, (2) prevention of the spread of infectious droplet nuclei into the general air circulation by applying effective isolation methods, (3) reduction of the number of infectious droplet nuclei in air by application of environmental control methods, and (4) systematic surveillance of personnel for tuberculous infection and evidence of continued risk of transmission.[20] Investigation of outbreaks of both sensitive and multidrug-resistant tuberculosis in recent years has shown that where inadequate attention is given to any of these approaches, the risk of tuberculosis transmission is increased.[20,16-19,37-40] See Chapter 3, this volume.

Specific elements of hospital control programs include (1) screening patients for active tuberculosis and tuberculous infection on admission, (2) provision of rapid diagnostic services (e.g., 24 h or less AFB smear reading time), (3) prescription of appropriate curative and preventive therapy, (4) provision and use of isolation rooms for persons with or suspected of having infectious tuberculosis, (5) maintenance of physical measures to reduce microbial contamination in the air, particularly in

areas where procedures are done in which respiratory aerosols are generated, (6) enforced systematic screening of health-care facility personnel for tuberculous infection and tuberculosis, (7) prompt investigation and control of outbreaks, and (8) continued assessment of the extent to which these elements are in place and effective.[20]

More detailed information on isolation and physical measures to reduce transmission can be found in Chapter 3 (this volume). The Centers for Disease Control published detailed guidelines for preventing transmission in health care settings in 1990.[20] An updated OSHA enforcement policy of a proposed revision to these guidelines has recently been developed (OSHA, Enforcement policy and procedures for occupational exposure to tuberculosis, OSHA memorandum, October 8, 1993, effective January 6, 1994).

2. Correctional Institutions

Correctional facilities, like acute care hospitals, have had particular problems with transmission of tuberculosis, including multidrug-resistant strains.[17] Conditions of crowding and poor ventilation combined with a particularly high-risk population (HIV infected) make it necessary that a systematic approach be applied to institutional tuberculosis control. Guidelines for such programs recently have been published.[21] These call for (1) rapid and aggressive identification and initiation of isolation and treatment of persons with infectious tuberculosis, (2) routine, systematic tuberculin screening and preventive therapy programs for all inmates and staff, beginning at admission and using directly observed preventive therapy, (3) centralized record keeping to ensure continuity of therapy on transfer or discharge, (4) identification of appropriate isolation facilities for persons suspected of being infectious, (5) establishment of means to disinfect air where ventilation is poor and cannot be improved (e.g., by use of ultraviolet lights), and (6) periodic assessment of tuberculous infection and disease rates and continuity of therapy and preventive therapy, particularly among those who are transferred from institution to institution. In addition, HIV counseling and testing expertise should be readily available so that HIV-antibody testing can be offered to all inmates found to be tuberculin positive.

3. Homeless Shelters

Homeless shelters have long been recognized as places where high-risk groups for tuberculosis reside and where tuberculosis transmission is common.[149-155] Nonetheless, tuberculosis control in homeless shelters continues to be problematic, in part because staff with medical expertise often are not available and shelter users often are transient.

Recently, guidelines have been published that take into account these facts and that advocate collaboration among health-care providers, health departments, shelter operators, and social service agencies to achieve certain basic tuberculosis control elements.[23] These include (1) detection, evaluation, and reporting of homeless persons who have current symptoms of active tuberculosis, (2) ensuring completion of an appropriate course of therapy in those diagnosed with active tuberculosis, (3) maintenance of high levels of ventilation, possibly supplemented as needed by appropriately installed ultraviolet light,[156] and (4) routine tuberculin skin testing for staff and regular volunteers. Tuberculin screening and preventive therapy initiatives among homeless persons generally have been unproductive because of poor patient adherence to follow-up visits and treatment regimens.[23] Screening should be undertaken only if there is a reasonable possibility that most infected persons will complete preventive treatment. Priority groups for screening initiatives include those with HIV infection and recent contacts of persons with infectious tuberculosis.[23]

IV. TUBERCULOSIS ELIMINATION

In 1987, an Advisory Committee for Elimination of Tuberculosis was established to provide recommendations to the U.S. Department of Health and Human Services for developing new technology, applying prevention and control methods, and managing state and local tuberculosis programs targeted at eliminating tuberculosis as a public health problem. In 1989 a strategic plan was published.[1] At that time the committee urged the nation to establish a goal of tuberculosis elimination (less than one case per million population) by the year 2010.

The basis for creating a strategic plan was threefold. First, tuberculosis incidence had been steadily declining and remained a significant problem in fewer and fewer geographic areas and in limited demographically defined pockets. In the remaining pockets, however, it continued to be a significant problem. It was felt that existing methods of tuberculosis control often were underapplied, particularly the use of screening and preventive therapy. Second, the biotechnical revolution had yet to be applied to tuberculosis research: there was substantial potential for generating better diagnostic, treatment, and prevention modalities with which to hasten the decline of tuberculosis. Finally, computer, telecommunications, and other technologies had the potential to allow rapid dissemination and application of new information and new methods for tuberculosis control.

The plan calls for a three-step effort: (1) more effective and intensive use of existing prevention and control methods, especially prevention in high-risk populations; (2) research, both basic science and applied, that will lead to the development and evaluation of new technologies for treatment, diagnosis, and prevention; and (3) rapid assessment and transfer of any newly developed technologies into clinical and public health practice. All three steps are essential if tuberculosis is to be eliminated in the near future. Significant delays in accomplishment of any of them are likely to result in postponement of elimination. In the published plan, it also was recognized that the effect of present tuberculosis control efforts is fragile. It was stated that tuberculosis had the potential for spreading more widely in the community.[1] Indeed, that statement appears to have been borne out.

Whether tuberculosis can be eliminated in the United States in the next 20 years without major scientific breakthroughs in the diagnosis and treatment of latent infection and substantial efforts to eliminate it worldwide remains a matter for conjecture. It is clear, however, that both the existence of the plan and the changing epidemiology of tuberculosis have raised public and professional consciousness about the need for intensified tuberculosis control efforts. The Strategic Plan for the Elimination of Tuberculosis[1] as supplemented by the National Action Plan to Combat Multidrug-Resistant Tuberculosis[15] provide a blueprint for action.

REFERENCES

1. Centers for Disease Control, A strategic plan for the elimination of tuberculosis in United States, *MMWR*, 38 (No. S-3), 1, 1989.
2. Centers for Disease Control, Tuberculosis and human immunodeficiency virus infection: Recommendations of the advisory committee for the elimination of tuberculosis, *MMWR*, 38, 236, 1989.
3. Rieder, H. L., Cauthen, G. M., Comstock, G. W., Snider, D. E., Jr., Epidemiology of tuberculosis in the United States, *Epidemiol. Rev.*, 11, 79, 1989.
4. Rieder, H. L., Cauthen, G. M., Kelly, G. D., Bloch, A. B., Snider, D. E., Jr., Tuberculosis in the United States, *J. Am. Med. Assoc.*, 262, 385, 1989.

5. Barnes, P. F., Bloch, A. B., Davidson, P. T., Snider, D. E., Jr., Tuberculosis in patients with human immunodeficiency virus infection, *N. Engl. J. Med.*, 324, 1644, 1991.

6. Daley, C. L., Small, P. M., Schechter, G. F., Schoolnik, G. K., McAdam, R. A., Jacobs, W. R., Jr., Hopewell, P. C., An outbreak of tuberculosis with accelerated progression among persons infected with the human immunodeficiency virus: an analysis using restriction-fragment-length-polymorphisms, *N. Engl. J. Med.*, 326, 231, 1992.

7. Centers for Disease Control, Nosocomial transmission of multidrug-resistant tuberculosis among HIV-infected persons — Florida and New York, 1988–1991, *MMWR*, 40, 585, 1991.

8. Nelson, A. M., Kayembe, M., Okonda, L., Mulanga, K., Hassig, S., Kalengayi, M., et al., HIV seroprevalence in 500 deaths at University Hospital, Kinshasa, Zaire (abstract), in *IV International Conference on AIDS*, Book 1, Stockholm, June 12–16, 1988, 323.

9. Slutkin, G., The impact of HIV/TB on health care systems: Interventions to meet the global challenge (abstract 2-D), in *World Congress on Tuberculosis, Program and Abstracts*, Bethesda, MD, November 16–19, 1992, 2.

10. Chum, H. L., Graf, P., O'Brien, R. J., Enarson, D., Styblo, K., The impact of HIV infection on tuberculosis in Tanzania (abstract 13-02), in *World Congress on Tuberculosis, Program and Abstracts*, Bethesda, MD, November 16–19, 1992, 41.

11. Aisu, T., Raviglione, M. C., Narain, J. P., Eriki, P., Namaara, W., Adatu, F., ten Dam, H. G., Kochi, A., Monitoring HIV-associated tuberculosis in Uganda (abstract 13-12), in *World Congress on Tuberculosis, Program and Abstracts*, Bethesda, MD, November 16–19, 1992, 43.

12. Slutkin, G., Leowski, J., Mann, J., Tuberculosis and AIDS: the effects of the AIDS epidemic on the tuberculosis problem and tuberculosis programs, *Bull. Int. Union Tuberc. Lung Dis.*, 63, 21, 1988.

13. Harries, A. D., Tuberculosis and human immunodeficiency virus infection in developing countries, *Lancet*, 335, 387, 1990.

14. Centers for Disease Control, Meeting the challenge of multidrug-resistant tuberculosis: Summary of a conference, *MMWR*, 41 (No. RR-11), 51, 1992.

15. Centers for Disease Control, National action plan to combat multidrug-resistant tuberculosis, *MMWR*, 41 (No. R-11), 1, 1992.

16. Centers for Disease Control, Nosocomial transmission of multidrug-resistant tuberculosis to health-care workers and HIV infected patients in an urban hospital — Florida, *MMWR*, 39, 718, 1990.

17. Centers for Disease Control, Transmission of MDR-TB among persons in a correctional system — New York, 1991, *MMWR* 41, 507, 1991.

18. Dooley, S. W., Villarino, M. E., Mercedes, L., Salinas, L., Amil, S., Rullan, J. V., Jarvis, W. R., Bloch, A. B., Cauthen, G. M., Nosocomial transmission of tuberculosis in a hospital unit for HIV-infected patients, *J. Am. Med. Assoc.*, 267, 2632, 1992.

19. Edlin, B. R., Tokars, J. I., Grieco, M. H., Crawford, J. T., Williams, J., Sordillo, E. M., Ong, K. R., Kilburn, J. O., Dooley, S. W., Castro, K. G., Jarvis, W. R., Holmberg, S. D., An outbreak of multidrug-resistant tuberculosis among hospitalized patients with the acquired immunodeficiency syndrome, *N. Engl. J. Med.*, 326, 1514, 1992.

20. Centers for Disease Control, Guidelines for preventing the transmission of tuberculosis in health-care settings, with specal focus on HIV-related issues, *MMWR*, 39 (No. RR-17), 1, 1990.

21. Centers for Disease Control, Prevention and control of tuberculosis in correctional institutions: recommendations of the Advisory Committee for the Elimination of Tuberculosis, *MMWR*, 38, 313, 1989.

22. Centers for Disease Control, Screening for tuberculosis and tuberculous infection in high-risk populations: recommendations of the Advisory Committee for the Elimination of Tuberculosis, *MMWR*, 39 (No. RR-8), 1, 1990.

23. Centers for Disease Control, Prevention and control of tuberculosis among homeless persons: recommendations of the Advisory Council for the Elimination of Tuberculosis, *MMWR*, 41 (No. RR-5), 13, 1992.

24. Centers for Disease Control, Prevention and control of tuberculosis in facilities providing long-term care to the elderly, *MMWR*, 39 (No. RR-10), 7, 1990.

25. Centers for Disease Control, Initial therapy for tuberculosis in the era of multidrug resistance: recommendations of the Advisory Council for the Elimination of Tuberculosis, *MMWR*, 42 (No. RR-7), 1, 1993.

26. City of New York, Tuberculosis blueprint: Goals and objectives (draft, October 8, 1992), 1, 1992.

27. Centers for Disease Control, The use of preventive therapy for tuberculous infection in the United States: recommendations of the Advisory Committee for the Elimination of Tuberculosis, *MMWR*, 39 (No. RR-8), 9, 1990.

28. Selwyn, P. A., Hartel, D., Lewis, V. A., Schoenbaum, E. E., Vermund, S. H., Klein, R. S., Walker, A. T., Friedland, G. H., A prospective study of the risk of tuberculosis among intravenous drug users with human immunodeficiency virus infection, *N. Engl. J. Med.*, 320, 545, 1989.

29. Villarino, M. E., Dooley, S. W., Geiter, L. J., Castro, K. G., Snider, D. E., Jr., Management of persons exposed to multidrug-resistant tuberculosis, *MMWR*, 41 (No. RR-11), 61, 1992.

30. World Health Organization, World Health Organization Expert Committee on Tuberculosis, Ninth report, Technical Report Service WHO 552, 1974.

31. Horne, N. W., Eradication of tuberculosis in Europe — so near and yet so far, *Bull. Int. Union Tuberc.*, 59, 107, 1985.

32. Styblo, K., Tuberculosis control and surveillance, in *Recent Advances in Respiratory Medicine*, Fenley, D. C., Petty, T. L., Eds., Churchill Livingston, London, 1986, chap. 6.

33. Kopanoff, D. E., Kilburn, J. O., Glassroth, J. L., Snider, D. E., Jr., Farer, L. S., Good, R. C., A continuing survey of tuberculosis primary drug resistance in the United States: March 1975 to November 1977. A United States Public Health Service cooperative study, *Am. Rev. Resp. Dis.*, 118, 835, 1978.

34. Centers for Disease Control, Primary resistance to antituberculosis drugs — United States, *MMWR*, 32, 521, 1983.

35. Snider, D. E., Jr., Cauthen, G. M., Farer, L. S., Kelly, G. D., Kilburn, J. O., Good, R. C., Dooley, S. W., Drug-resistant tuberculosis (letter to editor), *Am. Rev. Resp. Dis.*, 144, 732, 1991.

36. Simone, P., Centers for Disease Control, unpublished data, 1992.

37. Beck-Sague, C., Dooley, S. W., Hutton, M. D., Otten, J., Breeden, A., Crawford, J. T., Pitchenik, A. E., Woodley, C., Cauthen, G., Jarvis, W. R., Hospital outbreak of multidrug-resistant *Mycobacterium tuberculosis* infections: factors in transmission to staff and HIV-infected patients, *J. Am. Med. Assoc.*, 268, 1280, 1992.

38. Pearson, M. L., Jereb, J. A., Frieden, T. R., Crawford, J. T., Davis, B. J., Dooley, S. W., Jarvis, W. R., Nosocomial transmission of multidrug-resistant *Mycobacterium tuberculosis*: a risk to patients and health care workers, *Ann. Intern. Med.*, 117, 191, 1992.

39. Fischl, M. A., Uttamchandani, M. D., Daikos, G. L., Poblete, R. B., Moreno, J. N., Reyes, R. R., Boota, A. M., Thompson, L. M., Cleary, T. J., Lai, S., An outbreak of tuberculosis caused by multiple-drug-resistant tubercle bacilli among patients with HIV-infection, *Ann. Intern. Med.*, 117, 177, 1992.

40. Dooley, S. W., Jarvis, W. R., Martone, W. J., Snider, D. E., Jr., Multidrug-resistant tuberculosis, *Ann. Intern. Med.*, 117, 257, 1992.

41. Wadhawan, D., Hira, S., Mwansa, N., Tembo, G., Perine, P., Preventive tuberculosis chemotherapy with isoniazid among persons infected with human immunodeficiency virus (abstract W.B.2261), *Proceedings of the Seventh International Conference on AIDS*, Florence, Italy, June 16–21, 1992.

42. Minga, A., Elliot, A., Halwindii, B., Pobee, J., Luo, N., Porter, J., McAdam, K. P. W. J., One year follow-up on patients in a pilot study to determine efficacy of chemoprophylaxis in the prevention of HIV-related tuberculosis in Zambia (abstract 7-06), in *World Congress on Tuberculosis, Program and Abstracts*, Bethesda, MD, November 16–19, 1992, 35.

43. Aisu, T., Raviglione, M. C., Von Praag, E., Eriki, P., Narain, J. P., Adatu, F., Tembo, G., O'Brien, R., Feasibility of isoniazid preventive chemotherapy for HIV-associated tuberculosis in Uganda: Preliminary results (abstract 8-04), in *World Congress on Tuberculosis, Program and Abstracts*, Bethesda, MD, November 16–19, 1992, 36.

44. Centers for Disease Control, Use of BCG vaccines in the control of tuberculosis: a joint statement by the ACIP and the Advisory Committee for Elimination of Tuberculosis, *MMWR*, 37, 663, 1988.

45. Advisory Council for the Elimination of Tuberculosis, personal communication, 1992.

46. Bloch, A. B., Centers for Disease Control, personal communication, 1992.

47. Bloch, A. B., personal communication, 1992.

48. American Thoracic Society, Control of tuberculosis, *Am. Rev. Resp. Dis.*, 128, 336, 1983.

49. National Institute of Occupational Safety and Health, NIOSH recommended guidelines for personal respiratory protection of workers in health-care facilities potentially exposed to tuberculosis, U.S. Department of Health and Human Services, Public Health Service, Centers for Disease Control, September 14, 1992.

50. Maloney, S. A., Pearon, M., Gordon, M., Del Castillo, R., Boyle, J., Jarvis, W., The efficacy of recommended infection control measures in preventing nosocomial transmission of multidrug-resistant tuberculosis (abstract 15-10), in *World Congress on Tuberculosis, Program and Abstracts*, Bethesda, MD, November 16–19, 1992, 51.

51. Otten, J., Chan, J., Cleary, T., Successful control of an outbreak of multidrug-resistant tuberculosis in an urban teaching hospital (abstract 15-11), in *World Congress on Tuberculosis, Program and Abstracts*, Bethesda, MD, November 16–19, 1992, 51.

52. Wenger, P., Beck-Sague, C., Otten, J., Breeden, A., Orfas, D., Jarvis, W., Efficacy of control measures in preventing nosocomial transmission of multidrug-resistant *Mycobacterium tuberculosis* among patients and health-care workers (abstract 15-16), in *World Congress on Tuberculosis, Program and Abstracts*, Bethesda, MD, November 16–19, 1992, 53.

53. Small, P., unpublished data, 1992.

54. Nolan, C. M., unpublished data, 1992.

55. Centers for Disease Control, Division of Tuberculosis Elimination, 1990 Case Management Reports, unpublished data, 1992.

56. U.S. Department of Health and Human Services, *1987 Tuberculosis Statistics in the United States*, HHS Publication No.(CDC) 89-8322, 1989.

57. Hinman, A. R., Centers for Disease Control, unpublished data, 1992.

58. Hayden, C. R., HIV-related tuberculosis prevention in drug treatment centers and correctional facilities (abstract 11-02), in *World Congress on Tuberculosis, Program and Abstracts*, Bethesda, MD, November 16–19, 1992, 38.

59. Centers for Disease Control, Prevention and control of tuberculosis in migrant farm workers: recommendations of the Advisory Council for the Elimination of Tuberculosis, *MMWR*, 41 (No. RR-10), 1, 1992.

60. Centers for Disease Control, Tuberculosis among foreign-born persons entering the United States: recommendations of the Advisory Committee for Elimination of Tuberculosis, *MMWR*, 39 (No. RR-18), 1, 1990.

61. Centers for Disease Control, Drug-resistant tuberculosis among the homeless — Boston, *MMWR*, 34, 429, 1985.

62. Barry, M. A., Wall, C., Shirley, L., Bernardo, J., Schwingl, P., Brigandi, E., Lamb, G. A., Tuberculosis screening in Boston's homeless shelters, *Public Health Rep.*, 101, 487, 1986.

63. Slutkin, G., Management of tuberculosis in urban homeless indigents, *Public Health Rep.*, 101, 481, 1986.

64. McAdam, J., Brickner, P. W., Glicksman, R., Edwards, D., Fallon, B., Yanowitch P., Tuberculosis in the SRO/homeless population, in *Health Care of Homeless People*, Brickner, P. W., Scharer, L. K., Conanan, B., Elvy, A., Savarese, M., Eds., Springer, New York, 1985, 155.

65. Cielsielski, S. D., Seed, J. R., Esposito, P. H., Hunter, N., The epidemiology of TB among North Carolina migrant farm workers, *J. Am. Med. Assoc.*, 265, 1715, 1991.

66. American Thoracic Society, Treatment of tuberculosis and tuberculous infection in adult and children, *Am. Rev. Resp. Dis.*, 134, 355, 1986.

67. American Thoracic Society, Control of tuberculosis in the United States, *Am. Rev. Resp. Dis.*, 146, 1623, 1992.

68. Cohn, D. L., Catlin, B. J., Peterson, K. L., Judson, F. N., Sbarbaro, J. A., A 62-dose, 6 month therapy for pulmonary and extrapulmonary tuberculosis: a twice-weekly, directly observed and cost-effective regimen, *Ann. Intern. Med.*, 112, 407, 1990.

69. Combs, D. L., O'Brien, R. J., Geiter, L. J., United States Public Health Service tuberculosis short course chemotherapy trial 21: effectiveness, toxicity and acceptability, *Ann. Intern. Med.*, 112, 397, 1990.

70. Mugerwa, R., Okwera, A., Viecha, M., Aisu, T., Huebner, R., Ellner, J., Morrissey, A., Drug toxicity and mortality in HIV-infected Ugandan patients treated for pulmonary tuberculosis (abstract 13-11), in *World Congress on Tuberculosis, Program and Abstracts*, Bethesda, MD, November 16–19, 1992, 43.

71. Chintu, C., Bhat, G. T., Luo, C., Kabika, Raviglione, M. C., O'Brien, R. J., HIV seroprevalence and fatal skin reactions in children treated for tuberculosis in Lusaka, Zambia (abstract 13-13), in *World Congress on Tuberculosis, Program and Abstracts*, Bethesda, MD, November 16–19, 1992, 44.

72. Ireland, H. D., Outpatient chemotherapy for tuberculosis, *Am. Rev. Resp. Dis.*, 82, 378, 1960.

73. Preston, D. F., Miller, F. L., The tuberculosis outpatient's defection from therapy, *Am. J. Med. Sci.*, 247, 55, 1964.

74. Moulding, T., New responsibilities for health departments and public health nurses in tuberculosis — keeping outpatients on therapy, *Am. J. Public Health*, 56, 416, 1966.

75. Addington, W. W., Patient compliance: the most serious remaining problem in the control of tuberculosis in the United States, *Chest*, 76, 741, 1979.

76. Sbarbaro, J. A., Public health aspects of tuberculosis: supervision of therapy, *Clin. Chest Med.*, 1, 253, 1980.

77. Reichman, L., Compliance in developed nations, *Tuberculosis*, 68(Suppl.), 25, 1987.

78. Brudney, K., Dobkin, J., Resurgent tuberculosis in New York City: human immunodeficiency virus, homelessness, and the decline of tuberculosis control programs, *Am. Rev. Resp. Dis.*, 144, 745, 1991.

79. Styblo, K., How should a tuberculosis control program be evaluated?, unpublished talk at the World Congress on Tuberculosis, Bethesda, MD, November 17, 1992.

80. Meichembaum, D., Turk, D. C., *Facilitating Treatment Adherence: A Practitioner's Guidebook*, Plenum, New York, 1987.

81. Gerber, K. E., Nehemkis, A. M., Eds., *Compliance: The Dilemma of the Chronically Ill*, Springer, New York, 1986.

82. DiMatteo, M. R., DiNicola, D. D., *Achieving Patient Compliance: The Psychology of the Medical Practitioner's Role*, Pergamon Press, New York, 1982.

83. Haynes, R. B., Taylor, D. W., Sackett, D. L., Eds., *Compliance in Health Care*, The Johns Hopkins University Press, Baltimore, 1979.

84. Kirscht, J. P., Rosenstock, I. M., Patients' problems in following recommendations of health experts, in *Health Psychology: A Handbook*, Stone, G. C., Cohen, F., Adler, N. E., Eds., Jossey-Bass, San Francisco, 1979, 189.

85. Sumartojo, E., When tuberculosis treatment fails: a social behavioral account of patient adherence, *Am. Rev. Resp. Dis.*, 147, 1311, 1993.

86. Alcabes, P., Vossenas, P., Cohen, R., Braslow, C., Micheals, D., Zoloth, S., Compliance with isoniazid prophylaxis in jail, *Am. Rev. Resp. Dis.*, 140, 1194, 1989.

87. Corcoran, R., Compliance with chemotherapy for tuberculosis, *Irish Med. J.*, 79, 87, 1986.

88. Barnhoorn, F., Adriaanse, H., In search of factors responsible for noncompliance among tuberculosis patients in Wardha District, India, *Social Sci. Med.*, 34, 291, 1992.

89. Shears, P., Tuberculosis control in Somali refugee camps, *Tubercle*, 65, 111, 1984.

90. Morisky, D. E., Malotte, C. K., Choi, P., Davidson, P., Rigler, S., Sugland, B., Langer, M., A patient education program to improve adherence rates with antituberculosis drug regimens, *Health Ed. Quart.*, 17, 253, 1990.

91. Wurtele, S. K., Galanos, A. N., Roberts, M. C., Increasing return compliance in a tuberculosis detection drive, *J. Behav. Med.*, 3, 311, 1980.

92. Seetha, M. A., Srikantaramu, N., Aneja, K. S., Singh, H., Influence of motivation of patients and their family members on the drug collection by patients, *Indian J. Tuberc.*, 28, 182, 1981.

93. Wobeser, W., To, T., Hoeppner, V. H., The outcome of chemoprophylaxis on tuberculosis prevention in the Canadian Plains Indian, *Clin. Invest. Med.*, 12, 149, 1989.

94. Snider, D. E., Hutton, M. D., *Improving Patient Compliance in Tuberculosis Treatment Programs*, Centers for Disease Control, Atlanta, GA, 1, 1989.

95. Curry, F. J., Neighborhood clinics for more effective outpatient treatment of tuberculosis, *N. Engl. J. Med.*, 279, 1262, 1968.

96. McAdam, J. M., Brickner, P. W., Scharer, L. L., Crocco, J. A., Duff, A. E., The spectrum of tuberculosis in a New York City men's shelter clinic (1982–1988), *Chest*, 97, 798, 1990.

97. McDonald, R. J., Memon, A. M., Reichman, L. B., Successful supervised ambulatory management of tuberculosis treatment failures, *Ann. Intern. Med.*, 96, 297, 1982.

98. Werhane, M. J., Snukst-Torbeck, G., Schraufnagel, D. E., The tuberculosis clinic, *Chest*, 96, 815, 1989.

99. Adler, J. J., Ruggiero, D., Langhorne, W., Heetderks, A., Nivin, B., Residential facility for homeless tuberculosis patients (abstract), *Am. Rev. Resp. Dis.*, 141, A458, 1990.

100. Sbarbaro, J. A., Compliance: Inducements and enforcements, *Chest*, 76(Suppl.), 750, 1979.

101. Hopewell, P. C., Judd, K., Miller, R., Luft, H., Strategies for treating tuberculosis: Costs and outcomes, Centers for Disease Control, unpublished, 1988.

102. Centers for Disease Control, Drug-resistant tuberculosis — Mississippi, *MMWR*, 26, 417, 1977.

103. Centers for Disease Control, Follow-up on drug-resistant tuberculosis — Mississippi, *MMWR*, 27, 355, 1978.

104. Hotchkiss, R. L., Directly observed therapy in Mississippi, in TB Notes Fall/Summer Issue, Centers for Disease Control, 1992, 8.

105. Holcombe, R., Mississippi Department of Health, personal communication, 1992.

106. Sbarbaro, J. A., Iseman, M., Baby needs a new pair of shoes, *Chest*, 90, 754, 1986.

107. Division of Tuberculosis Control, South Carolina Department of Health and Environmental Control, *Enablers and Incentives*, American Lung Association of South Carolina, 1989.

108. Snider, D. E., Jr., Anders, H. M., Pozsik, C. J., Incentives to take up health services (letter), *Lancet*, 2, 812, 1986.

109. Marino, J. P., Connecticut Department of Health Services, personal communication, 1992.

110. Burkhardt, K. R., Nel, E. E., Monitoring regularity of drug intake in tuberculous patients by means of simple urine tests, *S. Afr. Med. J.*, 57, 981, 1980.

111. Ellard, G. A., Greenfield, C., A sensitive urine-test method for monitoring the ingestion of isoniazid, *J. Clin. Pathol.*, 30, 84, 1977.

112. Kilburn, J. O., Beam, R. E., David, H. L., Sanches, E., Corpe, R. F., Dunn, W., Reagent-impregnated paper strip for detection of metabolic products of isoniazid in urine, *Am. Rev. Resp. Dis.*, 106, 923, 1972.

113. Henderson, W. T., The development and use of the Potts-Cozart tube test for the detection of isoniazid metabolites in urine, *J. Arkansas Med. Soc.*, 82, 445, 1986.

114. Schraufnagel, D. E., Stoner, R., Whiting, E., Snukst-Torbeck, G., Werhane, M. J., Testing for isoniazid: an evaluation of the Arkansas method, *Chest*, 98, 314, 1990.

115. Moulding, T., Onstad, G. D., Sbarbaro, J. A., Supervision of outpatient drug treatment with the medication monitor, *Ann. Intern. Med.*, 73, 559, 1970.

116. Cheung, R., Dickins, J., Nicholson, P. W., Thomas, A. S. C., Smith, H. H., Larson, H. E., Desmukh, A. A., Dobbs, R. J., Dobbs, S. M., Compliance with anti-tuberculous therapy: A field trial of a pill-box with a concealed electronic recording device, *Eur. J. Clin. Pharmacol.*, 35, 401, 1988.

117. Moulding, T., Medication monitors for selecting tuberculosis patients who need directly observed therapy (abstract 8-01), in *World Congress on Tuberculosis, Program and Abstracts*, Bethesda, MD, November 16–19, 1992, 35.

118. Etkind, S., Boutotte, J., Ford, J., Singleton, L., Nardell, E. A., Tracking hard-to-treat tuberculosis patients in Massachusetts, *Sem. Resp. Infect.*, 6, 273, 1991.

119. Yeager, H., Medinger, A., Tuberculosis long-term care beds: have we thrown out the baby with the bath water?, *Chest*, 90, 752, 1986.

120. Glassroth, J., Bailey, W. C., Hopewell, P. C., Schecter, G., Harden, J. W., Why tuberculosis is not prevented, *Am. Rev. Resp. Dis.*, 141, 1236, 1990.

121. Mehta, J. B., Dutt, A. K., Harvill, L., Henry, W., Isoniazid preventive therapy for tuberculosis: are we losing our enthusiasm?, *Chest*, 94, 138, 1988.

122. Hadler, J., Connecticut Department of Health Services, personal communication, 1991.

123. Centers for Disease Control, Purified protein derivative (PPD)-tuberculin anergy and HIV infection: guidelines for anergy testing and management of anergic persons at risk of tuberculosis, *MMWR*, 40 (No. RR-5), 27, 1991.

124. Jordan, T. J., Lewit, E. M., Montgomery, R. L., Reichman, L. B., Isoniazid as preventive therapy in HIV-infected intravenous drug abusers, *J. Am. Med. Assoc.*, 265, 2987, 1991.

125. Shaw, J. B., Wynn-Williams, N., Infectivity of pulmonary tuberculosis in relation to sputum status, *Am. Rev. Tuberc.*, 69, 724, 1954.

126. Loudon, R. G., Spohn, S. K., Cough frequency and infectivity in patients with pulmonary tuberculosis, *Am. Rev. Resp. Dis.*, 99, 109, 1969.

127. Hutton, M. D., Stead, W. W., Cauthen, G. M., Bloch, A. B., Ewing, W. M., Nosocomial transmission of tuberculosis associated with a draining abscess, *J. Infect. Dis.*, 161, 286, 1990.

128. Cantanzaro, A., Nosocomial transmission of tuberculosis, *Am. Rev. Resp. Dis.*, 125, 559, 1982.

129. Centers for Disease Control, Crack cocaine use among persons with tuberculosis — Contra Costa County, California, 1987–1990, *MMWR*, 40, 485, 1991.

130. Nolan, C. M., unpublished data, 1992.

131. Centers for Disease Control, Transmission of multidrug-resistant tuberculosis from an HIV-positive client in a residential substance-abuse treatment facility — Michigan, *MMWR*, 40, 129, 1991.

132. Fine, L. B., Rwambuya, D. S., Siegel, P. L., Hadler, J. L., Tuberculosis screening policy and practices in urban Connecticut hospitals, April, 1992, unpublished, 1992.

133. Centers for Disease Control, Prevention and control of tuberculosis in U.S. communities with at-risk minority populations: Recommendations of the Advisory Council for the Elimination of Tuberculosis, *MMWR*, 41 (No. RR-5), 1, 1992.

134. Braun, M. M., Truman, B. I., Maguire, B., Increasing incidence of tuberculosis in a prison inmate population, *J. Am. Med. Assoc.*, 261, 393, 1989.

135. Stead, W. W., Lofgren, J. P., Warren, E., Thomas, C., Tuberculosis as an endemic and nosocomial infection among the elderly in nursing homes, *N. Engl. J. Med.*, 312, 1483, 1985.

136. Stead, W. W., To, T., The significance of the tuberculin skin test in elderly persons, *Ann. Intern. Med.*, 107, 833, 1987.

137. Stead, W. W., To, T., Harrison, R. W., Abraham, J. H., III, Benefit risk considerations in preventive therapy for tuberculosis in elderly persons, *Ann. Intern. Med.*, 107, 843, 1987.

138. City of Philadelphia Health Department, unpublished data, 1992.

139. Truman, B. I., Morse, D., Mikl, J., Lehman, S., Forte, A., Broaddus, R., Stevens, R., HIV seroprevalence and risk factors among prison inmates entering New York State prisons (abstract no.4207), in *IVth International Conference on AIDS,* Book I, Stockholm, June 12–16, 1988, 311.

140. Barrett-Conner, E., The epidemiology of tuberculosis in physicians, *J. Am. Med. Assoc.*, 241, 33, 1979.

141. Brennen, C., Muder, R. R., Muraca, P. W., Occult endemic tuberculosis in a chronic care facility, *Infect. Control Hosp. Epidemiol.*, 9, 548, 1988.

142. Goldman, K. P., Tuberculosis in hospital doctors, *Tubercle*, 69, 237, 1988.

143. Ehrenkranz, N. J., Kicklighter, J. L., Tuberculosis outbreak in a general hospital: evidence of airborne spread of infection, *Ann. Intern. Med.,* 77, 377, 1972.

144. Kantor, H. S., Poblete, R., Pusateri, S. L., Nosocomial transmission of tuberculosis from unsuspected disease, *Am. J. Med.*, 84, 833, 1988.

145. Lundgren, R., Norrman, E., Asberg, I., Tuberculous infection transmitted at autopsy, *Tubercle*, 68, 147, 1987.

146. Fraser, V., Kilo, C. M., Bailey, T., Medoff, G., Dunagan, W. C., Incidence and prevalence of tuberculosis among physicians (abstract 15-20), in *World Congress on Tuberculosis, Program and Abstracts*, Bethesda, MD, November 16–19, 1992, 54.

147. Rudnick, J., Kroc, K., Manangan, L., Banerjee, S., Pugliese, G., Jarvis, W., How prepared are U.S. hospitals to control nosocomial transmission of tuberculosis? (abstract 15-13), in *World Congress on Tuberculosis, Program and Abstracts*, Bethesda, MD, November 16–19, 1992, 52.

148. Hinman, A., Centers for Disease Control, personal communication, 1992.

149. Marsh, K., Tuberculosis among the residents of hostels and lodging houses in London, *Lancet*, 1, 1136, 1957.

150. Elmwood, P. C., Tuberculosis in a common lodging house, *Br. J. Prevent. Social Med.*, 15, 89, 1961.

151. Hurford, J. V., The "homeless" male with pulmonary tuberculosis, *Tubercle*, 43, 192, 1962.

152. Patel, K. R., Pulmonary tuberculosis in residents of lodging houses, night shelters and common hostels in Glasgow: a 5-year prospective survey, *Br. J. Dis. Chest*, 79, 60, 1985.

153. Centers for Disease Control, Drug-resistant tuberculosis among the homeless — Boston, *MMWR*, 34, 429, 1985.

154. Nardell, E., McInnis, B., Thomas, B., Weidhaas, S., Exogenous reinfection with tuberculosis in a shelter for the homeless, *N. Engl. J. Med.*, 315, 1570, 1986.

155. Nolan, C. M., Elarth, A. M., Barr, H., Saeed, A. M., Risser, D. R., An outbreak of tuberculosis in a shelter for homeless men, *Am. Rev. Resp. Dis.,* 143, 257, 1991.

156. Riley R. L., Nardell, E. A., Clearing the air: The theory and application of ultraviolet air disinfection, *Am. Rev. Resp. Dis.*, 139, 1286, 1989.

157. Frieden, T. R., Sterling, T., Pablos-Mendez, A., Kilburn, J. O., Cauthen, G. M., Dooley, S. W., The emergence of drug-resistant tuberculosis in New York City, *N. Engl. J. Med.,* 328, 521, 1993.

Chapter 15

BCG Vaccine

Robin E. Huebner, Ph.D., M.P.H., and George W. Comstock, M.D., Dr.P.H., F.A.C.E.

CONTENTS

I. THE HISTORY OF BCG

The discovery of *Mycobacterium tuberculosis* by Robert Koch in 1882 laid the foundation for a rational search for effective means to treat and prevent tuberculosis, a disease that at that time was the leading cause of death in much of the western world. Much research focused on the development of a vaccine; the approaches included the use of sterilized tuberculous tissue, the vaccination of cattle with human *M. tuberculosis* strains to which they were believed to be resistant, as well as the search for low virulence strains of mycobacteria.[1] In 1891 Edward Trudeau successfully attenuated a strain of *M. tuberculosis* isolated from a patient who had fatal miliary disease by inoculating the strain into a rabbit and then repeatedly subculturing the reisolated organisms on solid media.[2] While the use of these attenuated bacilli as a potential vaccine was never explored, the technique of subculturing eventually proved successful for Albert Calmette and Camille Guérin.

The history of what is known today as the bacillus of Calmette and Guérin (BCG) begins in 1908 when Calmette and Guérin began their work with "Lait Nocard," a virulent bovine strain of *M. tuberculosis* isolated by Nocard from a cow that had tuberculous mastitis. The French investigators observed that the addition of bile, a natural detergent, to the laboratory media to prevent clumping of the organisms appeared also to result in attenuation in virulence. Calmette and Guérin began subculturing the organism every 3 weeks on a glycerinated beef–bile–potato medium. In 1921, after 13 years and 230 subcultures, BCG had lost its virulence for animals. Skepticism prompted attempts to restore the virulence of the now predominantly rough colony types by selecting the smooth colony types that were indicative of the original, virulent strain. These attempts proved unsuccessful.[1-3]

The original strain of BCG maintained at the Pasteur Institute in Lille, France, produced hundreds of "daughter" strains and is the progenitor of the most commonly used vaccines, the Copenhagen strain, originating in 1931 as the 423rd transfer, the Tokyo strain, sent from France as a seed culture in 1925, and the Glaxo strain, derived from the 1077th transfer of the Copenhagen strain.[4]

II. VACCINE PRODUCTION AND STANDARDIZATION

Early BCG strains, maintained as freshly prepared cultures, were propagated in hundreds of laboratories using culture methods routine to the particular laboratory. Most laboratories maintained the organisms through serial passage on potato–bile or potato–Sauton media. This method of cultivation continued into the 1960s, when such repeated subculturing was discovered to have resulted in BCG strains that differed markedly from each other. Heterogeneous *in vitro* characteristics such as colony morphology (spreading versus nonspreading), viability on culture medium,[5] biochemical composition and activity,[6-8] drug resistance,[9] immunogenicity in animals and humans,[5,10,11] and virulence in animals[12] have been found among currently available vaccines. In 1950, the World Health Organization (WHO), in an effort to limit the genetic variability among strains of BCG, issued the first in a series of recommendations for BCG production. Since 1960 the availability of lyophilized vaccine has allowed laboratories worldwide to produce seed lots, or quantities of bacteria that are processed together and are of uniform composition, to inoculate working vaccine cultures. The homogeneity of the vaccine strain can be maintained by the use of organisms that are no more than four generations from the primary seed lot.[13,14] In 1982 the responsibility for the international quality control of BCG vaccines was given to the Statens Seruminstitut in Copenhagen, Denmark. The Statens Seruminstitut provides training in vaccine production, distributes reference and seed lots, and oversees the standardization of BCG strains. Three parent strains (Glaxo, Tokyo, and Pasteur) now account for more than 90% of the vaccines used worldwide. The Pasteur strain of BCG currently serves as the international reference strain of vaccine.[15]

While no *in vitro* test has been found to correlate with protection in humans, factors such as the dose of BCG and the proportion of viable bacilli to nonviable bacilli in the preparation are thought to be important factors in the efficacy of the vaccine.[13] The World Health Organization recommends that in addition to ensuring the absence of viable virulent mycobacteria in the preparation, quality control tests for BCG strains include measurements of the total bacterial content (dry weight), the number of viable organisms in the vaccine, the heat stability of the vaccine after incubation for 28 days at 37°C, and the ability of the vaccine to produce tuberculin sensitivity in guinea pigs.[14,15]

In the United States, production standards for BCG vaccines, set by the Food and Drug Administration, specify that they be freeze-dried preparations of live bacilli from a primary or secondary seed lot of a BCG strain identified by complete historical records. The manufacturer must provide estimates of the total bacillary mass by opacity and dry weight, viability as determined by oxygen uptake, germination rate or colony counts, and heat stability. Production lots must be incapable of producing progressive tuberculosis in guinea pigs and must be tested for potency by determination of the number of colony-forming units and by placement

of the intradermal guinea pig test (Jensen's test). In addition, the vaccine must induce tuberculin reactivity in guinea pigs and in 90% of previously tuberculin-nonreactive persons.[16]

III. MECHANISM OF PROTECTIVE IMMUNITY

Immunity to tuberculosis and the mechanism of action of BCG have been investigated in different animal models using different species of animals, as well as varying routes of vaccination and challenge. An estimated 19,683 vaccine test systems are available for evaluating BCG and the events leading to protective immunity.[17] Early work examining the role of humoral immunity showed that although rabbits immunized with BCG were protected against challenge with virulent *M. bovis*, the passive transfer of sera from such animals did not confer protection to *M. bovis*-naive rabbits.[17] That the induction of cell-mediated immunity results in protection against tuberculosis was demonstrated by experiments in which decreased numbers of mycobacteria were recovered from the lungs and spleens of *M. tuberculosis*-challenged mice given T-lymphocytes from BCG-vaccinated animals.[18]

Thus BCG may be useful as a vaccine because it is able to elicit protective cell-mediated immune responses in the absence of progressive disease. Where in the chain of events following exposure to *M. tuberculosis* does BCG interfere? Levy et al.[19] demonstrated that the BCG vaccination of mice did not prevent infection or the establishment of primary foci. These findings were confirmed by Smith et al. who found that the number of organisms recovered from the lung, spleen, and lymph node of vaccinated guinea pigs was not significantly different from those isolated from unvaccinated animals until 14 days postchallenge.[20] Vaccinated animals showed fewer organisms in the spleen and no evidence of dissemination of bacilli to lobes of the lungs not infected at the time of challenge. These data suggest that vaccination with BCG does not protect against infection itself, but rather against uncontrolled replication and dissemination of *M. tuberculosis* from the primary foci to other parts of the lung and body.

IV. ROUTES AND METHODS OF VACCINE ADMINISTRATION

The first child immunized with BCG in July 1921 was a newborn whose grandmother had tuberculosis. Since then, more than 1 billion children in more than 182 countries throughout the world have been vaccinated with BCG. The original BCG strain was given as an oral vaccine to newborns within the first 10 days of life. The oral route of vaccine administration was soon abandoned, however, as most of the infants failed to show tuberculin skin test conversions, which were thought to correlate with the development of protective immunity. The misconception that the bacilli could not penetrate the intestinal mucosa in older children and adults limited vaccination to infants. In addition, higher doses of the vaccine were required for oral immunization, causing an unacceptably high incidence of cervical lymphadenitis and damaging middle-ear infections. Administration of the vaccine by the subcutaneous method produced large abscesses; therefore, the intradermal method was chosen as the best technique for BCG vaccination as it resulted in only superficial abscesses.[21] Currently, the vaccine is most commonly administered by the intradermal method with 0.1 ml of the vaccine delivered into the upper layers of the skin through a 27-gauge syringe.

A second method used to administer BCG is percutaneous scarification or multiple puncture. This technique involves placing several drops of the vaccine on the arm and then introducing the vaccine into the skin through multiple small needles on the puncture device. Though simpler and faster than the intradermal method, this procedure requires a stronger concentration of vaccine. Furthermore, because of the nature of the technique, it is impossible to determine the actual dose of the vaccine administered.[21]

Regardless of the method of administration, vaccination causes a host immune response and eventual scar formation. With the intradermal method, an indurated papule forms within 2–3 weeks of BCG administration. A pustule develops by 6–8 weeks and heals in 3 months, leaving a scar at the vaccination site.[22] With the multiple puncture technique, 2- to 3-mm papules develop within 2 weeks and begin to subside by 6 weeks after vaccination. After 3–4 months the lesions disappear, leaving only discoloration of the skin or slight pitting.[21]

V. TUBERCULIN REACTIVITY AFTER VACCINATION

Tuberculin reactivity develops after vaccination with BCG. Sensitivity appears as early as 10 days after vaccination; maximal responses develop after 6–12 weeks.[23] The size of the reaction depends on a number of factors related both to the vaccine and the host. Edwards and Gelting found that a progressive decrease in the number of viable bacilli in the vaccine resulted in a quantitative decrease in the postvaccination allergy.[24] A 1:2 dilution of vaccine reduced the average tuberculin reaction size by approximately 1 mm[25] while higher concentrations

of vaccine increased the number of tuberculin reactors following vaccination.[26] One study using the Copenhagen 1331 strain found that a 10-fold increase in the dose of the vaccine reduced by 75% the number of children with negligible tuberculin reactivity 12 weeks after vaccination.[27]

Host factors also influence tuberculin reactivity after vaccination with BCG. Familial similarities influence the degree of postvaccination sensitivity in children.[28] Age at vaccination may be important in determining subsequent tuberculin reactivity. In some studies, infants who weighed less than the third percentile for their gestational age showed poor tuberculin conversions if vaccinated at birth,[29] while in other studies rates of conversion were similar for preterm infants and infants whose weight was appropriate for their gestational age.[30] Of Canadian infants vaccinated at 3 months of age, 33% developed sensitivity to tuberculin after vaccination. Only 14% of those vaccinated at birth developed tuberculin sensitivity.[31] These results agree with *in vitro* lymphocyte studies in Cree Indian children, which showed greater responses in lymphocytes from children vaccinated after 9 months of age than in those from children vaccinated at an earlier age.[32] Malnutrition also has been found to influence tuberculin reactivity after vaccination.[33]

Postvaccination sensitivity in BCG-vaccinated children ranges in size from 3 to 19 mm; this reactivity wanes with time. One study of Danish schoolchildren found that initially small postvaccination tuberculin reactions decreased by 1–2 mm after 5 years. In contrast, initial reaction sizes of 10 mm or greater remained unchanged over the same time period.[34] In Sri Lanka, BCG-induced sensitivity waned after 5–7 years.[35] Sixty-five percent of Navy recruits in the United States showed decreases in tuberculin reactivity within 8–15 years after vaccination.[36] Finally, in a study in Chicago, more than 90% of vaccinated infants were tuberculin reactive by 3 months after vaccination; the prevalence of tuberculin reactivity declined rapidly by 18 months after vaccination.[37]

Repeated tuberculin skin testing may prolong sensitivity in BCG-vaccinated persons. BCG-vaccinated children in Denmark who were tuberculin skin tested within 5 years of vaccination had significantly larger tuberculin reactions than those BCG-vaccinated children who had never been skin tested during the 5-year interval.[38] Young found the prevalence of 5 mm or greater induration in Canadian Indian children age 1–15 years to increase with the number of documented Mantoux tests.[39] Repeated tuberculin testing also can increase the reaction size of skin tests in vaccinated persons (the booster effect). After repeated skin testing an increase in duration of 6 mm or greater was noted in 13% of children attending day care centers in South Africa.[40] Finally, revaccination with BCG also can increase the size of tuberculin reactions.[41]

After BCG vaccination it is not possible on an individual basis to distinguish between a tuberculin skin test reaction caused by virulent mycobacterial infection or by vaccination itself. When interpreting skin tests, several factors increase the probability that a reaction was caused by virulent mycobacterial infection: large reaction size, a history of close contact with a person with active tuberculosis, residence in an area with a high prevalence of tuberculosis, and a long time interval since vaccination.[42] For more information on this matter, please refer to Chapter 13 (this volume).

Although tuberculin sensitivity occurs after BCG vaccination, there is poor correlation between tuberculin reactivity and protection against active tuberculosis.[43] Some studies have shown that high tuberculin conversion rates correlate with little protective efficacy, while other studies with low conversion rates have found good protection after vaccination.[43,44] Nevertheless, in most developed countries where BCG is used, children are revaccinated if their tuberculin skin test reactions fail to convert to positive within 2–3 months of vaccination.

VI. SAFETY OF BCG VACCINE

The safety of early BCG vaccines was questioned in 1930 when active tuberculosis developed in 72 of 251 children given oral vaccination during a mass vaccination program in Lubeck, Germany. All 72 children died.[45] Investigations into the tragedy later showed that a culture of virulent *M. tuberculosis* had been mistaken for the BCG strain, which had been kept in the same incubator. The directors and others in the laboratory subsequently were tried and convicted of negligence and malpractice.

Today BCG is considered to be one of the safer vaccines available. The most frequent side effects after BCG vaccination are regional suppurative adenitis and osteitis.

A. REGIONAL LYMPHADENITIS

In a review of literature published between 1921 and 1982, Lotte et al.[46] found 6000 reported cases of regional lymphadenitis. The majority occurred within the first 5 months after vaccination. *M. bovis* BCG was cultured from 7% of the lesions. For those vaccinated, the risk of lymphadenitis ranged from 0.0006 per 1000 to 38 per 1000. In 1983, a prospective survey of 2 million infants vaccinated between 1979 and 1981 in six European countries (Denmark, German Democratic Republic, Hungary, Romania, and four areas within Croatia and the Federal Republic of Germany) found the risk of lymphadenitis to be 0.025 per 1000.[47]

Several factors contribute to the occurrence of regional lymphadenitis: the vaccine strain, the total number of viable and nonviable bacilli in the vaccine preparation, and the dose of BCG given. The age of the persons vaccinated also is important; for newborns the risk of lymphadenitis is 5–10 times greater than that for preschool and school-age children.[47] Outbreaks of lymphadenitis associated with the use of the Pasteur vaccine in Africa and the Caribbean prompted the 1988 revision of the recommended dosages to be used in newborns and older children. Newborns and infants younger than 1 year old should receive 0.05 ml of vaccine; 0.1 ml is recommended for older children. The technical skill of the personnel who gave the intradermal vaccinations also was implicated in one outbreak in Zimbabwe.[48]

Opinions differ on the treatment of BCG adenitis; options range from administering no treatment, to providing antibiotic chemotherapy, to surgically excising the nodes. Data on the efficacy of treatment are not available from statistically proven and controlled studies; however, one prospective study compared antibiotic treatment to no active treatment.[49] No significant differences in the incidence of spontaneous drainage and suppuration were found between any of the groups. In those individuals receiving no treatment, the early onset of lymphadenitis was more likely to cause drainage and suppuration than were lesions that developed more slowly; these differences were not seen in the group receiving antibiotic treatment. While the authors conclude that medical therapy may have some beneficial effect if given to those in whom lymphadenitis develops rapidly after vaccination, there is no consensus in the medical community about what treatment is appropriate.

B. OSTEITIS

As with regional lymphadenitis, the risk of developing osteitis after BCG vaccination varies from country to country. Between 1948 and 1974, 291 cases of disseminated BCG involving lesions of the musculoskeletal system were reported from 13 countries.[47] Japan showed the lowest risk (0.01 per 1,000,000); Sweden and Finland showed the highest risks (32.5 and 43.4 per 1,000,000, respectively). Investigations in Sweden found that the incidence of BCG osteitis had increased significantly from 1 per 100,000 to 2.5 per 100,000 in the years from 1950 to 1969 to an annual rate of 25 per 100,000 to 33 per 100,000 between 1972 and 1975.[50] Osteitis developed within 4–144 months of vaccination; most cases occurred within 7–24 months. The most frequent site affected was the epiphysis of the long bones, particularly in the legs. Similar results were seen in Finland.[51] Explanations for the increases in BCG osteitis in both countries remain unclear, although cases appeared to coincide with a change in vaccine production. The Gothenburg strain, prepared in Sweden, had been used in both countries; in 1971 vaccine production was transferred to the Statens Seruminstitut in Copenhagen. Other countries also have experienced increases in BCG osteitis after changes in either the vaccine strain or the method of production.[15] In addition to the change in the vaccine manufacturer, the compulsory notification of BCG reactions to the Swedish Adverse Drug Reaction Committee, mandated in 1972, and the dissemination of information concerning the untoward reactions most likely prompted the expanded surveillance and reporting of cases of osteitis in both countries. As a result of these findings, Sweden discontinued the routine vaccination of neonates in 1975. Finland continued immunization using the Glaxo strain of vaccine.

Antituberculosis therapy, coupled in some cases with surgical curettage and debridement, usually results in healing of the skeletal lesions.

C. DISSEMINATED FATAL BCG DISEASE

The most serious complication of BCG vaccination is disseminated BCG disease. Although rare, "BCGitis" usually is fatal. Hematogenous dissemination of the bacilli after vaccination has been demonstrated. In most persons, the spread of the organisms is relatively benign and does not cause overt disease; however, at least 35 fatalities were reported between 1948 and 1972. BCGitis is seen most frequently in children with concomitant immunodeficiencies, such as severe combined immunodeficiency syndrome or chronic granulomatous disease. In only a few cases does disease develop in the presence of an intact immune system. Recently Tardieu et al. reported two cases of culture-confirmed BCG meningitis in immunocompetent children immunized 1.5–5 years previously.[52]

Although most cases of BCGitis occur within the first 6 months after vaccination, longer latent periods have been noted. In one instance, culture-confirmed BCG disease with widespread lymph node, liver, bone, and lung involvement developed in an 18-year-old boy 6 years after vaccination.[53] The patient subsequently was found to have several immunological defects, including abnormal macrophage and T-lymphocyte functions. The patient died despite prolonged antimycobacterial treatment.

Treatment for disseminated BCG disease is similar to the treatment for active tuberculosis with one exception; pyrazinamide is not used to treat BCGitis because all BCG strains are resistant to this antibiotic. Even when treated with potentially effective chemotherapeutic agents, many cases of disseminated BCG are fatal, particularly if the patient has underlying immunosuppression.

VII. VACCINE EFFICACY

A total of 17 controlled trials of the efficacy of BCG vaccine in humans have been carried out.[54-70] These trials are summarized in Table 15-1; the eight major trials are described in detail.

The first large field trial of BCG efficacy began in 1935 among eight North American Indian tribes.[58] The efficacy of a vaccine prepared by the Henry Phipps Institute of Philadelphia was evaluated in tuberculin-negative children and adolescents aged 0–20 years. The duration of follow-up was 9–11 years for the development of active tuberculosis; tuberculosis mortality was assessed after 20 years. Roentgenographic evidence of pulmonary tuberculosis was found in 238 of the 1457 unvaccinated persons; 64 of the 1551 given BCG vaccination developed active tuberculosis. The protective efficacy against active tuberculosis was 75%. There was an 82% reduction in deaths resulting from tuberculosis.

In their study of high-risk infants in Chicago, Rosenthal and colleagues[59] also found that BCG conferred a high degree of protection. Between 1937 and 1948, 3381 children born at Cook County Hospital were randomly assigned to receive either the Tice strain of BCG or to remain unvaccinated. The length of follow-up ranged from 12 to 23 years; during this time, 59 cases of tuberculosis occurred in the 1665 unvaccinated persons while only 16 of 1716 vaccinated individuals developed evidence of active disease (efficacy = 75%).

The Medical Research Council of Great Britain (MRC) conducted a large controlled trial of the Copenhagen strain of vaccine.[67] Between 1950 and 1952, a total of 14,100 tuberculin-negative schoolchildren between the ages of 14 and 16 were vaccinated; 13,300 children were randomized to the unvaccinated control group. The protective efficacy of the vaccine was 84% during the first 5 years of the study. By 15 years after vaccination, 243 cases of tuberculosis had developed in the unvaccinated group, compared with only 56 cases in those who had received BCG (efficacy = 77%). The prevalence and incidence of tuberculosis in Great Britain decreased significantly during the study period. The number of cases in the unvaccinated control group was so small during the 15 through 19 year follow-up that the trial was discontinued.

The growing support for BCG vaccination by WHO and the belief that preventive measures could significantly contribute to the control of tuberculosis

Table 15-1   **Controlled trials of BCG efficacy against tuberculosis**

Population	Vaccine	Year	Years of Follow-up	Percent Reduction in cases	Reference
237 infants — Philadelphia	King	1927	3–48	83 (deaths)	54
1,092 infant contacts — New York	IC	1933	5–11	8 (deaths)	55
609 newborns — Saskatchewan	Frappie	1933	15	81	56
41,301 newborns — Algiers	Oral	1935	1–11	11 (deaths)	57
2996 Indian children — United States	Phipps	1935	9–11	75	58
3,381 newborns — Chicago	Tice	1937	12–23	75	59
262 Indian newborns — United States	Phipps	1938	6–8	59	60
451 newborn contacts — Chicago	Tice	1941	19	75	61
4,839 children — Georgia	Tice	1947	20	−57	62
1,025 children — Illinois	Tice	1947	13	−40	63
77,972 children — Puerto Rico	Birkhaug	1949	18–20	29	64
13,914 adults — Georgia/Alabama	Tice	1950	20	33	65
21,000 villagers — Madanapalle	Danish	1950	16–21	20	66
27,400 adolescents — England	Danish	1950	18–20	77	67
16,314 miners — South Africa	Glaxo	1965	3	38	68
2,174 villagers — Haiti	Frappier	1965	3	67	69
260,000 villagers — Chingleput	Danish French	1968	15	−2	70

prompted the U.S. Public Health Service to sponsor a series of controlled trials examining the efficacy of BCG. The first study began in 1947. A total of 2948 tuberculin-negative schoolchildren in Muscogee County, GA, were vaccinated with the Tice strain of vaccine; 2341 tuberculin-negative children were left unvaccinated.[62] Allocation to vaccine group was done by even or odd year of birth. Eight cases of tuberculosis developed during the 20-year study period; three cases occurred in unvaccinated persons and five occurred in those given BCG. No protective efficacy was detected in this study.

When it became clear that the incidence of tuberculosis in schoolchildren in Muscogee County was not as high as originally expected, a second study was begun in adults in the county as well as in the neighboring Russell County, AL.[65] The 20-year evaluation, published in 1976, again found no protection after vaccination with BCG; equal numbers of cases were found in the vaccinated and control groups.

A 29% reduction in tuberculosis incidence was observed in another U.S. Public Health Service-sponsored study of Puerto Rican children aged 1–18 years who were given a vaccine prepared by the New York State Department of Health (Birkhaug strain).[64]

Finally, a study in a rural population in southern India found a 60% reduction in the incidence of tuberculosis in the vaccinated group as compared with the unvaccinated group 7 years after

vaccination.[66] By 20 years after vaccination, the vaccine efficacy had declined to 20%.

The variable results of the published trials of BCG efficacy and the concern that the vaccines used in previous studies were so heterogeneous that they might not be of uniform potency prompted what became the largest controlled community trial ever designed to examine the efficacy of BCG vaccine. The trial, cosponsored by the Indian Council of Medical Research, WHO, and the U.S. Public Health Service, began in 1968. During the course of 3 years, 265,172 villagers older than 1 month of age and living in the Chingleput district near Madras were enrolled in the study.[70] Participants were randomized to receive either a low or high dose of the French or Danish vaccine or dextran placebo without regard to tuberculin sensitivity or radiographic findings. These two vaccines were selected for the study as they had demonstrated the best test activity in animal models and were available as freeze-dried preparations. Follow-up data were analyzed according to the degree of initial skin test sensitivity. During the 15-year follow-up period, 533 cases of pulmonary tuberculosis developed in those persons with less than 7 mm induration to tuberculin at enrollment; the number of cases was divided evenly among those receiving the placebo or the low or high doses of vaccine. Vaccination did provide some protection (17%) against pulmonary tuberculosis in children aged 0–14 years; adult vaccinees had more tuberculosis than the unvaccinated controls.

An additional finding of the Chingleput trial has gone unnoticed. For several decades, it had been standard practice to vaccinate without a prior tuberculin test for the purpose of excluding persons already infected with *M. tuberculosis*. However, the safety of this procedure was established largely by casual and anecdotal evidence that vaccination reactions among positive tuberculin reactors did not seem sufficiently severe to contraindicate direct vaccination. The follow-up of the Chingleput trial established for the first time that BCG vaccine could be given to positively reacting children, to adults with abnormal chest radiographs, and even to persons with sputum positive for *M. tuberculosis* without demonstrable harm.[71]

Rather than resolving the issue of the efficacy of BCG, the Chingleput study brought forward even more questions about the usefulness of vaccination. The lack of protective efficacy observed in the study disappointed the public health community and forced a reevaluation of the WHO policy on the use of BCG in developing countries. Other than the two southern India trials,[66,70] none of the controlled studies was conducted in Africa or Asia, areas of the world where the incidence and prevalence of tuberculosis are highest and where BCG vaccination might be of greatest value. Another randomized, placebo-controlled trial of the efficacy of BCG would not be economically or logistically feasible and would require many years of follow-up to reach a statistically valid endpoint. In an effort to gain information on the impact of BCG on the tuberculosis burden in developing countries, WHO sponsored several case-control studies of BCG vaccination. The studies, conducted in Brazil, Burma, Sri Lanka, and Argentina, concentrated on childhood tuberculosis and used a variety of control populations, such as patients hospitalized for diseases other than tuberculosis and neighbors or siblings of tuberculosis patients.[72] As in the previous controlled prospective trials, the results varied widely: the effectiveness of the vaccination programs ranged from 2–84%. Protection conferred by vaccination was highest against disseminated forms of tuberculosis, such as meningitis. In recent years, numerous other case-control investigations have found similarly variable results.[73-76] Again, the majority of studies focused on vaccine effectiveness in children and have found protection ranging from 16 to 80%. A small number of cohort studies of children who are contacts of persons with newly diagnosed, culture-confirmed tuberculosis have been funded through WHO. In these studies, the incidence of tuberculosis decreased by 53–66% in children who were given BCG prior to exposure to tuberculosis, compared to those who were not vaccinated with BCG.[77,78]

VIII. EXPLANATIONS FOR VARIABILITY IN EFFICACY

Several hypotheses have been put forward to explain the variability in results of field trials with BCG. These hypotheses have been reviewed by Fine.[79] One hypothesis is that prior infection with nontuberculous mycobacteria could confer some protection against active tuberculosis. Natural infection with these mycobacteria could mask the effects of BCG vaccination by decreasing the susceptibility of the unvaccinated control group, thereby diluting the protective effects in the vaccinated groups. Indeed, studies in both animals and humans have found that infection with environmental mycobacteria can increase immunity to tuberculosis.[80] This hypothesis is supported by the fact that the trials showing the lowest BCG efficacy were in areas such as the southeastern United States where infection with the nontuberculous mycobacteria is common. However, data from studies in Puerto Rico showed no difference in protection after vaccination of persons who reacted only to a large dose (10 tuberculin units) of tuberculin, indicative of infection with nontuberculous mycobacteria.[64] In addition, two trials in the United States that excluded reactors to the large dose of tuberculin, showed the worst efficacy estimates of all of the trials.

There have been continued suggestions that the efficacy of BCG vaccination may be either enhanced or opposed by previous infection with environmental mycobacteria. Two types of cell-mediated immune responses may occur as a result of mycobacterial infection.[81] The first is the so-called "Koch phenomenon," which, in animals, develops 4–6 weeks after infection with *M. tuberculosis* and causes necrosis at the site of tuberculin skin testing. The second, described by Mackaness as a listeria-type response, occurs within days of infection, correlates with the appearance of macrophage-activating T-lymphocytes, and does not produce necrosis upon skin testing. Different species of mycobacteria have been demonstrated in animal models to produce varying levels of these two immune responses. Rook and his colleagues[81] postulate that prior infection with *M. vaccae* or any of the nontuberculous mycobacteria that produce the listeria-type response may enhance the protective effect of subsequent vaccination with BCG. In contrast, infection with *M. scrofulaceum* or those organisms that induce the Koch phenomenon may not only inhibit the development of protective immunity following BCG but actually increase susceptibility to disease from *M. tuberculosis*. It is unlikely, however, that exposure to nontuberculous mycobacteria accounts for all of the observed variability in the efficacy of BCG.

Differences in the potency and immunogenicity of individual vaccine strains also may contribute to the variability in the efficacy of BCG. No animal model has been found to predict the efficacy of vaccination in humans; therefore, protection can be assessed only in field trials in humans. While microbiological differences between the vaccine strains do exist, studies using the same vaccines in different settings have shown both similar and varying efficacies, as have studies using different vaccines in the same setting.[79]

The efficacy of BCG is believed by some to be influenced by differences in the risk of infection of the study populations, differences in the virulence of *M. tuberculosis* isolates or differences in the pathogenesis of disease. Some *M. tuberculosis* isolates from the Chingleput area have been found to be of low virulence for guinea pigs. One hypothesis is that BCG may not be able to protect against these "South Indian variants." This hypothesis has not been supported by laboratory data, which show that protection may be influenced by the virulence of the challenge strain of *M. tuberculosis*, but do not show evidence of poor protection against low-virulence South Indian variants.[82]

Host genetics also have been suggested to play a role in the efficacy of BCG. The immune response to BCG in mice has been found to be regulated by a gene on chromosome 1; this gene also has been found on chromosome 2 in man.[83] However, no statistically significant differences in the efficacy of BCG have been found between racial groups in field trials to suggest that genetic variability is an important factor in protection following vaccination.

Although chronic moderate dietary protein deficiency has been shown to impair the ability of BCG vaccine to protect guinea pigs against challenge with virulent *M. tuberculosis*,[84] data from human trials have failed to support nutrition as a cause of variability in BCG efficacy.

BCG has been shown in animal models to protect against dissemination of organisms from the primary site of infection. Therefore, the efficacy of BCG may depend on whether disease is due to endogenous reactivation or exogenous reinfection. In the latter, the progression to disease would depend on the new primary infection. Thus, in areas where the probability of reinfection is high, such as in southern India, the efficacy of BCG may be lower than in areas where reactivation disease predominates. This hypothesis is supported by data from the Chingleput trial, which showed a high risk of infection in the study area, but a low incidence of tuberculosis in the uninfected, a high incidence of tuberculosis in the infected population, and a long interval between tuberculin conversion and evidence of disease.[85] Data from the earlier trial in Puerto Rico would appear to contradict this hypothesis. The infection rate in Puerto Rico among children initially 1–3 years of age was approximately 2.5% per year. At the time of study recruitment, the area also had a high tuberculosis rate and, in the study population, the uninfected had a relatively low tuberculosis rate and those found to be infected had a relatively high rate. During the 20 year follow-up, the rate of infection decreased, yet the efficacy of BCG remained constant.[86]

Finally, the different study methodologies used in the controlled studies have been blamed for the variable study results. Differences in susceptibility to tuberculosis, follow-up surveillance, diagnostic testing and interpretation, and detection of active disease in the eight major controlled trials have been reviewed by Clemens and colleagues.[87]

It is likely that a combination of some or all of the above hypotheses has influenced the observed variation in the efficacy of BCG. As Fine says, "there is no simple global answer to the problem of BCG's efficacy."[79] Current technologies may provide the tools to unravel the mysteries of protective immunity to *M. tuberculosis* and the role of BCG vaccination.

IX. RECOMMENDATIONS FOR USE OF BCG IN THE CONTROL OF TUBERCULOSIS

Given the high incidence of tuberculosis in many developing countries and the inability to control the spread of infection through chemoprophylaxis and the prompt diagnosis and effective treatment of infectious cases, WHO continues to recommend the use of BCG vaccine on a worldwide basis. BCG vaccine is given as part of the WHO Expanded Programme on Immunization; the vaccine is administered to infants as soon as possible after birth.[88]

In the United States, the general population is at low risk for acquiring tuberculous infection. In most population groups, prevention of tuberculosis is most reliably accomplished by periodic Mantoux testing with tuberculin for high-risk children and adults and with administration of preventive therapy to selected persons with positive tuberculin tests. Therefore, a BCG vaccination policy for the entire population is not indicated. The Immunization Practices Advisory Committee and the Advisory Committee for the Elimination of Tuberculosis have recommended that BCG vaccination be considered only for children with negative tuberculin skin tests who cannot be placed on isoniazid preventive therapy but who have continuous exposure to persons with active tuberculosis, particularly isoniazid and rifampin-resistant disease or who belong to groups with annual rates of infection of >1%.[89] BCG vaccination no longer is recommended for health-care workers; however, in view of recent nosocomial outbreaks of drug-resistant tuberculosis, these recommendations are currently under review (CDC, personal communication).

X. BCG AND THE HUMAN IMMUNODEFICIENCY VIRUS (HIV)

Infection with HIV is known to be the greatest risk factor for the development of active tuberculosis. In developing countries tuberculosis is one of the most frequent opportunistic infections in HIV-infected persons.[90] WHO has recommended BCG vaccination as part of the Expanded Programme on Immunization; however, there now is concern that many children in developing countries may be infected with HIV. For example, more than 6% of AIDS cases and more than 3% of HIV infections in Uganda occurred in children.[91] These children may face an increased risk of disseminated BCG disease after vaccination. Initial reports from Africa suggested that a higher risk of regional lymphadenitis and local abscesses occurred in HIV-infected children after BCG administration. In Zaire an outbreak of local abscesses occurred in 19 children; however, all of the children were found to be HIV seronegative, and the outbreak was attributed later to a change in the manufacturer of the vaccine.[92] Another study in Zaire found that lymphadenitis was 1.8 times as common and fistulas 2 times as common in HIV-infected children as in uninfected children.[93] A relatively high rate (10%) of post-BCG adenopathies was seen among 105 HIV-infected children, although in this study no uninfected children were included as controls.[94]

Two prospective studies of infants at risk for perinatal HIV infection found no increase in untoward reactions to BCG vaccination. La Coeur observed 64 children born to HIV-infected mothers and 130 control children born to HIV-seronegative mothers, looking for local and regional complications of vaccination during the first month of life.[95] After 40 months of follow-up, no significant differences in the risk of lymphadenitis were seen between the HIV-infected and uninfected children (24 vs. 18%, respectively). All the cases resolved spontaneously and there were no cases of disseminated BCG.

Another prospective study in Rwanda found 6 cases of suppuration at the injection site among 377 children vaccinated during the first week of life, 1 child was HIV infected, 1 was born to an HIV-infected mother but was seronegative at 15 months of age, and 4 were born to HIV-uninfected mothers. No other untoward reactions were reported.[96]

Dissemination of BCG and subsequent disease have been seen in HIV-infected persons. *M. bovis* BCG was cultured from the lymph node and cerebrospinal fluid of an HIV-infected child presenting with fever, adenitis, and diarrhea 4 months after vaccination.[97] The symptoms improved after antituberculosis treatment.

Culture-proven dissemination also occurred in a native American child vaccinated at 3 months of age. Organisms were isolated from blood, gastric and tracheal aspirates, and the lung.[98] The vaccination site was crusted and oozing and the child had symptoms of AIDS.

Complications of BCG vaccination also have been reported in adults who had either prior or subsequent HIV infection. Ulceration at the injection site and regional lymphadenopathy developed 4 months after vaccination of one AIDS patient; *M. bovis*, BCG strain, was identified in lesion and blood samples from this patient.[99] BCG adenitis and disseminated disease can occur from months to years after vaccination;[100-102] cases were reported to have occurred in two persons 30 years after they were vaccinated with BCG.[103,104]

To date there have been no controlled studies of the safety of BCG vaccination in adults infected with HIV nor of the efficacy of BCG in either HIV-infected adults or children. However, given the lack of data suggesting a harmful effect of BCG vaccination on HIV-infected children and the high risk this population faces of being infected with *M. tuberculosis* and developing disease, WHO recommends BCG vaccination for asymptomatic HIV-infected children who are at increased risk of tuberculous infection. The WHO does not recommend BCG vaccination for children or adults with symptomatic HIV infection, or for persons known or suspected to be infected with HIV, who have minimal risk of infection with *M. tuberculosis*.[105] The latter recommendation would apply to most populations in the United States for whom BCG might be considered. [89]

XI. FUTURE VACCINE RESEARCH

The logistical advantages of the simultaneous administration of two or more vaccines prompted a study of combined vaccination with a mixture of BCG and diphtheria and tetanus toxoids. This mixed vaccine was found to induce tuberculin reactivity equal to BCG alone and to produce similar antitoxoid antibody responses upon booster immunization.[106]

Recombinant vaccines, using BCG as a vector, also have been tested. BCG offers several advantages as a vector, including its low rate of side effects, its ability to be administered at birth or to older persons, and the fact that a single immunization with BCG is sufficient but multiple administrations are possible. BCG also is a highly effective adjuvant and is very inexpensive ($0.06/dose).[107] Foreign DNA has been inserted into the BCG genome through mycobacteriophages, thus allowing expression of foreign proteins. This technology will enable the development of recombinant BCG vaccines capable of serving as live vaccine vehicles to induce immune responses to other pathogens. For example, a recombinant BCG vaccine is being studied as a possible carrier for HIV proteins; HIV polypeptides have been introduced into and expressed in BCG recombinants. These polypeptides have been demonstrated to induce antibody and T-cell responses in mice.[108]

Other proteins are being examined for their use as potential vaccines against tuberculosis. Guinea pigs develop tuberculin sensitivity when immunized subcutaneously with extracellular proteins that are released when *M. tuberculosis* replicates. They also show fewer viable bacilli in their lungs following aerosol challenge with *M. tuberculosis,* and can survive a normally lethal dose of *M. tuberculosis.*[109] Identification of the proteins capable of inducing protection could lead to the development of a subunit vaccine. This idea is supported by data demonstrating the successful insertion of *M. tuberculosis* proteins into the vaccinia virus genome. Lyons et al.[110] found that vaccinia recombinants expressing *M. tuberculosis* proteins were able to induce antibody production when injected into mice. Research using animal models still is being completed to determine whether these recombinants can provide protection against challenge with virulent *M. tuberculosis.*

However, a final question must be answered before a new vaccine can be recommended for use in humans: does it protect people against tuberculosis? Future controlled trials seem unlikely. They cannot give an answer within a relatively short period unless they are very large and consequently very expensive. Observational studies, whether case-control or cohort, also will require huge numbers or long observation periods. Furthermore, in all observational studies it is difficult if not impossible to separate the effects of the vaccine from the effects of the characteristics of the people who are vaccinated. To make the situation more unsatisfactory, postvaccinal tuberculin sensitivity does not indicate efficacy and animal models appear to be unreliable.

There are, however, ways in which large numbers of persons can be followed at little expense. Suppose that several countries currently using different BCG strains could be persuaded to use their current vaccine strain and the new vaccine in alternate years for the vaccination of newborns. Although reported diagnosable cases of tuberculosis might well be infrequent for the first few years, the large numbers vaccinated each year should provide enough cases to indicate whether the new vaccine was safer and more efficacious than the old vaccine. Comparing the same new vaccine with several BCG strains also would make it possible to rank all of the vaccines with respect to efficacy. Testing the vaccines in a variety of animals models would indicate which animal model is most similar to the human model, thereby allowing that model to be used in evaluating all BCG strains in current use.

REFERENCES

1. Grange, J. M., Gibson, J., Osborn, T. W., What is BCG?, *Tubercle*, 64, 129, 1983.
2. Gardner, L. V., The history of the R1 strain of tubercle bacillus, *Am. Rev. Tuberc.*, 25, 577, 1932.
3. Crispen, R., History of BCG and its substrains, in *BCG in Superficial Bladder Cancer*, EORTC Genitourinary Group Monograph 6, 35, 1989.
4. Osborn, T. W., Changes in BCG strains, *Tubercle*, 64, 1, 1983.
5. Gheorghiu, M., LaGrange, P. H., Viability, heat stability and immunogenicity of four BCG vaccines prepared from four different BCG strains, *Ann. Immunol.*, 134C, 125, 1983.
6. Minnikin, D. E., Parlett, J. H., Magnusson, M., Ridell, M., Lind, A., Mycolic acid patterns of representatives of *Mycobacterium bovis* BCG, *J. Gen. Microbiol.*, 130, 2733, 1984.
7. Abou-Zeid, C., Smith, I., Grange, J., Steele, J., Rook, G., Subdivision of daughter strains of Bacille Calmette-Guérin (BCG) according to secreted protein patterns, *J. Gen. Microbiol.*, 132, 3047, 1986.
8. International Union against Tuberculosis, Phenotypes of BCG-vaccines seed lot strains: results of an International Cooperative Study, *Tubercle*, 59, 139, 1978.
9. Hesselberg, I., Drug resistance in the Swedish/Norwegian BCG strain, *Bull. WHO*, 46, 503, 1972.
10. Grange, J. M., Gibson, J. A., Strain to strain variation in the immunogenicity of BCG, *Dev. Biol. Stand.*, 58, 37, 1986.

11. Nyboe, J., Bunch-Christensen, K., Assay in man of different BCG products, *Bull. WHO*, 35, 645, 1966.

12. Jespersen, A., The potency of BCG vaccines determined on animals, Ph.D. thesis, University of Copenhagen, 1971.

13. WHO Technical Report Series No. 8, *WHO-Sponsored International Quality Control of BCG Vaccine*, 1977.

14. WHO Expert Committee on Biological Standardization, *Requirements for Dried BCG Vaccine* (requirements for biological substances No. 11), 1985.

15. Milstien, J. B., Gibson, J. J., Quality control of BCG vaccine by WHO: a review of factors that may influence vaccine effectiveness and safety, *Bull. WHO*, 68, 93, 1990.

16. *Federal Register*, 50, 50159, 1985.

17. Smith, D. W., Protective effect of BCG in experimental tuberculosis, *Adv. Tuberc. Res.*, 22, 66, 1985.

18. Lefford, M. J., Induction and expression of immunity after BCG immunization, *Infect. Immun.*, 18, 646, 1977.

19. Levy, F. M., Conge, G. A., Pasquier, J. F., Mauss, H., Dubos, R., Schaedler, R., The effect of BCG vaccination on the fate of virulent tubercle bacilli in mice, *Am. Rev. Resp. Dis.*, 84, 28, 1961.

20. Smith, D. W., McMurray, D. N., Wiegeshaus, E. H., Grover, A. A., Harding, G. E., Host-parasite relationships in experimental tuberculosis. IV. Early events in the course of infection in vaccinated and nonvaccinated guinea pigs, *Am. Rev. Resp. Dis.*, 102, 937, 1970.

21. Rosenthal, S. R., Routes and methods of administration, in *BCG Vaccine: Tuberculosis—Cancer*, PSG, Littleton, MA, 1980, chap. 11.

22. Myint, T. T., Yin, Y., Yi, M. M., Aye, H. H., BCG test reaction in previously BCG vaccinated children, *Ann. Trop. Paediatr.*, 5, 29, 1985.

23. Stewart, C. J., Skin sensitivity to human, avian and BCG PPDs after BCG vaccination, *Tubercle*, 49, 84, 1968.

24. Edwards, L. B., Gelting, A. S., BCG-vaccine studies, *Bull. WHO*, 3, 279, 1950.

25. Bunch-Christensen, K., Evaluation of BCG vaccines in children, the effect of strain and dose, *J. Biol. Stand.*, 5, 159, 1977.

26. Ashley, M. J., Siebenman, C. O., Tuberculin skin sensitivity following BCG vaccination with vaccines of high and low viable counts, *Can. Med. Assoc. J.*, 97, 1335, 1967.

27. Lehmann, H. G., Engelhardt, H., Freudenstein, H., Hennessen, W., Widmark, R., BCG vaccination of neonates, infants, schoolchildren and adolescents. I. Dose finding studies with BCG strain 1331 Copenhagen, *Dev. Biol. Stand.*, 43, 127, 1979.

28. Palmer, C., Meyer, S. N., Research contributions of BCG vaccination programs. I. Tuberculin allergy as a family trait, *Public Health Rep.*, 66, 259, 1951.

29. Manerikar, S. S., Malaviya, A. N., Singh, M. B., Rajgopalan, P., Kumar, R., Immune status and BCG vaccination in newborns with intrauterine growth retardation, *Clin. Exp. Immunol.*, 26, 173, 1976.

30. Dawodu, A. H., Tuberculin conversion following BCG vaccination in preterm infants, *Acta Paediatr. Scand.*, 74, 564, 1985.

31. Kathipari, K., Seth, V., Sinclair, S., Arora, N. K., Kukreja, N., Cell mediated immune response after BCG as a determinant of optimum age of vaccination, *Indian J. Med. Res.*, 76, 508, 1982.

32. Pabst, H. F., Gobel, J. C., Spandy, D. W., McKechnie, J., Grace, M., Prospective trial of timing of Bacillus Calmette-Guérin vaccination in Canadian Cree infants, *Am. Rev. Resp. Dis.*, 140, 1007, 1989.

33. Heyworth, B., Delayed hypersensitivity to PPD-S following BCG vaccination in African children — an 18-month field study, *Trans. Royal Soc. Trop. Med. Hyg.*, 71, 3, 1977.

34. Horwitz, O., Bunch-Christensen, K., Correlation between tuberculin sensitivity after 2 months and 5 years among BCG vaccinated subjects, *Bull. WHO*, 47, 49, 1972.

35. Karalliedde, S., Katugaha, L. P., Uragoda, C. G., Tuberculin response of Sri Lankan children after BCG vaccination at birth, *Tubercle*, 68, 33, 1987.

36. Comstock, G. W., Edwards, L. B., Nabangxang, H., Tuberculin sensitivity eight to fifteen years after BCG vaccination, *Am. Rev. Resp. Dis.*, 103, 572, 1971.

37. Rosenthal, S. R., Routes and methods of administration, in *BCG Vaccine: Tuberculosis—Cancer*, PSG, Littleton, MA, 1980, chap. 12.

38. Guld, J., Waaler, H., Sundaresan, T. K., Kaufmann, P. C., Ten Dam, H. G., The duration of BCG-induced tuberculin sensitivity in children, and its irrelevance for revaccination, *Bull. WHO*, 39, 829, 1968.

39. Young, T. K., Mirdad, S., Determinants of tuberculin sensitivity in a child population covered by mass BCG vaccination, *Tubercle Lung Dis.*, 73, 94, 1992.

40. Friedland, I. R., The booster effect with repeat tuberculin testing in children and its relationship to BCG vaccination, *S. Afr. Med. J.*, 77, 387, 1990.

41. Shaaban, M. A., Ati, A., M., Bahr, G. M., Stanford, J. L., Lockwood, D. N. J., McManus, I. C., Revaccination with BCG: its effects on skin tests in Kuwaiti senior school children, *Eur. Resp. J.*, 3, 187, 1990.

42. Snider, D. E., Bacille Calmette-Guérin vaccinations and tuberculin skin tests, *J. Am. Med. Assoc.*, 253, 3438, 1985.

43. Comstock, G. W., Identification of an effective vaccine against tuberculosis, *Am. Rev. Resp. Dis.*, 138, 479–480, 1988.

44. Hart, P.D'A., Sutherland, I., Thomas, J., The immunity conferred by effective BCG and vole bacillus vaccines in relation to individual variations in tuberculin sensitivity and to technical variations in the vaccines, *Tubercle*, 48, 201, 1967.

45. Wilson, G. S., *The Hazards of Immunization*, Athlone, London, 1967.

46. Lotte, A., Wasz-Hockert, O., Poisson, N., Dumitrescu, N., Verron, M., Couvet, E., BCG complications, *Adv. Tuberc. Res.*, 21, 107, 1984.

47. Lotte, A., Wasz-Hockert, O., Poisson, N., Engbaek, H., Landmann, H., Quast, U., Andrasofszky, B., Lugosi, L., Vadasz, I., Mihailescu, P., Pal, D., Sudic, D., Second IUATLD study on complications induced by intradermal BCG-vaccination, *Bull. Int. Union Tuberc. Lung Dis.*, 63, 47, 1988.

48. Ray, C. S., Pringle, D., Legg, W., Mbengeranwa, O. L., Lymphadenitis associated with BCG vaccination: a report of an outbreak in Harare, Zimbabwe, *Cent. Afr. J. Med.*, 34, 281, 1988.

49. Caglayan, S., Yegin, O., Kayran, K., Timocin, N., Kasirga, E., Gun, M., Is medical therapy effective for regional lymphadenitis following BCG vaccination?, *Am. J. Dis. Child.*, 141, 1213, 1987.

50. Bottiger, M., Romanus, V., de Verdier, C., Boman, G., Osteitis and other complications caused by generalized BCG-itis, *Acta Paediatr. Scand.*, 71, 471, 1982.

51. Peltola, H., Salmi, I., Vahvanen, V., Ahlqvist, J., BCG vaccination as a cause of osteomyelitis and subcutaneous abscess, *Arch. Dis. Child.*, 59, 157, 1984.

52. Tardieu, M., Carriere, J. P., Truffot-Pernot, C., Dupic, Y., Tuberculous meningitis due to BCG in two previously healthy children, *Lancet*, 440, 1988.

53. MacKay, A., Alcorn, M. J., Macleod, I. M., Stack, B. H. R., Macleod, T., Laidlaw, M., Millar, J. S., White, R.G., Fatal disseminated BCG infection in an 18-year-old boy, *Lancet*, 1332, 1980.

54. Aronson, J. D., Dannenberg, A. M., Effect of vaccination with BCG on tuberculosis in infancy and in childhood, *Am. J. Dis. Child.*, 50, 1117, 1935.

55. Levine, M. I., Sackett, M. F., Results of BCG immunization in New York City, *Am. Rev. Tuberc.*, 53, 517, 1946.

56. Ferguson, R. S., Simes, A. B., BCG vaccination of Indian infants in Saskatchewan, *Tubercle*, 30, 5, 1949.

57. Sergent, E., Catanei, A., Ducros-Rougebief, H., Premunition anti-tuberculeuse par le BCG. Campagne controlee poursuivie a Alger depuis 1935. Troisieme note, *Arch. Inst. Pasteur Alger.*, 38, 131, 1960.

58. Aronson, J. D., Aronson, C. F., Taylor, H. C., A twenty-year appraisal of BCG vaccination in the control of tuberculosis, *Arch. Intern. Med.*, 101, 881, 1958.

59. Rosenthal, S. R., Loewinsohn, E., Graham, M., Liveright, D., Thorne, M., Johnson, V., BCG vaccination against tuberculosis in Chicago. A twenty-year study statistically analyzed, *Pediatrics*, 28, 622, 1961.

60. Aronson, J. D., Protective vaccination against tuberculosis with social references to BCG vaccination, *Am. Rev. Tuberc.*, 58, 275, 1948.

61. Rosenthal, S. R., Loewinsohn, E., Graham, M., Liveright, D., Thorne, M., Johnson, V., BCG vaccination in tuberculous households, *Am. Rev. Resp. Dis.*, 84, 690, 1961.

62. Comstock, G. W., Webster, R. G., Tuberculosis studies in Muscogee County, Georgia. VII. A twenty-year evaluation of BCG vaccination in a school population, *Am. Rev. Resp. Dis.*, 100, 839, 1969.

63. Bettag, O. L., Kaluzny, A. A., Morse, D., Radner, D. B., BCG study at a state school for mentally retarded, *Dis. Chest*, 45, 503, 1964.

64. Comstock, G. W., Livesay, V. T., Woolpert, S. F., Evaluation of BCG vaccination among Puerto Rican children, *Am. J. Public Health*, 64, 283, 1974.

65. Comstock, G. W., Woolpert, S. F., Livesay, V. T., Tuberculosis studies in Muscogee County, Georgia. Twenty-year evaluation of a community trial of BCG vaccination, *Public Health Rep.*, 91, 276, 1976.

66. Frimodt-Moller, J., Acharyulu, G. S., Kesava Pillai, K., Observations on the protective effect of BCG vaccination in a south Indian rural population: fourth report, *Bull. Int. Union Tuberc.*, 48, 40, 1973.

67. Hart, P. D., Sutherland, I., BCG and vole bacillus vaccines in the prevention of tuberculosis in adolescence and early adult life, *Br. Med. J.*, 2, 293, 1977.

68. Coetzee, A. M., Berjak, J., BCG in the prevention of tuberculosis in an adult population, *Proc. Mine Med. Officers' Assoc.*, 48, 41, 1968.

69. Vandiviere, H. M., Dworski, M., Melvin, I., Watson, K., Begley, J., Efficacy of bacillus Calmette-Guérin and isoniazid-resistant bacillus Calmette-Guérin with and without isoniazid chemoprophylaxis from day of vaccination, *Am. Rev. Resp. Dis.*, 108, 301, 1973.

70. Tripathy, S. P., Fifteen-year follow-up of the Indian BCG prevention trial, *Bull. Int. Union Tuberc.*, 62, 69, 1987.

71. Narain, R., Vallishayee, R. S., BCG vaccination of tuberculous patients and of strong reactors to tuberculin, *Bull. Int. Union Tuberc.*, 51, 243, 1976.

72. Smith, P. G., Case-control studies of the efficacy of BCG against tuberculosis, *Bull. Int. Union Tuberc.*, 62, 73, 1987.

73. Shapiro, C., Cook, N., Evans, D., Willett, W., Fajardo, I., Koch-Weser, D., Bergonzoli, G., Bolanos, O., Guerroero, R., Hennekens, C., A case-control study of BCG and childhood tuberculosis in Cali, Colombia, *Int. J. Epidemiol.*, 14, 3, 1985.

74. Young, T. K., Hershfield, E. S., A case-control study to evaluate the effectiveness of mass neonatal BCG vaccination among Canadian Indians, *Am. J. Public Health*, 76, 7, 783, 1986.

75. Houston, S., Fanning, A., Soskolne C. L., The effectiveness of bacillus Calmette-Guérin (BCG) vaccination against tuberculosis: a case-control study in Treaty Indians, Alberta, Canada, *Am. J. Epidemiol.*, 340, 1990.

76. Blin, P., Delolme, H. G., Heyraud, J. D., Charpak, Y., Sentilhes, L., Evaluation of the protective effect of BCG vaccination by a case-control study in Yaounde, Cameroon, *Tubercle*, 67, 283, 1986.

77. Padungchan, S., Konjanart, S., Kasiratta, S., The effectiveness of BCG vaccination of the newborn against childhood tuberculosis in Bangkok, *Bull. WHO*, 247, 1986.

78. Tidjani, O., Amedome, A., Ten Dam, H. G., The protective effect of BCG vaccination of the newborn against childhood tuberculosis in an African community, *Tubercle*, 67, 269, 1986.

79. Fine, P. E. M., BCG vaccination against tuberculosis and leprosy, *Br. Med. Bull.*, 44, 691, 1988.

80. Palmer, C. E., Long, M. W., Effect of infection with atypical mycobacteria on BCG vaccination and tuberculosis, *Am. Rev. Resp. Dis.*, 94, 553, 1966.

81. Rook, G. A. W., Bahr, G. M., Stanford, J. L., The effect of two distinct forms of cell-mediated response to mycobacteria on the protective efficacy of BCG, *Tubercle*, 62, 63, 1981.

82. Hank, J. A., Chan, J. K., Edwards, M. L., Muller, D., Smith, D. W., Influence of the virulence of *Mycobacterium tuberculosis* on protection induced by Bacille-Calmette-Guérin in guinea pigs, *J. Infect. Dis.*, 143, 734, 1981.

83. Blackwell, J. M., Bacterial infections, in *Genetics of Resistance to Bacterial and Parasitic Infections*, Wakelin D., Blackwell, J. M., Eds., Taylor and Francis, London, 1988.

84. McMurray, D. N., Carlomagno, M. A., Mintzer, C. L., Tetzlaff, C. L., *Mycobacterium bovis* BCG vaccine fails to protect protein-deficient guinea pigs against respiratory challenge with virulent *Mycobacterium tuberculosis, Infect. Immun.*, 50, 555, 1985.

85. Ten Dam, H. G., Pio, A., Pathogenesis of tuberculosis and effectiveness of vaccination, *Tubercle*, 63, 223, 1982.

86. Comstock, G. W., Edwards, P. Q., An American view of BCG vaccination, illustrated by results of a controlled trial in Puerto Rico, *Scand. J. Resp. Dis.*, 53, 207, 1972.

87. Clemens, J. B., Chuong, J. J. H., Feinstein, A. R., The BCG controversy: a methodological and statistical reappraisal, *J. Am. Med. Assoc.*, 249, 236, 1983.

88. WHO Study Group, BCG vaccination policies, *WHO Tech. Rep. Ser.*, 652, 1980.

89. Centers for Disease Control, Recommendations of the Immunization Practices Advisory Committee (ACIP). Use of BCG vaccines in the control of tuberculosis: a joint statement by the ACIP and the Advisory Committee for Elimination of Tuberculosis, *MMWR*, 37, 1, 1988.

90. Colebunders, R., Mann, J. M., Francis, H., Bila, K., Izaley, L., Kakonde, N., Kabasele, K., Ifoto, L., Nzilambi, N., Quinn, T. C., Van der Groen, G., Curran, J., Vercauteren, G., Piot, P., Evaluation of a clinical case-definition of acquired immunodeficiency syndrome in Africa, *Lancet*, 1, 492, 1987.

91. Ten Dam, H. G., BCG vaccination and HIV infection, *Bull. Int. Union Tuberc. Lung Dis.*, 65, 38, 1990.

92. Colebunders, R. L., Izaley, L., Musampu, M., Pauwels, P., Francis, H., Ryder, R., BCG vaccine abscesses are unrelated to HIV infection, *J. Am. Med. Assoc.*, 259, 3521, 1988.

93. Mvula, M., Ryder, R. W., Manzila, T., Response to childhood vaccinations in African children with HIV infection, *IV Int. Conf. AIDS*, Stockholm, Abstract 5112, June, 1988.

94. Bregere, P., BCG vaccination and AIDS, *Bull. Int. Union Tuberc. Lung Dis.*, 63, 40, 1988.

95. Lallemant-Le Coeur, S., Lallemant, M., Cheynier, D., Nzingoula, S., Drucker, J., Larouze, B., Bacillus Calmette-Guérin immunization in infants born to HIV-1-seropositive mothers, *AIDS*, 5, 195, 1991.

96. Centers for Disease Control, BCG vaccination and pediatric HIV infection — Rwanda, 1988–1990, *MMWR*, 40, 833, 1991.

97. Ninane, J., Grymonprez, A., Burtonboy, G., Francois, A., Cornu, G., Disseminated BCG in HIV infection, *Arch. Dis. Child.*, 63, 1268, 1988.

98. Houde, C., Dery, P., *Mycobacterium bovis* sepsis in an infant with human immunodeficiency virus infection, *Ped. Infect. Dis. J.*, 7, 810, 1988.

99. Centers for Disease Control, Disseminated *Mycobacterium bovis* infection from BCG vaccination of a patient with acquired immunodeficiency syndrome, *MMWR*, 34, 227, 1985.

100. Lumb, R., Shaw, D., *Mycobacterium bovis* (BCG) vaccination. Progressive disease in a patient symptomatically infected with the human immunodeficiency virus, *Med. J. Aust.*, 156, 286, 1992.

101. Smith, E., Thybo, S., Bennedsen, J., Infection with *Mycobacterium bovis* in a patient with AIDS: a late complication of BCG vaccination, *Scand. J. Infect. Dis.*, 24, 109, 1992.

102. Blondon, H., Guez, T., Paul, G., Truffot-Pernot, C., Sicard, D., Adenite a BCG 6 ans apres la vaccination au cours d'un SIDA, *La Presse Med.*, 20, 1091, 1991.

103. Reynes, J., Perez, C., Lamaury, I., Janbon, F., Bertrand, A., Bacille Calmette-Guérin adenitis 30 years after immunization in a patient with AIDS, *J. Infect. Dis.*, 160, 727, 1989.

104. Armbruster, C., Junker, W., Vetter, N., Jaksch, G., Disseminated Bacille Calmette-Guérin infection in an AIDS patient 30 years after BCG vaccination, *J. Infect. Dis.*, 162, 1216, 1990.

105. WHO/IUATLD, Tuberculosis and AIDS. Statement on AIDS and tuberculosis, *Bull. Int. Union Tuberc. Lung Dis.*, 64, 8, 1989.

106. Guld, J., Ladefoged, A., Ramhoj, W., Combined vaccination with BCG and toxoid antigens, *Bull. WHO*, 56, 957, 1978.

107. Barletta, R. G., Snapper, B., Cirillo, J. D., Connell, N. D., Kim, D. D., Jacobs, W. R., Bloom, B. R., Recombinant BCG as a candidate oral vaccine vector, *Res. Microbiol.*, 141, 931, 1990.

108. Aldovoni, A., Young, R., Humoral and cell-mediated immune responses to live recombinant BCG-HIV vaccines, *Nature(London)*, 351, 479, 1991.

109. Pal, P. G., Horwitz, M. A., Immunization with extracellular proteins of *Mycobacterium tuberculosis* induces cell-mediated immune responses and substantial protective immunity in a guinea pig model of pulmonary tuberculosis, *Infect. Immun.*, 60, 4781, 1992.

110. Lyons, J., Sinos, C., Destree, A, Caiazzo, T., Havican, K., McKenzie, S., Panicali, D., Mahr, A., Expression of *Mycobacterium tuberculosis* and *Mycobacterium leprae* proteins by vaccinia virus, *Infect. Immun.*, 58, 4098, 1990.

INDEX